The IMAGE PROCESSING Handbook

Fifth Edition

John C. Russ

North Carolina State University
Materials Science and Engineering Department
Raleigh, North Carolina

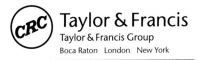

Taylor & Francis
Taylor & Francis Group
Boca Raton London New York

CRC is an imprint of the Taylor & Francis Group,
an informa business

CRC Press
Taylor & Francis Group
6000 Broken Sound Parkway NW, Suite 300
Boca Raton, FL 33487-2742

© 2007 by Taylor & Francis Group, LLC
CRC Press is an imprint of Taylor & Francis Group, an Informa business

No claim to original U.S. Government works
Printed in Canada
10 9 8 7 6 5 4 3 2 1

International Standard Book Number-10: 0-8493-7254-2 (Hardcover)
International Standard Book Number-13: 978-0-8493-7254-4 (Hardcover)

This book contains information obtained from authentic and highly regarded sources. Reprinted material is quoted with permission, and sources are indicated. A wide variety of references are listed. Reasonable efforts have been made to publish reliable data and information, but the author and the publisher cannot assume responsibility for the validity of all materials or for the consequences of their use.

No part of this book may be reprinted, reproduced, transmitted, or utilized in any form by any electronic, mechanical, or other means, now known or hereafter invented, including photocopying, microfilming, and recording, or in any information storage or retrieval system, without written permission from the publishers.

For permission to photocopy or use material electronically from this work, please access www.copyright.com (http://www.copyright.com/) or contact the Copyright Clearance Center, Inc. (CCC) 222 Rosewood Drive, Danvers, MA 01923, 978-750-8400. CCC is a not-for-profit organization that provides licenses and registration for a variety of users. For organizations that have been granted a photocopy license by the CCC, a separate system of payment has been arranged.

Trademark Notice: Product or corporate names may be trademarks or registered trademarks, and are used only for identification and explanation without intent to infringe.

Library of Congress Cataloging-in-Publication Data

Russ, John C.
   The image processing handbook / by John C. Russ.-- 5th ed.
      p. cm.
   Includes bibliographical references and index.
   ISBN 0-8493-7254-2
   1. Image processing--Handbooks, manuals, etc. I. Title.

TA1637.R87 2006
621.36'7--dc22   2006040469

**Visit the Taylor & Francis Web site at
http://www.taylorandfrancis.com**

**and the CRC Press Web site at
http://www.crcpress.com**

Preface

Image processing is used in a wide variety of applications for two somewhat different purposes:

Improving the visual appearance of images to a human viewer, including their printing and transmission
Preparing images for the measurement of the features and structures that they reveal

The techniques that are appropriate for each of these tasks are not always the same, but there is considerable overlap. This book covers methods that are used for both tasks.

To do the best possible job, it is important to know about the uses to which the processed images will be put. For visual enhancement, this means having some familiarity with the human visual process and an appreciation of what cues the viewer responds to in an image. In this edition of the book, a chapter on that subject has been added. It also is useful to know about the printing or display process, since many images are processed in the context of reproduction or transmission. Printing technology for images has advanced significantly with the consumer impact of digital cameras, and up-to-date information is provided.

The measurement of images is often a principal method for acquiring scientific data, and generally requires that features or structure be well defined, either by edges or unique brightness, color, texture, or some combination of these factors. The types of measurements that can be performed on entire scenes or on individual features are important in determining the appropriate processing steps. Several chapters deal with measurement in detail.

It may help to recall that image processing, like food processing or word processing, does not reduce the amount of data present but simply rearranges it. Some arrangements may be more appealing to the senses, and some may convey more meaning, but these two criteria do not necessarily overlap and may not call for identical methods.

This handbook presents an extensive collection of image-processing tools, so that the user of computer-based systems can both understand those methods provided in packaged software and program those additions that may be needed for particular applications. Comparisons are presented for different algorithms that can be used for similar purposes, using a selection of representative pictures from various microscopy techniques as well as macroscopic, remote sensing, and astronomical images. The emphasis throughout continues to be on explaining and illustrating methods so that they can be clearly understood, rather than providing dense mathematics. With the advances in computer speed and power, tricks and approximations in search of efficiency are not as important as they once were, so the examples based on exact implementation of methods with full precision can generally be implemented on today's desktop systems.

For many years, in teaching this material to students, I have described achieving mastery of these techniques as being much like becoming a skilled journeyman carpenter. The number of distinct woodworking tools — saws, planes, drills, etc. — is relatively small, and although there are some variations — slotted vs. Phillips-head screw drivers, for example — knowing how to use each type of tool is closely linked to understanding what it does. With a set of these tools, the skilled carpenter can produce a house, a boat, or a piece of furniture. So it is with image processing tools, which are conveniently grouped into only a few classes, such as histogram modification, neighborhood operations, Fourier-space processing, and so on, and can be used to accomplish a broad range of purposes. Visiting your local hardware store and purchasing the appropriate tools does not imply having the skills to use them, any more than purchasing a modern digital camera, computer, and software. Understanding their use requires practice, which develops the ability to visualize beforehand what each will do.

In revising the book for this new edition, I have again tried to respond to some of the comments and requests of readers and reviewers. New chapters on the measurement of images and the subsequent interpretation of the data were added in the second edition, and a section on surface images was added in the third. The fourth edition added the stereological interpretation of measurements on sections through three-dimensional structures, and the various logical approaches to feature classification. In this fifth edition, all of these areas have been strengthened with more than 600 new and revised figures introduced to add clarity and better illustrate techniques, and the reference list has been expanded by more than 20% with the latest citations. The reader will find expanded discussions on deconvolution, extended-dynamic-range images, and multichannel imaging, the latter including new material on principal-components analysis. The sections on the ever-advancing hardware for image capture and printing have been expanded and information added on the newest technologies.

As in past editions, I have resisted suggestions to put "more of the math" into the book. There are excellent texts on image processing, compression, mathematical morphology, etc., that provide as much rigor and as many derivations as may be needed. Many of them are referenced here. But the thrust of this book remains teaching by example. Few people learn the principles of image processing from the equations. Just as we use images to communicate ideas and to "do science," so most of us use images to learn about many things, including imaging itself. The hope is that, by seeing and comparing what various operations do to representative images, you will discover how and why to use them. Then, if you need to look up the mathematical foundations, they will be easier to understand.

The reader is encouraged to use this book in concert with a real source of images and a computer-based system, and to freely experiment with different methods to determine which are most appropriate for his or her particular needs. Selection of image processing tools to explore images when you don't know the contents beforehand is a much more difficult task than using tools to make it easier for another viewer or a measurement program to see the same things you have discovered. It places greater demand on computing speed and on the interactive nature of the interface. But it particularly requires that you become a very analytical observer of images. If you can learn to see what the computer sees, you will become a better viewer and obtain the best possible images, suitable for further processing and analysis.

To facilitate this hands-on learning process, I have collaborated with my son, Chris Russ, to produce a CD-ROM that can be used as a companion to this book. The Fovea Pro CD contains more than 200 images, many of them the examples from the book, plus an extensive set of Photoshop-compatible plug-ins that implement many of the algorithms discussed here. These can be used with Adobe Photoshop® or any of the numerous programs that implement the Photoshop plug-in interface, on either Macintosh or Windows computers. Information about the CD-ROM is available online at http://ReindeerGraphics. com.

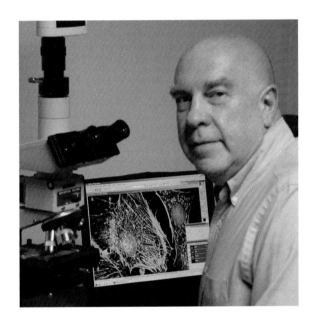

Acknowledgments

All of the image processing and the creation of the resulting figures included in this book were performed on an Apple Macintosh® or a Sony VAIO® computer using Adobe Photoshop® CS2 with the Fovea Pro plug-ins. Many of the images were acquired directly from various microscopes and other sources that provided digital output directly to the computer. Others were captured using a variety of digital cameras (Sony, Nikon, Canon, and Polaroid), and some were obtained using flatbed and slide scanners (Agfa, Nikon, and Epson), often from images supplied by coworkers and researchers. These are acknowledged wherever the origin of an image could be determined. A few examples, taken from the literature, are individually referenced.

The book was delivered to the publisher in digital form (on a writable DVD), without intermediate hard copy, negatives, or prints of the images, etc. Among other things, this means that the author must bear full responsibility for any typographical errors or problems with the figures. Every effort has been made to show enlarged image fragments that will reveal pixel-level detail when it is important. The process has also forced me to learn more than I ever hoped to know about some aspects of publishing technology! However, going directly from disk file to print also shortens the time needed in production and helps to keep costs down while preserving the full quality of the images. Grateful acknowledgment is made of the efforts by the editors at CRC Press to educate me and to accommodate the unusually large number of illustrations in this book (more than 2000 figures and more than a quarter of a million words).

Special thanks are due to Chris Russ (Reindeer Graphics Inc., Asheville, NC), who has helped to program many of these algorithms and contributed invaluable comments, and to Helen Adams, who has proofread many pages, endured many discussions about ways to present information effectively, and provided the support (and the occasional glass of wine) that makes writing projects such as this possible.

John C. Russ
Raleigh, NC

Contents

8 Processing Binary Images 443

9 Global Image Measurements. 511

10 Feature-Specific Measurements 543

11 Feature Recognition and Classification. 599

12 Tomographic Imaging 629

13 3-D Image Visualization 667

1

Acquiring Images

Human reliance on images for information

Humans are primarily visual creatures. As discussed in **Chapter 2**, not all animals depend on their eyes, as we do, for most of the information received about their surroundings. This bias in everyday life extends to how we pursue more technical goals as well. Scientific instruments commonly produce images to communicate their results to the operator, rather than generating audible tones or emitting a smell. Space missions to other planets and equally arduous explorations of the ocean depths always include cameras as major components, and we judge the success of those missions by the quality of the images returned. This suggests a few of the ways in which we have extended the range of our natural vision. Simple optical devices such as microscopes and telescopes allow us to see things that are vastly smaller or larger than we could otherwise. Beyond the visible portion of the electromagnetic spectrum (a narrow range of wavelengths between about 400 and 700 nm), we now have sensors capable of detecting infrared and ultraviolet light, X-rays, and radio waves, and perhaps soon even gravity waves. **Figure 1.1** shows an example, an image presenting radio-telescope data in the form of an image in which color represents the Doppler shift in the radio signal. Such devices and presentations are used to further extend our imaging capability.

Signals other than electromagnetic radiation can be used to produce images, too. Novel types of microscopes that use atomic-scale probes to "feel" a specimen surface present their data as images. Acoustic waves at low frequency produce sonar images, while at gigahertz frequencies the acoustic microscope produces images with resolution similar to that of the light microscope, but with image contrast that is produced by local variations in the attenuation and refraction of sound waves rather than light. **Figure 1.2** shows an acoustic microscope image of a composite material, and **Figure 1.3** shows a sonogram of a baby in the womb.

Some images such as holograms or electron diffraction patterns are recorded to show brightness as a function of position, but such images are unfamiliar to the observer. **Figure 1.4** and **Figure 1.5** show electron diffraction patterns from a transmission electron microscope, in which the atomic structure of the samples is revealed (but only to those who know how to interpret the image). Other kinds of data — including weather maps with specialized symbols, graphs of business profit and expenses, and charts with axes representing time, family income, cholesterol level, or even more obscure parameters — have become part of our daily lives.

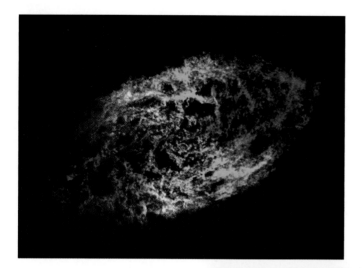

Figure 1.1 Radio astronomy produces images such as this view of Messier 33. These are often displayed with false colors to emphasize subtle variations in signal or, as in this example, Doppler shift. (This image was generated with data from telescopes of the National Radio Astronomy Observatory, a National Science Foundation Facility managed by Associated Universities, Inc. With permission.)

Figure 1.2 Scanning acoustic microscope image (with superimposed signal profile along one scan line) of a polished cross section through a composite. The central white feature is a fiber intersecting the surface at an angle. The peaks on either side are interference patterns that can be used to measure the fiber angle.

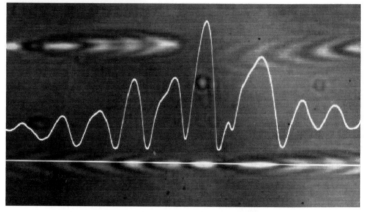

Figure 1.6 shows a few common examples. The latest developments in computer interfaces and displays make extensive use of graphics, again to take advantage of the large bandwidth of the human visual pathway. Tufte (1990, 1997, 2001) in particular has demonstrated the power of appropriate graphics to communicate complex information.

There are some important differences between human vision, the kind of information it extracts from images, and the ways in which it seems to do so, as compared with the use of imaging devices based on computers for technical purposes. Humans are especially poor at judging color or brightness of features within images unless they can be exactly compared by making them adjacent. Human vision is inherently comparative rather than quantitative, responding to the relative size, angle, or position of several objects but unable to supply numeric measures unless one of the reference objects is a measuring device. Overington (1976, 1992) disagrees with this widely accepted and documented conclusion but presents no compelling counterevidence. **Chapter 2** shows some of the consequences of the characteristics of human vision as they affect what we see.

This book's purpose is not to study the human visual pathway directly, but the overview in **Chapter 2** can help us to understand how we see things so that we become better observers. Computer-based image processing and analysis use algorithms based on human vision methods in some cases, but also employ other methods that seem not to have direct counterparts

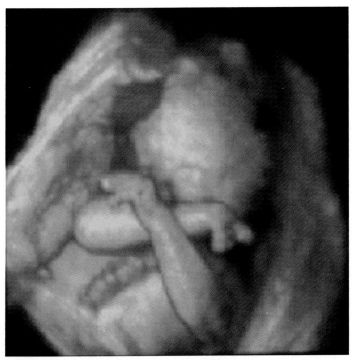

Figure 1.3 *Surface reconstruction of sonogram imaging showing a 26-week-old fetus in the womb.*

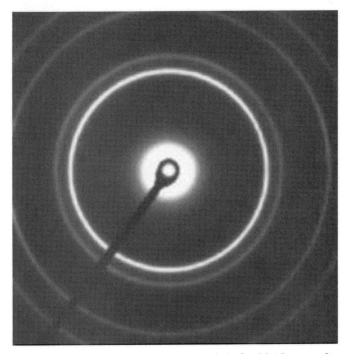

Figure 1.4 *An electron diffraction pattern from a thin foil of gold. The ring diameters correspond to diffraction angles that identify the spacings of planes of atoms in the crystal structure.*

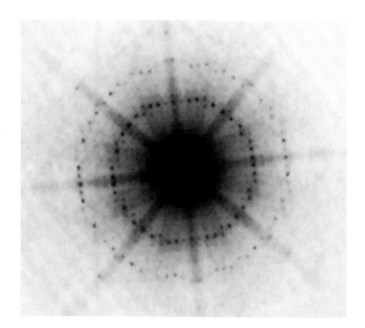

Figure 1.5 *A convergent-beam electron diffraction (CBED) pattern from an oxide microcrystal, vwhich can be indexed and measured to provide high accuracy values for the atomic unit cell dimensions.*

Figure 1.6 *Typical graphics used to communicate news information include one-dimensional plots such as stock market reports, two-dimensional presentations such as weather maps, and simplified charts using images.*

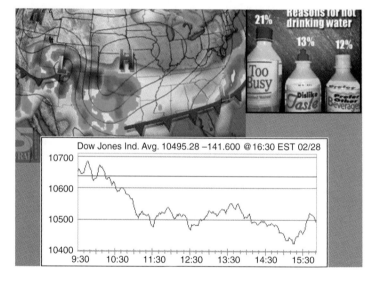

in human vision. In particular, some methods are based on the physics of the image formation and detection process (Sharma 2005).

Video cameras

When the first edition of this book was published in 1990, the most common and affordable way of acquiring images for computer processing was with a video camera. Mounted onto a microscope, or using appropriate optics to view an experiment, the camera sent an analog signal to a separate "frame grabber" or analog-to-digital converter (ADC) interface board in the computer, which then stored numeric values in memory (Inoué 1986; Inoué and Spring 1997).

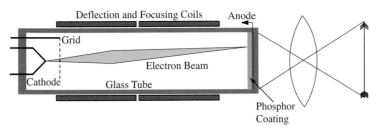

Figure 1.7 *Functional diagram of a vidicon tube. Light striking the phosphor coating changes its local resistance and hence the current that flows as the electron beam scans in a raster pattern.*

The basic form of the original type of video camera is the vidicon, illustrated in **Figure 1.7**. It functions by scanning a focused beam of electrons across a phosphor coating applied to the inside of an evacuated glass tube. The light enters the camera through the front glass surface (and a thin metallic anode layer) and creates free electrons in the phosphor. These vary the local conductivity of the layer, so the amount of current that flows to the anode varies as the beam is scanned, according to the local light intensity. This analog (continuously varying) electrical signal is amplified and, as shown in **Figure 1.8**, conforms to standards of voltage and timing. (The standards and timing are slightly different in Europe than the United States, but the basic principles remain the same.)

Digitizing the voltage is accomplished by sampling it and generating a comparison voltage. The child's game of "guess a number" illustrates that it takes only eight guesses to arrive at a value that defines the voltage to one part in 256 (the most widely used type of ADC). The first guess is 128, or half the voltage range. If this is (for example) too large, the second guess subtracts 64. Each successive approximation adds or subtracts a value half as large as the previous. In eight steps, the final (smallest) adjustment is made. The result is a number that is conveniently stored in the 8-bit memory of most modern computers.

The tube-type camera has several advantages and quite a few drawbacks. Scanning the beam with electromagnetic or electrostatic fields can produce a distorted scan (pincushion or barrel distortion, or more complicated situations) and is subject to degradation by stray fields from wiring or instrumentation. **Figure 1.9** shows an example of pincushion distortion as well as vignetting and loss of focus. Maintaining focus in the corners of the image takes special cir-

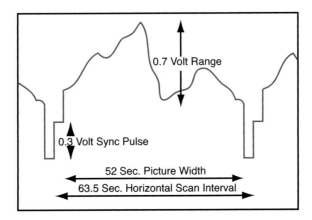

Figure 1.8 *Standard RS-170 video signal shows the brightness variation along one scan line (ranging between 0 volts = black and 0.7 volts = white).*

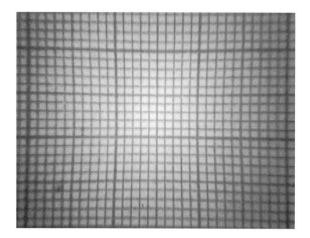

Figure 1.9 *Example of an image showing pincushion distortion as well as loss of focus and vignetting in the edges and corners.*

cuitry, and the corners can also be darkened by the additional thickness of glass through which the light must pass (vignetting). The sealed vacuum systems tend to deteriorate with time, and the "getter" used to adsorb gas molecules can flake and fall onto the phosphor if the camera is used in a vertical orientation. The response of the camera (voltage vs. brightness) approximates the logarithmic response of film and the human eye, but this varies for bright and dark scenes. Recovery from bright scenes and bright spots is slow, and blooming can occur, in which bright light produces spots that spread laterally in the coating and appear larger than the features really are, with "comet tails" in the scan direction.

There are, however, some advantages of the tube-type camera. The spatial resolution is very high, limited only by the grain size of the phosphor and the size of the focused beam spot. Also, the phosphor has a spectral response that can be made quite similar to that of the human eye, which sees color from red (about 0.7 μm wavelength) to blue (about 0.4 μm). Adaptations of the basic camera design with intermediate cathode layers or special coatings for intensification are capable of acquiring images in very dim light (e.g., night scenes, fluorescence microscopy).

CCD cameras

The tube-type camera has now been largely supplanted by the solid-state chip camera, the simplest form of which is the CCD (charge-coupled device). The camera chip contains an array of diodes that function as light buckets. Light that enters the semiconductor raises electrons from the valence to the conduction band, so the number of electrons is a direct linear measure of the light intensity. The diodes are formed by photolithography, so they have a perfectly regular pattern, with no image distortion or sensitivity to the presence of stray fields. The devices are also inexpensive and rugged, compared with tube cameras. CCDs were first invented and patented at Bell Labs (in 1969); have been strongly involved in the NASA-JPL space program, since they provide a reliable way of acquiring images from satellites and space probes; and now are even displacing film in consumer and professional still cameras.

The basic operation of a CCD is illustrated in **Figure 1.10**. Each bucket represents one "pixel" in the camera (this word has a lot of different meanings in different contexts, as will be explained below, so it must be used with some care). With anywhere from a few hundred thousand to several million detectors on the chip, it is impractical to run wires directly to each one to read out the signal. Instead, the electrons that accumulate in each bucket due to incident

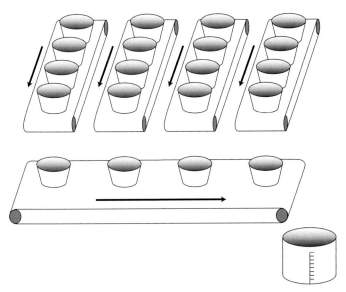

Figure 1.10 *The basic principle of CCD operation, illustrated as a set of buckets and conveyors. (After* Janesick, J.R., Scientific Charge-Coupled Devices, *SPIE Press, Bellingham, WA, 2001.)*

photons are transferred, one line at a time, to a readout row. On a clock signal, each column of pixels shifts the charge by one location. This places the contents of the buckets into the readout row, and that row is then shifted, one pixel at a time but much more rapidly, to dump the electrons into an amplifier, where the information can be sent out as an analog signal from a video camera or measured immediately to produce a numeric output from a digital camera.

The simplest way of shifting the electrons is shown in **Figure 1.11**. Every set of three electrodes on the surface of the device constitutes one pixel. By applying a voltage to two of the electrodes, a field is set up in the semiconductor that acts like a bucket. Electrons are trapped

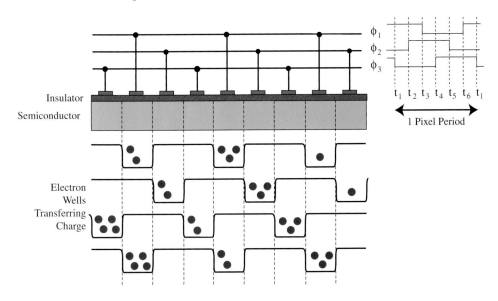

Figure 1.11 *Varying voltages on a set of three electrodes shifts electrons from one pixel to another.*

in the central region by the high fields on either side. Note that this does not reduce the area sensitive to incoming photons, because electrons generated in the high-field regions will quickly migrate to the low-field bucket, where they are held. By changing the voltage applied to the regions in six steps or phases, as shown in the figure, the electrons are shifted by one pixel. First one field region is lowered and the electrons spread into the larger volume. Then the field on the other side is raised, and the electrons have been shifted by one-third of the pixel height. Repeating the process acts like a conveyor belt, and this is the reason for the name "charge-coupled device."

One significant problem with the chip camera is its spectral response. Even if the chip is reversed and thinned so that light enters from the side opposite the electrodes, very little blue light penetrates into the semiconductor to produce electrons. On the other hand, infrared light penetrates easily, and these cameras have red and infrared (IR) sensitivity that far exceeds that of human vision, usually requiring the installation of a blocking filter to exclude it (because the IR light is not focused to the same plane as the visible light and would produce blurred or fogged images). **Figure 1.12** shows this spectral response, which can be further tailored and extended by using materials other than silicon. The chip can reach quite high total efficiency when antireflective coatings are applied, limited primarily by the "fill factor" — the area frac-

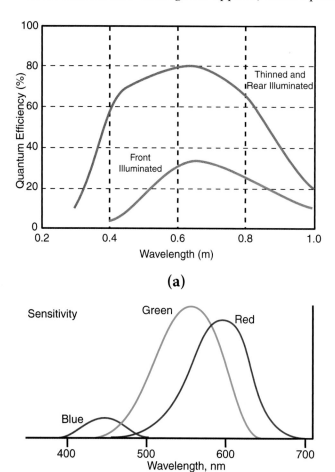

Figure 1.12
    (a) Spectral response of a silicon-based chip, compared with
    (b) the color sensors in the human eye, which are commonly identified as red, green-, and blue-sensitive but actually cover a range of long, medium, and short wavelengths.

tion of the chip that contains active devices between the narrow ditches that maintain electrical separation. Also, the chip camera has an output that is linearly proportional to the incident light intensity, convenient for some measurement purposes but very different from human vision, the vidicon, and photographic film, which are logarithmic.

Human vision notices brightness differences of a few percent, i.e., a constant ratio of change rather than a constant increment. Film is characterized by a response to light exposure that (after chemical development) produces a density-vs.-exposure curve such as that shown in **Figure 1.13**. The low end of this curve represents the fog level of the film, the density that is present even without exposure. At the high end, the film saturates to a maximum optical density, for instance based on the maximum physical density of silver particles. In between, the curve is linear, with a slope that represents the contrast of the film. A steep slope corresponds to a high-contrast film that exhibits a large change in optical density with a small change in exposure. Conversely, a low-contrast film has a broader latitude to record a scene with a greater range of brightnesses. The slope of the curve is usually called "gamma," and some chip cameras, particularly those used for consumer video camcorders and pocket digital cameras, may include circuitry that changes their output from linear to logarithmic so that the image contrast is more familiar to viewers. More expensive consumer cameras and most professional cameras include the possibility of reading the "raw" linear data as well as the converted image.

When film is exposed directly to electrons, as in the transmission electron micrograph, rather than photons (visible light or X-rays), the response curve is linear rather than logarithmic. Many light photons are needed to completely expose a single halide particle for development, but only a single electron. Consequently, electron image films and plates are often very high in density (values of optical density greater than 4, which means that 9,999/10,000 of incident light is absorbed), which creates difficulties for many scanners and requires more than 8 bits to record.

The trend in camera chips has been to make them smaller and to increase the number of pixels or diodes present. Some scientific cameras, such as those used in the Hubble telescope, occupy an entire wafer. But for consumer devices, making each chip one-third, one-quarter, or even two-tenths of an inch in overall (diagonal) dimension places many devices on a single wafer and provides greater economic yield. Putting more pixels into this reduced chip area (for more spatial resolution, as discussed below) makes the individual detectors small, but the ditches between them have to remain about the same size to prevent electrons from diffusing laterally. The result markedly reduces the total efficiency. Some devices place small lenses over the diodes to capture light that would otherwise fall into the ditches, but these add cost and also are not as uniform as the diodes themselves (which are typically within 1% across the entire chip).

Figure 1.13 *Response of photographic film. The central portion of the curve shows a linear increase in density (defined as the base-ten logarithm of the fraction of incident light that is transmitted) with the logarithm of exposure. High film contrast ("hard" contrast) corresponds to a steep curve, while "soft" (low contrast, less steep curve) films have a greater dynamic range.*

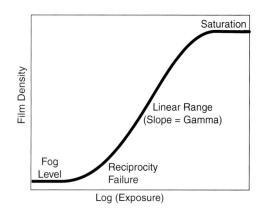

The other, and more important, effect of making the detectors small is to reduce their capacity for electrons, called the well capacity. A typical 15-μm pixel in a scientific-grade CCD has a capacity of about 500,000 electrons, which, with low readout noise (as can be achieved in special situations) of a few electrons, gives a dynamic range greater than photographic film. Even larger well capacity and dynamic range can be achieved by combining more detectors in each pixel (binning) by using more steps in the phase shifting during readout. Conversely, reducing the area of the detector also reduces the well size and, with it, the dynamic range. Increasing the noise, for instance by reading out the signal at video rates (each horizontal line in 52 μsec for U.S. video), dramatically reduces the dynamic range, and a typical consumer-grade video camera has no more than about 64 distinguishable brightness levels (expensive studio cameras meet the broadcast video specification of 100 levels). Since these levels are linear with brightness with the chip camera, they produce even fewer viewable gray levels, as shown in **Figure 1.14**. This performance is much inferior to film, which can distinguish thousands of brightness levels.

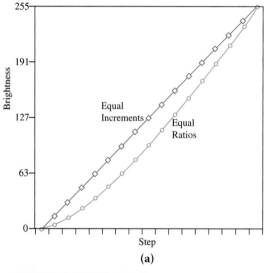

(a)

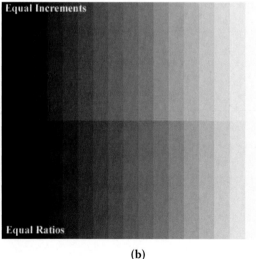

(b)

Figure 1.14 *Comparison of visibility of gray-level steps from linear (equal steps) and logarithmic (equal ratios) detectors:* *(a)* *plots of intensity;* *(b)* *display of the values from* ***a***.

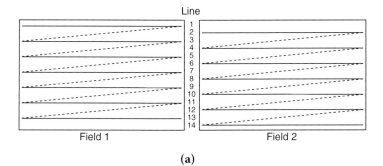

Line

Field 1   Field 2

(a)

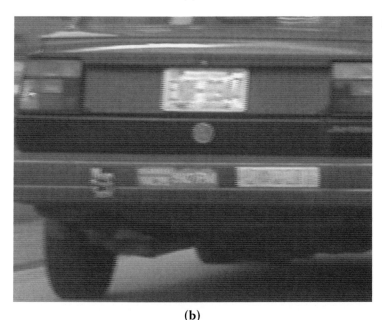

(b)

Figure 1.15
  (a) *Interlace scan covers even-numbered lines in 1/60-sec field and even-numbered lines in a second field.*
  (b) *When motion is present, this produces an offset in the complete image.*

Camera artifacts and limitations

There are several problems with video cameras using chips, and these contribute to specific types of defects in the images that must be dealt with by subsequent processing. One is the fact that video signals are interlaced (**Figure 1.15**). This clever trick to minimize visual flicker in broadcast television images was accomplished with tube cameras simply by scanning the electron beam in the same interlace pattern as the display television set. With a chip camera, the array must be read out twice for every frame (at 30 frames per second), once to collect the even-numbered lines and again for the odd-numbered lines. In fact, many cameras combine two lines to get better sensitivity, averaging lines 1 and 2, 3 and 4, 5 and 6, and so on, in one interlaced field, and then 2 and 3, 4 and 5, 6 and 7, etc., in the other. This reduces vertical resolution, but for casual viewing purposes this is not noticeable. Motion can cause the even and odd fields of a full frame to be offset from each other, producing a significant degradation of the image, as shown in the figure. A similar effect occurs with stationary images if the horizontal retrace signal is imprecise or difficult for the electronics to lock onto; this is a particular problem with signals played back from consumer videotape recorders.

During the transfer and readout process, unless the camera is shuttered either mechanically or electrically, photons continue to produce electrons in the chip. This produces a large background signal that further degrades dynamic range and may produce blurring. Electronic shuttering is usually done a line at a time, so that moving images are distorted. Some designs avoid shuttering problems by doubling the number of pixels, with half of them opaque to incoming light. A single transfer shifts the electrons from the active detectors to the hidden ones, from which they can be read out. Of course, this reduces the active area (fill factor) of devices on the chip, costing 50% in sensitivity.

The high speed of horizontal-line readout can produce horizontal blurring of the signal, again reducing image resolution. This is partially due to inadequate time for the electrons to diffuse along with the shifting fields and to the time needed to recover electrons from traps (impurities in the silicon lattice), and partially to the inadequate frequency response of the amplifier, which is a trade-off to reduce amplifier noise. Even though the individual electron transfers are very efficient, better than 99.999% in most cases, the result of being passed through many such transfers before being collected and amplified increases the noise. This varies from one side of the chip to the other, and from the top to the bottom, and can be visually detected in images if there is not a lot of other detail or motion to obscure it.

Many transfers of electrons from one detector to another occur during readout of a chip, and this accounts for some of the noise in the signal. Purely statistical variation in the production and collection of charge is a relatively smaller effect. The conversion of the tiny charge to a voltage and its subsequent amplification is the greatest source of noise in most systems. Readout and amplifier noise can be reduced by slowing the transfer process so that fewer electrons are lost in the shifting process and the amplifier time constant can integrate out more of the noise, producing a cleaner signal. Cooling the chip to about −40°C also reduces the noise from these sources and from dark current, or thermal electrons. Slow readout and cooling are used only in nonvideo applications, of course. Digital still-frame cameras use the same chip technology as solid-state video cameras, but produce higher quality images because of the slower readout. Janesick (2001) discusses the various sources of noise and their control in scientific-grade CCDs of the type used in astronomical imaging (where they have almost entirely replaced film) and in space probes.

Color cameras

Color cameras can be designed in three principal ways, as shown in **Figure 1.16**, **Figure 1.17**, and **Figure 1.18**. For stationary images (which include many scientific applications such as microscopy, but exclude "real-time" applications such as video), a single detector array can be used to acquire three sequential exposures through red, green, and blue filters, respectively, which are then combined for viewing (**Figure 1.16**). The advantages of this scheme include low cost and the ability to use different exposure times for the different color bands, which can compensate for the poorer sensitivity of the CCD chip to blue light.

Many high-end consumer- and most professional- and scientific-grade video cameras use three sensors (**Figure 1.17**). A prism array splits the incoming light into red, green, and blue components, which are recorded by three different sensors whose outputs are combined electronically to produce a standard video image. This approach is more costly, since three chips are needed, but for video applications they need not be of particularly high resolution (fewer pixels). The optics and hardware to keep everything in alignment add some cost, and the depth of the prism optics makes it impractical to use short-focal-length (wide angle) lenses. This design is rarely used in digital still cameras.

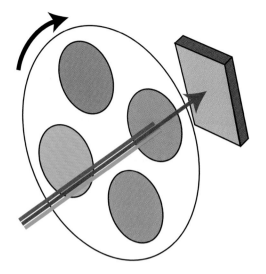

Figure 1.16 Schematic diagram of a color-wheel camera. The fourth filter position is empty, allowing the camera to be used as a monochrome detector with greater sensitivity for dim images (e.g., fluorescence microscopy).

Figure 1.17 Schematic diagram of a three-chip color camera.

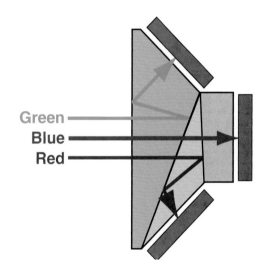

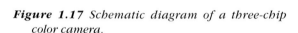

Video images are often digitized into a 640 × 480 array of stored pixels, but this is not the actual resolution of the image. The broadcast bandwidth limits the high frequencies and eliminates any rapid variations in brightness and color. A video image has no more than 330 actual elements of resolution in the horizontal direction for the brightness (luminance) signal, and about half that for the color (chrominance) information. Color information is intentionally reduced in resolution because human vision is not very sensitive to blurring of color beyond boundary lines.

Of course, video signals can be further degraded by poor equipment. Recording video on consumer-grade tape machines can reduce the resolution by another 50% or more, particularly if the record head is dirty or the tape has been used many times before. Video images are just not very high resolution, although some forms of HDTV (high-definition television) may improve things in the future. Consequently, video technology is usually a poor choice for scientific imaging unless there is some special need to capture "real-time" images (i.e., 25 to 30 frames per second) to record changes or motion. Digital cameras have largely replaced them now, as they produce much higher resolution images and at lower cost.

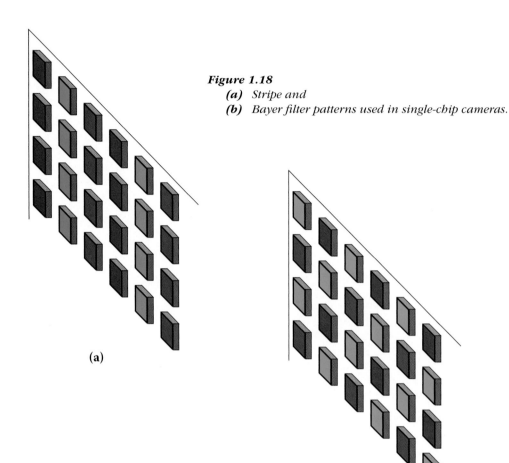

Figure 1.18
(a) *Stripe and*
(b) *Bayer filter patterns used in single-chip cameras.*

(a)

(b)

Most digital cameras use a single-pixel array, often of very high pixel (detector) count, with a color filter that allows red, green, and blue light to reach specific detectors. Different patterns can be used (**Figure 1.18**), with the Bayer pattern being very common. Notice that it assigns twice as many detectors for green as for red or blue, which mimics to some extent the human eye's greater sensitivity to green. The problem with the single-chip camera, of course, is that the image resolution in each color channel is reduced. The red intensity at some locations must be interpolated from nearby sensors, for example. It is also necessary to design the filters to give the same brightness sensitivity in each channel. If this is not done well, a herringbone pattern will appear in images of a uniform gray test card, and color fringes will appear along edges in the picture.

Interpolation techniques for Bayer pattern color filters reduce the image resolution as compared with the number of individual detectors in the camera (which is generally the specification advertised by the manufacturer). The quality of the interpolation, judged by its ability to preserve sharp boundaries in brightness while minimizing the introduction of color artifacts, varies inversely with the computational requirements. A comparison of several patented methods can be found in Ramanath (2000) and Shao et al. (2005).

Another approach to color camera design, developed by Foveon Corp. and used in a few cameras, creates three transistors at each pixel location, with the transistors stacked on top of each other. Blue light penetrates the shortest distance in silicon, and is detected in the topmost transistor. Green light penetrates to the second transistor, and red light penetrates to the bottom one. The output signals are combined to produce the color information. This approach does not suffer from loss of spatial resolution due to interpolation, but it does have potential problems with consistent or accurate color fidelity.

Camera resolution

The signal coming from the chip is an analog voltage, even if the digitization takes place within the camera housing, so the interpolation is done in the amplifier stage through the use of appropriate time constants. This means that the voltage cannot vary rapidly enough to correspond to brightness differences for every pixel. Because of this interpolation, the actual image resolution with a single-chip camera and filter arrangement will, in most cases, be one-half to two-thirds the value that might be expected by the advertised number of pixels in the camera. And some cameras record images with many more stored pixels than the chip resolution would warrant in any case. Such interpolations and empty magnification contribute no additional information to the image.

Comparing cameras based on actual resolution rather than the stated number of recorded pixels can be quite difficult. It is important to consider the multiple meanings of the word "pixel." In some contexts, it refers to the number of light detectors in the camera (without regard to any color filtering, and sometimes including ones around the edges that do not contribute to the actual image but are used to measure dark current). In other contexts, it describes the number of recorded brightness or color values stored in the computer, although these may represent empty magnification. In other situations, the term is used to describe the displayed points of light on the computer monitor, even if the image is shown in a compressed or enlarged size. It makes much more sense to separate these various meanings and to talk about resolution elements when considering real image resolution. This refers to the number of discrete points across the image that can be distinguished from each other, and is sometimes described in terms of the number of line pairs that can be resolved. This is half the number of resolution elements, since one element is needed for the line and one for the space between lines, and it depends on the amount of brightness contrast between the lines and the spaces and, of course, the amount of noise (random variations) present in the image.

The situation is even more complicated with some digital still cameras that shift the detector array to capture multiple samples of the image. The most common method is to use a piezo-electric device to offset the array by half the pixel spacing in the horizontal and vertical directions, capturing four images that can be combined to more or less double the resolution of the image as data are acquired from the gaps between the original pixel positions. For an array with colored filters, additional shifts can produce color images with resolution approaching that corresponding to the pixel spacing. And some studio cameras displace the entire sensor array to different regions of the film plane to collect tiles that are subsequently assembled into an image several times as large as the detector array. Of course, the multiple exposures required with these methods means that more time is required to acquire the image.

With either the single-chip or three-chip camera, the blue channel is typically the noisiest due to the low chip sensitivity to blue light and the consequent need for greater amplification. In many cases, processing software that reduces image noise using one of the averaging or median filters discussed in **Chapter 4** can be applied separately to each color channel, using different parameters according to the actual noise content, to best improve image appearance.

Because of the longer exposure times, which collect more electrons and so reduce noise due to statistics and amplification, and because of the much slower readout of the data from the chip, which can take several seconds instead of 1/30th of a second, digital cameras using the same chip technology as a video camera can produce much better image quality. Digital still cameras read out the data in one single pass (progressive scan), not with an interlace. By cooling the chip and amplifier circuitry to reduce dark currents, integration (long exposures up to tens of seconds or, for some astronomical applications, many minutes) can be used to advantage because of the high dynamic range (large well size and large number of bits in the digitizer) of some chip designs. In addition, the ability to use a physical rather than an electronic shutter simplifies chip circuitry and increases fill factor. The number of pixels in video cameras need not be any greater than the resolution of the video signal, which as noted above is quite poor. In a digital still camera, very high pixel counts can give rise to extremely high resolution, which is beginning to rival film in some cases.

There is also an interesting crossover occurring between high-end consumer- and professional scientific-grade cameras. In addition to dedicated cameras for attachment to microscopes or other separate optics, manufacturers are producing consumer-grade cameras with enough resolution (up to 16 million pixels at the time of this writing) that it is becoming practical to use them in technical applications, and simple optical attachments are making it easy to connect them to microscopes. **Figure 1.19** shows one of the cameras in routine use in the author's laboratory. It is portable, with internal memory for images, and useful for many other

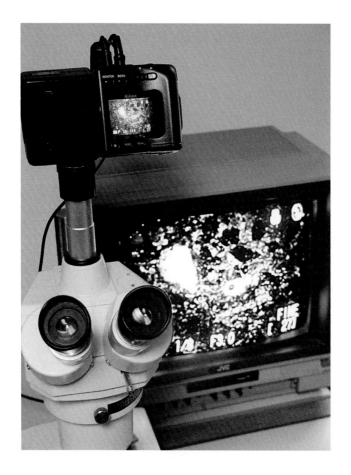

Figure 1.19 A digital camera mounted on the trinocular head of a microscope. This model (Nikon Coolpix 4500) produces a small preview display on its own LCD (liquid-crystal display) as well as a video output for display on a monitor that can be used for field selection and focusing. The digital images are stored as 4-megapixel TIFF (tagged image file format) files on removable memory cards that can be read by a computer. Other camera models also store the RAW image data. (RAW files are the full precision unmodified sensor data before any color corrections, noise reduction, nonlinear gamma adjustments, or other adjustments are made; there is no standard industry-wide format.)

applications. Professional digital cameras with extremely high-resolution detector arrays, interchangeable lenses, etc., are providing capabilities that compete with traditional 35-mm and larger film cameras. Every manufacturer of cameras has recognized the shift away from film and toward digital recording, and an incredibly wide variety of cameras is now available, with new developments appearing frequently.

CMOS cameras

A competitor to the CCD design for chips is the CMOS type (complementary metal oxide semiconductor), which uses a different fabrication approach that promises several potential advantages. The most important is cost, because the manufacturing process is similar to that used for other common chips such as computer memory, whereas CCDs require separate fabrication lines. It is also possible to incorporate additional circuitry on the CMOS chip, such as the amplifier's electronics, the readout and control electronics, and the digitizer, leading to the possibility of a single-chip camera. This can lead to less expensive systems but with more costly development procedures. The devices will also be more compact and possibly more rugged. CMOS devices also require lower voltages and have lower power requirements, which can be important for portable devices.

In the CMOS design (**Figure 1.20**), the chip is organized much like a computer memory chip. At each "pixel" location a detector responds to incoming photons, as in the CCD type. The electrons from the detector are read out by addressing the pixel based on its row and column position. One potential advantage of the CMOS design is windowing, the possibility to read out a portion of the array rather than the entire array, since row-column addressing (just like memory chips) can be used to access any pixel. This can provide rapid updating for focusing, measurement of regions of interest, etc.

On the other hand, CMOS devices have higher noise than CCDs. Partly, this is due to the fact that the CCD has less on-chip circuitry and uses a common output amplifier for less variability.

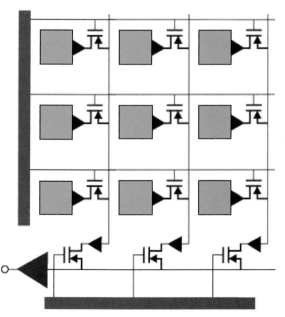

Figure 1.20 Schematic diagram of a typical CMOS detector. Each active light sensor (green) has additional transistors that are connected to addressing and output lines.

CMOS has higher dark currents, and hence more noise. Also there is more capacitance in the output wiring, which degrades amplifier noise characteristics. CMOS uses amplifiers for each pixel, producing a unique nonuniformity for each chip called fixed-pattern noise (FPN). FPN can in principle be removed by recording the pattern and postprocessing with software to remove it, but this further reduces the useful dynamic range. The additional transistors used for amplification and readout also take up more area on the chip, further reducing fill factor, and with it well capacity and dynamic range. Each pixel requires at least two or three transistors to control the detector in addition to the amplifier, and fill factors are often less than 30% (light-collecting lenses on each pixel are often used to compensate). The sensitivity and dynamic range of the CCD is much greater due to the larger size of the detector, lower noise, etc.

While CMOS detector production facilities are similar in principle to those used for computer memory and other devices, in fact the quest for lower noise has led to the use of special fabrication processes and techniques to reduce trapping and other defects, which largely eliminates this commonality. CMOS is expected to continue to dominate in the low-end consumer market for camcorders and snapshot cameras, toys, cell phones, and other specialty applications such as surveillance video cameras. It is being used in some professional digital still cameras, particularly ones with very large chip areas (e.g., the size of a full-frame 35-mm film negative), because four chips can be combined into a single array by carefully cutting away two adjacent sides of each (the addressing circuitry resides entirely along the other two sides). CMOS is not expected to challenge CCDs for most scientific and technical applications requiring high fidelity, resolution, and dynamic range for several more years, and it is generally expected that both will continue to enjoy a significant market and further technical developments (Nakamura 2006).

Focusing

Regardless of what type of camera is employed to acquire images, it is important to focus the optics correctly to capture the fine details in the image. Often the human eye is used to perform this task manually. In some situations, such as automated microscopy of pathology slides or surveillance tracking of vehicles, automatic focusing is required. This brings computer processing into the initial step of image capture. Sometimes, in the interest of speed, the processing is performed in dedicated hardware circuits attached to the camera. But in many cases the algorithms are the same as might be applied in the computer, and the focusing is accomplished in software by stepping the optics through a range of settings and choosing the one that gives the "best" picture.

Several different approaches to automatic focus are used. Cameras used for macroscopic scenes may employ methods that use some distance-measuring technology, e.g., using high-frequency sound or infrared light, to determine the distance to the subject so that the lens position can be adjusted. In microscopy applications this is impractical, and the variation with focus adjustment in the image itself must be used. Various algorithms are used to detect the quality of image sharpness, and all are successful for the majority of images in which there is good contrast and fine detail present. Each approach selects some implementation of a high-pass filter output that can be realized in various ways, using either hardware or software, but that must take into account the effect of high-frequency noise in the image and the optical-transfer function of the optics (Boddeke et al. 1994; Buena-Ibarra 2005; Bueno et al. 2005; Firestone et al. 1991; Green et al. 1985; Sun et al. 2004).

Electronics and bandwidth limitations

Video cameras of either the solid-state chip or tube type produce analog voltage signals corresponding to the brightness at different points in the image. In the standard RS-170 signal convention, the voltage varies over a 0.7-volt range from minimum to maximum brightness, as shown previously in **Figure 1.8**. The scan is nominally 525 lines per full frame, with two interlaced 1/60th-sec fields combining to make an entire image. Only about 480 of the scan lines are actually usable, with the remainder lost during vertical retrace. In a typical broadcast television picture, more of these lines are lost due to overscanning, leaving about 400 lines in the actual viewed area. The time duration of each scan line is 62.5 μsec, part of which is used for horizontal retrace. This leaves 52 μsec for the image data, which must be subdivided into the horizontal spacing of discernible pixels. For PAL (European) television, these values are slightly different, based on a 1/25th-sec frame time and more scan lines, and the resulting resolution is slightly higher.

Broadcast television stations are given only a 4-MHz bandwidth for their signals, which must carry color and sound information as well as the brightness signal we have so far been discussing. This narrow bandwidth limits the number of separate voltage values that can be distinguished along each scan line to a maximum of 330, as mentioned previously, and this value is reduced if the signal is degraded by the electronics or by recording using standard videotape recorders. Consumer-quality videotape recorders reduce the effective resolution substantially; in "freeze frame" playback, they display only one of the two interlaced fields, so that only about 200 lines are resolved vertically. Using such equipment as part of an image-analysis system makes choices of cameras or digitizer cards on the basis of resolution quite irrelevant.

Even the best system can be degraded in performance by such simple things as cables, connectors, or incorrect termination impedance. Another practical caution in the use of standard cameras is to avoid automatic gain or brightness-compensation circuits. These can change the image contrast or linearity in response to bright or dark regions that do not even lie within the digitized portion of the image, and they can increase the gain and noise for a dim signal.

Figure 1.21 shows a micrograph with its brightness histogram. This is an important tool for image analysis, which plots the number of pixels as a function of their brightness values. It will be used extensively in subsequent chapters. The histogram is well spread out over the available 256 brightness levels, with peaks corresponding to each of the phases in the metal sample. If a bright light falls on a portion of the detector in the solid-state camera that is not part of the image area of interest (e.g., due to internal reflections in the optics), automatic gain circuits in the camera may alter the brightness-voltage relationship so that the image changes. This same effect occurs when a white or dark mask is used to surround images placed under a camera on a copy stand. The relationship between structure and brightness is changed, making subsequent analysis more difficult.

Issues involving color correction and calibration will be dealt with below, but obtaining absolute color information from video cameras is impossible because of the broad range of wavelengths passed through each filter, the variation in illumination color (e.g., with slight voltage changes on an incandescent bulb), and the way the color information is encoded. Matching colors so that the human impression of color is correct requires calibration, discussed in **Chapter 4**.

The analog voltage signal is usually digitized with an 8-bit "flash" ADC (analog-to-digital converter). This is a chip using successive approximation techniques (described previously) to rapidly sample and measure the voltage in less than 100 nsec, producing a number value from 0 to 255 that represents the brightness. This number is immediately stored in memory

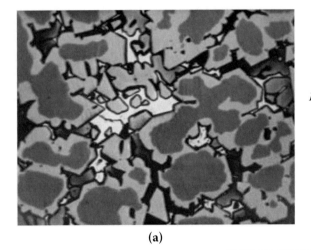

(a)

Figure 1.21 A gray-scale image digitized from a metallographic microscope and its brightness histogram, which plots the number of pixels with each possible brightness value.

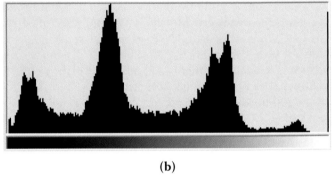

(b)

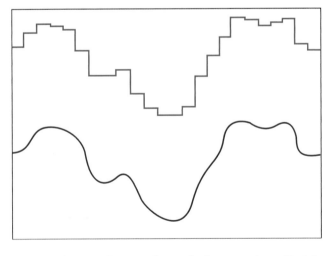

Figure 1.22 Digitization of an analog voltage signal such as one line in a video image (blue) produces a series of numbers that represent a series of steps (red) equal in time and rounded to integral multiples of the smallest measurable increment.

and another reading made, such that a series of brightness values is obtained along each scan line. **Figure 1.22** illustrates the digitization of a signal into equal steps both in time and value. Additional circuitry is needed to trigger each series of readings on the retrace events so that positions along successive lines are consistent. Digitizing several hundred points along each scan line, repeating the process for each line, and storing the values into memory while adjusting for the interlace of alternate fields produces a digitized image for further processing or analysis.

This process is essentially identical for a "digital" camera, except that it takes place inside the camera housing; thus the numbers rather than the voltages are transmitted to the computer (or simply stored in memory for later readout). Because the readout is slower for a still camera, the noise is reduced and the measurement precision is greater. Many high-end digital still cameras use 12-bit ADCs (one part in 4096) rather than 8-bit (one part in 256). Also, of course, there are many more pixels in most digital still cameras than in a video camera.

Pixels

It is most desirable to have the spacing of the pixel values be the same in the horizontal and vertical directions (i.e., square pixels), as this simplifies many processing and measurement operations. There are some theoretical advantages to having pixels arranged as a hexagonal grid, but because of the way that all acquisition hardware actually functions, and to simplify the addressing of pixels in computer memory, this is almost never done.

Accomplishing the goal of square pixels requires a well-adjusted clock to control the acquisition. Since the standard video image is not square, but has a width-to-height ratio of 4:3, the digitized image may represent only a portion of the entire field of view. Digitizing boards, also known as frame grabbers, were first designed to record 512 × 512 arrays of values, since the power-of-two (2^9) dimension simplified design and memory addressing. Most of the current generation of boards acquire a 640-wide × 480-high array, which matches the image proportions and the size of standard VGA display monitors while keeping the pixels square. Because of the variation in clocks between cameras and digitizers, it is common to find distortions of several percent in pixel squareness. This can be measured and compensated for after acquisition by resampling the pixels in the image, as discussed in **Chapter 4**. Most digital still cameras acquire images that have a width-to-height ratio of 4:3 or 3:2, and have square pixels.

Of course, digitizing 640 values along a scan line that is limited by electronic bandwidth and only contains 300+ meaningfully different values produces an image with unsharp or fuzzy edges and "empty" magnification. Cameras that are capable of resolving more than 600 points along each scan line can sometimes be connected directly to the digitizing electronics to reduce this loss of horizontal resolution. Digital camera designs bypass the analog transmission altogether, sending digital values to the computer or to internal memory, but digital still cameras are slower than standard video systems, as discussed previously.

Since pixels have a finite area, those that straddle a boundary in the scene effectively average the brightness levels of two regions and have an intermediate brightness that depends on how the pixels lie with respect to the boundary. This means that a high lateral-pixel resolution and a large number of distinguishable gray levels are needed to accurately locate boundaries. **Figure 1.23** shows several examples of an image with varying numbers of pixels across its width, and **Figure 1.24** shows the same image with varying numbers of gray levels.

For the most common types of image-acquisition devices, such as cameras, the pixels represent an averaging of the signal across a finite area of the scene or specimen. However, there are other situations in which this is not so. At low magnification, for example, the scanning electron microscope (SEM) beam samples a volume of the specimen much smaller than the dimension of a pixel in the image. So does the probe tip in a scanned-probe microscope. Range imaging of the moon from the Clementine orbiter read the elevation of points about 10 cm in diameter using a laser range finder, but the points were spaced apart by 100 m or more.

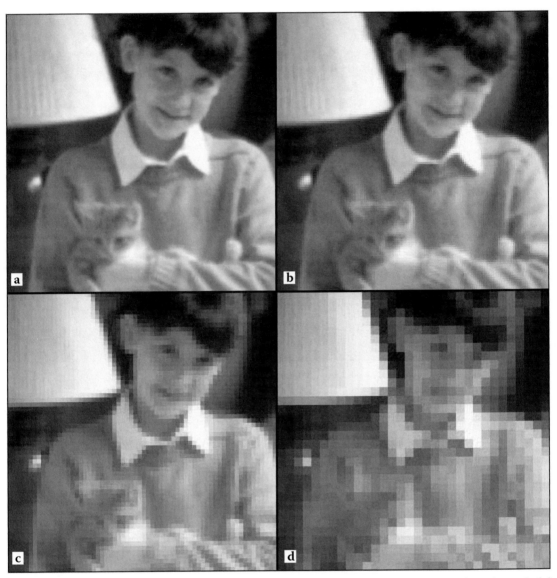

Figure 1.23 *Four representations of the same image, with variation in the number of pixels used:* **(a)** *256 × 256;* **(b)** *128 × 128;* **(c)** *64 × 64;* **(d)** *32 × 32. In all cases, the full set of 256 gray values is retained. Each step in coarsening of the image is accomplished by averaging the brightness of the region covered by the larger pixels.*

In these cases, the interpretation of the relationship between adjacent pixels is slightly different. Instead of averaging across boundaries, the pixels sample points that are discrete and well separated. Cases of intermediate or gradually varying values from pixel to pixel are rare, and the problem instead becomes how to locate a boundary between two sampled points on either side. If there are many points along both sides of the boundary, and if the boundary can be assumed to have some geometric shape (such as a locally straight line), then fitting methods can be used to locate it to a fraction of the pixel spacing. These methods are discussed further in **Chapter 10** on image measurements.

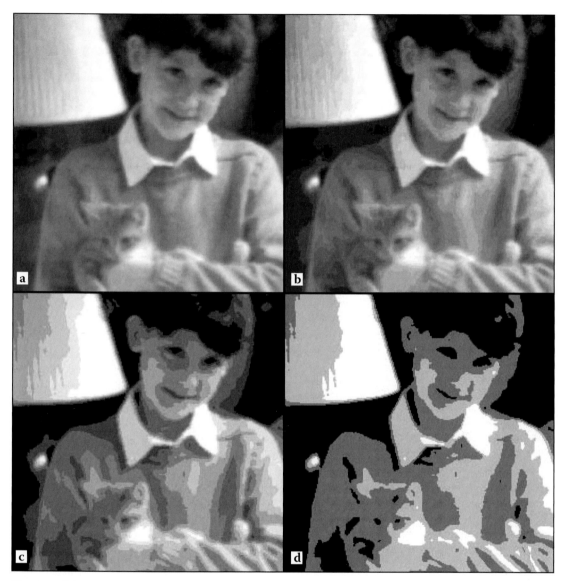

Figure 1.24 *Four representations of the same image, with variation in the number of gray levels used: (a) 32; (b) 16; (c) 8; (d) 4. In all cases, a full 256 × 256 array of pixels is retained. Each step in the coarsening of the image is accomplished by rounding the brightness of the original pixel value.*

Gray-scale resolution

In addition to defining the number of sampled points along each scan line, and hence the resolution of the image, the design of the ADC also controls the precision of each measurement. Inexpensive commercial flash analog-to-digital converters usually measure each voltage reading to produce an 8-bit number from 0 to 255. This full range may not be needed for an actual image, e.g., one that does not vary from full black to white. Also, the quality of most cameras and other associated electronics rarely produces voltages that are free enough from electronic noise to justify full 8-bit digitization anyway. A typical "good" camera specification of a 49-dB signal-to-noise ratio implies that only 7 bits of real information are available and that the eighth bit is random noise. But 8 bits corresponds nicely to the most common organization of computer memory into bytes, so that 1 byte of storage can hold the brightness value from one pixel in the image.

High-end digital still cameras and most scanners produce more than 256 distinguishable brightness values, and for these it is common to store the data in 2 bytes or 16 bits, giving a possible range of 65,536:1, which exceeds the capability of any current imaging device (but not some other sources of data that can be displayed as images, such as surface elevation measured with a scanned probe, as discussed in **Chapter 14**). For a camera with a 10- or 12-bit output, the values are simply shifted over to the most significant bits, and the low-order bits are either zero or random values. For display and printing purposes 8 bits is enough, but the additional depth can be very important for processing and measurement, as discussed in subsequent chapters. In many systems the histogram of values is still expressed as 0 to 255 for compatibility with the more common 8-bit range, but instead of being restricted to integers the brightness values have real or floating-point values.

Figure 1.25 shows an image that appears to be a uniform gray. When the contrast range is expanded, we can see the faint lettering present on the back of this photographic print. Also evident is a series of vertical lines that is due to the digitizing circuitry, in this case electronic noise from the high-frequency clock used to control the time base for the digitization. Nonlinearities in the ADC, electronic noise from the camera itself, and degradation in the amplifier circuitry combine to make the lowest 2 bits of most standard video images useless, so that only about 64 gray levels are actually distinguishable in the data. As noted previously, higher performance cameras and circuits exist, but do not generally offer "real-time" video speed (30 frames per second).

When this stored image is subsequently displayed from memory, the numbers are used in a digital-to-analog converter to produce voltages that control the brightness of a display monitor, often a cathode-ray tube (CRT) or liquid crystal display (a flat-screen LCD). This process is comparatively noise free and high resolution, since computer display technology has been developed to a high level for other purposes. These displays typically have 256 steps of brightness for the red, green, and blue signals, and when equal values are supplied to all three, the result is perceived as a neutral gray value.

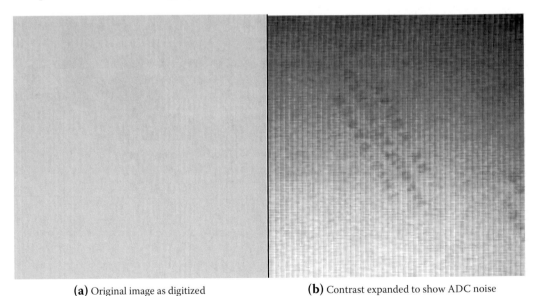

(a) Original image as digitized   (b) Contrast expanded to show ADC noise

Figure 1.25 *Digitized camera image of the back of a photographic print, showing the periodic noise present in the lowest few bits of the data from the electronics (especially the clock) in the analog-to-digital converter:* *(a)* *original;* *(b)* *expanded contrast.*

The human eye cannot distinguish all 256 different levels of brightness in this type of display, nor can they be successfully recorded or printed using ink-jet or laser printers, as discussed in **Chapter 3**. About 20 to 30 gray levels can be visually distinguished on a CRT, LCD, or photographic print, suggesting that the performance of the digitizers in this regard is more than adequate, at least for those applications where the performance of the eye was enough to begin with and where the purpose of the imaging is to produce prints.

A somewhat different situation that results in another limitation arises with images that cover a very large dynamic range. Real-world scenes often include brightly lit areas and deep shade. Scientific images such as SEM pictures have very bright regions corresponding to edges and protrusions and very dark ones such as the interiors of depressions. Astronomical pictures range from the very bright light of stars to the very dark levels of dust clouds. If only 256 brightness levels are stretched to cover this entire range, there is not enough sensitivity to small variations to reveal detail in either bright or dark areas. Capturing images with higher bit depth, for instance 12 bits (4096 brightness levels, which is approximately the capability of a film camera), can record the data, but it cannot be viewed successfully on a display screen or in a print. Processing methods that can deal with such high-dynamic-range images to facilitate visual interpretation are shown in **Chapter 5**.

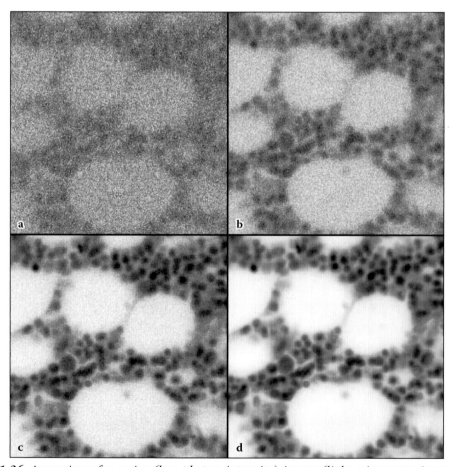

Figure 1.26 *Averaging of a noisy (low photon intensity) image (light-microscope image of bone marrow):* ***(a)*** *one frame;* ***(b)*** *averaging of 4 frames;* ***(c)*** *averaging of 16 frames; and* ***(d)*** *averaging of 256 frames.*

Images acquired in very dim light, or some other imaging modalities such as X-ray mapping in the SEM, impose another limitation of the gray-scale depth of the image. When the number of photons (or other particles) collected for each image pixel is low, statistical fluctuations become important. **Figure 1.26a** shows a fluorescence microscope image in which a single video frame illustrates extreme statistical noise, which would prevent distinguishing or measuring the structures present.

Noise

Images in which the pixel values vary within regions that are ideally uniform in the original scene can arise either because of limited counting statistics for the photons or other signals, losses introduced in the shifting of electrons within the chip, or electronic noise in the amplifiers or cabling. In any case, the variation is generally referred to as noise, and the ratio of the contrast that is actually due to structural differences represented by the image to the noise level is the signal-to-noise ratio. When this is low, the features present may be invisible to the observer. **Figure 1.27** shows an example in which several features of different size and shape are superimposed on a noisy background with different signal-to-noise ratios. The ability to discern the presence of the features is generally proportional to their area, and independent of shape.

In the figure, a smoothing operation is performed on the image with the poorest signal-to-noise ratio, which somewhat improves the visibility of the features. The methods available for smoothing noisy images by image processing are discussed in the chapters on spatial- and

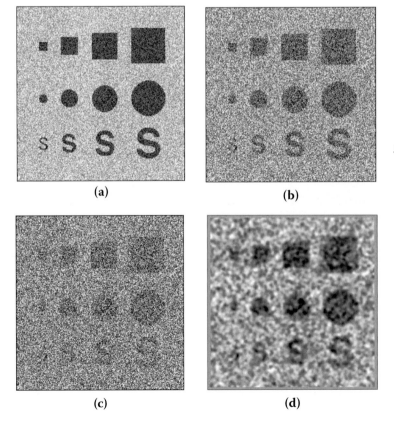

(a)

(b)

(c)

(d)

Figure 1.27 Features on a noisy background:
(a) signal-to-noise ratio 1:1;
(b) signal-to-noise ratio 1:3;
(c) signal-to-noise ratio 1:7;
(d) image *c* after spatial smoothing.

frequency-domain methods (**Chapter 4** and **Chapter 6**, respectively). However, the best approach to noisy images, when it is available, is simply to collect more signal and improve the statistics.

The effect of adding together more video frames is shown in **Figure 1.26**. The improvement in quality is proportional to the square root of the number of frames. Since each frame is digitized to 8 bits, adding together up to 256 frames as shown requires a total image storage capability that is 16 bits (2 bytes) deep. Acquiring frames and adding together the pixels at video rates generally requires specialized hardware, and performing the operation in a general-purpose computer limits the practical acquisition to only a few of the video frames per second. This limitation discards a large percentage of the photons that reach the detector. It is more efficient to use a camera capable of integrating the signal directly for the appropriate length of time (provided that the detector has a sufficient well size to hold the charge), and then to read the final image to the computer, which also reduces the noise due to readout and digitization. Digital still cameras (as contrasted with video cameras) provide this capability, and with cooled chips they can reduce electronic noise during long acquisitions of many minutes. Most uncooled camera chips will begin to show unacceptable pixel noise due to dark current with integration times of more than a few seconds.

Acquiring images from a video camera is sometimes referred to as "real time" imaging, but of course this term should properly be reserved for any imaging rate that is adequate to reveal temporal changes in a particular application. For some situations, time-lapse photography may only require one frame to be taken at periods of many minutes. For others, very short exposures and high rates are needed. Special cameras that do not use video frame rates or bandwidths can achieve rates up to ten times that of a standard video camera for full frames, and even higher for small image dimensions. These cameras typically use a single line of detectors and optical deflection (e.g., a rotating mirror or prism) to cover the image.

For many applications, the repetition rate does not need to be that high. Either stroboscopic imaging or simply a fast shutter speed may be enough to stop the important motion to provide a sharp image. Electronic shutters can be used instead of a mechanical shutter to control solid-state imaging devices. Exposure times under 1/1000th of a second can easily be achieved, but of course this short exposure requires plenty of light intensity.

High-depth images

Other devices that produce data sets that are often treated as images for viewing and measurement produce data with a much greater range than a camera. For instance, a scanned stylus instrument that measures the elevation of points on a surface can have a vertical resolution of a few nanometers with a maximum vertical travel of hundreds of micrometers, for a range-to-resolution value of 10^5. This would require storing data in a format that preserved the full-resolution values, and such instruments typically use 4 bytes per pixel.

In some cases with cameras having a large brightness range, the entire 12- or 14-bit depth of each pixel is stored. However, since this depth exceeds the capabilities of most CRTs to display, or of the user to see, reduction may be appropriate. If the actual brightness range of the image does not cover the entire possible range, scaling (either manual or automatic) to select just the range actually used can significantly reduce storage requirements. In other cases, especially when performing densitometry, a nonlinear conversion table is used. For densitometry, the desired density value varies as the logarithm of the brightness; this is discussed in detail in

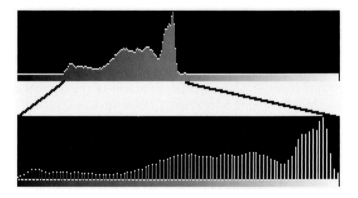

Figure 1.28 Linear expansion of a histogram to cover the full range of storage or display.

Chapter 10. A range of 256 brightness steps is not adequate to cover a typical range from 0 to greater than 3 in optical density with useful precision, because at the dark end of the range, 1 part in 256 represents a very large step in optical density. Using a digitization with 12 bits (1 part in 4096) solves this problem, but it is efficient to convert the resulting value with a logarithmic lookup table to store an 8-bit value (occupying a single computer byte) that is the optical density.

Lookup tables (LUTs) can be implemented either in hardware or software. They simply use the original value as an index into a stored or precalculated table, which then provides the derived value. This process is fast enough that acquisition is not affected. The LUTs discussed here are used for image acquisition, converting a 10-, 12-, or 14-bit digitized value with a nonlinear table to an 8-bit value that can be stored. LUTs are also used for displaying stored images, particularly to substitute colors for gray-scale values to create pseudocolor displays, but also to apply correction curves to output devices (displays and printers) in order to match colors. This topic is discussed later in this chapter and in **Chapter 3**.

Many images do not have a brightness range that covers the full dynamic range of the digitizer. The result is an image whose histogram covers only a portion of the available values for storage or for display. **Figure 1.28** shows a histogram of such an image. The flat (empty) regions of the plot indicate brightness values at both the light and dark ends that are not used by any of the pixels in the image. Expanding the brightness scale by spreading the histogram out to the full available range, as shown in the figure, may improve the visibility of features and the perceived contrast in local structures. The same number of brightness values are missing from the image, as shown by the gaps in the histogram, but now they are spread uniformly throughout the range. Other ways to stretch the histogram nonlinearly are discussed in **Chapter 4**.

The contrast range of many astronomical images is too great for photographic printing, and special darkroom techniques have been developed to solve this problem. These techniques have since been adapted to other applications and to computer software. "Unsharp masking" (**Figure 1.29**) increases the ability to show local contrast by suppressing the overall brightness range of the image. The suppression is done by first printing a "mask" image, slightly out of focus, onto another negative. This negative is developed and then placed on the original to make the final print. This superposition reduces the exposure in the bright areas so that the detail can be shown. The same method can also be used in digital image processing, either by subtracting a smoothed version of the image or by using a Laplacian operator or high-pass filter (discussed in **Chapter 5** and **Chapter 6**). When the entire depth of a 12- or 14-bit image is stored, such processing may be needed to display the image for viewing on a CRT.

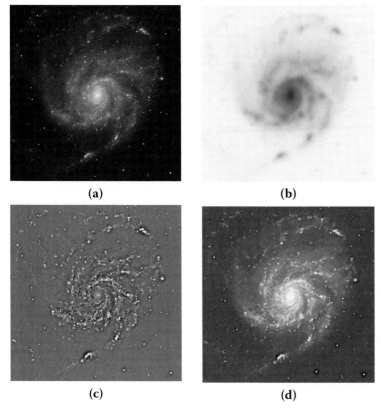

Figure 1.29 Unsharp masking:
(a) original telescope image of M101 (NGC5457);
(b) the "out-of-focus" negative;
(c) combining images **a** and **b** produces an image of just the local contrast;
(d) adding image **c** back to image **a** produces the classic unsharp-mask result.

Some perspective on camera performance levels is needed. While a standard video camera has about 300,000 sensors and a high-performance digital still camera can have a few million, the human eye has about 1.5×10^8. Furthermore, these are clustered particularly tightly in the fovea, the central area where we concentrate our attention. While it is true that only a few dozen brightness levels can be distinguished in a single field, the eye adjusts automatically to overall brightness levels, covering about nine orders of magnitude, to select the optimal range (although color sensitivity is lost in the darkest part of this range). **Chapter 2** further explores the capabilities of human vision.

Some cameras use a single-line CCD instead of a two-dimensional array. This gives high resolution but requires physically scanning the line across the film plane, much like a flatbed scanner. Most of these systems store the image digitally, converting the signal to a full-color image (for instance with 8 to 12 bits each of red, green, and blue data).

There is a major difference between the interlace scan used in conventional television and a noninterlaced or "progressive" scan. The latter gives better quality because there are no line-to-line alignment or shift problems. Most high-definition television (HDTV) modes use progressive scan. The format requires a higher rate of repetition of frames to fool the human eye into seeing continuous motion without flicker, but it has many other advantages. These include simpler logic to read data from the camera (which can be incorporated directly on the chip), more opportunity for data compression because of redundancies between successive lines, and simpler display or storage devices. Most scientific imaging systems such as digital cameras, direct-scan microscopes (the scanning electron microscope or SEM, scanning tunneling microscope or STM, the atomic force microscope or AFM, etc.), flatbed scanners, film or slide digitizers, and similar devices use progressive rather than interlaced scan.

HDTV modes include many more differences from conventional television than the use of progressive scan. The pixel density is much higher, with a wider aspect ratio of 16:9 (instead of the 4:3 used in NTSC [National Television Systems Committee] television), and the pixels are square. A typical HDTV mode presents 1920 × 1080-pixel images at the rate of 30 full scans per second, for a total data rate exceeding 1 gigabit per second, several hundred times as much data as current broadcast television. One consequence of this high data rate is the interest in data-compression techniques, discussed in **Chapter 3**, and the investigation of digital transmission techniques using cable or optical fiber instead of broadcast channels. Whatever the details of the outcome in terms of consumer television, the development of HDTV hardware is likely to produce spin-off effects for computer imaging, such as high-pixel-density cameras with progressive scan output, high-bandwidth recording devices, and superior CRT displays. For example, color cameras being designed for HDTV applications output digital rather than analog information by performing the analog-to-digital conversion within the camera, with at least 10 bits each for red, green, and blue.

It is also interesting to compare camera technology with other kinds of image-acquisition devices. The scanning electron (SEM) or scanned probe microscopes (such as the AFM) typically use from a few hundred to about 1000 scan lines. Those that digitize the signals use 8 or sometimes 12 bits, and so are similar in image resolution and size to many camera systems. **Figure 1.30** shows schematically the function of an SEM. The focused beam of electrons is scanned over the sample surface in a raster pattern while various signals generated by the electrons are detected. These include secondary and backscattered electrons, characteristic X-rays, visible light, and electronic effects in the sample.

Other point-scanning microscopes, such as the AFM, the confocal scanning light microscope (CSLM), and even contact profilometers, produce very different signals and information. All provide a time-varying signal that is related to spatial locations on the sample by knowing the scanning speed and parameters, which allows storing the data as an image. Many of these devices have noise and resolution characteristics that are different in directions parallel and perpendicular to the scanning direction.

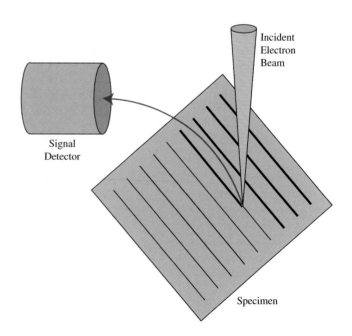

Figure 1.30 The SEM focuses a fine beam of electrons on the specimen, producing various signals that can be used for imaging as the beam is scanned in a raster pattern.

Significantly larger arrays of pixels are available from flatbed scanners. These devices use a linear solid-state detector array and can typically scan areas at least 8 × 10 in., and sometimes up to several times that size. While primarily intended for the desktop publishing market, they are readily adapted to scan electrophoresis gels used for protein separation, or photographic prints or negatives. A high-quality negative can record several thousand distinguishable brightness levels and several thousand points per inch (both values are much better than prints). Scanners are also used for digitizing photographic negatives such as medical X-rays and 35-mm slides. Commercial scanners are used in publishing and to convert films to digital values for storage (for instance in Kodak's Photo-CD format). At the consumer level, scanners with 1000 to as many as 2400 pixels per inch are common for large-area reflective originals, and 3000 to 4000 pixels per inch are common for 35-mm slide film. Most scanners digitize full-color red, green, and blue (RGB) images.

These devices are quite inexpensive but rather slow, taking tens of seconds to digitize the scan area. Another characteristic problem they exhibit is pattern noise in the sensors: if all of the detectors along the row are not identical in performance, a "striping" effect will appear in the image as the sensor is scanned across the picture. If the scan motion is not perfectly smooth, it can produce striping in the other direction. This latter effect is particularly troublesome with handheld scanners that rely on the user to move them and sense the motion with a contact roller that can skip, but these devices should not be used for inputting images for measurement anyway (they are marketed for reading text) because of their tendency to skip or twist in motion.

By far the greatest difficulty with such scanners arises from the illumination. There is often a drop-off in intensity near the edges of the scanned field because of the short length of the light source. Even more troublesome is the warm-up time for the light source to become stable. In scanners that digitize color images in a single pass by turning colored lights on and off, stability and consistent color are especially hard to obtain. On the other hand, making three separate passes for red, green, and blue often causes registration difficulties. Even for monochrome scanning, it can take several minutes before the light source and other electronics become stable enough for consistent measurements.

Scanning technology is also impacting conventional light microscopy. Devices are now available (some adapted from 35-mm film scanners) that scan conventional light-microscope slides directly to produce medium- or high-resolution images of the entire slide area. Other microscopes have been designed with motorized stages and digital cameras to acquire a mosaic of conventional images that are stitched together in memory to produce a single large image of the entire slide. There are even designs for microscopes that use multiple optical paths and cameras to rapidly image entire slide areas. In all of these cases, the goal is to obtain a stored digital image representing the entire slide, which can then be examined on a display screen rather than "live" through the microscope (Bacus and Bacus 2000, 2002). Special software is required to efficiently access the stored array (which can be a single enormous file) and to interactively deliver the selected portion of the image data as the user varies position and magnification. Network access to such stored images also presents bandwidth challenges, but facilitates collaboration and teaching.

Color imaging

Most real-world images are color rather than monochrome. The light microscope produces color images, and many biological specimen preparation techniques make use of color to

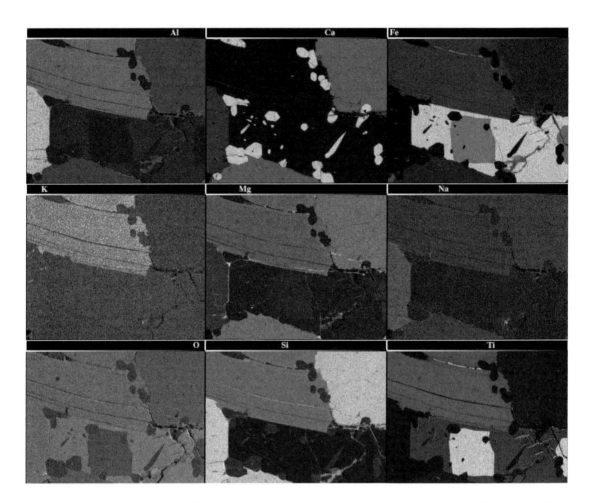

Figure 1.31 *SEM images of a polished sample of mica. The individual X-ray images or "dot maps" show the localization of the corresponding elements within various minerals in the sample.*

identify structure or localize chemical activity in novel ways. Even for inorganic materials, the use of polarized light or surface oxidation produces color images to delineate structure. The SEM is usually a strictly monochromatic imaging tool, but color can be introduced based on X-ray energy or backscattered electron energy. **Figure 1.31** shows individual gray-scale images from the X-ray signals from a mineral sample imaged in the SEM. The X-ray images show the variation in composition of the sample for each of nine elements (Al, Ca, Fe, K, Mg, Na, O, Si, Ti). There are more individual images than the three red, green, and blue display channels, and no obvious "correct" choice for assigning colors to elements. **Figure 1.32** shows a few possibilities, but it is important to keep in mind that no single color image can show all of the elements at once. Assigning several of these arbitrarily, e.g., to the red, green, and blue planes of a display, may aid the user in judging the alignment of regions and areas containing two or more elements. **Chapter 4** introduces methods for processing multiple-channel images to find principal components. Colored X-ray maps are now fairly common with the SEM, as are similar concentration maps based on measured intensities from ion microprobes, but other uses of color such as energy loss in the transmission electron microscope (TEM) are still experimental.

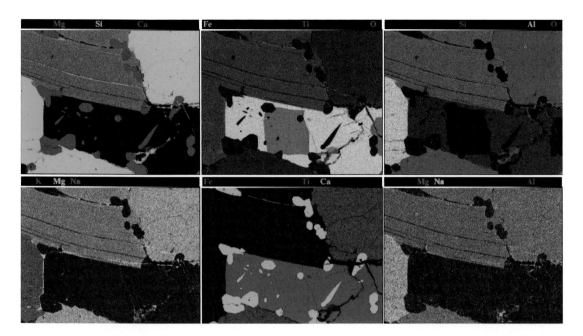

Figure 1.32 Composite color images made by assigning various images from **Figure 1.31** to the red, green, or blue channels of the display. This assists in the identification and discrimination of the various minerals.

Similar use of color is potentially useful with other kinds of microscopes, although in many cases these possibilities have not been exploited in commercial instruments. This is also true for macroscopic imaging tools. A simple example is the use of color to show altitude in air traffic control displays. This use of color increases the bandwidth for communicating multidimensional information to the user, but the effective use of these methods requires some education of users and would benefit from some standardization. Of course, it also requires that users possess full-color vision capability.

The use of color to encode richly multidimensional information must be distinguished from the very common use of false color or pseudocolor to substitute colors for brightness in a monochrome image. Pseudocolor is used because of the limitation mentioned before in our visual ability to distinguish subtle differences in brightness. Although we can only distinguish about 20 to 30 shades of gray in a monochrome image, we can distinguish hundreds of different colors. Also, it may aid communication to describe a particular feature of interest as "the dark reddish-orange one" rather than "the medium-gray one."

The use of color scales as a substitute for brightness values allows us to show and see small changes locally and to identify the same brightness values globally in an image. This should be a great benefit, since these are among the goals for imaging discussed below. Pseudocolor has been used particularly for many of the images returned from space probes. It would be interesting to know how many people think that the rings around Saturn really are brightly colored, or that comet Halley really is surrounded by a rainbow-colored halo! The danger in the use of pseudocolor is that it can obscure the real contents of an image. The colors force us to concentrate on the details of the image, and to lose the gestalt information. Examples of image processing in this book will use pseudocolor selectively to illustrate some of the processing effects and the changes in pixel values that are produced, but often pseudocolor distracts the human eye from seeing the real contents of the enhanced image.

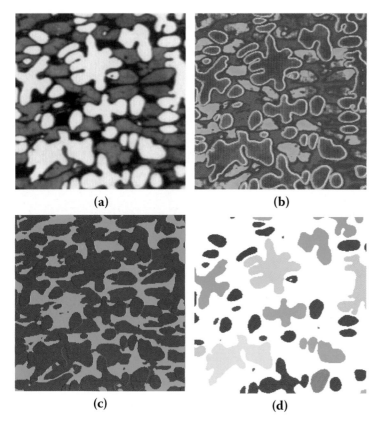

(a)   **(b)**

(c)   **(d)**

Figure 1.33 Different uses for pseudocolor displays.
- **(a)** *Portion of a gray-scale microscope image of a polished metallographic specimen with three phases having different average brightnesses.*
- **(b)** *Image a with pseudocolor palette or LUT that replaces gray values with colors. (Note the misleading colors along boundaries between light and dark phases.)*
- **(c)** *Image with colors assigned to phases. This requires segmentation of the image by thresholding and other logic to assign each pixel to a phase based on gray-scale brightness and neighboring pixel classification.*
- **(d)** *Lightest features from the original image with colors assigned based on feature size. This requires the steps to create image **c**, plus collection of all touching pixels into features and the measurement of the features.*

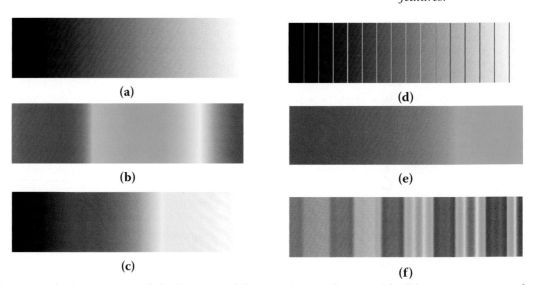

(a)   **(d)**

(b)   **(e)**

(c)   **(f)**

*Figure 1.34 Six examples of display LUTs: **(a)** monochrome (gray scale); **(b)** spectrum or rainbow (variation of hue, with maximum saturation and constant intensity); **(c)** heat scale; **(d)** monochrome with contour lines (rainbow colors substituted every 16th value); **(e)** tricolor blend of three primary colors; **(f)** sinusoidal variation of hue with linear variation of saturation and intensity.*

Pseudocolor displays as used in this context simply substitute a color from a stored or precalculated table for each discrete stored brightness value. As shown in **Figure 1.33**, this should be distinguished from some other uses of color displays to identify structures or indicate feature properties. These also rely on the use of color to communicate rich information to the viewer, but require considerable processing and measurement of the image before this information becomes available.

Color can be used to encode elevation of surfaces (see **Chapter 14**). In scientific visualization it is used for velocity, density, temperature, composition, and many less obvious properties. These uses generally have little to do with the properties of the image and simply take advantage of the human ability to distinguish more colors than gray-scale values.

Most computer-based imaging systems make it easy to substitute various lookup tables (LUTs) of colors for the brightness values in a stored image. These work in the same way as input lookup tables, described before. The stored gray-scale value is used to select a set of red, green, and blue brightnesses in the LUT that controls the voltages sent to the display tube. Many systems also provide utilities for creating tables of these colors, but there are few guidelines to assist in constructing useful ones. All I can do here is advise caution. One approach is to systematically and gradually vary color along a path through color space. Examples (**Figure 1.34**) are a rainbow spectrum of colors or a progression from brown through red and yellow to white, the so-called heat scale. This gradual variation can help to organize the different parts of the scene. Another approach is to rapidly shift colors, for instance by varying the hue sinusoidally. This enhances gradients and makes it easy to see local variations, but may completely hide the overall contents of some images (**Figure 1.35**).

Another application of color to images that were originally monochrome is the artistic manual colorization or tinting of features. This is typically done to distinguish different types of objects, according to the understanding and recognition of a human observer. **Figure 1.36** shows an example. Such images certainly have a value in communicating information, especially to

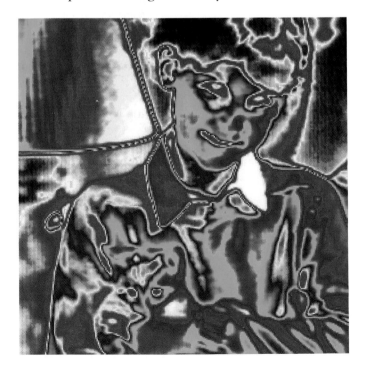

Figure 1.35 The same image used in Figure 1.23 and Figure 1.24 with a pseudocolor or display LUT. The gestalt contents of the image are obscured.

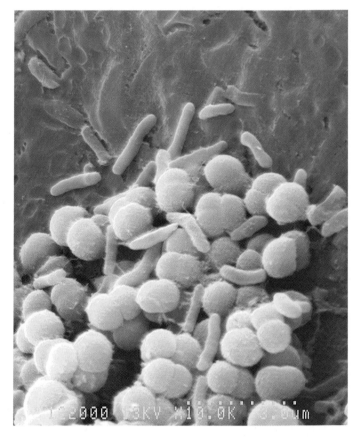

Figure 1.36 Manually colorized SEM image of bacteria, in which color tints have been applied to distinguish rod-shaped bacilli and spherical cocci from the background. (Courtesy of T. Carvalho, Pacific Biomedical Research Center, University of Hawaii at Manoa.)

people who are not familiar with either the subject matter or the functioning of the imaging device, and some may qualify as art, but this type of procedure is outside the scope of this book.

Some image sources use color to encode a variety of different kinds of information, such as the intensity and polarization of radio waves in astronomy. However, by far the most common type of color image is that produced by recording the intensity at three different wavelengths of visible light. Video deserves mention as a medium for this type of image, since standard broadcast television uses color in a way that is visually satisfactory. The NTSC color-encoding scheme used in the U.S. was developed as a compatible add-on to existing monochrome television broadcasts. It adds the color information within the same, already narrow bandwidth limitation. The result is that the color has even less lateral resolution than the brightness information.

Color subsampling reduces the amount of data in an image by representing color data with lower resolution than luminance (brightness) data. This is done in the YUV color space (Y = luminance or brightness, U and V = chrominance or color), described later in this chapter. Uncompressed YUV color is represented as 4:4:4. The common subsampling options are 4:2:2, 4:2:0, 4:1:1, and YUV-9:

> *4:2:2:* Full-bandwidth sampling of Y and 2:1 horizontal sampling of U and V. This is the sampling scheme most commonly used in professional and broadcast video and in tape formats such as D-1 and Digital Betacam. It looks good, but the data-compression ratio is only 33%.

4:2:0: Full-bandwidth sampling of Y and 2:1 sampling of U and V in both the horizontal and vertical dimensions. That is, for every four luminance samples, there are two chrominance samples every other line. This yields a 50% reduction in data. 4:2:0 is the color space used in MPEG (Moving Pictures Expert Group) compression.

4:1:1: Full-bandwidth sampling of Y and 4:1 horizontal sampling of U and V. This is the color space of the digital video (DV) formats. It uses U and V samples four pixels wide and one pixel tall, so color bleeding is much worse in the horizontal than in the vertical direction.

YUV-9: This is the color format used in most of the video compression on the Internet. For every 16 luminance Y samples in a 4 × 4-pixel block, there is only one U and one V sample, producing smaller files with correspondingly lower color fidelity. YUV-9 subsampling often results in noticeable color artifacts around the edges of brightly colored objects, especially red.

Such limitations are acceptable for television pictures, since the viewer tolerates colors that are less sharply bounded and uses the edges of features defined by the brightness component of the image where they do not exactly correspond. The same tolerance has been used effectively by painters and may be familiar to parents whose young children have not yet learned to color "inside the lines." **Figure 1.37** shows an example in which the bleeding of color across boundaries or variations within regions is not confusing to the eye.

The poor spatial sharpness of NTSC color is matched by its poor consistency in representing the actual color values (a common joke is that NTSC means "never the same color" instead of "National Television Systems Committee"). Videotape recordings of color images are even less useful for analysis than monochrome ones. But the limitations imposed by the broadcast channel do not necessarily mean that the cameras and other components may not be useful. An improvement in the sharpness of the color information in these images is afforded by Super-VHS or S-video recording equipment, also called component video, in which the brightness or luminance and color or chrominance information are transmitted and recorded separately, without subsampling of data.

Some color cameras intended for technical purposes bring out the red, green, and blue signals separately so that they can be individually digitized. Recording the image in computer

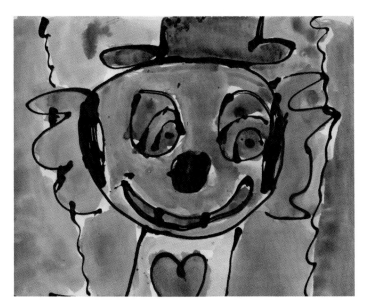

Figure 1.37 A child's painting of a clown. Notice that the colors are unrealistic but their relative intensities are correct, and that the painted areas are not exactly bounded by the lines. The dark lines nevertheless give the dimensions and shape to the features, and we are not confused by the colors that extend beyond their regions.

memory then simply involves treating each signal as a monochrome one, converting it to a set of numbers, and storing it in memory. If the signals have first been combined, the encoding scheme used is likely to be YIQ or YUV (defined below), which are closely related to the NTSC broadcasting scheme. Much better fidelity in the image can be preserved by not mixing together the color and brightness information. Instead of the composite signal carried on a single wire, some cameras and recorders separate the chrominance (color) and luminance (brightness) signals onto separate wires. This so-called component, Y-C or S-video format is used for high-end consumer camcorders (Hi-8 and S-VHS formats). Many computer interfaces accept this format, which gives significant improvement in the quality of digitized images, as shown in **Figure 1.38**.

Another important development in video is digital video (DV) recording. Like analog videotape recorders, digital video writes each scan line onto the tape at an angle using a moving head that rotates as the tape moves past it (**Figure 1.39**). The signal is encoded as a series of digital bits that offers several advantages. Just as CD technology replaced analog audio tapes, the digital video signal is not subject to loss of fidelity as images are transmitted or copies are made. More important, the high-frequency information that is discarded in analog recording because

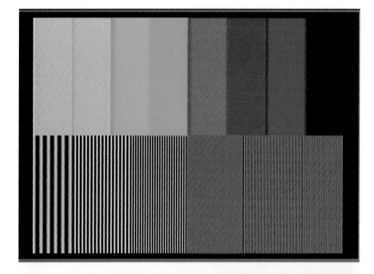

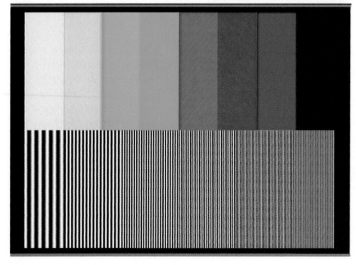

Figure 1.38 *Comparison of*
(a) *composite and*
(b) *component video*
  signals from a signal
  generator, digitized
  using the same
  interface board.
  Note the differences in
  resolution of the black
  and white stripes and
  the boundaries between
  different colors.

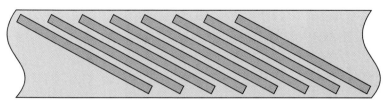

Figure 1.39 In digital video, each video frame is recorded digitally in 10 tracks on metal-coated magnetic tape (12 tracks for the larger PAL format). Each track contains video, audio, and timing information.

of the 4-MHz upper-frequency limit imposed by conventional broadcast TV is preserved in DV. Digital video records up to 13.5 MHz for the luminance (brightness) information and up to one-fourth that for the chrominance (color) information. This produces much sharper edge delineation, particularly for the brightness data in the image, and greatly improves the usefulness of the resulting images. The digital video signal is fully preserved on the tape recording, unlike conventional analog recorders, which impose a further bandwidth reduction on the data and are susceptible to quality loss due to dirty heads, worn tape, or making successive copies from an original.

The result is that DV images have about 500 × 500-pixel resolution and nearly 8 bits of contrast, and can be read into the computer without a separate digitizer board, since they are already digital in format. The IEEE 1394 standard protocol for digital video (also known as "firewire") establishes a standard serial interface convention that is available on consumer-priced cameras and decks and is being supported by many computer manufacturers as well. Inexpensive interface boards are available, and the capability is built into the basic circuitry of some personal computers, even laptops. Most of these digital cameras can be controlled by the computer to select individual frames for transfer. They can also be used to record single frames annotated with date and time, turning the digital videotape cartridge into a tiny but high-fidelity storage format for hundreds of single images. Some DV video cameras are now replacing the tape cartridge with flash (solid state) memory to store the data, but the same format is used.

Digital camera limitations

The current development of the digital still-frame cameras for the consumer market involves practically every traditional maker of film cameras and photographic supplies. Many of these are unsuitable for technical applications because of limitations in the optics (fixed-focus lenses with geometric distortions) and limited resolution (although even a low-end 320 × 240-pixel camera chip in a cell phone offers resolution as good as conventional analog video recording). Some cameras interpolate between the pixels on the chip to create images with empty magnification. In most cases this produces artifacts in the image that are serious impediments to quantitative measurement.

However, it is the use of image compression that creates the most important problem. In an effort to pack many images into the smallest possible memory, JPEG (Joint Photographers Expert Group) and other forms of image compression are used. As discussed in **Chapter 3**, these are lossy techniques that discard information from the image. The discarded data is selected to minimally impact the human interpretation and recognition of familiar images — snapshots of the kids and the summer vacation — but the effect on quantitative image analysis can be severe. Edges are broken up and shifted, color and density values are altered, and fine details can be eliminated or moved. The important advantage of the higher-end consumer and

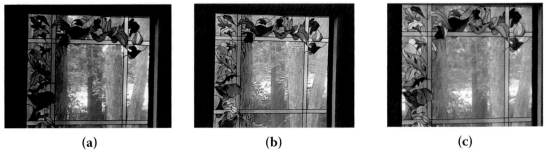

Figure 1.40 *Images of the same scene (see text) recorded using:* **(a)** *a three-chip video camera and analog-to-digital converter;* **(b)** *an inexpensive consumer digital camera; and* **(c)** *a research-grade digital camera.*

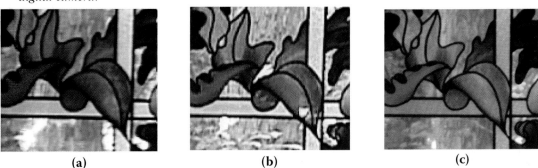

Figure 1.41 *Enlarged regions of the images in* **Figure 1.40**, *showing the greater resolution and fidelity in the high-end digital camera image.*

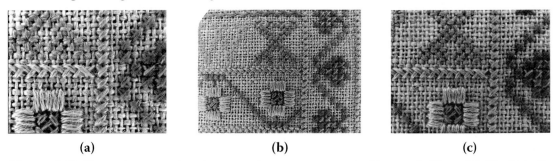

Figure 1.42 *Macro images using the same three cameras as in* **Figures 1.40** *and* **1.41**. *Note the variations in resolution and color rendition.*

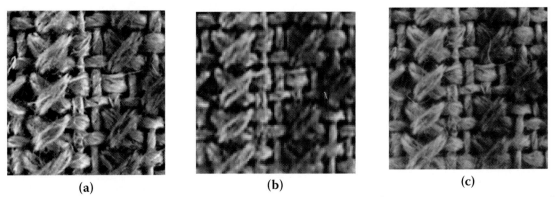

Figure 1.43 *Enlargement of a portion of the images in* **Figure 1.42**, *showing the appearance of individual fibers.*

professional cameras is that they offer storage or transfer to the computer without any lossy compression, and this is much preferred for technical applications.

Figure 1.40 and **Figure 1.41** compare images of the same scene using three different cameras. The subject is a difficult view through a stained glass window, with a dark interior and bright daytime exterior. This produces a very high-contrast range, with some regions that are saturated in color and others with low saturation, subtle differences, and fine detail. The first image is video from a three-chip color video camera acquired using a high-quality analog-to-digital converter producing a 640 × 480-pixel image and averaging eight frames to reduce noise. The second image was acquired with a consumer digital camera, also as a 640 × 480-pixel image, using the highest quality compression setting (least compression). The third image was acquired with a research-grade digital camera as a 1600 × 1200-pixel image.

The original colors are represented with greater fidelity in the third image. In addition to color shifts, the first two images have brightness values that are clipped to eliminate the brightest and darkest values, and the video image does not produce 256 distinct values of red, green, and blue, so that the image has missing values within the range. The consumer digital camera apparently applies a high-pass or sharpening filter that exaggerates contrast at edges, producing dark and light borders. There are other artifacts present in the first two images as well: scan-line noise in the video image and square blocks resulting from the JPEG compression in the consumer digital camera image. Enlarging the image to see fine details makes apparent the far higher resolution of the research-grade digital image. In **Figure 1.41** a region is expanded to show fine details in each of the images. The research-grade digital camera image renders these with greater fidelity in both the high-brightness and high-saturation regions.

The high-resolution digital still camera offers the same advantages for recording of images in microscope and other technical applications. **Figure 1.42** shows three images obtained with the same three cameras using a low-power microscope to view an antique cross-stitch fabric specimen. Identification of individual characteristics (and occasional errors) in the formation of the stitches and tension on the threads is of interest to cultural anthropologists to identify individual handiwork. This requires a low enough magnification to see the overall pattern, while identification of the threads and dyes used requires a high enough resolution to see individual fibers as well as good color fidelity to represent the dyes. **Figure 1.43** shows an enlargement of one small region of the three images. The difference in resolution and color fidelity between these images is another demonstration of the importance of using a high-quality camera.

A few words of caution may be useful. The slower readout from digital cameras makes focusing more difficult unless there is special provision for a real-time image, or independent optics to view the image, because the camera produces a preview image that updates several times a second. This is fine for selecting fields of view, but for convenient focusing it is important to adjust the optics so that the camera is truly parfocal with the eyepiece image. Some digital cameras also put out a live video signal that can be connected to a monitor for previews, albeit with only video resolution. Some digital cameras do not have a useful preview image but instead rely on a separate viewfinder that is of little practical use. There are also professional digital still cameras with single-lens-reflex designs that allow viewing through the camera optics and that replace the film with a sensing chip. In most of these, the chip is smaller in area than the film, and the resulting image is clipped (or, equivalently, the effective lens focal length is increased by a factor between 1.5 and 2.0).

On the other hand, it is possible in some instances with very low-end cameras to acquire useful images. For instance, digital cameras intended for video conferencing are available that deliver 64 gray levels or 32 levels of red, green, and blue with 320 × 240-pixel resolution (about as good as many examples of digitized video!) at about ten frames per second via a simple serial interface to the computer. No digitizer or separate power supply is required, and the digitization is built into the camera chip, requiring no hardware to be added to the computer. Such cameras cost well under $100 and can be quite useful for such purposes as capturing an image for videoconferencing.

The illustration in **Figure 1.44** was obtained by holding one such camera directly onto the eyepiece of a microscope with duct tape. The automatic gain control in the software was turned off, as the black area around the image confused the automatic adjustment. **Figure 1.45** shows another example of the use of the same camera. Placing it on an 8× loupe allows direct capture of images when (as in this forensic case) it was essential to collect images, and the only equipment available was the camera and a laptop computer. The biggest flaws with this setup were the difficulty in controlling the specimen illumination and the distortion caused by the very wide angle view from the optics. But there are situations in which any image is better than no image.

Color spaces

Conversion from RGB (the brightness of the individual red, green, and blue signals, as captured by the camera and stored in the computer) to YIQ/YUV and to the other color encoding schemes is straightforward and loses no information except for possible round-off errors. Y, the "luminance" signal, is just the brightness of a panchromatic monochrome image that would be displayed by a black-and-white television receiver. It combines the red, green, and blue signals in proportion to the human eye's sensitivity to them. The I and Q (or U and V) components of the color signal are chosen for compatibility with the hardware used in broadcasting; the I signal is essentially red minus cyan, while Q is magenta minus green. The relationship between YIQ and RGB is shown in **Table 1.1**. An inverse conversion from the encoded YIQ signal to RGB simply requires inverting the matrix of values.

RGB (and the complementary CMY [cyan, magenta, yellow] subtractive primary colors used for printing) and YIQ are both hardware-oriented schemes. RGB comes from the way camera

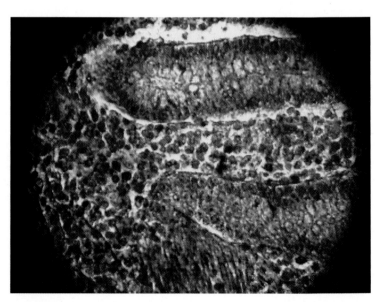

Figure 1.44 View of a biological thin section using a videoconferencing camera placed on the eyepiece of a bench microscope. Despite significant vignetting, the main details of the slide are visible.

Table 1.1. Interconversion of RGB and YIQ Color Scales

Y =	0.299 R	+ 0.587 G	+ 0.114 B	R =	1.000 Y	+ 0.956 I	+ 0.621 Q
I =	0.596 R	− 0.274 G	− 0.322 B	G =	1.000 Y	− 0.272 I	− 0.647 Q
Q =	0.211 R	− 0.523 G	+ 0.312 B	B =	1.000 Y	− 1.106 I	+ 1.703 Q

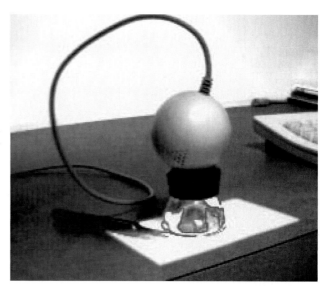

Figure 1.45 Using the same camera as in Figure 1.44 with a loupe to record an image for forensic examination.

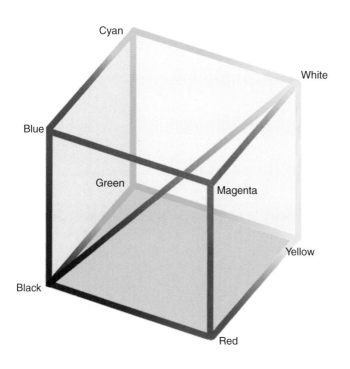

Figure 1.46 RGB color space, showing the additive progression from black to white. Combining red and green produces yellow, green plus blue produces cyan, and blue plus red produces magenta. Grays lie along the cube diagonal, with equal proportions of red, green, and blue. Cyan, yellow, and magenta are subtractive primaries used in printing, which if subtracted from white leave red, blue, and green, respectively.

sensors and display phosphors work, while YIQ or YUV stem from broadcast considerations. **Figure 1.46** shows the "space" defined by RGB signals: it is a Cartesian cubic space, since the red, green, and blue signals are independent and can be added to produce any color within the cube. There are other encoding schemes that are more useful for image processing and are more closely related to human perception.

The CIE (Commission Internationale de L'Éclairage) chromaticity diagram is a two-dimensional plot defining color, shown in **Figure 1.47**. The third (perpendicular) axis is the luminance, which corresponds to the panchromatic brightness which, like the Y value in YUV, produces a monochrome (gray scale) image. The other two primaries, called x and y, are always positive (unlike the U and V values) and combine to define any color that we can see.

Instruments for color measurement utilize the CIE primaries, which define the dominant wavelength and purity of any color. Mixing any two colors corresponds to selecting a new point in the diagram along a straight line between the two original colors. This means that a triangle on the CIE diagram, with its corners at the red, green, and blue locations of emission phosphors used in a cathode-ray tube (CRT), defines all of the colors that the tube can display. Some colors cannot be created by mixing these three phosphor colors, shown by the fact that they lie outside the triangle. The range of possible colors for any display or other output device is called the "gamut"; hard-copy printers generally have a much smaller gamut than display tubes, as discussed in **Chapter 3**. The edge of the bounded region in the diagram corresponds to pure colors and is marked with the wavelength in nanometers.

Complementary colors are shown in the CIE diagram by drawing a line through the central point, which corresponds to white light. Thus, a line from green passes through white to magenta. One of the drawbacks of the CIE diagram is that it does not indicate the variation in color that can be discerned by eye. Sometimes this is shown by plotting a series of ellipses on the diagram. These are much larger in the green area, where small changes are poorly perceived, than elsewhere. Variation in saturation (distance out from the center toward the edge) is usually more easily discerned than variation in hue (position around the diagram).

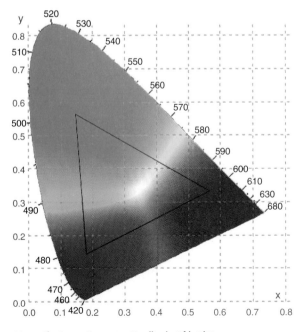

Figure 1.47 The CIE chromaticity diagram. The colors are fully saturated along the edge. Numbers give the wavelength of light in nanometers. The inscribed triangle shows the colors that typical color CRTs can produce by mixing of red, green, and blue light from phosphors.

The CIE diagram provides a tool for color definition, but corresponds neither to the operation of hardware nor directly to human vision. An approach that does is embodied in the HSV (hue, saturation, and value), HSI (hue, saturation, intensity), and HLS (hue, lightness, and saturation) systems. These are closely related to each other and to the artist's concept of tint, shade, and tone. In this system, hue is the color as described by wavelength, for instance the distinction between red and yellow. Saturation is the amount of the color that is present, for instance the distinction between red and pink. The third axis (called lightness, intensity, or value) is the amount of light, the distinction between a dark red and light red or between dark gray and light gray.

The space in which these three values is plotted can be shown as a circular or hexagonal cone or double cone, or sometimes as a cylinder. It is most useful to imagine the space as a double cone, in which the axis of the cone is the gray-scale progression from black to white, distance from the central axis is the saturation, and the direction is the hue. **Figure 1.48** shows this concept schematically.

This space has many advantages for image processing and for understanding color. For instance, if the algorithms discussed in **Chapter 4**, such as spatial smoothing or median filtering, are used to reduce noise in an image, applying them to the RGB signals separately will cause color shifts in the result, but applying them to the HSI components will not. Also, the use of hue (in particular) for distinguishing features in the process called segmentation (**Chapter 7**) often corresponds to human perception and ignores shading effects. On the other hand, because the HSI components do not correspond to the way that most hardware works (either for acquisition or display), it requires computation to convert RGB-encoded images to HSI and back.

Conversion between RGB space and hue-saturation-intensity coordinates can be performed in several ways, depending on the shape of the HSI space that is used. The most common choices are a sphere, cylinder, or double cone. In all cases the intensity axis is aligned along the body diagonal of the RGB cube, but none of the HSI space geometries exactly fits the shape of that cube. This means that, to represent colors in both spaces, the satu-

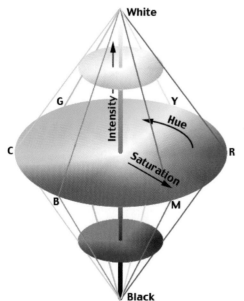

Figure 1.48 Biconic representation of hue-saturation-intensity space. Grays lie along the central axis. Distance from the axis gives the saturation, while direction (angle) specifies the hue.

ration values must be distorted somewhat in the conversion process. This can be seen in the example of **Figure 1.69** (presented later in this chapter), in which a high-resolution panchromatic satellite image is used to replace the intensity channel in an image constructed by merging three lower resolution R, G, B images.

The HSI spaces are useful for image processing because they separate the color information in ways that correspond to the human visual system's response, and also because the axes correspond to many physical characteristics of specimens. One example of this is the staining of biological tissue. To a useful approximation, hue represents the stain color, saturation represents the amount of stain, and intensity represents the specimen density. But these spaces are mathematically awkward: not only does the hue value cycle through the angles from 0 to 360° and then wrap around, but the conical spaces mean that increasing the intensity or luminance can alter the saturation. A geometrically simpler space that is close enough to the HSI approach for most applications and easier to deal with mathematically is the spherical L*a*b* model. L* as usual is the gray-scale axis, or luminance, while a* and b* are two orthogonal axes that together define the color and saturation (**Figure 1.49**). The a* axis runs from red (+a*) to green (–a*) and the b* axis from yellow (+b*) to blue (–b*). Notice that the hues do not have the same angular distribution in this space as in the usual color wheel. These axes offer a practical compromise between the simplicity of the RGB space that corresponds to hardware and the more physiologically based spaces such as HSI, which are used in many color management systems, spectrophotometers, and colorimeters.

The CIELab color space is considered to be "perceptually uniform," meaning that a just-detectable visual difference constitutes a constant distance in any location or direction within the space. Despite the apparent precision of the six-digit numerical values in the equations below, this is somewhat oversimplified, since the numbers are based on a limited number of human testers, and technically this space applies to the viewing of a hard-copy print under specific illuminating conditions, not to emissive displays such as a computer monitor. Nevertheless, CIELab is widely used as a standard space for comparing colors. It has several additional shortcomings, the most important of which is that simple radial lines do not maintain a constant hue. The transformation from RGB to CIELab requires an intermediate step, called XYZ:

Figure 1.49 L*a*b* color space. Gray values lie along a vertical north–south line through the sphere.

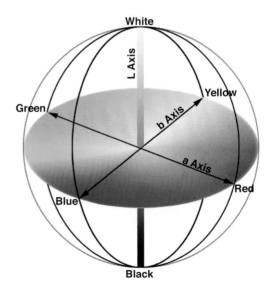

$$X = 0.412453 \cdot R + 0.357580 \cdot G + 0.180423 \cdot B$$

$$Y = 0.212671 \cdot R + 0.715160 \cdot G + 0.072169 \cdot B \qquad (1.1)$$

$$Z = 0.019334 \cdot R + 0.119193 \cdot G + 0.950227 \cdot B$$

Based on these XYZ values, the L*, a*, b* components are

$$L^* = 116 \cdot f\left(\frac{Y}{Y_n}\right) - 16$$

$$a^* = 500 \cdot \left[f\left(\frac{X}{X_n}\right) - f\left(\frac{Y}{Y_n}\right) \right]$$

$$b^* = 200 \cdot \left[f\left(\frac{Y}{Y_n}\right) - f\left(\frac{Z}{Z_n}\right) \right] \qquad (1.2)$$

in which the function f is defined as

$$f(q) = q^{\left(\frac{1}{3}\right)} \qquad \text{if } (q > 0.008856) \qquad (1.3)$$

$$f(q) = 7.787 \cdot q + 0.137931 \quad \text{otherwise}$$

and where X_n, Y_n, Z_n are calculated for a reference white point that depends on the illumination of the scene. This is usually described by the color temperature of the lamp; for instance, the standard D65 illuminant (6500K) corresponds to R = G = B = 100. The notations D65 or D50 describe the color spectrum of the illumination as being similar (but not quite identical) to the color spectrum of light emitted by an ideal black body radiator, which is a pinhole opening in a cavity held at a temperature of 6500K or 5000K.

It is interesting to compare this to the television YUV model. For an 8-bit (256 value) image, the conversion from RGB to YUV is simply:

$$Y = (0.299 \cdot R) + (0.587 \cdot G) + (0.114 \cdot B)$$
$$U = 128 - (0.169 \cdot R) - (0.331 \cdot G) + (0.500 \cdot B) \qquad (1.4)$$
$$V = 128 + (0.500 \cdot R) - (0.418 \cdot G) - (0.081 \cdot B)$$

Note that the Y (luminance) expression is the same as the YIQ conversion in **Table 1.1**. The 128 values in the U and V expressions are offsets to keep the results within the 0 to 255 range of positive integers. Note also that the Y value weights the red, green, and blue to approximate the human visual response to brightness, while the U and V values represent approximately yellow-blue and red-cyan differences.

A much simpler spherical color model than this can be used as a medium for image processing that retains the essential character of CIELab and is simpler than a true HSI space because it uses orthogonal axes instead of representing color as an angle. In this spherical space the luminance (intensity) value L* is simply the average of R, G, and B, and the a* and b* values are coordinates along two orthogonal directions. A typical conversion is:

$$\begin{bmatrix} L \\ a \\ b \end{bmatrix} = \begin{bmatrix} 1/3 & 1/3 & 1/3 \\ -\sqrt{2}/6 & -\sqrt{2}/6 & -\sqrt{2}/6 \\ 1/\sqrt{2} & -1/\sqrt{2} & 0 \end{bmatrix} \cdot \begin{bmatrix} R \\ G \\ B \end{bmatrix}$$

(1.5)

From these values, values for hue and saturation can be calculated as:

$$H = \tan^{-1}\left(\frac{b}{a}\right)$$

$$S = \sqrt{a^2 + b^2}$$

(1.6)

Alternatively, the conversion can be performed for a conical space:

$$I = \frac{R+G+B}{3}$$

$$S = 1 - \frac{3 \cdot \min(R,G,B)}{R+G+B}$$

$$H = \begin{cases} \cos^{-1}(z) & if \, (G \geq R) \\ 2\pi - \cos^{-1}(a) & if \, (G \leq R) \end{cases}$$

$$z = \frac{(2B - G - R)/2}{\sqrt{(B-G)^2 + (B-R)/(G-R)}}$$

(1.7)

Ledley et al. (1990) showed that the difference between these various RGB-HSI conversions lies principally in the saturation values. A fuller analysis of how this affects combinations of RGB images such as the satellite imagery in **Figure 1.69** can be found in Tu et al. (2001), where ways to compensate for the saturation changes are proposed. It is also possible to modify the intensity scale of either L*a*b* or HSI spaces to correspond to perceptual response to different colors. A typical model used for this is shown in **Equation 1.8**. Other weight factors that are shown with great apparent precision, such as ([0.212671 × R] + [0.715160 × G] + [0.072169 × B]), originally were derived from the specific phosphors used in television tubes to convert color video signals to monochrome, and even then were properly applied only to linear (not gamma corrected) intensities, but they have since come to be used in many cases to represent the approximate roles of the various color channels. In real cases, the actual weights depend on the color filters used in a particular camera, and they also probably vary from individual to individual and depend on illumination conditions.

$$I = 0.25 \cdot R + 0.65 \cdot G + 0.10 \cdot B$$

(1.8)

Hardware for digitizing color images accepts either direct RGB signals from the camera, or the Y-C component signals, or a composite signal (e.g., NTSC) and uses electronic filters to separate the individual components and extract the red, green, and blue signals. As for the monochrome case discussed previously, these signals are then digitized to produce values, usually 8-bit ones ranging from 0 to 255 each for R, G, and B. This takes 3 bytes of storage per pixel, so a 640 × 480-pixel image would require nearly 1 megabyte of storage space in the computer. With most video cameras and electronics, the signals do not contain this much information, and the lowest 2 or more bits are noise. Consequently, some systems keep only 5 bits each for R, G, and B, which can be fit into 2 bytes. This reduction is often adequate for Internet graphics and some desktop-publishing applications, but when packed this way, the color information is hard to get at for processing or analysis operations.

Color images are typically digitized as 24-bit RGB, meaning that 8 bits or 256 (linear) levels of brightness for red, green, and blue are stored. This is enough to allow display on video or computer screens, or for printing purposes, but, depending on the dynamic range of the data, it may not be enough to adequately measure small variations within the image. Since photographic film can capture large dynamic ranges, some scanners intended for transparency or film scanning provide greater range, typically 12 bits (4096 linear levels) for R, G, and B. Professional-quality digital still cameras also capture this much data in their "raw" images. These 36-bit images can be reduced to an "optimum" 8 bits per channel when the image is stored in the computer. One of the problems with converting the "raw" dynamic range of color or grayscale storage is that the brightness values measured by solid-state detectors are linear, whereas film (and human vision) are logarithmic, so that in the dark regions of an image the smallest brightness step that can be stored is quite large and may result in visual artifacts or poor measurement precision for density values.

Further reduction of color images to 256 colors — using a lookup table to select the best 256 colors matching the contents of the image — can be used for computer images to reduce the file size. The lookup table itself requires only 3×256 bytes to specify the R, G, B values for the 256 colors, which are written to the display hardware. Only a single byte per pixel is needed to select from this palette of colors. The most common technique for selecting the optimum palette is the Heckbert or median-cut algorithm, which subdivides color space based on the actual RGB values of the pixels in the original image. For visual purposes, such a reduction often provides a displayed image that is satisfactory, but this should be avoided for image-analysis purposes.

In many situations, although color images are acquired, the "absolute" color information is not useful for image analysis. Instead, it is the relative differences in color from one region to another that can be used to distinguish the structures and features present. In such cases, it may not be necessary to store the entire color image. Various kinds of color separations are available. Calculation of the RGB components (or the complementary CMY values) is commonly used in desktop publishing, but this is not often useful for image analysis. Separating the image into hue, saturation, and intensity components (often called channels) can also be performed. **Figure 1.50** and **Figure 1.51** show two examples, one a real-world image of flowers, and the second a microscope image of stained biological tissue. Note that some structures are much more evident in one separation than another (e.g., the pink spots on the white lily petals are not visible in the red image, but are much more evident in the green or saturation images). Also, note that for the stained tissue, the hue image shows where the stains are, and the saturation image shows how much of the stain is present. This distinction is also evident in the stained tissue sample shown in **Figure 1.52**.

It is possible to compute the amount of any particular "color" (hue) in the image. This calculation is equivalent to the physical insertion of a transmission filter in front of a monochrome camera. The filter can be selected to absorb a complementary color (for instance, a blue filter will darken yellow regions by absorbing the yellow light) and transmit light of the same color, so that the resulting image contrast can be based on the color distribution in the image. Photographers have long used yellow filters to darken the blue sky and produce monochrome images with dramatic contrast for clouds, for example. The same color filtering can be used

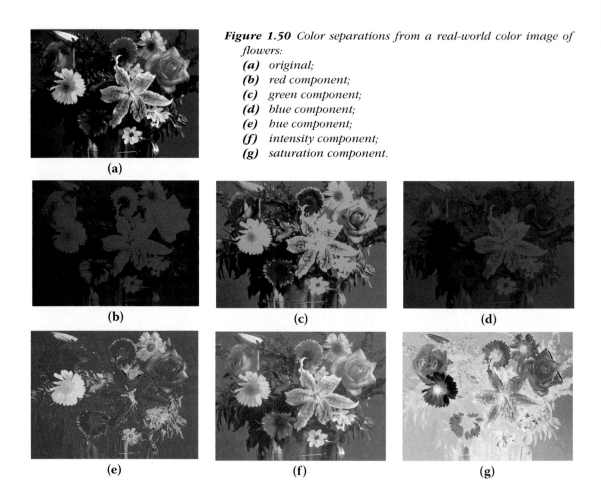

Figure 1.50 *Color separations from a real-world color image of flowers:*
(a) *original;*
(b) *red component;*
(c) *green component;*
(d) *blue component;*
(e) *hue component;*
(f) *intensity component;*
(g) *saturation component.*

(a)

(b) (c) (d)

(e) (f) (g)

to convert color images to monochrome (gray scale). **Figure 1.53** and **Figure 1.54** show examples in which the computer is used to apply the filter. This method offers greater flexibility than physical filters, since the desired wavelength can be specified; the operation can be performed later, using a stored image; and a drawer full of physical filters is not needed.

Reducing a color image to gray scale is useful in many situations and can be accomplished in many ways in addition to the obvious methods of selecting an R, G, B or H, S, I image channel, or applying a selected color filter. If obtaining the maximum gray-scale contrast between structures present in the image is desired to facilitate gray-scale image thresholding and measurement, then a unique function can be calculated for each image that fits a line through the points representing all of the pixels' color coordinates in color space. This least-squares fit or principal-components line gives the greatest separation of the various pixel color values, and the position of each pixel's coordinates as projected onto the line can be used as a gray-scale value that gives the optimum contrast (Russ 1995e). **Chapter 5** discusses this method at greater length and provides examples.

Figure 1.51 *Color separations from a light-microscope image of stained biological tissue (1 μm section of pancreas, polychromatic stain):*

(a) *original;*
(b) *hue;*
(c) *intensity;*
(d) *saturation;*
(e) *luminance (Y);*
(f) *U image (green-magenta);*
(g) *V image (blue-yellow).*

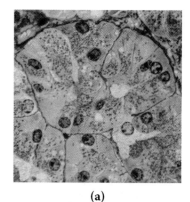

(a)

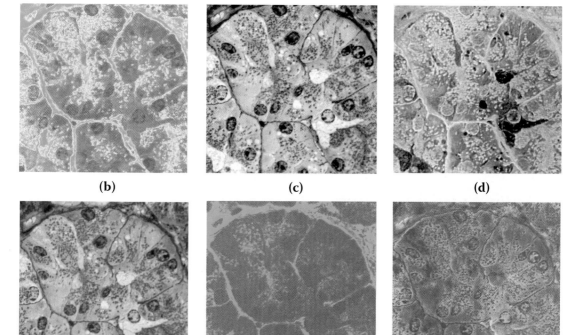

(b)   **(c)**   **(d)**

(e)   **(f)**   **(g)**

Color correction

When images are acquired under different lighting conditions, the color values recorded are affected. Human vision is tolerant of considerable variation in lighting, apparently using the periphery of the viewing field to normalize the color interpretation. Some cameras, especially video cameras, have an automatic white-point correction that allows recording an image from a gray card with no color, and using that to adjust subsequent colors. This same correction can be applied in software by adjusting the relative amount of red, green, and blue to set a region that is known to be without any color to pure gray. As shown in **Figure 1.55**, the method is straightforward, but works only for images that have regions that correspond to white, black, and neutral gray.

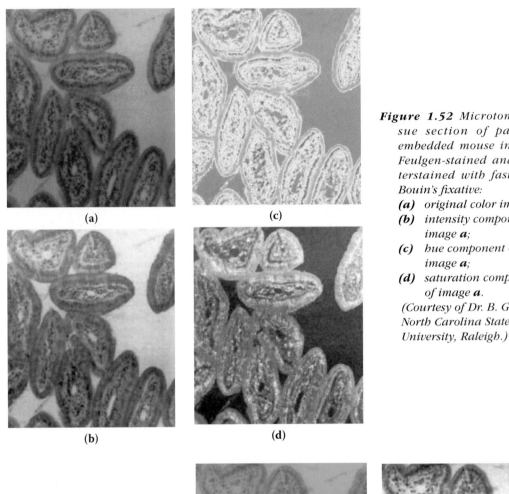

(a)

(c)

(b)

(d)

Figure 1.52 *Microtomed tissue section of paraffin-embedded mouse intestine, Feulgen-stained and counterstained with fast green, Bouin's fixative:*
(a) *original color image;*
(b) *intensity component of image a;*
(c) *hue component of image a;*
(d) *saturation component of image a.*
(Courtesy of Dr. B. Grimes, North Carolina State University, Raleigh.)

Figure 1.53 *Filtering of the image in* **Figure 1.52**:
(a) *application of a 480-nm filter to the original color image;*
(b) *monochrome intensity from image* **1.52c**.

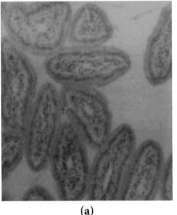

(a)

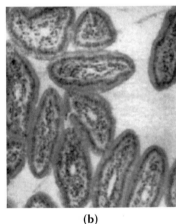

(b)

This approach can be extended to produce stored calibration curves that allow matching of colors for several devices. With a color target containing many known colors, it is possible to make adjustments that produce color matching between a camera or scanner, various CRT and LCD monitors, printers of various types, and even projectors. The typical procedure is to photograph or scan a known array of colors in order to construct the calibration curves for the acquisition devices (which includes, of course, the characteristics of the illumination used).

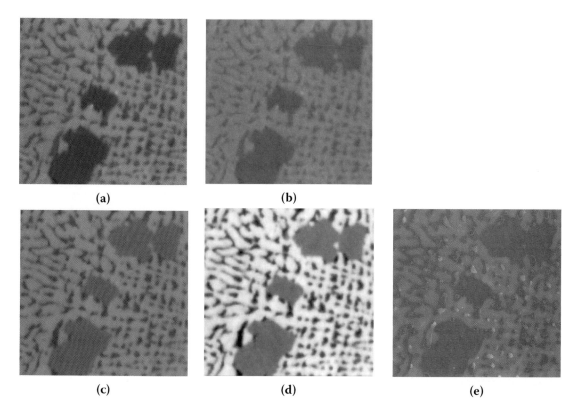

Figure 1.54 *Cast aluminum alloy containing 7.4% Ca, 0.8%Si, 0.2%Ti, showing two intermetallic phases (Al$_4$Ca in blue, CaSi$_2$ in reddish violet): **(a)** original color image; **(b)** the panchromatic intensity component of image **a**, showing inability to distinguish two of the phases; **(c)** application of a 590-nm filter; **(d)** monochrome intensity from image **c**; **(e)** the hue component of image **a**. (From Bühler, H.-E. and Hougardy, H.P.,* Atlas of Interference Layer Metallography, *Deutsche Gesellschaft für Metallkunde, Oberursel, Germany, 1980. With permission.)*

Printing a similar array from a stored file and then measuring each color with a spectrophotometer makes it possible to construct similar curves for the printer (which, as discussed in **Chapter 3,** will be specific to the inks and paper being used). Displaying colors on the screen and measuring them with the spectrophotometer produces another calibration curve, which is used to adjust values sent to the display.

The result is images that have matching visual colors everywhere. Several such devices are on the market, one of which (GretagMacbeth Eye-1, GretagMacbeth Corp, New Windsor, CT) consists of a single spectrophotometer that can be used on both emissive (CRT, LCD displays) and reflective (printed hard copy), a color target (**Figure 1.56**), and suitable software that performs the necessary actions and calculations with minimal user attention. Since the phosphors in CRTs and the backlight used for LCD displays age over time, printers use different inks and papers from time to time, and lighting changes alter camera color response, it is necessary to repeat the calibration from time to time.

A simpler, but quite accurate approach to color adjustment for image acquisition is tristimulus correction. This requires measuring a test image with areas of pure red, green, and blue color, such as the calibration card shown in **Figure 1.57**. In practical situations, such a card can be included in the scene being digitized. The camera (or scanner) will record some intensity

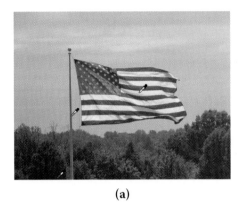

(a)

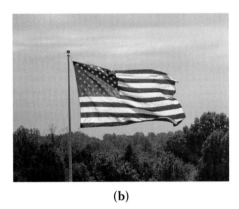

(b)

Figure 1.55 Color adjustment by selecting neutral points:

(a) original image with markers showing three points selected to have neutral dark, medium gray, and light values;

(b) result of adjustment;

(c) color adjustment for red, green, and blue showing the original values for the three selected points (horizontal axis) and the curves that produce new displayed values (vertical axis).

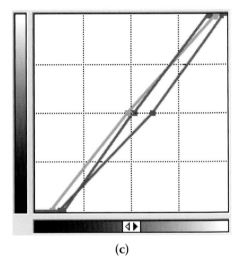

(c)

Figure 1.56 The GretagMacbeth color target consists of carefully controlled color patches designed to cover a range of colors that can be used to calibrate cameras and other devices. Note that the reproduction of the colors in this printed book will not be accurate, and that the illustration serves only to demonstrate the idea behind the calibration approach.

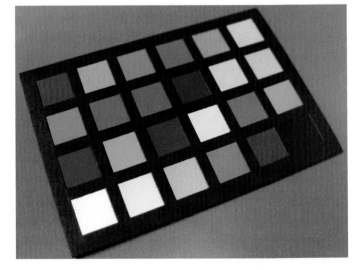

for red, green, and blue in each of the areas because of the fact that the color filters cover wide and overlapping ranges of wavelengths. This produces a matrix of values as shown in **Table 1.2**, which can be inverted to generate the tristimulus correction matrix. Calculating new red, green, and blue values by multiplication of this matrix times the measured R, G, B

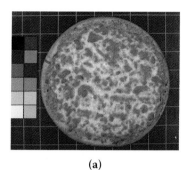
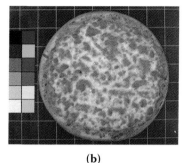

Figure 1.57 *Tristimulus color correction using RGB values:*
(a) *original image;*
(b) *corrected image using the tristimulus matrix calculated in* *Table 1.2.*

Table 1.2. Color Correction Using Tristimulus Values

Measure the RGB intensities from three target areas that are to be corrected to pure red, green, and blue; enter the intensities in the matrix

Measured intensity:		Red	Green	Blue
Area:	Red	131.91	43.08	69.16
	Green	72.91	152.66	53.74
	Blue	56.34	63.74	125.98

Intermediate normalized intensity matrix (the above values divided by 255)

		0.5173	0.1689	0.2712
		0.2859	0.5987	0.2107
		0.2209	0.2500	0.4940

Inverse matrix calculated by Excel (MINVERSE function)

Channel:		Red	Green	Blue
Result:	Red	2.6066	−0.1680	−1.3593
	Green	−1.0154	2.0978	−0.3375
	Blue	−0.6520	−0.9863	2.8027

values for each pixel produces an image in which the calibration areas are adjusted to pure red, green, and blue, and other colors in the image are also corrected, as shown.

For microscope images, a suitable set of color targets can be constructed by depositing known stains or dyes on a slide (Hoffmann et al. 2005). It is not necessary to have pure red, green, or blue. As long as the three colors are known and well separated in color space, a correction matrix can be computed.

Color displays

Of course, color is also important as a vehicle for communicating with the computer user. Most computers use color monitors that have much higher resolution than a television set but operate on essentially the same principle. Smaller phosphor dots, a higher frequency scan and higher bandwidth amplifiers, and a single progressive scan (rather than interlaced) produce much greater sharpness and color purity.

Besides color video monitors, other kinds of displays can be used with desktop computers. For example, many notebook computers and flat-panel monitors for desktop computers use a liquid crystal display (LCD). The passive type of LCD display, now declining in use, has much poorer saturation and is also slower than the active-matrix type that uses a separate transistor to control each pixel (or, actually, each of the RGB cells that together make up a pixel in a color display). However, most active-matrix color LCDs are inferior to most CRTs because of their lower brightness and narrower viewing angle. They also have an inferior brightness and contrast range for each color, which reduces the number of distinct colors that can be displayed.

LCDs are also used in projection devices used to show images on a screen. The most common design uses a very bright (and color-corrected) light source with small LCD panels and appropriate optics. High-brightness projectors generally use three separate CRTs with red, green, and blue filters. With these projectors, the resolution is potentially higher because the individual CRTs have continuous phosphor coatings. However, careful alignment of the optics is needed to keep the three images in registration; readjustment may be needed every time the equipment is moved or even as it heats up. Getting enough brightness for viewing large images in rooms with imperfect light control is also a challenge.

A third class of displays uses the digital light-modulation principle developed by Texas Instruments. An array of tiny mirrors produced by photolithography on silicon wafers is used to reflect light from the illumination source through appropriate optics to a viewing screen. The mirrors can be flipped from the "on" to the "off" position in nanoseconds. Moving each mirror back and forth rapidly to control the fraction of the time that it is in the "on" position controls the brightness of each pixel. A rotating filter wheel allows the array to sequentially project the red, green, and blue channels, which the eye perceives as a color display.

Other kinds of flat-panel computer displays, including electroluminescence and plasma (gas discharge), are fundamentally monochrome but can be filtered to produce color images. Arrays of red, green, and blue LEDs can, in principle, be arranged to make a flat-panel display, but the difficulty of generating blue light with these devices and the prohibitive cost of such devices has so far prevented their common use. Arrays of colored light bulbs are used to show images in some sports stadia.

It takes combinations of three color phosphors (RGB) to produce the range of colors displayed on the CRT. The brightness of each phosphor is controlled by modulating the intensity of the electron beam in the CRT that strikes each phosphor. Using a separate electron gun for each color and arranging the colored dots as triads is the most common method for achieving this control. To prevent stray electrons from striking the adjacent phosphor dot, a shadow mask of metal with holes for each triad of dots can be used. Each of the three electron beams passes through the same hole in the shadow mask and strikes the corresponding dot. The shadow mask increases the sharpness and contrast of the image, but reduces the total intensity of light that can be generated by the CRT.

A simpler design that increases the brightness applies the phosphor colors to the CRT in vertical stripes. It uses either a slotted pattern in the shadow mask or no mask at all. The simplicity of the Sony Trinitron design makes a tube with lower cost, no curvature of the glass in the vertical direction, high display brightness, and fewer alignment problems. However, the vertical extent of the phosphor and of the electron beam tends to blur edges in the vertical direction on the screen. While this design has become fairly common for home television, most high-performance computer CRTs use triads of phosphor dots because of the greater sharpness it affords the image, particularly for lines and edges. A high-resolution computer monitor can have a pitch (the spacing from one triad to the next) of 200 μm. At normal viewing distances, this is not visually resolved, producing a continuous image.

Image types

The brightness of each point in a simple image depends in part on the strength, location, and color of the illumination. It also is a function of the orientation, texture, color and other characteristics of the surface that reflect or scatter the light. Human interpretation of such images takes all of these factors into account. These "surface" or "real-world" images are actually rather difficult to interpret using computer algorithms because of their three-dimensional (3-D) nature and the fact that some surfaces may obscure others. Even for relatively flat scenes in which precedence is not a problem and the light source is well controlled, the combination of effects of surface orientation and the color, texture, and other variables make it difficult to quantitatively interpret these parameters independently. In the case of a carefully prepared flat and polished surface (as in the typical metallographic microscope), interpretation of contrast as delineating phases, inclusions, grains, or other structures is more successful. For additional background on image formation and on the role of lighting and optics, see Jahne (1997).

A second class of images that commonly arises in microscopy shows the intensity of light (or other radiation) that has come through the sample. (For additional background on light microscopes and their use for imaging, see texts such as R. Smith [1990], Bracegirdle and Bradbury [1995], Bradbury and Bracegirdle [1998], and Heath [2005].) Transmission images start with a uniform light source, usually of known intensity and color. The absorption of the light at each point is a measure of the density of the specimen along that path. For some kinds of transmission images, such as those formed with electrons and X-rays, diffraction effects due to the coherent scattering of the radiation by atomic or molecular structures in the sample may also be present. These often complicate analysis, because diffraction is strongly dependent on the exact orientation of the crystalline lattice or other periodic microstructure.

To illustrate the complications that factors other than simple density can cause, **Figure 1.58** shows a transmission electron microscope (TEM) image of a thin cobalt foil. The evident structure is the magnetic domains in this ferromagnetic material. In each striped domain, the electron spins on the atoms have spontaneously aligned. There is no change in the atomic

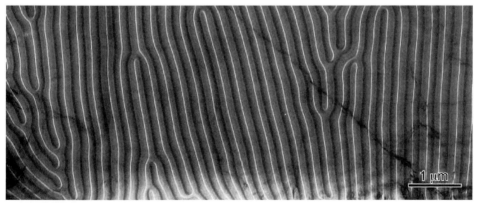

Figure 1.58 *TEM image of a thin metal foil of cobalt. The striped pattern reveals ferromagnetic domains in which the electron spins of the atoms are aligned in one of two possible directions. (Courtesy of Hitachi Scientific Instrument, Pleasanton, CA.)*

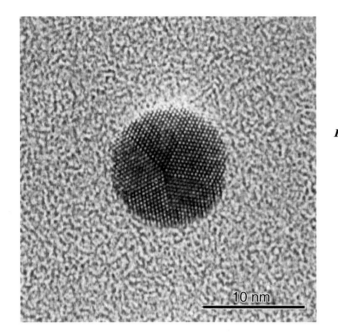

Figure 1.59 TEM image of colloidal gold particle on an amorphous carbon substrate, used to show very high microscope resolution. (Courtesy of Hitachi Scientific Instruments, Pleasanton, CA.)

structure, sample density, or thickness, although the image certainly can fool the viewer into thinking such variations may be present.

Likewise, **Figure 1.59** shows an image of a colloidal gold particle on an amorphous carbon film viewed in a high-resolution TEM. The so-called atomic resolution shows a pattern of dark spots on the substrate that appear more or less random, while within the gold particle they are regularly arranged. The arrangement is a result of the crystalline structure of the particle, and the spots are related to the atom positions. However, the spots are not simply the atoms; the relationship between the structure and the image is very complex and depends strongly on the microscope parameters and on the amount of defocus in the lens. Calculating the expected image contrast from a predicted structure is possible and can be done routinely for simple structures. The inverse calculation (structure from image) is more interesting, but can only be accomplished by iteration.

In another subclass of transmission images, some colors (or energies) of radiation may be selectively absorbed by the sample according to its chemical composition or the presence of selective stains and dyes. Sometimes, these dyes themselves also emit light of a different color that can be imaged to localize particular structures. In principle, this is very similar to the so-called X-ray maps made with the SEM, in which electrons excite the atoms of the sample to emit their characteristic X-rays. These are imaged using the time-base of the raster scan of the microscope to form a spatial image of the distribution of each selected element, since the wavelengths of the X-rays from each atom are unique. In many of these emission images, density variations, changes in the thickness of the specimen, or the presence of other elements can cause at least minor difficulties in interpreting the pixel brightness in terms of concentration or amount of the selected target element or compound.

A third major class of images uses the pixel brightness to record distances. For example, an atomic force microscope image of a surface shows the elevation of each point on the surface, represented as a gray-scale (or pseudocolor) value. Range images are produced by raster-scan microscopes, such as the scanning tunneling microscope (STM) and atomic force microscope

(AFM), or by physical scanning with a profilometer stylus. They are also produced by inter-ferometric light microscopes and, at larger scales, by laser ranging, synthetic aperture radar, side-scan sonar, and other techniques. Additional methods that present an image in which pixel brightness values represent range information obtained indirectly by other means include stereoscopy, shape-from-shading, and motion blur.

Range imaging

Most of the measurement tools available for very flat surfaces provide a single-valued eleva-tion reading at each point in an *x,y* raster or grid. **Chapter 14** discusses the processing and measurement of surface-range images in detail. This set of data is blind to any undercuts that may be present. Just as radar and sonar have wavelengths in the range of centimeters to me-ters (and thus are useful for measurements of large objects such as geologic landforms), so a much shorter measuring scale is needed for high precision on very flat surfaces. Attempts to use SEM, conventional light microscopy, or confocal scanning light microscopy (CSLM) either on the original surfaces, or on vertical sections cut through them, have been only partially satisfactory. The lateral resolution of the SEM is very good, but its depth resolution is not. Stereo-pair measurements are both difficult to perform and time-consuming to convert to an elevation map or range image of the surface, and the resulting depth resolution is still much poorer than the lateral resolution.

Conventional light microscopy has a lateral resolution of better than 1 μm, but the depth of field is neither great enough to view an entire rough surface nor shallow enough to isolate points along one isoelevation contour line. The CSLM improves the lateral resolution slightly and greatly reduces the depth of field while rejecting scattered light from out-of-focus loca-tions. The result is an instrument that can (a) image an entire rough surface by moving the sample vertically and keeping only the brightest light value at each location or (b) produce a range image by keeping track of the sample's vertical motion when the brightest reflected light value is obtained for each point in the image. The latter mode is most interesting for surface measurement purposes. The resolution is better than 1 μm in all directions.

Figure 1.60 shows a reconstructed view of the surface of a fracture in a brittle ceramic. It is formed from 26 planes, each separated by 1 μm in the *z* direction, and each of which records a pixel only if that location is brighter than any other plane. The perspective view can be rotated

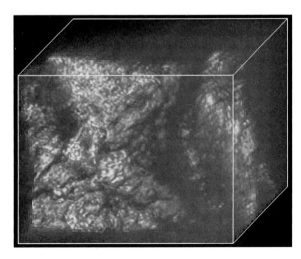

Figure 1.60 Reconstructed 3-D image of a brittle fracture surface in a ceramic that was imaged with a confocal scanning light microscope.

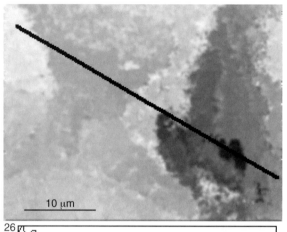

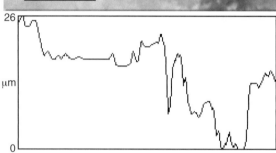

Figure 1.61 Range image produced from the data in Figure 1.60, with an elevation profile along an arbitrary line.

to present a very realistic image of the surface. However, plotting the same information in the form of a range image (in which each pixel brightness corresponds to the plane in which the brightest reflection was recorded) is more useful for measurement. **Figure 1.61** shows this presentation of the same surface with an elevation profile along an arbitrary line across the surface.

This method is interesting for many macroscopically rough samples, such as fractures and some deposited coatings, but it is not adequate for the really flat surfaces that are currently being produced in many applications. The surface irregularities on a typical polished silicon wafer or precision-machined mirror surface are typically on the order of nanometers.

Three principal methods have been applied to such surfaces. Historically, the profilometer provided a tool that would accurately measure vertical elevation with a resolution approaching a nanometer. Although it has been widely used, the profilometer has two serious disadvantages for many surface applications. The first is that it determines elevations only along a single profile. While the analysis of such elevation profiles is straightforward, their relevance to complex surfaces that may have anisotropic properties is questionable. The second limitation is the large tip size, which makes it impossible to follow steep slopes or steps accurately.

This leaves the interferometric light microscope and the AFM as the methods of choice for studying very flat surfaces. Both are somewhat novel instruments. One is a modern implementation of the principles of light interference discovered more than a century ago, while the other is a technology invented and rapidly commercialized only within the past few decades.

The interferometric light microscope (see the review by Robinson et al. [1991]) reflects light from the sample surface as one leg in a classic interferometer, which is then combined with light from a reference leg. **Figure 1.62** shows a schematic diagram. According to the usual principles of phase-sensitive interference, changes in path length (due to different elevations

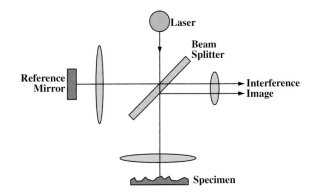

Figure 1.62 *Schematic diagram of an interference microscope.*

Laser

Beam Splitter

Reference Mirror

Interference Image

Specimen

of points on the surface) produce changes in the intensity of the light. This image is then digitized using an appropriate CCD detector array and analog-to-digital conversion, and a brightness value (and from it a derived elevation value) is recorded for each point on the surface. Although the wavelength of light used is typically about 630 nm, phase differences between the two legs of the interferometer of one-thousandth of the wavelength produce a change in intensity, so that the vertical resolution is a few angstroms. The lateral resolution, however, is still on the order of one micrometer, limited by the wavelength of the light used and the design of the optics.

The interferometric light microscope suffers if the surface has high slopes or a highly specular finish, since no light is reflected back to the detector. Such points become dropouts in the final image. For visual purposes, it is satisfactory to fill in such missing points with a median or smoothing filter (**Chapter 4**), but of course this may bias subsequent measurements.

The vertical resolution of the interferometric microscope is very high, approaching atomic dimensions. Although the lateral resolution is much lower, it should be quite suitable for many purposes. The absolute height difference between widely separated points is not measured precisely because the overall surface alignment and the shape or "figure" of the part is not known. It is common to deal with the problems of alignment and shape by fitting a function to the data. Determining a best-fit plane or other low-order polynomial function by least-squares fitting to all of the elevation data and then subtracting it is called "detrending" the data or "form

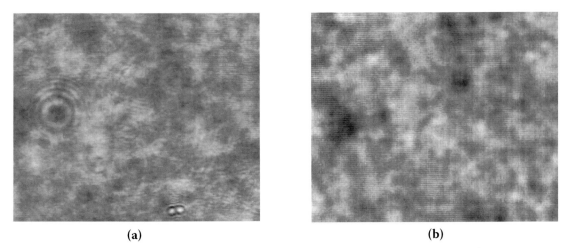

(a)   (b)

Figure 1.63 *Comparison of interferometric range images on a flat polished silicon wafer using Fizeau (a) and Mirau (b) optics.*

removal." It is then possible to display the magnitude of deviations of points from this surface. However, the absolute difference between points that are widely separated is affected by the detrending plane, and the ability to distinguish small differences between points that are far apart is reduced.

Figure 1.63 shows a very flat surface (produced by polishing a silicon wafer) imaged in a commercial interferometric light microscope (Zygo Corp.) using both Fizeau and Mirau sets of optics. The field of view is the same in both images, and the total vertical range of elevations is only about 2 nm. The two bright white spots toward the bottom of the image are probably due to dirt somewhere in the optics. These artifacts are much less pronounced with the Mirau optics. In addition, the ringing (oscillation or ripple pattern) around features that can be seen in the Fizeau image is not present with the Mirau optics. These characteristics are usually interpreted as indicating that the Mirau optics are superior for the measurement of very flat surfaces. On the other hand, the Mirau image has less lateral resolution (it appears to be "smoothed"). A pattern of horizontal lines can be discerned that could come from the misalignment of the diffuser plate with the raster scan pattern of the camera.

The AFM is, in essence, a profilometer that scans a complete raster over the sample surface, but with a very small tip (see the review by Wickramasinghe [1989]). The standard profilometer tip cannot follow very small or very steep-sided irregularities on the surface because of its dimensions, which are on the order of micrometers. The AFM tip can be much smaller and sharper, although it is still not usually fine enough to handle the abrupt steps (or even undercuts) present in microelectronic circuits and some other surfaces. The tip can be operated in either an attractive or repulsive mode of interaction between the electrons around the atom(s) in the tip and those in the surface. Usually, repulsive mode (in which the tip is pressed against the surface) does a somewhat better job of following small irregularities, but it can also deform the surface and displace atoms.

There are other modalities of interaction for these scanned-tip microscopes. The STM was the original, but it can only be used for conductive specimens and is strongly sensitive to surface electronic states, surface contamination, and oxidation. Lateral force, tapping mode, and other modes of operation developed within the last few years offer the ability to characterize many aspects of surface composition and properties, but the straightforward AFM mode, which is most often used to determine surface geometry, presents quite enough complexities for understanding.

As indicated in the schematic diagram of **Figure 1.64**, the classic mode of operation for the AFM is to move the sample in the x, y, and z directions. The x,y scan covers the region of interest, while the z motion brings the tip back to the same null position as judged by the reflection

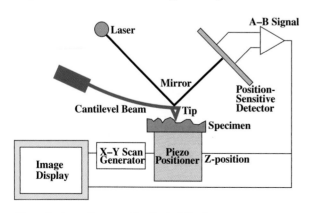

Figure 1.64 Schematic diagram of an atomic force microscope (AFM).

of a laser beam. The necessary motion is recorded in a computer to produce the resulting image. Modifications that move the tip instead of the sample, or that use a linear-array light sensor to measure the deflection of the tip rather than wait for the specimen to be moved in z, do not change the basic principle. The motion is usually accomplished with piezoelectric elements whose dimensions can be sensitively adjusted by varying the applied voltage. However, there is a time lag or creep associated with these motions that appears in the modulation transfer function (MTF) of the microscope as a loss of sensitivity at the largest or smallest dimensions (lowest and highest frequencies). Locating the x,y coordinates of the tip interferometrically instead of based on the piezodriver voltages can overcome some of these problems, but this adds complexity to the instrument.

Although the AFM has, in principle, a lateral resolution of a few angstroms as well as a vertical sensitivity within this range, it is not always possible to realize that performance. For one thing, the adjustment of scan speeds and amplifier time constants to obtain the best visual picture can eliminate some of the fine-scale roughness and thus bias subsequent analysis. Conversely, it can introduce additional noise from electrical or mechanical sources. Special care must also be taken to eliminate vibration.

Most of the attention to the performance of the AFM, STM, and related instruments has been concerned with the high-resolution limit (Denley 1990a, 1990b; Grigg et al. 1992). This is generally set by the shape of the tip, which is not easy to characterize. Many authors (Aguilar et al. [1992], Pancorbo et al. [1991]) have shown that it may be possible to deconvolve the tip shape and improve the image sharpness in exactly the same way that it is done for other imaging systems. This type of deconvolution is discussed in **Chapter 6** and **Chapter 14**.

Figure 1.65 shows a sample of polished silicon (traditional roughness values indicate 0.2- to 0.3-nm magnitude, near the nominal vertical resolution limit for interferometry and AFM) with a hardness indentation. One limitation of the AFM can be seen by generating a rendered or isotropic display of the indentation, which shows that the left side of the indentation appears to be smoother than the right. This difference is an artifact of the scanning, since the tip-response dynamics are different when following a surface down (where it may lag behind the actual surface and fail to record deviations) or up (where contact forces it to follow irregularities). In addition, the measured depth of the indentation is much less than the actual depth. This discrepancy occurs because the tip cannot follow the deepest part of the indentation and

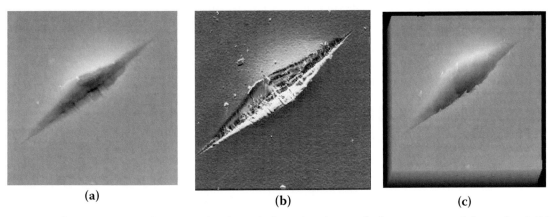

| (a) | (b) | (c) |

Figure 1.65 AFM image of a Knoop hardness indentation in metal, shown as range **(a)**, rendered **(b)**, and isometric **(c)** presentations.

because the calibration of the AFM in the vertical direction is less precise than in the x, y directions.

Tools with sufficient lateral and vertical resolution for application to a variety of surface-range measurements are available. The interferometer is more convenient to use than the AFM, operates over a wide range of magnifications, and accepts large samples. It also introduces less directional anisotropy due to the instrument characteristics. The AFM, on the other hand, has higher lateral resolution, which may be required for the metrology of the very fine features that are becoming commonplace in the fabrication of integrated circuits and in nanotechnology.

It is important to keep in mind that the signal produced by many microscopes is only indirectly related to the surface elevation. In some cases, it may represent quite different characteristics of the sample, such as compositional variations or electronic properties. In **Figure 1.66**, the apparent step in surface elevation provides an example. The surface is actually flat, but the electronic properties of the sample (a junction in a microelectronic device) produce variation in the signal.

Multiple images

For many applications, a single image is not enough. Multiple images can constitute a series of views of the same area using different wavelengths of light or other signals. Examples include the images produced by satellites, such as the various visible and infrared wavelengths recorded by the *Landsat Thematic Mapper* (TM) satellite, and SEM images in which as many as a dozen different elements can be represented by their X-ray intensities. These images may each require processing; for example, X-ray maps are usually very noisy. The processed images are then often combined either by using ratios, such as the ratio of different wavelengths used to identify crops in TM images, or Boolean logic, such as locating regions that contain both iron and sulfur in an SEM image of a mineral. **Figure 1.67** shows an example in which two satellite color photographs of the same region, one covering the usual visual range of wavelengths and one extending into the near infrared, are combined by constructing the ratio of infrared to

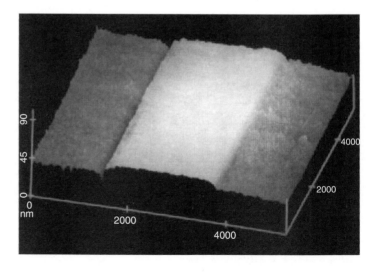

Figure 1.66 Scanning tunneling microscope (STM) image. The specimen actually is flat-surfaced silicon, with apparent relief showing altered electron levels in a 2-µm-wide region with implanted phosphorus. (Courtesy of J. Labrasca, North Carolina State University, Raleigh, and R. Chapman, Microelectronics Center of North Carolina, Research Triangle.)

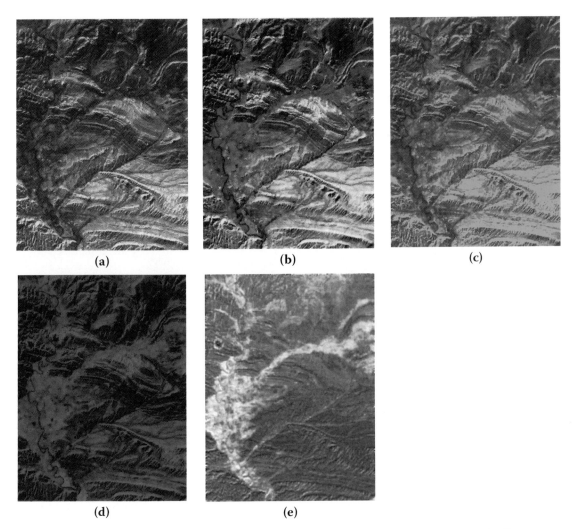

Figure 1.67 Landsat Thematic Mapper *images in visual and infrared color of a 20-km² region at Thermopolis, WY:* **(a)** *visible light;* **(b)** *infrared light;* **(c)** *result of filtering the visible image at 520 nm;* **(d)** *filtering the infrared image at 1100 nm;* **(e)** *the ratio of the green (visible) to red (IR) filtered intensities. (From Sabins, F.F., Jr.,* Remote Sensing: Principles and Interpretation, *2nd ed., W.H. Freeman, New York, 1987. With permission.)*

green intensity as a vegetation index, insensitive to the local inclination of the surface to the sun. Combinations reduce, but only slightly, the amount of data to be stored.

Satellite images are typically acquired in several wavelengths, covering the visible and near-infrared bands. *Landsat* images, for example, can be combined to generate a "true color" image by placing bands 1, 2, and 3 into the blue, green, and red channels of a color image, respectively. Other satellites produce images with higher resolution, although without color sensitivity. **Figure 1.68** shows three color channels with ground resolution of about 15 m and one panchromatic gray-scale image (from a different satellite) with ground resolution of 5 m. Combining the three low-resolution channels to produce a color image, converting this to HSI, and then replacing the intensity channel with the higher-resolution image produces the result shown in **Figure 1.69**, which shows both color information and high spatial resolution. The

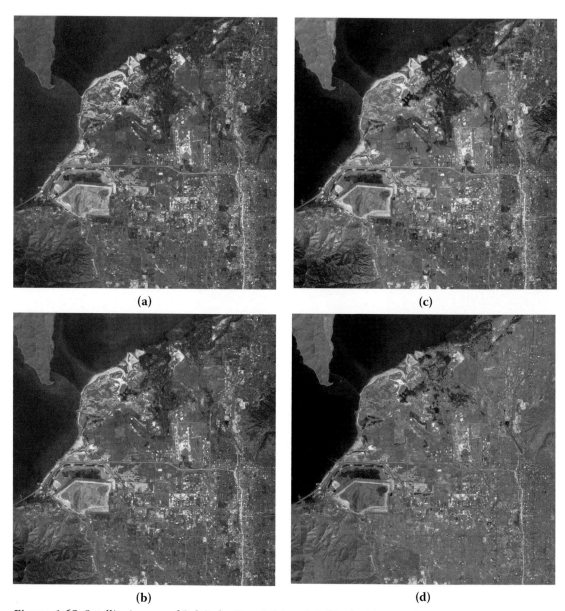

Figure 1.68 *Satellite images of Salt Lake City: **(a)** band 1 (blue), 15-m resolution; **(b)** band 2 (green), 15-m resolution; **(c)** band 3 (red), 15-m resolution; **(d)** panchromatic, 5-m resolution. (Courtesy of Y. Siddiqul, I-Cubed Corp., Ft. Collins, CO.)*

fact that the color data are not as sharp as the brightness data does not hinder viewing or interpretation, as discussed previously.

Another example of a multiple-image situation is a time sequence. This could be a series of satellite image of parallel slice images through a solid object (**Figure 1.70**). Medical imaging methods such as computed tomography (CT) and magnetic resonance images (MRI) can produce this sort of data. So can some seismic imaging techniques. Even more common are various serial-section methods used in microscopy. The classic method for producing such a series

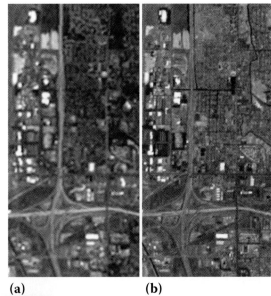

Figure 1.69 *Combination of planes:*
(a) *RGB composite using 15-m resolution*
images, **Figure 1.68a,b,c**;
(b) *replacement of the intensity channel*
of **Figure 1.68a** *with the higher*
resolution panchromatic image from
Figure 1.68d.

(a)   **(b)**

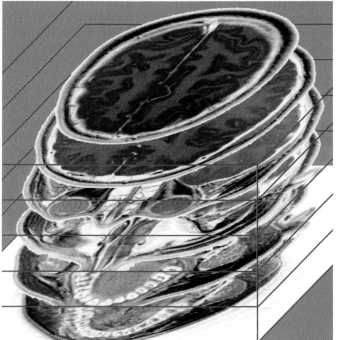

Figure 1.70 *Multiple planes of*
pixels (sections through a
human head) fill three-dimen-
sional space. Voxels (volume
elements) are ideally cubic for
processing and measurement
of 3-D images.

of images is to microtome a series of sections from the original sample, image each separately in the light or electron microscope, and then align the images afterward.

Optical sectioning, especially with the CSLM, which has a very shallow depth of field and can collect images from deep within partially transparent specimens, eliminates the problems of alignment. **Figure 1.71** shows several focal-section planes from a CSLM. Some imaging methods, such as the SIMS (secondary ion mass spectrometry), produce a series of images in depth by physically eroding the sample, which also preserves alignment. **Figure 1.72** shows an example of SIMS images. Sequential polishing of harder

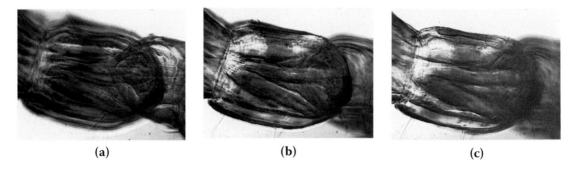

(a)   (b)   (c)

Figure 1.71 *Serial-section images formed by transmission CSLM. These are selected views from a series of sections through the leg joint of a head louse, with optical section thickness about 0.5 μm.*

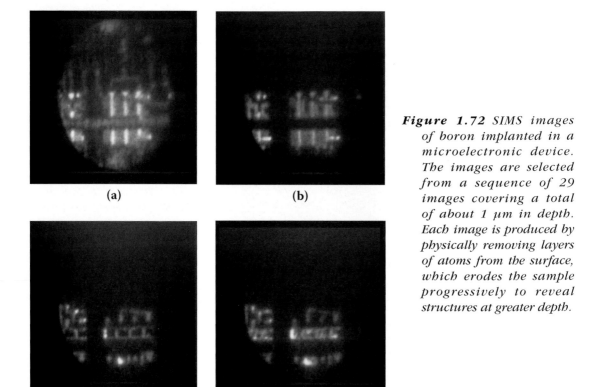

Figure 1.72 *SIMS images of boron implanted in a microelectronic device. The images are selected from a sequence of 29 images covering a total of about 1 μm in depth. Each image is produced by physically removing layers of atoms from the surface, which erodes the sample progressively to reveal structures at greater depth.*

samples such as metals also produces new surfaces for imaging, but it is generally difficult to control the depth in order to space them uniformly. Focused-ion beam (FIB) machining, which can be performed inside an SEM so that the specimen remains fixed in position and can be examined to control the process, provides another way of preparing multiple surfaces for viewing.

The ideal situation for three-dimensional interpretation of structure calls for the lateral resolution of serial-section image planes to be equal to the spacing between the planes. This produces cubic "voxels" (volume elements), which have the same advantages for processing and

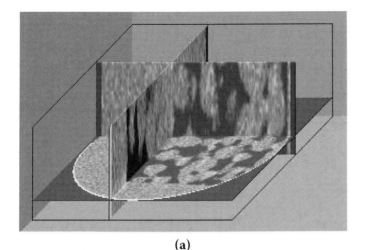

(a)

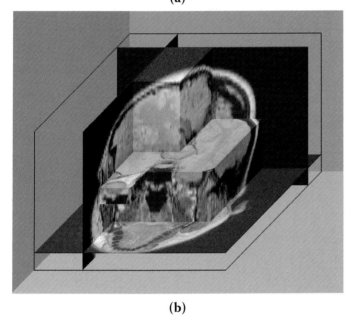

(b)

Figure 1.73 Examples of three-dimensional data sets formed by a series of planar images.

(a) *A sintered ceramic imaged by X-ray tomography (CAT), with a characteristic dimension of a few micrometers; the dark regions are voids. The poorer resolution in the vertical direction is due to the spacing of the image planes, which is greater than the lateral pixel resolution within each plane.*

(b) *A human head imaged by magnetic resonance (the same data set as shown in Figure 1.70), with characteristic dimension of centimeters. The section planes can be positioned arbitrarily and moved to reveal the internal structure.*

measurement in three dimensions that square pixels have in two. However, it is usually the case that the planes are spaced apart by much more than their lateral resolution, and special attention is given to interpolating between the planes. In the case of the SIMS, the situation is reversed, and the plane spacing (as little as a few atom dimensions) is much less than the lateral resolution in each plane (typically about 1 µm).

There are techniques that directly produce cubic voxel images, such as three-dimensional tomography. In this case, a series of projection images, generally using X-rays or electrons, is obtained as the sample is rotated to different orientations, and then mathematical reconstruction calculates the density of each voxel. The resulting large, three-dimensional image arrays can be stored as a series of planar slices. When a three-dimensional data set is used, a variety of processing and display modes are available. These are discussed in more detail in **Chapter 13**. **Figure 1.73** shows examples of sectioning through a series of X-ray tomographic and magnetic resonance images (MRI) in the *x*, *y*, and *z* planes.

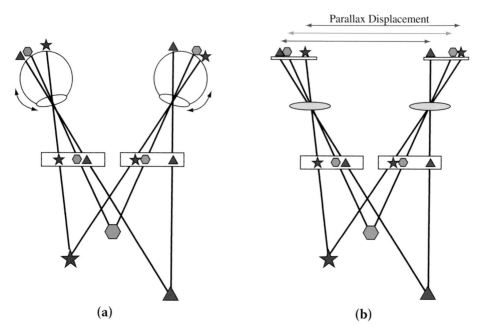

Figure 1.74 *Stereoscopic depth perception. (a) The relative distance to each feature identified in both the left- and right-eye views is given by differences in the vergence angles by which the eyes must rotate inward to bring each feature to the central fovea in each eye. This is accomplished one feature at a time. Viewing stereo-pair images provides the same visual cues to the eyes and produces the same interpretation. (b) Measurement of images to obtain actual distances uses the different parallax displacements of the features in two images. The distance between the two viewpoints must be known. Locating the same feature in both images is the hardest part of the task for automated analysis.*

Stereoscopy

Three-dimensional information can also be obtained from two images of the same scene, taken from slightly different viewpoints. Human stereoscopy gives us depth perception, although we also get important data from relative size, precedence, perspective, atmospheric haze, and other cues, all of which were discovered and used very effectively by artists during the Renaissance. Like other aspects of human vision, stereoscopy is primarily comparative, with the change of vergence angle of the eyes as we shift attention from one feature to another indicating to the brain which is closer. **Figure 1.74** shows schematically the principle of stereo fusion, in which the images from each eye are compared to locate the same feature in each view. The eye muscles rotate the eye to bring this feature to the fovea, and the muscles provide the vergence information to the brain. Notice that this implies that stereoscopy is only applied to one feature in the field of view at a time, and not to the entire scene. From the amount of vergence motion needed, the relative distance of the object is ascertained. Since only comparative measurements are made, only the direction or relative amount of motion required to fuse the images of each object is required.

Not all animals use this method. The owl, for instance, has eyes that are not movable in their sockets. Instead, the fovea has an elongated shape along a line that is not vertical, but angled toward the owl's feet. The owl tilts its head to accomplish fusion (bringing the feature of interest to the fovea) and judges the relative distance by the tilt required.

Although the human visual system makes only comparative use of the parallax, or vergence, of images of an object, it is straightforward to measure the relative displacement of two objects in the field of view to calculate their relative distance, or to measure the angle of vergence of one object to calculate its distance from the viewer. This is routinely done at scales ranging from aerial photography and mapmaking to scanning electron microscopy.

Measurement of range information from two views is a straightforward application of trigonometry. The lateral position of objects in these two views is different, depending on their distance. From these parallax displacements, the distance can be computed by a process called stereoscopy or photogrammetry. However, computer fusion of images is a difficult task that requires locating matching points in the images. Brute-force correlation methods that try to match many points based on local texture are fundamentally similar to the motion flow approach. This produces many false matches, but these are assumed to be removed by subsequent noise filtering. The alternative approach is to locate selected points in the images that are "interesting" based on their representing important boundaries or feature edges, which can then be matched more confidently. The areas between the matched points are then assumed to be simple planes.

However fusion is accomplished, the displacement of the points in the two images, or parallax, gives the range. This method is used for mapping surface elevation, ranging from satellite or aerial pictures used to produce topographic maps (in which the two images are taken a short time apart as the position of the satellite or airplane changes) to scanning electron microscope metrology of semiconductor chips (in which the two images are produced by tilting the sample). **Figure 1.75** shows an example of a stereo pair from an SEM; **Figure 1.76** shows two aerial photographs and a complete topographic map drawn from them.

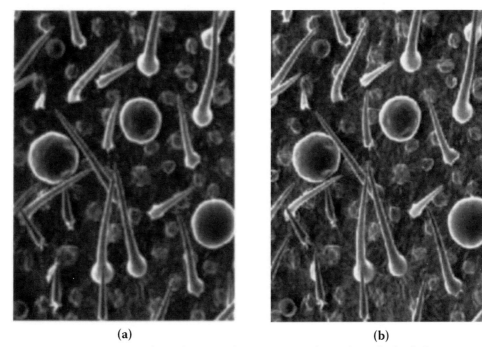

(a)   (b)

Figure 1.75 *Stereo-pair images from the SEM. The specimen is the surface of a leaf; the two images were obtained by tilting the beam incident on the specimen by 8° to produce two points of view. (Courtesy of Japan Electron Optics Laboratory, Peabody, MA.)*

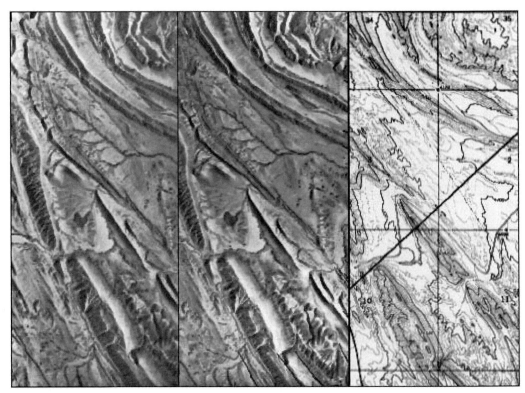

Figure 1.76 *Stereo-pair images from aerial photography, and the topographic map showing isoelevation contour lines derived from the parallax in the images. The scene is a portion of the Wind River in Wyoming. (From Sabins, F.F., Jr.,* Remote Sensing: Principles and Interpretation, *2nd ed., W.H. Freeman, New York, 1987. With permission.)*

The utility of a stereoscopic view of the world to communicate depth information re-sulted in the use of stereo cameras to produce "stereopticon" slides for viewing, which were very popular more than 50 years ago. Stereo movies (requiring the viewer to wear polarized glasses) have enjoyed brief vogues from time to time. Publication of stereo-pair views to illustrate scientific papers is now relatively common. The most common for-mats are (a) the presentation of two side-by-side images about 7.5 cm apart (the distance between human eyes), which an experienced viewer can see without optical aids by looking straight ahead and allowing the brain to fuse the two images, and (b) the use of different col-ors for each image. Overprinting the same image in red and green (or red and blue) allows a viewer with colored glasses to see the correct image in each eye, and again the brain can sort out the depth information (**Figure 1.77**). Some SEMs display true stereo views of surfaces using this method. Of course, this only works for gray-scale images. Computer displays using polarized light and glasses are also used to display three-dimensional data, usually synthesized from calculations or simulations rather than direct imaging.

There are several different measurement geometries (Boyde 1973; Piazzesi 1973). In all cases, the same scene is viewed from two different locations, and the distance between those loca-tions is precisely known. Sometimes this is accomplished by moving the viewpoint, for in-stance the airplane carrying the camera. In aerial photography, the plane's speed and direction are known, and the time of each picture is recorded to obtain the distance traveled.

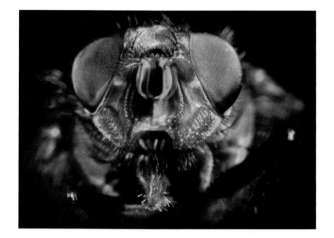

Figure 1.77 Red/cyan stereo image of a fly's head. This image was captured as two separate SEM images, which were then superimposed as different color planes. To view the image, use glasses with a red filter in front of the left eye, and either a green or blue filter in front of the right eye.

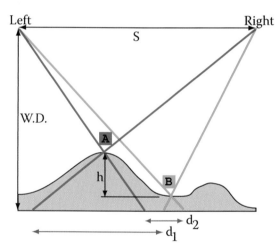

Figure 1.78 Geometry used to measure the vertical height difference between objects viewed in two different images obtained by shifting the sample or viewpoint (typically used for aerial photography).

In **Figure 1.78**, S is the shift distance (either the distance the plane has traveled or the distance the SEM stage was translated), and WD is the working distance or altitude. The parallax ($d_1 - d_2$) from the distances between two points as they appear in the two different images (measured in a direction parallel to the shift) is proportional to the elevation difference between the two points. For the case of d_1 and d_2 much smaller than S, the simplified relationship is:

$$h = WD \cdot \frac{(d_1 - d_2)}{S}$$

(1.9)

If the vertical relief of the surface being measured is a significant fraction of WD, then foreshortening of lateral distances as a function of elevation will also be present in the images. The x and y coordinates of points in the images can be corrected with the following equations. This means that rubber-sheeting to correct the foreshortening is needed to allow fitting or "tiling" together a mosaic of pictures into a seamless whole.

$$X' = X \cdot (WD - h) / WD$$

$$Y' = Y \cdot (WD - h) / WD$$

(1.10)

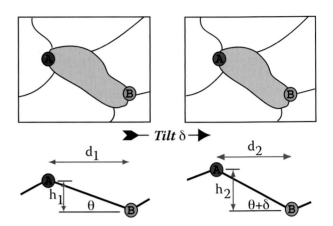

Figure 1.79 *Geometry used to measure the vertical height difference between points viewed in two different images obtained by tilting the sample (typically used for microscopy).*

Much greater displacement between the two eyepoints can be achieved if the two views are not in parallel directions, but are instead directed inward toward the same central point in each scene. This is rarely done in aerial photography because it is impractical when trying to cover a large region with a mosaic of pictures, and it is not usually necessary to obtain sufficient parallax for measurement. However, when examining samples in the SEM, it is very easy to accomplish this by tilting the sample between two views. In **Figure 1.79**, the two images represent two views obtained by tilting the specimen about a vertical axis. Points A and B are separated by a horizontal distance d_1 or d_2 that is different in the two images. From this parallax value and the known tilt angle δ applied between the two images, the height difference *h* and the angle θ of a line joining the points (usually a surface defined by the points) can be calculated (Boyde 1973) as:

$$\theta = \tan^{-1}\left\{\frac{(\cos\delta - d_2 / d_1)}{\sin\delta}\right\}$$

$$h_1 = \frac{(d_1 \cdot \cos\delta - d_2)}{\sin\delta} \tag{1.11}$$

Notice that the angle θ is independent of the magnification, since the distances enter as a ratio.

When two angled views of the same region of the surface are available, the relative displacement or parallax of features can be made quite large relative to their lateral magnification. This makes it possible to measure relatively small amounts of surface relief. Angles of 5 to 10° are commonly used; for very flat surfaces, tilt angles as great as 20° can sometimes be useful. When large angles are used with rough surfaces, the images contain shadow areas where features are not visible in both images, and locating matching points becomes very difficult. Also, when the parallax becomes too great in a pair of images, it can be difficult for the human observer to fuse the two images visually if this step is used in the measurement operation.

Many of the measurements made with stereo-pair photographs from both SEM and aerial photography are made using extensive human interaction. The algorithms that have been developed for automatic fusion require many of the image processing operations that will be described in later chapters to make possible the identification of the same features in each image. For the moment, it is enough to understand the principle that identifying the same points in left and right images, and measuring the parallax, gives the elevation. With data for many different pairs of points, it is possible to construct a complete map of the surface. The elevation data can then be presented in a variety of formats, including a range image encoding elevation as the brightness or color of each pixel in the array. Other display modes, such as contour maps, isometric views, or shaded renderings, can be generated to assist the viewer in interpreting these images, which are not common to our everyday experience. The range image data are in a suitable form for many types of image processing and for the measurement of the surface area or the volume above or below the surface.

The majority of elevation maps of Earth's surface being made today are determined by the stereoscopic measurement of images taken either from aerial photography or satellite remote imaging. Of course, two-thirds of Earth is covered by water and cannot be measured this way. Portions of the sea bottom have been mapped stereoscopically by side-scanned sonar. The technology is very similar to that used for the radar mapping of Venus, except that sonar uses sound waves (which can propagate through water) and radar uses high-frequency (millimeter length) electromagnetic radiation that can penetrate the opaque clouds covering Venus.

The synthetic aperture radar (SAR) used by the Magellan probe to map Venus does not directly give elevation data to produce a range image. The principle of SAR is not new, nor is it restricted to satellites and space probes. Aerial mapping of desert regions has been used to penetrate through the dry sand and map the underlying land to find ancient watercourses, for instance. The principle of SAR is that the moving satellite (or other platform) emits a series of short pulses directed downward and to one side of the track along which it is moving. Direction parallel to the track is called the azimuth, and the direction perpendicular to it is called the range (not to be confused with the range image that encodes the elevation information). The name "synthetic aperture" refers to the fact that the moving antenna effectively acts as a much larger antenna (equal in size to the distance the antenna moves during the pulse) that can more accurately resolve directions in the azimuth.

The radar records the intensity of the returning pulse, the travel time, and the Doppler shift. The intensity is a measure of the surface characteristics, although the radar (or sonar) reflectivity is not always easy to interpret in terms of the surface structure and is not directly related to the albedo (or reflectivity) for visible light. The travel time for the pulse gives the range. For a perfectly flat surface, there would be an arc of locations on the surface that would have the same range from the antenna. Because of the motion of the satellite or airplane, each point along this arc produces a different Doppler shift in the signal frequency. Measuring the Doppler shift of each returned pulse provides resolution along the arc. Each point on the ground contributes to the return pulse with a unique range and Doppler shift, which allows a range map of the ground to be reconstructed.

However, since the surface is not flat, there are multiple possible combinations of location and elevation that could produce the same return signal. Combining the measurements from several overlapping sweeps (for Magellan, several sequential orbits) allows the elevation data to be refined. The database for Venus resolves points on the ground with about 120-m spacing and has elevation data with resolutions that vary from 120 to 300 m (depending on where along the track, and how far from the center of the track, they were located). For each point, the elevation and the reflectivity are stored (**Figure 1.80**). In many of the published renderings of these data, the elevation values are used to construct the surface shape, and the reflectivity values are used to color the surface (**Figure 1.81**). Of course, the colors do not reflect the actual visual appearance of the surface.

Synthetic aperture ranging with either radar or sonar is not the only way these signals can be used to construct a range map. Directing a beam straight down and measuring the echo, or return time, gives the range at a single point. Many such measurements can be used to construct a map or image. The simple "fish-finder" type of sonar can be used to construct a map of a lake

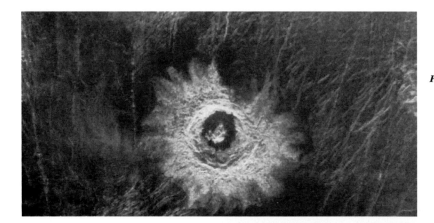

Figure 1.80 Range image
of Venus obtained from
SAR data. (Courtesy of Jet
Propulsion Laboratory,
Pasadena, CA.)

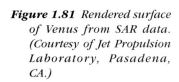

Figure 1.81 Rendered surface
of Venus from SAR data.
(Courtesy of Jet Propulsion
Laboratory, Pasadena,
CA.)

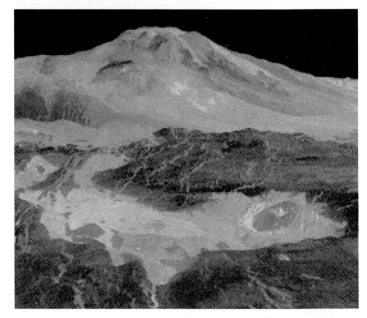

bottom in this way by steering the boat back and forth in a raster pattern to cover the whole surface. Other signals can be used, as well. The Clementine mission to the moon used a laser beam from the orbiting spacecraft in a similar fashion. By pulsing the laser and waiting for the echo, points were measured every few hundred meters across the entire lunar surface, with a vertical resolution of about 40 m.

Imaging requirements

Given the diversity of image types and sources described above, there are several general criteria we can prescribe for images intended for computer processing and analysis. The first is the need for global uniformity. The same type of feature should look the same wherever it appears in the image. This implies that brightness and color values should be the same and, consequently, that illumination must be uniform and stable for images acquired at different times. When surfaces are nonplanar, such as Earth as viewed from a satellite or a fracture surface in the microscope, corrections for the changing local orientation may be possible, but this usually requires extensive calculation or prior knowledge of the surface and source of illumination.

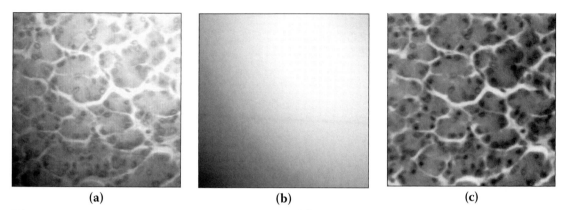

| (a) | (b) | (c) |

Figure 1.82 A microscope image (a) obtained with nonuniform illumination (due to a misaligned condenser lens). The "background" image (b) was collected under the same conditions, with no sample present (by moving to an adjacent region on the slide). Subtracting the background image and expanding the contrast of the difference produces a "leveled" image (c) with uniform brightness values for similar structures.

Figure 1.82 shows an example of a microscope image with nonuniform illumination. Storing a "background" image with no specimen present (by moving to a clear space on the slide) allows this nonuniformity to be leveled. The background image is either subtracted from or divided into the original (depending on whether the camera has a logarithmic or linear response). This type of leveling is discussed in **Chapter 4** on correcting image defects, along with other ways to obtain the background image when it cannot be acquired directly.

The requirement for uniformity limits the kinds of surfaces that are normally imaged. Planar surfaces, or at least simple and known ones, are much easier to deal with than complex surfaces. Simply connected surfaces are much easier to interpret than ones with arches, bridges, caves, and loops that hide some of the structure. Features that have precedence problems, in which some features hide entirely or in part behind others, present difficulties for interpretation or measurement. Illumination that casts strong shadows, especially to one side, is also undesirable in most cases. The exception occurs when well-spaced features cast shadows that do not interfere with each other. The shadow lengths can be used with the known lighting geometry to calculate feature heights. **Figure 1.83** shows an example in aerial photography. One form of sample preparation for the TEM deposits a thin film of metal or carbon from a point source, which also leaves shadow areas behind particles or other protrusions that can be used in the same way (**Figure 1.84**).

In addition to global uniformity, we generally want local sensitivity to variations. This means that edges and boundaries must be well delineated and accurately located. The resolution of the camera sensor was discussed previously. Generally, anything that degrades high frequencies in the signal chain will disturb the subsequent ability to identify feature boundaries or locate edges for measurement. On the other hand, such simple problems as dust on the optics can introduce local variations that can be mistaken for image features, causing serious errors.

Measurement of dimensions requires that the geometry of the imaging system be well known. Knowing the magnification of a microscope or the altitude of a satellite is usually straightforward. Calibrating the lateral scale can be accomplished either by knowledge of the optics or by using an image of a known scale or standard. When the viewing geometry is more complicated, either because the surface is not planar or the viewing angle is not perpendicular,

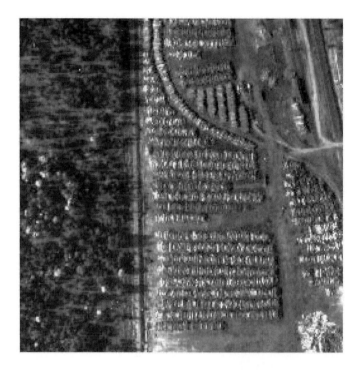

Figure 1.83 Aerial photograph in which length of shadows and knowledge of the sun's position permit calculation of the heights of trees and the height of the piles of logs in the lumberyard, from which the amount of wood can be estimated.

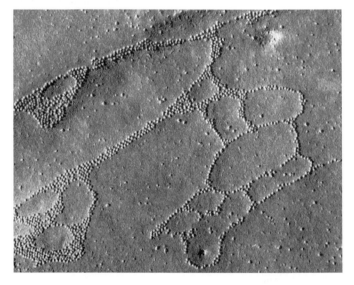

Figure 1.84 Electron microscope image showing shadowed particles delineating the gap junctions between cells, revealed by freeze-fracturing the tissue.

measurement is more difficult and requires determination of the geometry first, or the inclusion of a scale or fiducial marks on the object being viewed.

Figure 1.85 shows the simplest kind of distortion when a planar surface is viewed at an angle. Different portions of the image have different magnification scales, which makes subsequent analysis difficult. It also prevents combining multiple images of a complex surface into a mosaic. This problem is evident in two applications at very different scales. Satellite images of planet surfaces are assembled into mosaics covering large areas only with elaborate image warping to bring the edges into registration. This type of warping is discussed in **Chapter 4.** SEM images of rough surfaces are more difficult to assemble in this way because

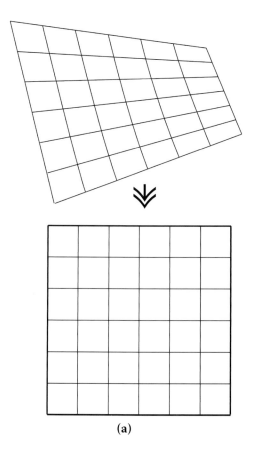

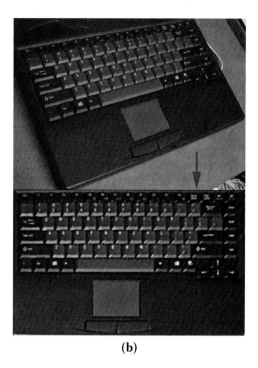

Figure 1.85 *Geometric distortion occurs when a surface is viewed from a position away from the surface normal. Correcting this distortion to obtain a rectilinear image that can be properly processed and measured, or fitted together with adjoining images, requires knowing the viewing geometry or including some known fiducial marks in the scene that can be used to determine the distortion.*

(a)

(b)

the overall specimen geometry is not so well known, and the required computer processing is more difficult.

Measuring brightness information, such as density or color values, requires a very stable illumination source and sensor. Color measurements are easily affected by changes in the color temperature of an incandescent bulb due to minor voltage fluctuations or as the bulb warms up or ages. Fluorescent lighting, especially when used in light boxes with X-ray films or densitometry gels, may be unstable or may introduce interference in solid-state cameras due to the high-frequency flickering of the fluorescent tube. Bright specular reflections can cause saturation, blooming, or shifts in the camera gain.

It will help to bear in mind what the purpose is when digitizing an image into a computer. Some of the possibilities are listed below, and these place different restrictions and demands on the hardware and software used. Subsequent chapters discuss these topics in greater detail. The emphasis throughout this book is on the results produced by various processing and measurement techniques, with plain English descriptions of the methods and illustrations comparing different approaches. There are numerous books that provide computer code that implements various algorithms (e.g., Lichtenbelt et al. 1998; Myler and Weeks 1993; Parker

1997; Pavlidis 1982; Ritter and Wilson 2001; Seul et al. 2000; Umbaugh 1998), with more rolling off the presses every month.

There are also a great many books on digital image processing, some of which delve deeply into the mathematical underpinnings of the science, while others concentrate on applications in a particular field. A representative selection of general texts includes Costa and Cesar (2001), Gonzalez and Woods (1993), Hader (1992), Kriete (1992), Nikolaidis and Pitas (2001), Pitas (2000), Pratt (1991), Rosenfeld and Kak (1982), Sanchez and Canton (1999), Sonka et al. (1999), Weeks 1996). Several application-specific texts discuss image processing and, to a lesser extent, image measurement as it applies to particular fields of study. A few examples include forensics (Russ 2002), food science (Russ 2004), geology (Francus 2004), and medical imaging (Costaridou 2004; Rangayyan 2005). The emphasis in this book is on the generality of the methods, showing that the same techniques apply to a broad range of types of images, and trying to educate the user in the performance and results rather than the theory.

Storing and filing of images becomes more attractive as massive storage devices (such as writable DVD disks) drop in price or where multiple master copies of images may be needed in more than one location. In many cases, this application also involves hard-copy printing of the stored images and transmission of images to other locations. If further processing or measurement is not required, then compression of the images may be acceptable. The advantage of electronic storage is that the images do not degrade with time and can be accessed by appropriate filing and cross-indexing routines. On the other hand, film storage is far cheaper and offers much higher storage density and higher image resolution, and it is likely that devices for examining film will still be available in 100 years, which probably will not be the case for DVD disks.

Enhancement of images for visual examination requires a large number of pixels and adequate pixel depth so that the image can be acquired with enough information to perform the filtering or other operations with fidelity and then display the result with enough detail for the viewer. Uniformity of illumination and control of geometry are of secondary importance. When large images are used, and especially for some of the more time-consuming processing operations, or when interactive experimentation with many different operations is intended, this application may benefit from very fast computers with large amounts of memory or specialized hardware.

Measurement of dimensions and density values can often be performed with modest image resolution if the magnification or illumination can be adjusted beforehand to make the best use of the image sensor. Processing may be required before measurement (for instance, derivatives are often used to delineate edges for measurement), but this can usually be handled completely in software. The most important constraints are tight control over the imaging geometry and the uniformity and constancy of illumination.

Quality control applications usually do not involve absolute measurements so much as detecting variations. In many cases, this is handled simply by subtracting a reference image from each acquired image, point by point, to detect gross changes. This can be done with analog electronics at real-time speeds. Preventing variation due to accidental changes in the position of camera or targets, or in illumination, is a central concern.

Microstructural research in either two or three dimensions usually starts with image measurement and has the same requirements as noted above, plus the ability to subject the measurement values to appropriate stereological and statistical analysis. Interpretation of images in terms of structure is different for images of planar cross sections or projections (**Figure 1.86**). The latter are familiar to human vision, while the former are not. However, section images, such as the one in **Figure 1.87**, contain rich information for

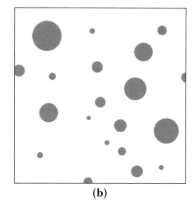

(a)   (b)

Figure 1.86 *Projection images, such as the spheres shown in* **(a)** *are familiar, showing the external surfaces of features. However, some features are partially or entirely obscured, and it is not easy to determine the number or size distribution of the spheres. Cross-section images, as shown in* **(b)** *are unfamiliar and do not show the maximum extent of features, but statistically it is possible to predict the size distribution and number of the spheres.*

Figure 1.87 *Light-microscope image of section through a colored enamel coating applied to steel. The spherical bubbles arise during the firing of the enamel. They are sectioned to show circles whose diameters are smaller than the maximum diameter of the spheres, but since the shape of the bubbles is known it is possible to infer the number and size distribution of the spheres from the data measured on the circles. (Courtesy of V. Benes, Research Institute for Metals, Panenské Brezany, Czechoslovakia.)*

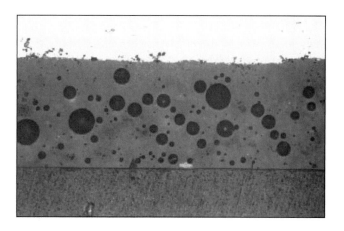

measurement in three dimensions that can be revealed by appropriate analysis. **Chapter 9** describes the methods. Projection images, such as the one in **Figure 1.88**, may present greater difficulties for interpretation.

Three-dimensional imaging utilizes large data sets, and in most cases the alignment of two-dimensional images is of critical importance. Some three-dimensional structural parameters can be inferred from two-dimensional images. Others, principally topological information, can only be determined from the three-dimensional data set. Processing and measurement operations in three dimensions place extreme demands on computer storage and speed. Displays of three-dimensional information in ways interpretable by, if not familiar to, human users are improving, but need further development. They also

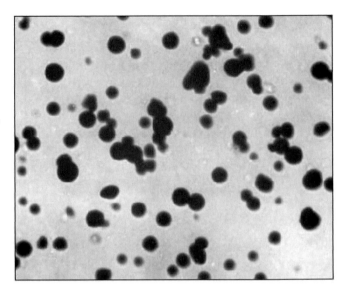

Figure 1.88 *Transmission electron microscope image of latex spheres in a thick, transparent section. Some of the spheres are partially hidden by others. If the section thickness is known, the size distribution and volume fraction occupied by the spheres can be estimated, but some small features may be entirely obscured and cannot be determined.*

place considerable demands on processor and display speed. **Chapter 12** and **Chapter 13** discuss three-dimensional imaging.

Classification and recognition is generally considered to be the high-end task for computer-based image analysis. It ranges in complexity from locating and recognizing isolated objects belonging to a few well-established classes to much more open-ended problems. Examples of the former are locating objects for robotic manipulation or recognizing targets in surveillance photos. An example of the latter is medical diagnosis, in which much of the important information comes from sources other than the image itself. Fuzzy logic, expert systems, and neural networks are all being applied to these tasks with some success. The methods are reviewed in **Chapter 11**. Extracting the correct information from the image to feed the decision-making process is more complicated than simple processing or measurement, because the best algorithms for a specific application must themselves be determined as part of the logic process.

These tasks all require a computer-based image processing and analysis system, and by inference the image-acquisition hardware, to duplicate some operations of the human visual system. In many cases they do so in ways that copy the algorithms we believe are used in vision, but in others quite different approaches are used. While no computer-based image system can come close to duplicating the overall performance of human vision in its flexibility or speed, there are specific tasks at which the computer-based system surpasses any human. It can detect many more imaging signals than just visible light; is unaffected by outside influences, fatigue, or distraction; performs absolute measurements rather than relative comparisons; can transform images into other spaces that are beyond normal human experience (e.g., Fourier, wavelet, or Hough space) to extract hidden data; and can apply statistical techniques to see through the chaotic and noisy data that may be present to identify underlying trends and similarities.

These attributes have made computer-based image analysis an important tool in many diverse fields. The image scale can vary from the microscopic to the astronomical, with substantially the same operations used. For the use of images at these scales, see especially Inoué (1986) and Sabins (1987). Familiarity with computer methods also makes most users better observers of images, able to interpret unusual imaging modes (such as cross sections) that are not encountered in normal scenes, and conscious of both the gestalt and details of images as well as their visual response to them.

Human Vision[1]

There are two main reasons for including a chapter on the characteristics of human vision in a book that is primarily concerned with computer processing and measurement of digital images. First, much of image processing is concerned with enhancing the visibility of details and features within images, and this depends upon some understanding of what people see in images (and what they overlook). Second, many of the algorithms described in subsequent chapters for image processing and for detecting objects in scenes are based to a greater or lesser extent on our understanding of how human visual processes work. Of course, that is not the only source of processing algorithms. Some are based on the physics of light (or other signals) interacting with specimens, and some are simply ad hoc procedures that have been found to be useful. In any event, the understanding gained from the study of human vision has been and continues to be an important source of methods for computer processing.

This chapter also seeks to broaden the reader's understanding of the similarities and differences between (a) the hardware of the human eye versus a digital camera and (b) the software of a computer versus the human neural system. Such knowledge should help to make us more thoughtful observers and better users of these new tools.

What we see and why

Human beings are intensely visual creatures. Most of the information we acquire comes through our eyes (and the related circuitry in our brains), rather than through touch, smell, hearing, or taste. For better or worse, that is also the way scientists acquire information from their experiments. But the skills in interpreting images developed by millions of years of evolution do not deal as well with scientific images as they do with "real world" experiences. Understanding the differences in the types of information to be extracted, and the biases introduced by our vision systems, is a necessary requirement for the scientist who would trust his or her results.

The percentage of environmental information that flows through visual pathways has been estimated at 90 to 95% for a typical human without any sensory impairment. Indeed, our dependence on vision can be judged from the availability of corrective means, ranging from eyeglasses to laser eye surgery, for those whose vision is not perfect or deteriorates with age.

---

[1] *Note*: Portions of this chapter first appeared as a series of articles in the *Proceedings of the Royal Microscopy Society* in 2004.

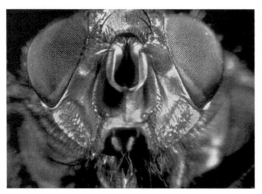

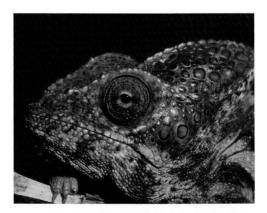

Figure 2.1 *Eyes come in many forms, optimized for different purposes. Insect eyes consist of many individual lenses and sensors, producing comparatively low resolution. The chameleon can swivel its eyes independently to track different objects in left and right visual fields. The horse has little stereo vision but a broad field of view. The eagle's acuity and resolution is extremely high. Primates are well adapted for stereo vision and also have greater sensitivity to red colors than most other animals. The eye of the octopus apparently evolved independently and has its neural circuitry on the opposite side of the retina, but it provides very good acuity and color sensitivity.*

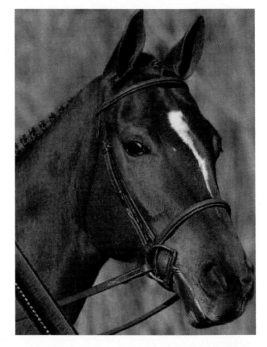

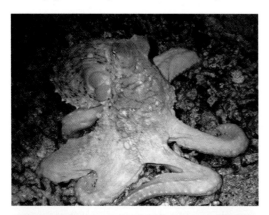

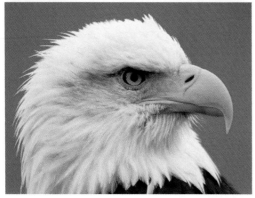

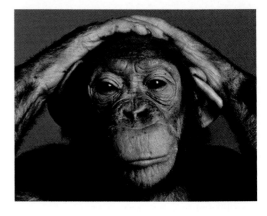

Hearing aids and cochlear implants are available (but underutilized) for those with severe hearing loss, but there are no palliatives for the other senses. As taste becomes less sensitive, the only solution is to sprinkle on more chili powder.

Not all animals, even all mammals, depend on or use sight to the extent that we do (**Figure 2.1**). Bats and dolphins use echolocation or sonar to probe the world about them. Pit vipers sense infrared radiation. Moles, living underground, trade sight for sensitive touch organs around their nose. Bloodhounds follow scents, and butterflies have taste organs so sensitive they can detect single molecules. Some eels generate and sense electric fields to interact with their surroundings. Fish and alligators have pressure sensors that detect very slight motions in their watery environment. Birds and bees both have the ability to detect the polarization of light as an aid to locating the sun's position on a cloudy day. Birds and some bacteria seem to be able to sense the orientation of Earth's magnetic field, another aid to navigation. And many birds and insects have vision systems that detect infrared or ultraviolet colors beyond our range of vision (Goldsmith 2006).

It is not easy for humans to imagine what the world looks like to a bat, eel, or mole. Indeed, even the word "imagine" demonstrates the problem. The root word "image" implies a picture, or scene, constructed inside the mind, reflecting our dependence on images to organize our perceptions of the world, and our language illustrates that bias. Even persons who have been blind from birth report that they construct a mental image of their surroundings from touch, sound, and other clues.

With two forward-facing eyes capable of detecting light over a wavelength range of about 400 to 700 nm (blue to red), we are descended from arboreal primates who depended on vision and stereoscopy for navigation and hunting. Many animals and insects have sacrificed stereoscopy for coverage, with eyes spaced wide to detect motion. A few, like the chameleon, can move their eyes independently to track different objects. But even in the category of hunters with stereo vision, there are many birds with much better sight than humans. Eagles have resolution that can distinguish a mouse at a range of nearly a mile. In fact, most birds devote a much larger portion of their head space to eyes than we do. In some birds, the eyes are so large that it affects other functions, such as using blinking to force the eyes down onto the throat to swallow food.

An oft-quoted adage states that "a picture is worth a thousand words," and is used as an illustration of the importance of images and their apparent rich information content. But the statement is wrong in many ways. First, a typical image, digitized and stored in a computer, occupies the space of several million words of text. Using this chapter as an example, 1000 words require an average of 6080 bytes to store, exclusive of formatting information, and can be compressed (zip format) without any loss of information to require about 2150 bytes per 1000 words. Furthermore, the resolution of modern digital cameras is far less than that of the human eye, which has about 160 million rods and cones. Second, as a means of communicating information from one person to another, the image is very inefficient. There is little reason to expect another person to derive the same information from a picture as we did without some supporting information to bring it to their attention and create a context for interpreting it. Arlo Guthrie describes this in the song "Alice's Restaurant" as "twenty-seven 8 × 10 color glossy pictures with circles and arrows and a paragraph on the back of each one." That is not a bad description of many typical scientific papers!

Research indicates that cultural differences strongly affect what we see in an image. Many westerners fix their attention on one (or a few) objects that are in the foreground or brightly colored, and ignore the surroundings. Many Asians pay much attention to the overall scene and the background details, noting the presence of objects in the foreground but not devoting any extra attention to studying their characteristics. And, of course, recognition of something in a scene that is familiar to the observer strongly influences where attention is focused.

Human vision can extract several different kinds of information from images, and much of the processing that takes place has been optimized by evolution and experience to perform very efficiently. But at the same time, other types of information are either ignored or suppressed and are not normally observed. Sherlock Holmes often criticized Watson for "seeing but not observing," which is as good a distinction as any between having photons fall upon the retina and the conscious mind becoming aware. This chapter examines some of the processes by which information is extracted and the conscious levels of the mind alerted while also noting that the extraction process overlooks some kinds of information or makes them very difficult to detect. And, of course, expectations color perception; we are more likely to find what we are looking for.

Recognition

The goal of much of human vision is recognition. Whether searching for food, avoiding predators, or welcoming a mate, the first thing that catches our attention in an image is something familiar. To be recognized, an object or feature must have a name, some label that our consciousness can assign. Behind that label is a mental model of the object that can be expressed either in words, images, memories of associated events, or perhaps in other forms. This model captures the important (to us) characteristics of the object. It is unfortunate that, in many scientific experiments, the task assigned to human vision is not the recognition of familiar objects, but the detection and description of unfamiliar ones, which is far more difficult.

Things for which we do not have an existing label are difficult to recognize or identify. In contrast, the stored representation of a recognized object is the example or instance that contains those characteristics and features that, in our individual memories, are the identifying hallmarks of the class of objects. Each person may have his or her own example, of course. To cite a trivial example, one person's "dolphin" may be the mammal ("Flipper") and another's the fish (mahi-mahi). Failing to specify which is intended opens the way for miscommunication. In addition, the remembered example that corresponds to the label will generally not represent any real object or any kind of statistically representative combination of real objects, but will instead contain those specific and particular features that have become important to each individual through accidents of prior experience. In other words, even if our labels for something are the same down to genus, species, and variety, they may not be supported by the same set of expected characteristics. In the days when scientists published papers illustrated by drawings, the drawings represented their personal model for the class of objects. Now that "real" images are used, the illustrations may actually be less representative because they show a particular member of the class that is not likely to be representative in any sense, corresponding neither to the writer's mental representation nor to a statistically meaningful prototype for the class.

The basic technique that lies at the root of human vision is comparison. Nothing in images is measured by the eye and mind; we have no rulers and protractors in our heads for size, and no spectrophotometers for color or brightness. Features that can be viewed next to each other with similar orientation, surroundings, and lighting can be compared most easily. Ones that must be mentally flipped or rotated are more difficult. **Figure 2.2** shows an example in which the length of time required to mentally turn each object over in the mind — to match align-

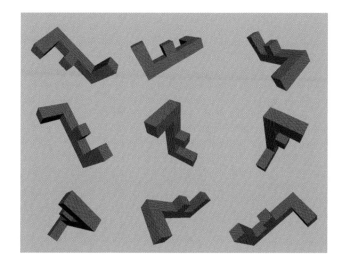

Figure 2.2 *Some of these objects are identical and some are mirror images. The length of time required to turn each one over in the mind for comparison is proportional to the angular difference.*

ments and determine which features are the same and which are mirror images — is proportional to the angular differences between them. Comparisons to memory work the same way, and they take time. If the remembered object is familiar, then the underlying model consists of a list of characteristics that can be swiftly compared. That is, after all, how recognition works.

If the perceived object is not familiar and has no label and model, then comparison depends on the remembered characteristics of the original view. The efficiency of the memory process as well as the features and characteristics selected for recall are themselves subject to comparison to yet other models. As an example, eyewitness accounts of crime and accident scenes are notoriously unreliable. Different observers select different attributes of the scene (or of the suspect) as being notable based on their similarity to or difference from other objects in memory, so of course each person's results vary. Police sketches of suspects rarely match well with actual photographs taken after capture. In some respects they are caricatures, emphasizing some aspect (often trivial) that seemed familiar or unusual to an individual observer (see, for example, Figure 37 in Chapter 2 of Russ [2002]). The message for a would-be bank robber is obvious: provide some easily remembered clues, like a tattoo, bandage, and limp, that can be discarded afterward.

A "threshold logic unit" implements the process that can signal recognition based on the weighted sum of many inputs. This process does not duplicate the exact functions of a real neuron, but is based on the McCulloch and Pitts (1943) "perceptron" model, which successfully describes the overall process (**Figure 2.3**). This idea appears again in **Chapter 11** as a tool for software that performs similar classification.

Recognition is frequently described in terms of a "grandmother cell." This is a theoretical construct, and not a single physical cell someplace in the brain, but it provides a useful framework to describe some of the significant features of the recognition process. The idea of the grandmother cell is that it patiently examines every image for the appearance of grandmother, and then signals the conscious mind that she is present. Processing of the raw image that reaches the eye proceeds in a parallel fashion in several places, including the retina and visual cortex. In the process, several characteristics that can roughly be described as color, size, position, and shape are extracted. Some of these can be matched with those in the stored model for grandmother (such as short stature, white hair, a smile, perhaps even a familiar dress). Clearly, some characteristics are more important than others, so there must be weighting of the inputs.

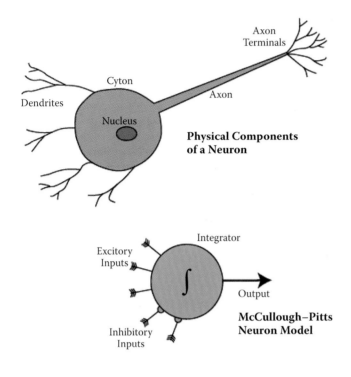

Physical Components
of a Neuron

Figure 2.3 Comparison of a physical neuron (the McCulloch and Pitts simplified model of a neuron) and its implementation as a threshold logic unit. If the weighted sum of many inputs exceeds a threshold, then the output (which may go to another logic unit) is turned on. Learning consists of adjusting the weights, which can be either positive or negative.

Integrator

Excitory Inputs

∫

Output

McCullough–Pitts
Neuron Model

Inhibitory Inputs

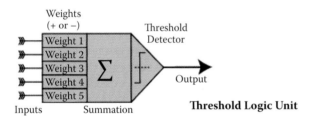

Weights
(+ or −)

Threshold
Detector

Weight 1
Weight 2
Weight 3
Weight 4
Weight 5

Σ

Output

Inputs   Summation

Threshold Logic Unit

If there are enough positive matches — in the absence of negative characteristics (such as a flaming red mustache) — then the "grandmother" signal is sent.

This simple model for a "threshold logic unit" has evolved into the modern neural network, in which several layers of these individual decision-making units are connected. Their inputs combine data from various sensors and the output from other units, and the final output is a decision, basically a recognition that the inputs match (well enough) some recognized circumstance or object. The characteristics of neural-network decisions, whether performed on images in the human mind or other types of data in a computer circuit, include very high speed (due to the extremely parallel way in which all of the small logic decisions happen at the same time), the ability to learn (by adjusting the weights given to the various inputs), and the tendency to make mistakes.

Many people have had the experience of thinking that they recognized someone ("grandmother") and then, on closer inspection, realized that it was not actually the right person at all. There were enough positive clues, and an absence of negative clues, to trigger the recognition process. Perhaps in a different situation, or with a different point of view, we would not have made that mistake. On the other hand, setting the threshold value on the weighted sum of positive inputs too high, while it would reduce false positives, would be inefficient, requiring too much time to collect more data. The penalty for making a wrong identification is a little minor embarrassment. The benefit of the fast and efficient procedure is the ability to perform recognitions based on incomplete data.

In some implementations of this logic, it is possible to assign a probability or a degree of confidence to an identification, but the utility of this value depends in high degree upon the quality of the underlying model. This can be represented as the weights in a neural network, as the rules in a fuzzy logic system, or in some other form. In human recognition, the list of factors in the model is not so explicit. Writing down all of the characteristics that help to identify grandmother (and especially the negative exclusions) is very difficult. In most scientific experiments, we try to enumerate the important factors, but there is always a background level of underlying assumptions that may or may not be shared by those who read the results.

It is common in scientific papers that involve imaging to present a picture, usually with the caption "typical appearance" or "representative view." Editors of technical journals understand that these pictures are intended to show a few of the factors in the model list that the author considers particularly significant (and hopefully describes in the text). But of course no one picture can be truly "typical." For one thing, most naturally occurring structures have some variability, and the chances of finding the mean value of all characteristics in one individual is small and, in any case, would not demonstrate the range of variation.

But even in the case of an individual like "grandmother," no one picture will suffice. Perhaps you have a photo that shows her face, white hair, rimless glasses, and she is even wearing a favorite apron. So you present that as the typical picture, but the viewer notices instead that she is wearing an arm sling, because on the day you took the picture she happened to have strained her shoulder. To you, that is a trivial detail, not the important thing in the picture. But the viewer cannot know that, so the wrong information is transmitted by the illustration.

Editors know that the usual meaning of "typical picture" is that "this is the prettiest image we have." Picture selection often includes an aesthetic judgment that biases many uses of images.

Technical specs

The human eye is a pretty good optical device (**Figure 2.4**). Based on the size of the lens aperture (5×10^{-3} m) and the wavelength of light (about 5×10^{-7} m for green), the theoretical resolution should be about 10^{-4} radians or 1/3 arc min. The lens focuses light onto the retina, and it is only in the fovea, the tiny portion of the retina (covering approximately 2°) in which the cones are most densely packed, that the highest resolution is retained in the sensed image. One arc min is a reasonable estimate for the overall resolution performance of the eye, a handy number that can be used to estimate distances. Estimate the size of the smallest objects you can resolve, multiply by 3000, and that is how far away you are in the same units. For example, a car about 13 ft long can be resolved from an airplane at 40,000 ft, and so on.

The number of 160 million rods and cones in the retina does not estimate the actual resolution of images. When we "look at" something, we rotate our head or our eyeballs in their sockets so that the image of that point falls onto the fovea, where the cone density is highest. The periphery of our vision has relatively fewer cones (which respond to color) as compared with rods (which sense only brightness), and is important primarily for sensing motion and for judging scene illumination so that we can correct for color balance and shading. To produce a digital

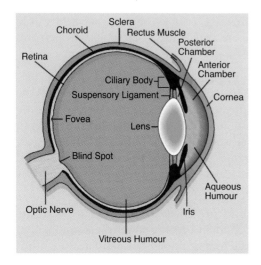

Figure 2.4 Simplified diagram of the eye, showing the lens, retina, fovea, optic nerve, etc.

camera that captured entire scenes (as large as the area we see) with resolution that would match human foveal vision, so that we could later look anywhere in the stored image and see the finest detail, would require several billion sensors.

Human vision achieves something quite miraculous by rapidly shifting the eye to look at many different locations in a scene and, without any conscious effort, combining those bits and pieces into a single perceived image. There is a blind spot in the retina without sensors, where the optic nerve connects. We do not notice that blind spot because the brain fills it in with pieces interpolated from the surroundings or stored from previous glances. Tests in which objects appear or disappear from the blind spot prove that we do not actually get any information from there — our minds make something up for us.

The eye can capture images over a very wide range of illumination levels, covering about nine or ten orders of magnitude ranging from a few dozen photons on a starlit night to a bright sunny day on the ski slopes. Some of that adaptation comes from changing the aperture with the iris, but most of it depends on processing in the retina. Adaptation to changing levels of illumination takes some time, up to several minutes, depending on the amount of change. In the darkest few orders of magnitude we lose color sensitivity and use only the rods. Since the fovea is rich in cones but has few rods, looking just "next to" what we want to see (averted vision) is a good strategy in the dark. It shifts the image over to an area with more rods to capture the dim image, albeit with less resolution.

Rods are not very sensitive to light at the red end of the visible spectrum, which is why red-light illumination is used by astronomers, submariners, and others who wish to be able to turn off the red light and immediately have full sensitivity in the dark-adapted rod vision. The cones come in three kinds, each of which responds over slightly different wavelength ranges (**Figure 2.5**). They are typically called long-, medium-, and short-wavelength receptors, or more succinctly but less accurately, red-, green-, and blue-sensitive cones. By comparing the response of each type of cone, the eye characterizes color. Yellow is a combination of red and green, magenta is the relative absence of green, and so on.

Because of the different densities of red-, green-, and blue-sensitive cones, the overall sensitivity of the eye is greatest for green light and poorest for blue light (shown in **Figure 1.12** of **Chapter 1**). But this sensitivity comes at a price: it is within this same range of green wavelengths that our ability to distinguish one color from another is poorest. A common technique

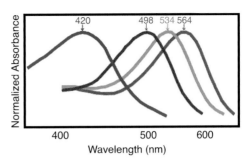

Figure 2.5 *Sensitivity of the rods (shown in gray) and three kinds of cones (shown in red, green, and blue) as a function of wavelength. Human vision detects roughly the range from about 400 nm (blue) to 700 nm (red).*

in microscopy uses filters to select just the green light because of the eye's sensitivity, but if detection of color variations is important, this is not a good strategy.

Like most of the things that the eye does, the perception of color is determined in a comparative rather than an absolute way. It is only by comparing something to a known color reference that we can really estimate color at all. The usual color reference is a white object, since that (by definition) has all colors. If the scene we are looking at contains something known to be a neutral gray in color, then any variation in the color of the illumination can be compensated for (as illustrated in **Chapter 1**). This is not so simple as it might seem, because many objects do not reflect light of all colors equally and appear to change color with angle or illumination. (This "metamerism" is often a problem with ink-jet printers as well.)

Because just three types of color-sensitive cone receptors are available, each with broad and overlapping wavelength response, there are many different combinations of wavelengths of light that evoke the same visual response, which may furthermore vary from individual to individual. Color matching, which is discussed further in **Chapter 3** as it relates to making printed images that visually match original scenes and to presentation of the same image on a computer monitor, is a specialized topic that depends on careful calibration.

A commonly asked question is "what RGB (red, green, blue) proportions correspond to a particular wavelength of light?" There is no answer to that question, for several reasons. Perceived color is dependent on human perception and to some extent varies from person to person, and it is also dependent on the viewing environment. The wide (and overlapping) wavelength range of sensitivities of the three kinds of cones means that the same perception of color can be produced by many different combinations of wavelengths. Generating colors using RGB components on different computer displays is difficult enough because of the different phosphors (and their aging) and the difference between CRTs (cathode-ray tubes), LCDs (liquid crystal displays), and other devices. For printing, the problems (as discussed in **Chapter 3**) are much worse and also depend on the paper and illumination under which the image is viewed. However, as a useful way to represent the variation of colors with wavelength, a model such as that shown in **Figure 2.6** can be used (Bruton 2005).

For viewing colors by reflected light, if the illumination is deficient in some portion of the color spectrum compared with daytime sunlight (under which our vision evolved), then the missing colors cannot be reflected or detected, and it is impossible to accurately judge the object's true colors. Under monochromatic yellow sodium lights, color is completely confused with albedo (total reflectivity), and we cannot distinguish color from brightness. Even with typical indoor lighting, colors appear different (which is why the salesperson suggests you might want to carry that shirt and tie to the window to see how they look in sunlight!).

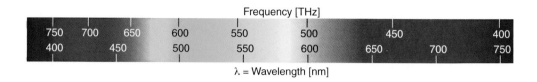

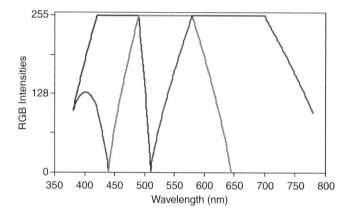

Figure 2.6 An approximate visual representation of the relationship between wavelength and RGB color components is constructed by adjusting the RGB intensities (shown on the usual 0 to 255 scale used for computer displays).

When Newton first split white sunlight into its component parts using a prism, he was able to show that there were invisible components beyond both ends of the visible spectrum by measuring the rise in temperature that was caused by the absorption of that light. Since sunlight extends well beyond the narrow 400- to 700-nm range of human vision, it is not surprising that some animals and insects have evolved vision systems that can detect components of sunlight that are invisible to humans. Plants, in particular, have developed signals that are visible only in these extended colors to attract birds and insects to pollinate them. Extending our human vision into these ranges and even beyond is possible with instrumentation. Ultraviolet (UV) microscopy, radio astronomy, and X-ray diffraction all use portions of the electromagnetic spectrum beyond the visible, and all produce data that is typically presented as images, with colors shifted into the narrow portion of the spectrum we can detect.

Being able to detect brightness or color is not the same thing as being able to measure it or detect small variations in either brightness or color. While human vision functions over some nine to ten orders of magnitude, we cannot view a single image that covers such a wide range, nor can we detect variations of one part in 10^9. A change in brightness of about 2 to 3% over a lateral distance of a few arc minutes is the limit of detectability under typical viewing conditions. It is important to note that the required variation is a percentage, so that a greater absolute change in brightness is required in bright areas than in dark ones. Anyone with photographic darkroom experience is aware that different details are typically seen in a negative than in a positive image.

Overall, the eye can detect only about 20 to 30 shades of gray in an image, and in many cases fewer will produce a visually satisfactory result. In an image dominated by large areas of different brightness, it is difficult to pick out the fine detail with small local contrast within each area. One of the common methods for improving the visibility of local detail is computer enhancement that reduces the global (long range) variation in brightness while increasing the local contrast. This is typically done by comparing a pixel to its local neighborhood. If the pixel is slightly brighter than its neighbors, it is made brighter still, and vice versa. This will be the basis for some of the enhancement techniques presented in **Chapter 5**.

Human vision deals with scenes that include a wide range of brightness by adapting to local regions and detecting the contrast locally. Such scenes cannot be recorded in their entirety by either film or digital cameras, which have limited dynamic range (a maximum of three to four orders of magnitude). By recording such scenes with different exposures, and combining them with appropriate software, it is possible to preserve local contrast by sacrificing long-range contrast, as shown in **Figure 2.7** (the exposure merging procedure is shown in **Chapter 5**). **Chapter 3** discusses related methods that process high-dynamic-range images so that they can be displayed or printed with reduced overall contrast while preserving local detail and contrast.

Local and abrupt changes in brightness (or color) are the most readily noticed details in images. Variations in texture often represent structural variations that are important, but these are more subtle. As shown in **Figure 2.8**, in many cases variations that are classified as textural actually represent changes in the average brightness level. When only a change in texture is present, visual detection is difficult. If the boundaries are not straight lines (and especially vertical or horizontal in orientation), they are much more difficult to see. **Chapter 5** includes methods that can distinguish regions based on textural differences.

Thirty shades of brightness in each of the red, green, and blue cones would suggest that 30^3 = 27,000 colors might be distinguished, but that is not so. Sensitivity to color changes at the ends of the spectrum is much better than in the middle (in other words, greens are hard to distinguish from each other). Only about a thousand different colors can be distinguished. Since computer displays offer 256 shades of brightness for the R, G, and B phosphors, or 256^3 = 16 million colors, we might expect that they could produce any color we can see. However, this

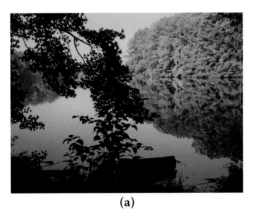

Figure 2.7
(a,b) Merging images photographed with different exposures to form a
(c) single image in which local contrast is preserved.

(a)

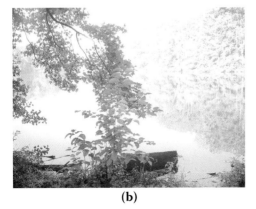

(b)

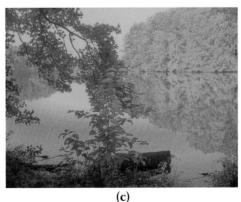

(c)

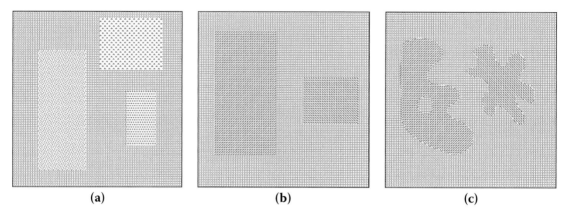

Figure 2.8 *Examples of textural differences: **(a)** regions are also different in average brightness; **(b)** no brightness difference but simple linear boundaries; **(c)** irregular boundaries.*

is not the case. Both computer displays and printed images suffer from limitations in gamut — the total range of colors that can be produced — as compared with what we can see. This is another reason that the "typical image" may not actually be representative of the object or class of objects.

Acuity

Many animals, particularly birds, have vision that produces much higher spatial resolution than humans. Human vision achieves its highest spatial resolution in just a small area at the center of the field of view (the fovea), where the density of light-sensing cones is highest. At a 50-cm viewing distance, details with a width of 1 mm represent an angle of slightly more than one-tenth of a degree. Acuity (spatial resolution) is normally specified in units of cycles per degree. The upper limit (finest detail) visible with the human eye is about 50 cycles per degree, which would correspond to a grating in which the brightness varied from minimum to maximum about five times over that same 1 mm. At that fine spacing, 100% contrast would be needed, in other words black lines and white spaces. This is where the common specification arises that the finest lines distinguishable without optical aid are about 100 μm.

Less contrast is needed between the light and dark locations to detect them when the features are larger. Brightness variations about 1-mm wide represent a spatial frequency of about nine cycles per degree, and under ideal viewing conditions can be resolved with a contrast of a few percent, although this assumes the absence of any noise in the image and a very bright image. (Acuity drops significantly in dark images or in ones with superimposed random variations, and is much poorer at detecting color differences than brightness variations.)

At a normal viewing distance of about 50 cm, 1 mm on the image is about the optimum size for detecting the presence of detail. On a typical computer monitor, that corresponds to about 4 pixels. As the spatial frequency drops (features become larger), the required contrast increases, so that when the distance over which the brightness varies from minimum to maximum is about 1 cm, the required contrast is about ten times greater. The variation of spatial resolution ("acuity") with contrast is called the modulation transfer function (**Figure 2.9**).

Enlarging images does not improve the ability to distinguish small detail, and in fact degrades it. The common mistake made by microscopists is to work at very high magnification expect-

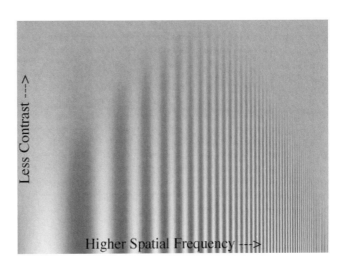

Figure 2.9 Illustration of the modulation transfer function for human vision, showing that the greatest ability to resolve low-contrast details occurs at an intermediate spatial frequency and becomes poorer for both smaller and larger details.

ing to see the finest details. That may be needed for details that are small in dimension, but it will make it more difficult to see larger features that have less contrast. For the same reason, enlarging the digitized image on the computer display does not improve, and often degrades, the ability to see details.

Because the eye does not "measure" brightness, but simply makes comparisons, it is very difficult to distinguish brightness differences unless the regions are immediately adjacent. **Figure 2.10a** shows four gray squares, two of which are 5% darker than the others. Because they are separated, the ability to compare them is limited. Even if the regions are adjacent, as in **Figure 2.10b**, if the change from one region to another is gradual it cannot be detected. Only when the step is abrupt, as in **Figure 2.10c**, can the eye easily determine which regions are different.

Even when the features have sizes and contrast that should be visible, the presence of variations in the background intensity (or color) can prevent the visual system from detecting them. In the example of **Figure 2.11**, the text has a local contrast of about 2% but is superimposed on a ramp that varies from white to black. Application of an image processing operation reveals the message. The "unsharp mask" routine (discussed in **Chapter 5**) subtracts a blurred

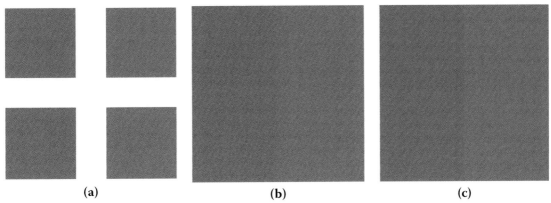

(a)   (b)   (c)

Figure 2.10 Comparison of regions with a 5% brightness difference: (a) separated; (b) adjacent but with a gradual change; (c) adjacent with an abrupt boundary.

 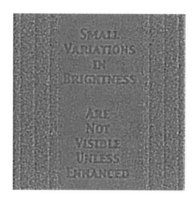

Figure 2.11 Intensity differences superimposed on a varying background are visually undetectable:
(a) *original;*
(b) *processed with an "unsharp mask" filter to suppress the gradual changes and reveal the detail.*

(smoothed) copy of the image from the original, suppressing large-scale variations in order to show local details.

It is easy to confuse resolution with visibility. A star in the sky is essentially a point; there is no angular size, and even in a telescope it does not appear as a disk. It is visible because of its contrast, appearing bright against the dark sky. Faint stars are not visible to the naked eye because there is not enough contrast. Telescopes make them visible by collecting more light into a larger aperture. A better way to think about resolution is the ability to distinguish as separate two stars that are close together. The classic test for this has long been the star Mizar in the handle of the Big Dipper. In Van Gogh's *Starry Night over the Rhone*, each of the stars in this familiar constellation is shown as a single entity (**Figure 2.12**). But a proper star chart shows that the second star in the handle is actually double. Alcor and Mizar are an optical double — two stars that appear close together but in fact are at different distances and have no gravitational relationship to each other. They are separated by about 11.8 min of arc, and being able to detect the two as separate has been considered by many cultures from the American Indians to the desert dwellers of the Near East as a test of good eyesight (as well as the need for a dark sky with little turbulence or water vapor, and without a moon or other light pollution).

But there is more to Mizar than meets the eye, literally. With the advent of the Galilean telescope, observers were surprised to find that Mizar itself is a double star. Giovanni Battista Riccioli (1598–1671), the Jesuit astronomer and geographer of Bologna, is generally supposed to have split Mizar, the first double star ever discovered, around 1650. The two stars Mizar-A and Mizar-B, are a gravitational double 14.42 arc sec apart, and any good modern telescope can separate them (**Figure 2.13**). But they turn out to be even more complicated; each star is itself a double as well, so close together that only spectroscopy can detect them.

There are many double stars in the sky that can be resolved with a backyard telescope, and many of them are familiar viewing targets for amateur astronomers who enjoy the color differences between some of the star pairs or the challenge of resolving them. This depends on more than just the angular separation. If one star is significantly brighter than the other, it is much more difficult to see the weaker star close to the brighter one.

What the eye tells the brain

Human vision is a lot more than rods and cones in the retina. An enormous amount of processing takes place, some of it immediately in the retina and some in the visual cortex at the rear of the brain, before an "image" is available to the conscious mind. The neural connections

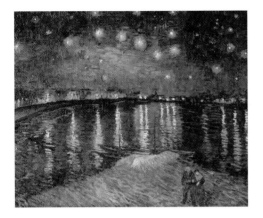

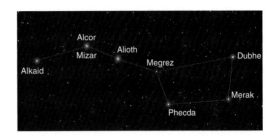

Figure 2.12 The Big Dipper, as depicted in Van Gogh's Starry Night over the Rhone and as shown in a star chart.

within the retina were first seen about a hundred years ago by Ramón y Cajal, and have been studied ever since. **Figure 2.14** shows a simplified diagram of the human retina. The light-sensing rods and cones are at the back, and light must pass through several layers of processing cells to reach them. Only about 10% of the photons that enter the human eye are detected; the rest is either reflected (about 3%), absorbed by nonsensing structures, or fall between the active molecules. In many nocturnal animals, the pigmented layer behind the rods and cones reflects light back so that the photons are twice as likely to be captured and detected (and some comes back out through the lens to produce the reflective eyes we see watching us at night). Incidentally, the eye of the octopus does not have this backward arrangement; evolution in that case put the light-sensing cells on top, where they can most efficiently catch the light.

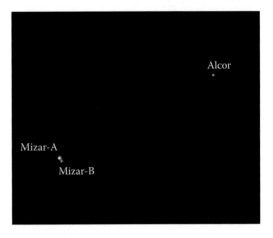

Figure 2.13 Photograph showing the relative separation of Alcor from Mizar A and B.

The first layer of processing cells, called horizontal cells, connect light-sensing cells in various size neighborhoods. The next layer, the amacrine cells, combine and compare the outputs from the horizontal cells. Finally the ganglion cells collect the outputs for transmission to the visual cortex. There are about 100 times as many sensors as there are neural connections in the optic nerve, implying a considerable processing to extract the meaningful information. This physical organization corresponds directly to the logical processes of inhibition, discussed below.

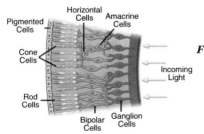

Figure 2.14 The principal layers in the retina. Light passes through several layers of processing neurons to reach the light-sensitive rod and cone cells. The horizontal, bipolar, and amacrine cells combine the signals from various size regions, compare them to locate interesting features, and pass that information on to higher levels in the visual cortex.

In many respects, the retina of the eye is actually part of the brain. The scientists who elucidated the early processing of image data and the extraction of the information transmitted from the eye to the visual cortex were awarded the Nobel Prize (in 1981, to David H. Hubel and Torsten N. Wiesel, for their discoveries concerning information processing in the visual system). A good summary of the physical structures and functions can be found in Hubel (1988).

Without elaborating the anatomical details of the retina or the visual cortex discovered by Hubel, Wiesel, and others (particularly a seminal paper "What the frog's eye tells the frog's brain," published in 1959 by Jerome Lettvin), it is still possible to summarize the logical and practical implications. Within the retina, outputs from the individual light sensors are combined and compared by layers of neurons. Comparing the output from one sensor or region with that from the surrounding sensors, so that excitation of the center is tested against the inhibition from the surroundings, is a basic step that enables the retina to ignore regions that are uniform or only gradually varying in brightness, and to efficiently detect locations where a change in brightness occurs. Testing over different size regions locates points and features of varying sizes.

Comparison of output over time is carried out in the same way to detect changes, which if they are either too rapid or too slow will not be seen. We do not notice the 60-Hz flickering of fluorescent lamps, although insects and some birds do, and adjustment to any change that takes place over more than tens of seconds prevents it from being noticed.

In the frog's eye, the retina processes images to find just a few highly specific stimuli. These include small dark moving objects (food) and the location of the largest, darkest region (safety in the pond). The eye is hardwired to detect "looming," the presence of something that grows rapidly larger and does not shift in the visual field. That represents something coming toward the eye, and causes the fly to avoid the swatter or the frog to jump into the water. In a human, the eyelid blinks for protection before we become consciously aware that an object was even seen.

The outputs from these primitive detection circuits are then further combined in the cortex to locate lines and edges. There are specific regions in the cortex that are sensitive to different orientations of lines and to their motion. The "wiring" of these regions is not built in, but must be developed after birth; cats raised in an environment devoid of lines in a specific orientation do not subsequently have the ability to see such lines. Detection of the location of brightness changes (feature edges) creates a kind of mental sketch of the scene, which is dominated by the presence of lines, edges, corners, and other simple structures. These in turn are linked together in a hierarchy to produce the understanding of the scene in our minds. "Image understanding" software attempts to do the same thing with scene images, constructing a model of the scene geometry and identifying and locating objects based on a sketch formed by edges.

The extraction of changes in brightness or color with position or with time explains a great deal about what we see in scenes, and about what we miss. Changes that occur gradually with position, such as shading of light on a wall, is ignored. We have to exert a really conscious effort to notice such shading, and even then we have no quantitative tools with which to estimate its magnitude. But even small changes in brightness of a few percent are visible when they occur abruptly, producing a definite edge. And when that edge forms a straight line (and particularly when it is vertical) it is noticed. Similarly, any part of a scene that is static over time tends to be ignored, but when something moves it attracts our attention.

These techniques for extracting information from scenes are efficient because they are highly parallel. For every one of the 160 million light sensors in the eye, there are as many as 50,000 neurons involved in processing and comparing. One of Hubel and Wiesel's contributions was showing how the connections in the network are formed shortly after birth and the dependence of that formation on providing imagery to the eyes during that critical period.

Mapping of the specific circuitry in the brain is accomplished by placing electrodes in various locations in the cortex and observing the output of neurons as various images and stimuli are presented to the eyes. At a higher level of scale and processing, functional scans using MRI (magnetic resonance imaging) or PET (positron emission tomography) can identify regions of the brain that become active in response to various activities and stimuli. But there is another source of important knowledge about processing of images in the mind: identifying the mistakes that are made in image interpretation. One important but limited resource is studying the responses of persons who have known specific damage, either congenital or as the result of illness or accident. A second approach studies the errors in interpretation of images resulting from visual illusions. Since everyone tends to make the same mistakes, those errors must be a direct indication of how the processing is accomplished. Several of the more revealing cases are presented in the sections that follow.

Spatial comparisons

The basic idea behind center-surround or excitation-inhibition logic is comparing the signals from a central region (which can be a single detector or progressively larger scales by averaging detectors together) to the output from a surrounding annular region. That is the basic analysis unit in the retina, and by combining the outputs from many such primitive units, the detection of light or dark lines, corners, edges, and other structures can be achieved. In the frog's eye, it was determined that a dark object of a certain size (corresponding to an insect close enough to be captured) generated a powerful recognition signal. In the cat's visual cortex there are regions that respond only to dark lines of a certain length and angle, moving in a particular direction. Furthermore, those regions are intercalated with regions that perform the same analysis on the image data from the other eye, which is presumed to be important in stereopsis or fusion of stereo images.

This fundamental center-surround behavior explains several very common illusions (**Figure 2.15**). A set of uniform gray steps (Mach bands) is not perceived as being uniform (Mach

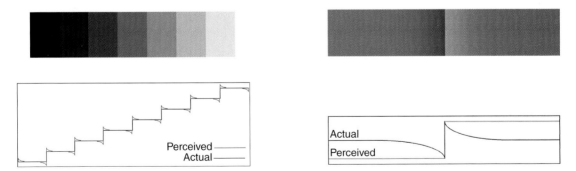

Figure 2.15 *Two common illusions based on inhibition: Mach bands (top) demonstrate that the visual system increases the perceived change in brightness at steps; the Craik–Cornsweet–O'Brien step (bottom) shows that providing the visual system with a step influences the judgment of values farther away.*

1906). The side of each step next to a lighter region is perceived as being darker, and vice versa, because it is the step that is noticed. In the case of the Mach bands, the visual response to the step aids us in determining which region is darker, although it makes it very difficult to judge the amount of the difference. But the same effect can be used in the absence of any difference to cause one to be perceived. In the Craik–Cornsweet–O'Brien illusion, two adjacent regions have the same brightness but the values are raised and lowered on either side of the boundary (Cornsweet 1970). The eye interprets this in the same way as for the Mach bands, and judges that one region is, in fact, lighter and one darker.

Similar excitation-inhibition comparisons are made for color values. Boundaries between blocks of color are detected and emphasized, while the absolute differences between the blocks are minimized. Blocks of identical color placed on a gradient of brightness or some other color will appear to be different.

Center-surround comparisons are used in several computer image processing algorithms, including the unsharp-mask and top-hat filters discussed in **Chapter 5**. Some implementations of edge-finding algorithms, also discussed there, are also emulations of the processing that seems to be performed in vision systems.

Whether described in terms of brightness, hue, and saturation or the artist's tint, shade, and tone, or various mathematical spaces, three parameters are needed. All of the color-space coordinate systems shown in **Chapter 1** require three values to define a color. Brightness is a measure of how light or dark the light is, without regard to any color information. For the artist, this is the shade, achieved by adding black to the pigment. Hue distinguishes the various colors, progressing from red to orange, yellow, green, blue, and magenta around the color wheel we probably encountered in kindergarten (or the ROY G BIV mnemonic for the order of colors in the rainbow). Hue corresponds to the artist's pure pigment. Saturation is the amount of color present, such as the difference between pink and red, or sky blue and royal blue. A fully saturated color corresponds to the artist's pure pigment, which can be tinted with neutral pigment to reduce the saturation (tone describes adding both white and black pigments to the pure color).

Even without formal training in color science (or art), this is how people describe color to themselves. Combination and comparison of the signals from the red-, green-, and blue-sensitive cones is used to determine these parameters. Simplistically, we can think of the sum of all three, or perhaps a weighted sum that reflects the different sensitivities of the red, green, and blue detectors, as being the brightness, while ratios of one to another are interpreted as hue, with the ratio of the greatest to the least corresponding to the saturation. It is important to remember that hue does not correspond directly to the wavelength range from red to blue. We interpret a color with reduced green but strong red and blue as being magenta, which is not a color in the wavelength sense but certainly is in terms of perception.

Relying on comparisons to detect changes in brightness or color rather than absolute values simplifies many tasks of image interpretation. For example, the various walls of a building, all painted the same color, will have very different brightness values because of shading, their angle to the sun, etc., but what we observe is a building of uniform color with well-defined corners and detail because it is only the local changes that count. The "light gray" walls on the shadowed side of the building in **Figure 2.16** are actually darker than the "black" shingles on the sunlit side, but our perception understands that the walls are light gray, the trim white, and the shingles black on all sides of the building.

The same principle of local comparisons applies to many other situations. Many artists have used something like the Craik–Cornsweet–O'Brien illusion to create the impression of a great range of light and shadow within the rather limited range of absolute brightness values that

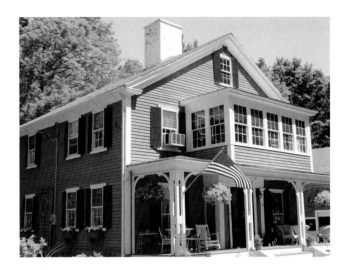

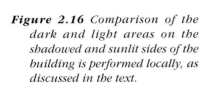

Figure 2.16 Comparison of the dark and light areas on the shadowed and sunlit sides of the building is performed locally, as discussed in the text.

can be achieved with paint on canvas (**Figure 2.17**). The effect can be heightened by adding colors, and there are many cases in which shadows on skin are tinted with colors such as green or magenta that have no physical basis, but increase the perception of a brightness difference.

Edwin Land (of Polaroid fame) studied color vision extensively and proposed a somewhat different interpretation than the tristimulus model described above (which is usually credited to Helmholtz). Also relying heavily on the excitation-inhibition model for processing signals, Land's opponent-color "retinex" theory predicts or explains several interesting visual phenomena. It is important to note that in Land's retinex theory the composition of light from one region in an image considered by itself does not specify the perceived color of that area, but rather that the color of an area is determined by a trio of numbers, each computed on a single waveband (roughly the long, medium, and short wavelengths usually described as red, green, and blue) to give the relationship on that waveband between that area and the rest of the areas in the scene.

One of the consequences Land's theory is that the spectral composition of the illumination becomes very much less important, and the color of a particular region can become relatively

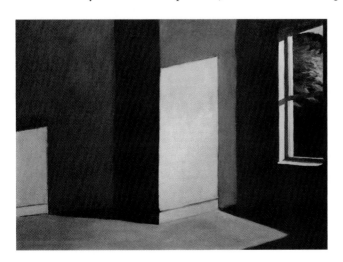

Figure 2.17 Edward Hopper painted many renderings of light and shadow. *His* Sunlight in an Empty Room *illustrates shading along uniform surfaces and steps at edges.*

independent of the light that illuminates it. Our eyes have relatively few cones to sense the colors in the periphery of our vision, but that information is apparently very important in judging colors in the center by correcting for the color of incident illumination. Land demonstrated that if a scene is photographed through red, green, and blue filters, and then projectors are used to shine colored and/or white light through just two of the negatives, the scene can be perceived as having full color. Another interesting phenomenon is that a spinning disk with black and white bars can be perceived as having color, depending on the spacing of the bars. Many of the questions about exactly how color information is processed in the human visual system have not yet been answered.

The discussion of center-surround comparisons above primarily focused on the processes in the retina, which compare each point with its surroundings. But as the extracted information moves up the processing chain, through the visual cortex, there is much evidences of other local comparisons. It was mentioned that there are regions in the visual cortex that respond to lines of a particular angle. They are located adjacent to regions that respond to lines of a slightly different angle. Comparison of the output from one region to its neighbor can thus be used to detect small changes in angle, and indeed that comparison is carried out.

We do not measure angles with mental protractors, but we do compare them and notice differences. Like the case for brightness variations across a step, a difference in angle is amplified to detect boundaries and increase the perceived change. In the absence of any markings on the dial of a wristwatch, telling time to the nearest minute is about the best we can do. One minute corresponds to a 6° motion of the minute hand. But if there are two sets of lines that vary by only a few degrees, we notice that difference (and usually judge it to be much larger).

Inhibition in the context of interpreting angles means that cross-hatching diagonal lines with short marks that are vertical or horizontal will alter our perception of the main line's orientation. As shown in **Figure 2.18**, this makes it difficult or impossible to correctly compare the angle of the diagonal lines (which are in fact parallel).

Local to global hierarchies

Interpretation of elements in a scene relies heavily on grouping them together to form features and objects. A very simple example (**Figure 2.19**) using just dots shows that the eye connects nearest neighbors to construct alignments. Similar grouping of points and lines is also used to connect parts of feature boundaries that are otherwise poorly defined to create the outlines of objects that we visually interpret (**Figure 2.20**). It is a simple extension of this grouping to

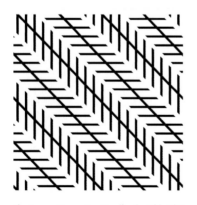

Figure 2.18 Zollner lines. The cross-hatching of the diagonal lines with short vertical and horizontal ones causes our visual perception of them to rotate in the opposite direction. In fact, the diagonal lines are exactly parallel.

include points nearest over time that produces the familiar "Star Trek" impression of motion through a star field. Temporal comparisons are discussed more fully below.

Our natural world does not consist of lines and points; rather, it consists of objects that are represented by connected lines and points. Our vision systems perform this grouping naturally, and it is usually difficult to deconstruct a scene or structure into its component parts. Again, illusions are very useful to illustrate the way this grouping works. **Figure 2.21** shows the same illustration as **Figure 2.18**, but with different colors used for the diagonal lines and the cross hatching. Because the vertical and horizontal lines are different in color than the diagonal ones, they are less strongly grouped with them and, consequently, their effect on the impression of line angles is significantly reduced.

Grouping is necessary for inhibition to work effectively. The common illusion of brightness alteration due to a surrounding, contrasting frame depends on the frame being grouped with the central region. In the example shown in **Figure 2.22**, the insertion of a black line separating the frame from the center alters the appearance of the image and reduces or eliminates the perceived difference in brightness of the central gray regions. Without the line, the brighter and darker frames are grouped with the center, and inhibition alters the apparent brightness, making the region with the dark surroundings appear lighter, and vice versa.

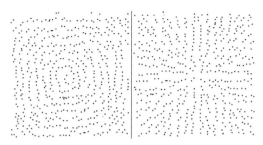

Figure 2.19 Visually connecting each point to its nearest neighbor produces radial or circumferential lines.

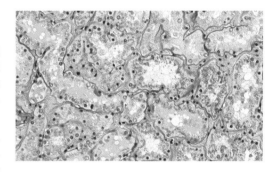

Figure 2.20 The cell boundaries in this tissue section are visually constructed by grouping the lines and points.

The combination of grouping with inhibition gives rise to the illusion shown in **Figure 2.23**. The angled shading causes the lines to appear slightly turned in the opposite direction, and the various pieces of line are connected by grouping, so that the entire figure is perceived as a spiral. But in fact, the lines are circles, as can be verified by tracing around one of them. This is an example of spatial grouping, but temporal grouping works in much the same way. A rotating spiral (**Figure 2.24**) is commonly seen as producing endless motion.

Grouping features in an image that are the same in color lies at the heart of the common tests for color blindness. In the Ishihara tests, a set of colored circles is arranged so that similar colors can be grouped to form recognizable numbers (**Figure 2.25**). For the person who cannot differentiate the colors, the same grouping does not occur and the interpretation of the numbers changes. The example shown is one of a set that diagnoses red-green deficiency, the most common

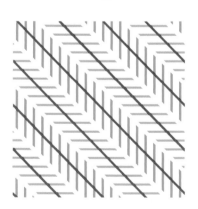

Figure 2.21 The illusion from Figure 2.18, with the cross-hatching in a different color from the lines, which reduces their visual effect.

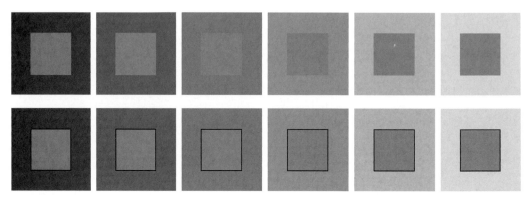

Figure 2.22 *In the top image the lighter and darker surrounds affect our visual comparison of the (identical) central gray regions. This effect is reduced in the bottom image by the separating border.*

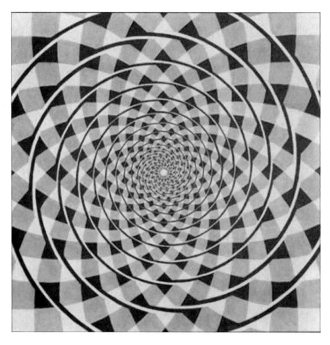

Figure 2.23 *Fraser's spiral. The circular rings are visually "tilted" and perceived to form a spiral.*

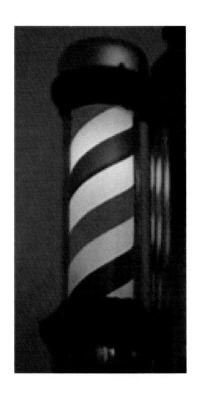

Figure 2.24 *Moving helical or spiral patterns, such as the barber pole, produce an illusion of motion of the background perpendicular to the lines.*

form of color blindness, which affects as many as one in ten males. This deficiency can be classed as either protanopia or deuteranopia. In protanopia, the visible range of the spectrum is shorter at the red end compared with that of the normal, and that part of the spectrum that appears blue-green in the normal appears as gray to those with protanopia. In deuteranopia the part of the spectrum that appears to the normal as green appears as gray. Purple-red (the complementary color of green) also appears as gray. In the example in **Figure 2.25**, those with normal color vision should read the number 74. Red-green color deficiency will cause the number to be read as 21. Someone with total color blindness will not be able to read any numeral.

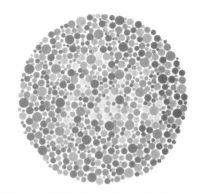

Figure 2.25 One of the Ishihara color blindness test images (see text).

Camouflage is used to hide objects; it works by interfering with our visual ability to group parts of the image together. The military discovered this before the First World War, when the traditional white of U.S. Navy ships (Teddy Roosevelt's "Great White Fleet") was replaced by irregular patterns of grays and blues to reduce their visibility. But nature figured it out long ago, and examples are plentiful. Predators wanting to hide from their prey, and vice versa, typically use camouflage as a first line of defense. There are other visual possibilities of course — butterflies whose spots look like the huge eyes of a larger animal (mimicry), or frogs whose bright colors warn of their poison — but usually (as in **Figure 2.26**) the goal is simply to disappear. Breaking the image up so that the brain does not group the parts together very effectively prevents recognition.

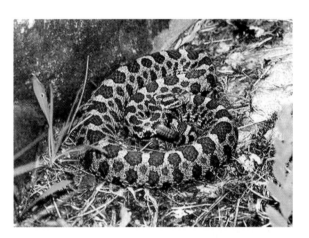

Figure 2.26 Natural camouflage: a pygmy rattlesnake hides very well on a bed of leaves.

Motion can destroy the illusion produced by camouflage, because moving objects (or portions of objects) attract notice; if several image segments are observed to move in coordinated ways, they are grouped, and the hidden object emerges. Human vision attempts to deal with moving features or points as rigid bodies, and easily connects separated pieces that move in a coordinated fashion. Viewing scenes or images with altered illumination, or through a colored filter, often reveals the objects as well. But in nature, the ability to keep still and rely on camouflage is a well-developed strategy.

Grouping operates on many spatial (and temporal) scales. In a typical scene there may be lines, edges, and other features that group to be perceived as an object; that object is then grouped with others to form a higher level of organization, and so on. Violations that occur in the grouping hierarchy give rise to conflicts that the mind must resolve. Sometimes this is done by seeing only one interpretation and ignoring another, and sometimes the mind switches back and forth between interpretations. **Figure 2.27** shows two examples. If the bright object is perceived as the foreground, it is seen as a vase with an irregular shape. If the background

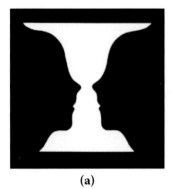
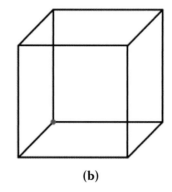

(a)   (b)

Figure 2.27 Illusions with two alternative interpretations:
(a) *either two facing profiles or a vase;*
(b) *the Necker cube is the corner marked in red closest to or farthest from the viewer.*

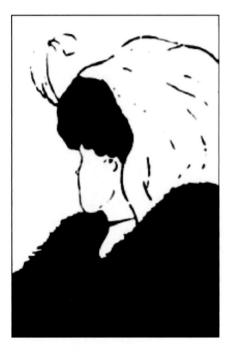

Figure 2.28 An illusion with alternative interpretations.

around the vase becomes the foreground, it emerges as two facing human profiles. An even simpler example is the drawing of a cube. The highlighted corner can be seen either as the point closest to the viewer or farthest away.

Figure 2.28 shows another familiar example of rivalrous interpretations. Is the drawing a young girl or an old woman? For all such images in which multiple interpretations or foreground-background reversal produce different perceptions, some people initially see only one or the other possibility and may have difficulty in recognizing the alternative. But once you manage to "see" both interpretations, it is impossible to see both at once, and for most people the two possibilities alternate every few seconds as the image is viewed.

As tricks that can provide some insight into how images are processed in the mind, these examples have some interest. But they also provide a warning for anyone who relies on visual inspection of images to obtain information about the subject. If you are to see past camouflage to connect the disparate parts of an object and recognize its presence, you must have a good stored model of what that object is. But when you approach an image with a strong model and try to connect the parts of the image to it, you are forced to ignore other interpretations. Anything in the image that does not conform to that model is likely to be ignored.

In one of Tony Hillerman's detective stories, his Navajo detective Joe Leaphorn explains how he looks for tracks. The FBI man asks, "What were you looking for?" and Leaphorn replies, "Nothing in particular. You're not really looking for anything in particular. If you do that, you don't see things you're not looking for." But learning how to look for everything and nothing is a hard skill to master. Most of us see only the things we expect to see, or at least the familiar things for which we have previously acquired labels and models.

The artist M. C. Escher created many drawings, in which grouping hierarchy was consistent locally but not globally, to create conflicts and rivalries that make the art very interesting.

Figure 2.29 shows diagrams and examples of some of his simpler conundrums. In one, lines that represent one kind of edge at the tip of the fork become something different at its base, exchanging inside for outside along the way. In the second, the front-to-rear order of edges changes. Edges that occlude others and are therefore perceived as being in front are grouped by angles that clearly place them at the back. In both of these cases, the local interpretation of the information is consistent, but no global resolution of the inconsistencies is possible.

Figure 2.30 shows another Escher drawing, *Climbing and Descending*. Locally, the stairs have a direction that is everywhere clear and obvious. However, by clever use of perspective distortion, the steps form a closed path without top or bottom, so the path is endless and always in one direction. Several other geometric rivalries are also present in this drawing.

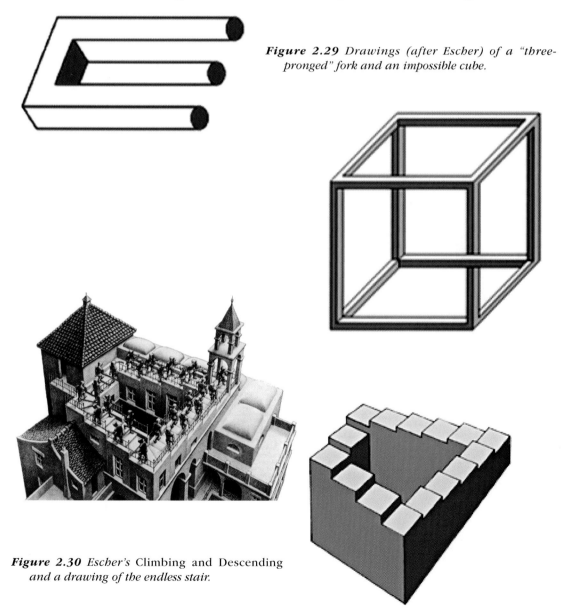

Figure 2.29 Drawings (after Escher) of a "three-pronged" fork and an impossible cube.

Figure 2.30 Escher's Climbing and Descending and a drawing of the endless stair.

It's about time

Comparison and inhibition operate temporally as well as spatially. The periphery of our vision is particularly well wired to detect motion. Comparison of a response at one point with that at a short time previously is accomplished by a short time delay. Slightly more complicated connections detect motion of edges, with the ability to distinguish edges at different orientations. Gradual changes of brightness and slow motion, like gradual spatial variations, are ignored and very difficult to detect.

Temporal inhibition is not the same thing as adaptation or depletion. It takes a little while for our eyes to adapt to changes in scene brightness. Part of this is the response of the iris to open or close the pupil, letting either more light or less light into the eye. The other part of the adaptation response involves a chemical action within the cells to amplify dim light signals. The former requires several seconds and the latter several minutes to operate fully.

Staring at a fixed pattern or color target for a brief time will chemically deplete the rods or cones. Then looking at a blank page will produce an image of the negative or inverse of the original. **Figure 2.31** shows a simple example. Stare fixedly at the center of the circle for about 60 seconds, and then look away. Because the color-sensitive cones have been depleted, the afterimage of a circle composed of opposing colors will appear (green for red, yellow for blue, and so on). The brighter the original image, the stronger the afterimage.

Motion sensing is obviously important. It alerts us to changes in our environment that may represent threats or opportunities. And the ability to extrapolate motion lies at the heart of tracking capabilities that enable us to perform actions such as catching a thrown ball. Tracking and extrapolation present a second-order opportunity to notice discontinuities of motion. If a moving feature suddenly changes speed or direction, that is also noticed. It is because of this ability to track motion and notice even subtle changes that the presentation of data as graphs is so useful, and why plots of the derivatives of raw data often reveal information visually.

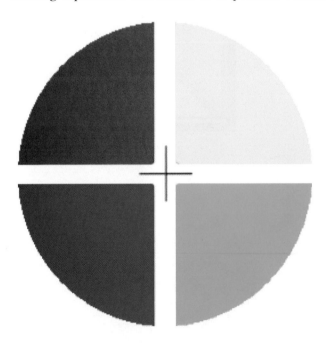

Sequences of images are interpreted very differently, depending on the speed of their presentation. If they are presented at a sufficiently slow rate, they are seen as a sequence of individual pictures, but a faster presentation of sequential images provides the illusion of continuous motion. Much of the credit (or blame) for motion pictures and television can be assigned to Eadweard Muybridge, a photographer who was asked to settle a bet for

Figure 2.31 *A target to demonstrate an afterimage. Stare at the central cross for about a minute and then look away toward a blank sheet of paper. The complementary colors will be seen.*

Leland Stanford as to whether a galloping horse ever had all four feet off the ground. Muybridge set up a row of cameras with trip wires to photograph a horse as it galloped past, producing a sequence of pictures. Viewing them individually was enough to settle the bet, but Muybridge discovered that flipping through them rapidly gave the visual illusion of continuous motion. The movie industry began almost immediately thereafter. **Figure 2.32** shows a sequence of twelve images of a trotting horse, taken by Muybridge.

In viewing a series of images, an important phenomenon called "aliasing" can occur. Generally we assume that a feature in one frame will correspond to a feature in the next if they are nearly the same in color and shape, and if they are close together (i.e., grouping). The familiar reversal of direction of the spokes on a turning wheel is an example of the visual error that results when a feature in one frame is matched to a different one in the next. From observing this phenomenon, it is but a short step to stroboscopic imaging in which a series of pictures is taken at time intervals that match, or nearly match, the repetition rate of some phenomenon. This is commonly used to study turning or vibrating objects, falling water drops, and so on. Each image shows almost the same thing, albeit with a different tooth on the gear or a different

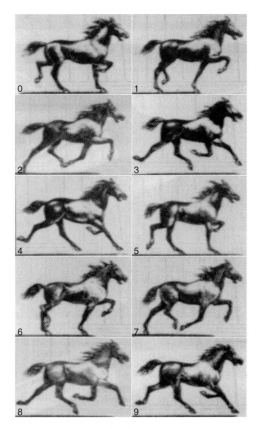

Figure 2.32 Muybridge's horse sequence.

water drop as the subject. We visually assume they are the same and perceive no change. By slightly varying the timing of the images (typically by controlling the rate at which the light source flashes), it is possible to extract subtle patterns and motions that occur within the faster repetitions.

If an image sequence is slower than about 15 frames per second, we do not perceive it as continuous. In fact, flickering images at 10 to 12 frames per second can induce epileptic fits in those with that affliction. But at higher rates, the temporal response of the eye and vision system sees continuous action. Movies are typically recorded at 24 frames per second, and television broadcasts either 25 (in Europe) or 30 (in the United States) frames per second. In all of these cases, we interpret the sequential images as continuous. Incidentally, that is one of the problems with most of the video surveillance systems in use today. To record a full day's activity on a single VHS tape, the images are not stored at 30 frames per second; instead, single frames (actually, single fields with only half the vertical resolution) are stored every few seconds. The result is a series of still images from which some important clues are absent. We recognize people not only by still images, but also by how they move, and the trajectories of motion are missing from the recording. We can observe posture, but not motion.

Just as human vision is best able to detect features or other causes of brightness or color variation over a relatively narrow range of sizes, so it deals best with events that occur over a relatively narrow range of times. Very short duration events are invisible to our eyes without techniques such as high-speed photography to capture them (**Figure 2.33**). Both high-speed

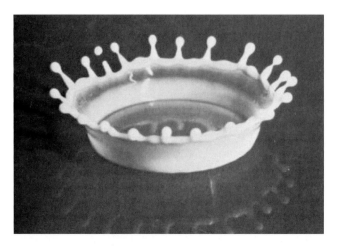

Figure 2.33 Doc Edgerton's famous high-speed photograph of a milk drop creating a splash.

imaging and stroboscopic imaging techniques were pioneered by Doc Edgerton at MIT (Massachusetts Institute of Technology).

Likewise, events that take a long time (minutes) to happen are not easy to examine visually to detect changes. Even side-by-side images of the clock face in **Figure 2.34** do not reveal all of the differences, and when one of the images must be recalled from memory, the results are even poorer. Capturing the images in a computer and calculating the difference shows clearly the motion of the minute hand and even the very slight shift of the hour hand.

Considering the sensitivity of vision to motion, it is astonishing that our eyes are actually in nearly constant motion. It is only in the fovea that high-resolution viewing is possible, and we rotate our eyes in their sockets so that this small, high-resolution region can view many individual locations in a scene, one after another. By flicking through the points in a scene that seem "interesting," we gather the information that our minds require for interpretation and judgment. Most of the scene is never actually examined unless the presence of edges, lines, colors, or abrupt changes in color, brightness, texture, or orientation make locations interesting and attract our attention.

Somehow, as our eyes move and different images fall onto the retina every few hundred milliseconds, our minds sort it all out and plug the information into the perceptual scene that is constructed in our head. Although the entire image shifts on the retina, it is only relative motion within the scene that is noticed. This motion of the eye also serves to fill in the blind spot, the location on the retina where the connection of the optic nerve occurs, and where there are no light sensors. Experiments that slowly move a light through the visual field while the eyes remain fixed on a single point easily demonstrate that this blind spot exists, but it is never noticed in real viewing because eye motion picks up enough information to fill the perceptual model of the scene that we actually interpret. But there may be a great deal of information in the actual scene that we do not notice. Clearly, there is a lot of interpretation going on.

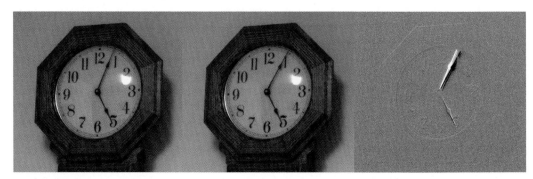

Figure 2.34 Pictures taken slightly over a minute apart of the clock on my office wall, and the difference between them.

The perceived image of a scene has very little in common with a photographic recording of the same scene. The latter exists as a permanent record, and each part of it can be examined in detail at a later time. The mental image of the scene is transitory, and much of it was filled with low-resolution information from our visual periphery, or was simply assumed from memory of other similar scenes. Scientists need to record images rather than just view them, because it is often not obvious until much later which are the really important features present (or absent).

The evolution of the structure and function of the eye and the brain connections that process the raw data have been a response to the environment and to the challenges of survival. Different animals clearly have different needs, and this has resulted in different types of eyes, as noted previously, and also different kinds of processing. Apparently the very few but extremely specific bits of information that the fly's eye sends to the fly's brain are enough to trigger appropriate and successful responses (for example, a looming surface triggers a landing reflex in which the fly reorients its body so the legs touch first). But for most of the "higher" animals, the types of information gathered by the visual system and the interpretations that are automatically applied are much more diverse.

For example, when people see a pencil placed in a glass of water, the pencil appears to be bent at an angle (**Figure 2.35**). Intellectually we know this is due to the difference in the refractive indices of water and air, but the view presented to our brain still has the bend. South Pacific islanders who have spent their lives fishing with spears in shallow water learn how to compensate for the bend, but the image that their eyes present to their brains still includes the optical effect. There is evidence that fishing birds like the heron have a correction for this offset built into their visual system and that from the point of view of the perceived image, they strike directly toward the fish to catch it. They "see" a corrected image, not the physical representation we observe. Conversely, there are species of fish that see bugs above the water; these fish spit water at the bugs to knock them down and then catch them for food. This requires a similar correction for the optics.

It may seem strange that computation in the brain could distort an image in exactly the proper way to correct for a purely optical effect such as the index of refraction of light in water. But this is different only in degree from the adjustments that we have already described, in which human vision corrects for shading of surfaces and illumination that can vary in intensity and color. The process combines the raw visual data with a lot of "what we know about the world" to create a coherent and usually accurate, or at least accurate enough, depiction of the scene.

Humans are very good at tracking moving objects and predicting their path, taking into account air resistance and gravity (for instance, an outfielder catching a fly ball). Most animals do not have this ability, but a few have learned it. My dog chases a thrown ball by always running toward its present position, which produces a path that is

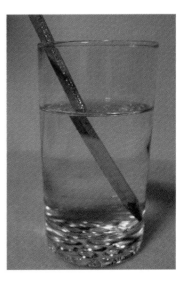

Figure 2.35 The apparent bend in the pencil and its magnification are familiar optical effects.

mathematically a tractrix. It works; it does not take much computation; but it is not optimum. My cat, on the other hand, runs in a straight line toward where the ball is going to be. She has solved the math of a parabola, but having pounced on the ball, she will not bring it back to me, as the dog will.

What we typically describe in humans as "eye–hand" coordination involves an enormous amount of subtle computation about what is happening in the visual scene. A professional baseball or tennis player who can track a ball moving at over 100 miles per hour well enough to connect with it and hit it in a controlled fashion has great reflexes, but it starts with great visual acuity and processing. In one exercise used to train young baseball players, a pitching machine is set up to shoot balls across the plate, and the player in the batter's box must identify the balls with different colored dots on them in time to react. From such exercises, they learn to spot the different rotations of the seams on a ball thrown as a fastball, curve, or slider. Since the total time of flight of the ball from pitcher to catcher is about 2 sec, and some time is required to activate the muscles in response, that calls for some very rapid visual processing. It was mentioned earlier that the human eye has some 150+ million light sensors, and for each of them some 25,000 to 50,000 processing neurons are at work extracting lots of information that evolution has decided we can use to better survive.

The third dimension

Most people have two functioning eyes and have at least a rudimentary idea that two eyes allow stereoscopic vision, which provides information on the distance of the objects that we see. However, many animals have eyes located on the sides of their heads (e.g., horses), where the overlap in the two fields of view is minimal. This configuration provides them with a broad range of view at the cost of information about the distance of perceived objects. Animals with forward-facing eyes are typically predators or those that live by leaping about in trees, with both modes demonstrating the importance of stereoscopic vision. However, stereoscopic vision is not the only way to determine distances, and it is not a particularly quantitative tool.

Humans use stereo vision by rotating the eyes in their sockets to bring the same feature to the fovea in each eye (as judged by matching that takes place in the visual cortex). It is the feedback from the muscles to the brain that tell us whether one feature is closer than another, depending on whether the eyes had to rotate in or out as we directed our attention from the first feature to the second. Notice that this is not a measurement of how much farther or closer the feature is, and that it works only for comparing one point with another. It is only by glancing around the scene and building up a large number of two-point comparisons that our brain constructs a map of the relative distances of many locations. Computer algorithms that match points between scenes and build up a similar map of distances are discussed in **Chapter 13** and **Chapter 14**.

Stereoscopy can become confused if there are several similar features in the image such that there are multiple matches (corresponding to different apparent distances). This happens rarely in natural scenes, but can create problems in imaging of repetitive structures.

One of the fascinating discoveries about stereopsis, the ability to fuse stereo-pair images by matching details from the left- and right-eye views, is the random-dot stereogram (**Figure 2.36**). Bela Julesz showed that the visual system was able to match patterns of dots that, to a single eye, appeared chaotic and without structure, to form stereo images. Slight lateral displacements of the dots are interpreted as parallax and produce depth information.

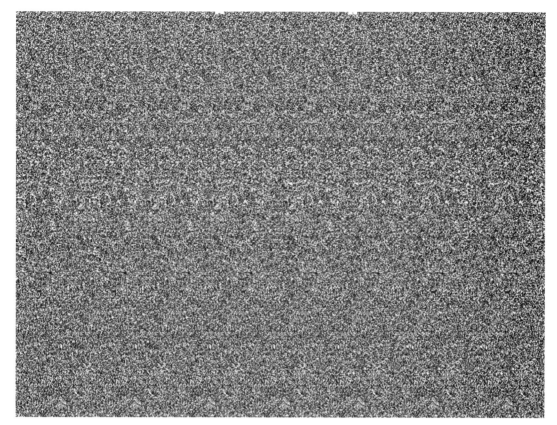

Figure 2.36 *Random-dot stereogram showing a torus on a plane. Stare at the image and the eyes will pick out the matching patterns and fuse them into an image.*

Sequential images produced by moving a single eye can also produce stereoscopic depth information. The relative sideways motion of features as we shift our head from side to side is inversely proportional to distance. One theory holds that snakes, whose eyes are not well positioned for stereo vision, move their heads from side to side to better triangulate the distance to strike.

Stereoscopy only works for things that are fairly close. At distances beyond about 100 ft, the angular differences become too small to notice. Furthermore, there are plenty of people who, for one reason or another, do not have stereo vision (for example, this is a typical consequence of childhood amblyopia), but who still function quite well in a three-dimensional world, drive cars, play golf, and so on. There are several other cues in images that are used to judge distance.

If one object obscures part of another, it must be closer to our eye. Precedence seems like an absolute way to decide the distance order of objects, at least those that lie along the same line of sight. But there are built-in assumptions of recognition and of the simple shape of objects, the violation of which creates an incorrect interpretation, as shown in the example in **Figure 2.37**.

Relative size also plays an important role in judging distance. Many of the things we recognize in familiar scenes have sizes — most typically heights — that fall into narrow ranges. Closely related is our understanding of the rules of perspective: parallel lines appear to converge as

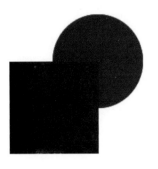

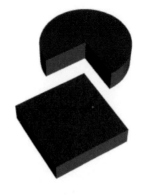

Figure 2.37 Left: Obviously the blue square is in front of the red circle. Right: But it may not be a circle, and viewed from another angle we see that the red object is actually in front of the blue one.

Figure 2.38 Converging lines are interpreted as parallel lines that converge according to the rules of perspective, and so the surface is perceived as receding from the viewer.
 (a) Straight lines imply a flat surface while
 (b) irregularities are interpreted as bumps or dips in the perceived surface.

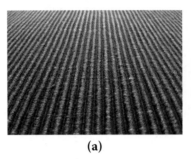

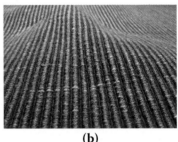

(a) (b)

they recede (**Figure 2.38**). In fact, the presence of such lines is interpreted visually as corresponding to a surface that extends away from the viewer, and irregularities in the straightness of the lines are interpreted as representing bumps or dips on the perceived surface. Driving through the countryside looking at plowed fields provides a simple example.

By comparing the apparent sizes of features in our visual field, we judge the relative distance of the objects and of things that appear to be close to them. But again, the underlying assumptions are vital to success, and violations of the straightness of alignments of features or the constancy of sizes produces mistaken interpretations (**Figure 2.39**).

A simple extension of the assumption of size constancy for major features uses the sizes of marks or features on surfaces to estimate distance and angle. It is logical, and indeed often correct, to assume that the marks or texture present on a surface are random and isotropic, and that visual changes in apparent size or aspect ratio indicate differences in distance or orientation (**Figure 2.40**). Once again, violations of the underlying assumptions can lead to the wrong conclusions.

There are other clues that may be present in real scenes, although they are less relevant to the viewing of images from microscopes or in the laboratory. For instance, atmospheric haze makes distant features appear more blue (or brown, if the haze is smog) and less sharp. Renaissance painters, who mastered all of these clues, represented atmospheric haze in scenes along with correct geometric perspective. Working from a known geometry to a realistic representation is a very different task than trying to extract geometric information from a scene whose components are only partially known, however.

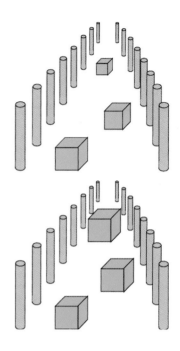

Figure 2.39 *In these illustrations, the expectation of distance is established by assuming the pink posts are constant in size and arranged in straight parallel lines, whose apparent convergence is a function of perspective. In the top illustration, the appearance of the green boxes is consistent with this interpretation. In the bottom illustration it is not, and we must either conclude that the boxes differ in size or that the posts do not conform to our expectation.*

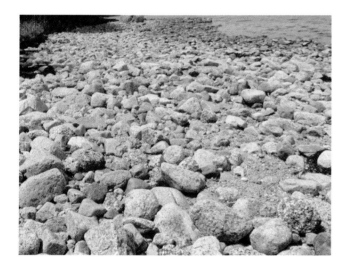

Figure 2.40 *Rocks on a beach. Assuming that the rocks are similar in size and round on the average informs us of the viewing angle and the distance to farther locations.*

How versus what

Several very plausible models have been put forward for the algorithms functioning in the eye and other portions of the visual pathway. The first few layers of neurons in the retina are connected in ways that can account for mechanisms behind local and temporal inhibition, and the interleaving of information from right and left eyes in the visual cortex is consistent with the fusion of two images for stereopsis. Such models serve several purposes: they can be tested by physiological probes and external stimuli, and they form the basis for computer techniques that attempt to extract the same information from images. In fact, they serve the latter purpose even if they turn out to be failures as actual descriptions of the functioning of the neurons. But while they may be effective at describing *how* at least some parts of the visual system work, because they work at the level of bits and pieces of the image and not at the gestalt or information level, they do not tell us much about *what* we see.

Several years ago I was retained as an expert witness in a major criminal trial. The issue at hand was whether a surveillance videotape from the scene of a murder was useful for the identification of the suspects. The images from the tape had been extensively computer-enhanced and were shown to the jury, who were invited to conclude that the current appearance of the defendants could not be distinguished from those images. In fact, the images were so poor in both spatial and tonal resolution that they could not be distinguished from a significant percentage of the population of the city in which the murders took place, and it was the job of the defense to remind the jury that the proper question was whether the pictures contained enough matching information to identify the defendants "beyond a reasonable doubt." It was very interesting in this case that none of the numerous witnesses to the crime were able to pick any of the defendants out from a lineup. The human eye is indisputably a higher resolution, more sensitive imaging device than a cheap black and white surveillance video camera. But for a variety of reasons the humans present could not identify the perpetrators.

In that trial I was accepted by the court as an expert both in the field of computer-based image processing (to comment on the procedures that had been applied to the camera images) and on human perception (to comment on what the people present might have been able to see, or not). The point was raised that my degrees and background are not in the field of physiology, but rather physics and engineering. How could I comment as an expert on the processes of human vision? The point was made (and accepted by the court) that it was not an issue of how the human visual system worked, at the level of rhodopsin or neurons, that mattered, but rather of what information human vision is capable of extracting from a scene. I do understand what can be seen in images because I have spent a lifetime trying to find ways for computers to extract some of the same information (using what are almost certainly very different algorithms). Accomplishing that goal, by the way, will probably require a few more lifetimes of effort.

In fact, there has often been confusion over the difference between the *how* and the *what* of human vision, often further complicated by questions of *why*. In describing a computer algorithm for some aspect of image analysis, the explanation of the steps by which information is extracted (the *how*) is intimately bound up in the computed result (the *what*). But in fact, the algorithm may not be (in fact usually is not) the only way that information can be obtained. Many of the important steps in image analysis have several more-or-less equivalent ways of extracting the same result, and moreover each of them can typically be programmed in quite a few different ways to take advantage of the peculiarities of different computer architectures. And, of course, no one claims that any of those implementations is identical to the processing carried out by the neurons in the brain.

In his final book *Vision*, David Marr (1982) has pointed out very forcefully and eloquently that confusing the *how* and the *what* had led many researchers, including himself, into some swampy terrain and dead ends in the quest for an understanding of vision (both human and animal). Mapping the tiny electrical signals in various parts of the visual cortex as a function of stimuli presented to the eye, or measuring the spectral response of individual rod or cone cells, are certainly important in eventually understanding the *how* of the visual system. And such experiments are performed at least in part because they can be done, but it is not clear that they tell us very much about the *what*. On the other hand, tests that measure the response of the frog's eye to a small dark moving target invite speculation about the *why* (e.g., to detect a moving insect: food).

Researchers have performed many experiments to determine what people see, usually involving the presentation of artificial stimuli in a carefully controlled setting and comparing the responses as small changes are introduced. This has produced some useful and interesting results, but it falls short of addressing the problem of visual interpretation of scenes. The key is not just that people can detect ("see") a certain stimulus, but that they can interpret its meaning in a complex scene. It might be better to substitute the word "interpret" for "see" to emphasize that the individual cues in images are only important for understanding the world when they are combined and processed to become a semantic representation. In other words, we do have to turn that picture into its "thousand word" equivalent. For that purpose, it is often more revealing to study the errors that humans make in looking at whole images. This includes, but is not limited to, various kinds of visual illusions.

There are also important clues in what artists have portrayed (or left out) of representational paintings and even cartoons. By exaggerating a few selected features into a caricature, for example, editorial cartoonists create very distorted but extremely recognizable representations of familiar political figures. For many people, such cartoons may represent a greater truth about the person than an actual photograph (**Figure 2.41**).

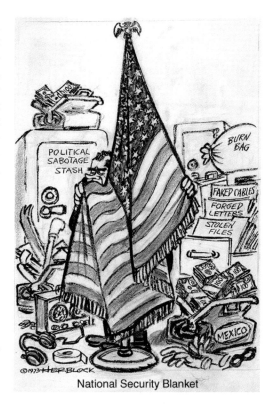

National Security Blanket

Figure 2.41 Richard Nixon's ski nose, dark eyebrows and shady eyes, receding hairline, and 5 o'clock-shadowed jowls were used by cartoonists to create an instantly recognizable caricature.

Seeing what isn't there, and vice versa

One problem that plagues eyewitness testimony and identification is that we tend to see (i.e., pick out from a scene) things that are familiar (i.e., already have mental labels). One facility that is hardwired into our brains, just like the ability of the frog to spot a bug, is finding faces. Babies find and track faces from birth. We are so good at it that even with just a few clues, like two eyes and a mouth, we see a face, whether it is real or not. The ubiquitous "smiley face" cartoon has enough information to be recognized as a face. So does a mountain on Mars, when illuminated and viewed a certain way (**Figure 2.42**).

But to recognize a particular face, for instance as grandmother, we need a lot more clues. Computer programs that perform facial recognition use ratios of dimensions, for instance the ratio of the distance between the eyes to that between the tips of the ears, or the distance between the mouth and chin to the distance from the tip of the nose to the chin. The advantage of ratios is that they are insensitive to the size of the image, and to a considerable extent to orientation or point of view. But that is an algorithm and so addresses the *how* rather than the *what*. It seems likely that human facial recognition uses more or different clues, but certainly altering those proportions by even a few percent changes a face so that it becomes unrecognizable (**Figure 2.43**).

Police artists routinely produce sketches from eyewitness descriptions. Comparing these pictures with actual photographs of perpetrators after capture suggests that only a few character-

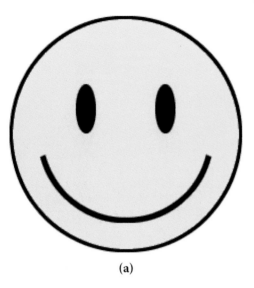

(a)

Figure 2.42 It takes very few cues to trigger the recognition of a face:
(a) the ubiquitous happy face;
(b) the "face on Mars," which appears only if the viewing angle and lighting are correct.

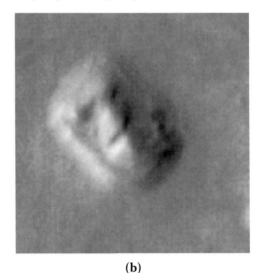

(b)

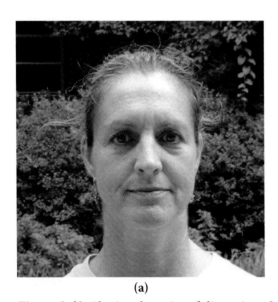

(a)

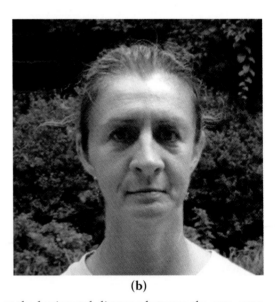

(b)

Figure 2.43 Altering the ratios of dimensions (such as the horizontal distance between the eyes, ears, width of mouth, etc., or vertical dimensions such as length of nose, distance from mouth to chin, height of forehead, etc.) strongly affects our ability to recognize faces.

istics of the face are likely to be noticed, and these are turned into a mental caricature rather than an actual representation. Differences in race between witness and perpetrator make it especially difficult to pick out those characteristics that are likely to identify the person. We learn to pick out the particular kinds of details that are most useful in identifying those familiar to us, and these are not very helpful for other races ("they all look alike").

Finally, when something or someone is recognized (rightly or wrongly) in an image, our minds mentally endow the semantic representation of that person or object with the full set of characteristics that we remember from past encounters. A typical example would be seeing a friend's face from the side, but "knowing" that there is a mole on the other cheek and believing we had seen it this time as well. That leads to a lot of eyewitness problems. If a witness thinks they have recognized someone or something, they will often testify with confidence and honesty that they have seen things that were actually not present. This can include even highly specific items like articles of clothing, tattoos, etc. One witness was sure that a car in a hit-and-run case had a particular bumper sticker on the back, when in fact she had not been in a position to see the back of the car, because she was familiar with a car of the same model and color that she believed was the vehicle in question, and which did have such a bumper sticker.

We all do this, unconsciously. When you pass a neighbor's house, if you glimpse someone mowing the lawn and you "expect" it to be the teenage son, you are likely to "see" details of his appearance, haircut, clothing, etc., that may not be visible, or may not even be there — it might not even be the right person. Usually this process is helpful because it gives us a sense of place and situation that is most often correct without requiring additional time or effort. A few mistakes will be made, but fortunately they are not usually serious ones, and the consequences are rarely more than momentary embarrassment. Many decades ago, when my eldest son was a preschooler, I shaved off a mustache that I had worn since before his birth. He did not notice for two days, until it was pointed out to him (and then he was upset at the change).

Seeing what we "know" is present, or at least expect to be present, is common. A colleague of mine, who for years helped in teaching courses on image analysis, has a favorite picture of herself holding a dearly loved pet, now deceased. Unfortunately the dog is black, she is wearing a black sweater, and the photographic print is very dark (and the negative, which would have a greater dynamic range, is not available). She has challenged us for years to process that image to show the dog that she sees when she looks at the picture, but we've failed because there is just nothing there in terms of the pixel values — they are all the same shade of near black. One of my students took a copy of the scanned print and painstakingly drew in a plausible outline of the correct breed of dog. Her immediate response was, "That's not the right dog!" She has a stored image in her mind that contains information not available to anyone else who looks at the image, and she believes she can see that information when she looks at the picture. Certainly her mind sees it, if not her eyes.

The extension of this process to scientific image analysis is obvious and should be of great concern. We see what we expect to see (things for which we have existing mental labels), fail to see or recognize things that are unfamiliar, misjudge things for which we do not have an appropriate set of stored clues, and truly believe that we have seen characteristics in one image that have been seen in other instances that are remembered as being similar. That's what it means to be human, and those are the tendencies that a careful scientific observer must combat in analyzing images.

Image compression

There are some important lessons about human vision to be found in the rapid acceptance of digital still-frame and video cameras. All consumer cameras and many higher-end cameras store images in a compressed format because memory is expensive and also because smaller files can be saved more quickly (more than enough improvement to make up for the time needed to carry out the compression). People seem willing to pay for high-resolution multimegapixel cameras and then try to compress the image by a factor of 10, 20, or more to produce a file that can be transmitted efficiently over the Internet.

Compression techniques such as MPEG for video and JPEG for still pictures are widely used and too-little questioned. In addition to MPEG (Moving Pictures Expert Group) compression, a variety of codecs (compressor-decompressor) are available for Apple's QuickTime and Macromedia's Flash software. The original JPEG (Joint Photographers Expert Group) technique using a discrete cosine transform has been joined by wavelet and fractal methods.

All of these methods achieve compression by leaving out some of the information in the original image, as discussed in **Chapter 1** and **Chapter 3**; technically, they are "lossy" compression techniques. The intent of the compression is to preserve enough information to enable people to recognize familiar objects. Most of the techniques depend to some extent on the characteristics of human vision to decide what should be kept and what can be modified or left out. Some, like fractal compression, replace the actual details with other detail "borrowed" from elsewhere in the image, on the theory that any fine detail will fool the eye.

Compression discards what people do not easily see in images. Human vision is sensitive to abrupt local changes in brightness, which correspond to edges. These are kept, although they may shift slightly in location and in magnitude. On the other hand, absolute brightness is not visually perceived, so it is not preserved. Since changes in brightness of less than a few percentage points are practically invisible, and even larger variations cannot be seen if they occur gradually over a distance in the image, compression can eliminate such details with minor effect on visual interpretation.

Color information is reduced in resolution because boundaries are primarily defined by changes in brightness. The first step in most compression schemes is to reduce the amount of color information, either by averaging it over several neighboring pixels or by reducing the number of colors used in the image, or both. Furthermore, color perception is not the same in all parts of the visible spectrum. We cannot discriminate small changes in the green range as well as we can other colors. Also, gradual changes in color, like those in brightness, are largely invisible; only sharp steps are noticed. So the reduction of color values in the image can be quite significant without being noticeable.

It is also possible to reduce the size of video or movie files by finding regions in the image that do not change, or do not change rapidly or very much. In some cases, the background behind a moving object can be simplified, even blurred, while the foreground feature can be compressed because we do not expect to see fine detail on a moving object. Prediction of the locations in an image that will attract the eye — sometimes called "interesting points" and usually associated with high local contrast or familiar subjects (where do your eyes linger when looking at a picture of a movie star? what parts of the image don't you notice?) — and cause it to linger in just a few areas allows other areas to be even further compressed.

Certainly it can be argued that this type of compression works below the threshold of visual discrimination most of the time and does not prevent people from recognizing familiar objects. But that is exactly the problem: compression works because enough information remains to apply labels to features in the image, and those labels in turn cause our memories to supply the details that are no longer present in the picture. The reason for recording images in scientific studies is not to keep remembrances of familiar objects and scenes, but to document the unfamiliar. If it is not possible to know beforehand what details may turn out to be important, it is not wise to discard them. And if measurement of features is contemplated (to measure size, shape, position, or color information), then lossy compression, which alters all of those values, must be avoided.

It is not the point of this section to just make the rather obvious case that compression of digital images is extremely unwise and should be avoided in scientific imagery. Rather, it is to shed illumination on the fact that compression is only acceptable for snapshots because human vision does not notice or depend upon very much of the actual contents of an image. Recognition requires only a few clues and ignores much of the fine detail.

A world of light

Our eyes are only one part of the overall system involved in producing the sensory input to the visual cortex. It is easy to overlook the importance of the light source and its color, location, and brightness. A few concerns are obvious. When shopping for clothes, furniture, or other items, it is best not to rely on their appearance under the artificial lighting in the store, but to see how the colors appear in sunlight. The difference in the color of the light source (sunlight, incandescent lighting, fluorescent lighting) can produce enormous differences in the visual appearance of colors. And don't even think about trying to guess at colors using the illumination from a sodium street light, which is essentially monochromatic and provides no clues to color at all.

In a laboratory setting, such as the use of a light microscope, color judgments can be similarly affected by small variations in the color temperature of the bulb, which depends very sensitively on the voltage applied to it (and also tends to change significantly over the first few and last few hours of use as the filament and its surface undergo physical alterations). Simply reducing the illumination (e.g., to take a photo) by turning down the voltage will change the colors in the image. This happens whether we are imaging the light that is transmitted (not reflected or absorbed) through a thin sample, as in the transmission light microscope, or the light reflected from a surface, as in macroscopic imaging. But generally it is the latter case that our brains are prepared to interpret.

For real-world scenes, there may be a single light source (e.g., sunlight or a single bulb), or there may be multiple sources. The source may be highly localized or it may be extended. Lighting may be direct or indirect, meaning that it may have been reflected or scattered from other surfaces between the time it leaves the source and reaches the object. All of these variables affect the way the object will appear in the final image.

The surface of the object also matters, of course. Most of the light that is not transmitted through or absorbed within the object is scattered from an extremely thin layer just at the surface of the object. For a perfect metal, this happens exactly at the surface, but most materials allow the light to penetrate at least a short distance beneath the surface. It is the variation of absorption within this thin layer for different light wavelengths, and the variation of penetration with wavelength, that give an object color. For instance, preferential absorption of green light will cause an object to appear purple. Ideal metals, for which there is no light penetration, have no color. (The colors of gold, copper, and silver result from a complex electronic structure that actually allows slight penetration.)

The fraction of the incident light that is reflected or scattered is measured by the surface albedo. A very dark object may absorb as much as 90% of the incident light, whereas a very bright one may absorb only a few percent. The interaction of the light with the object typically includes a mixture of diffuse and specular reflection. The diffuse component sends light in all directions, more or less following a cosine pattern, as discussed in **Chapter 13**. The specular component sends light in the particular direction of mirror reflection, with an angle to the local surface normal equal to the incident angle. The specularity of the surface is defined by the fraction of the light that reflects at the mirror angle and the narrowness of the reflected beam.

Computer programs that generate rendered-surface images from measurements and shape information use models that correspond to the behavior of typical materials. As shown by the examples in **Chapter 14**, it is possible to change the appearance of the surface and our judgment of its composition and nature by altering the specularity. From a series of images with different light-source locations, it is possible to interpret the geometry of the object from its appearance. We do this automatically, because our brains have evolved in a world that provides many opportunities to learn about the effect of tilting objects on their appearance, and the effect of coating a surface with different materials.

Changing the appearance of a surface from one material to another, or altering the light-source color or position, can help us to notice important details on an object. Partly this is due to enhancement of the reflections from particular features, and partly to violating the expectations we normally have when viewing a surface and consequently forcing our attention to all of the details in the image. A surface-imaging technique developed by Tom Malzbender et al. (2001) at Hewlett Packard Labs uses a series of images taken with a single, stationary camera but with lighting from many different (known) orientations to compute the orientation and albedo of the surface at each location on an object. This data set is then used to render an image of the surface with any characteristics, including those of an ideal metal, while the viewer interactively moves the light-source position. The example in **Chapter 14** shows the recovery of fine details from an ancient clay tablet.

The technique that underlies this calculation is called "shape from shading" or "photometric stereo." Instead of taking two or more pictures from different viewpoints, as in stereoscopy, photometric stereo uses multiple images from the same viewpoint but with different illumination. Shape from shading uses the known distributions of diffuse and specular reflections for a particular type of surface to estimate changes in the local slope of the surface with respect to the lines of sight from the light source and the viewpoint. The weakness of the shape-from-shading approach is that it deals only with differences in intensity (and hence in slope). Determining the actual surface elevation at each point requires integrating these slope values with an unknown constant of integration. Nevertheless, the method has numerous applications and also serves to illustrate a computation performed by the computer that our minds have been trained by years of practical observations to make automatically.

The mental shortcuts that enable us to interpret brightness variations as shape are convenient and often correct (or at least correct enough for purposes such as recognition and range finding). But an observer relying on such shortcuts also can also be easily fooled. Surface brightness can change for reasons other than geometry, such as the effect of intentional or unintentional coatings on the surface (e.g., oxidation, stains). There may also be nonuniformities in the illumination, such as shadows on the surface. If these are not recognized and compensated for, they will influence our judgment about the surface geometry.

One thing that we are conditioned to expect from real-world viewing is that lighting comes from above, whether it be the sun in the sky or lights above our desk surface. If that expectation is violated, our built-in shape-from-shading calculation reaches the wrong conclusion and we interpret peaks as pits, and vice versa (**Figure 2.44**). Such illusions are amusing when we recognize them, but sometimes we can remain fooled.

Images that come from novel modalities, such as the scanning electron microscope, appear to be familiar and readily interpretable because the brightness of surfaces varies with slope, just as in the true shape from shading situation. But different physical processes are involved, and the mathematical relationships between brightness and geometry are not quite the same, which can lead to misinterpretations. For one thing, the appearance of edges and fine protrusions is very bright in the SEM, which does not occur in normal light scattering from surfaces.

Many other types of images, such as the surface maps produced by the AFM (atomic force microscope) based on various tip–sample interactions, are commonly presented to the viewer as rendered-surface representations. These are typically generated using the strength of a measured signal as a measure of actual surface geometry, which it may or may not be. Electronic

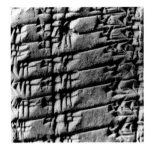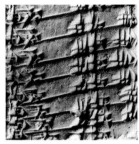

Figure 2.44 Rotating the same image (of cuneiform indentations in a clay tablet) by 180° makes the pits appear to be peaks.

or chemical effects become "visible" as though they were physical elevations or depressions of the surface. This is an aid to "visualization" of the effects, taking advantage of our ability to interpret surface images, but it is important (and sometimes difficult) to remember that it is not really physical geometry that is represented but some other, more abstract property (see, for example, **Figure 1.66** in **Chapter 1**).

Size matters

The size of features is determined by the location of the feature boundaries. The only problem with this rather obvious statement is in deciding where the boundary lies. Human vision works by finding many types of lines in images, which includes edges of features, based on locating places where brightness or color changes abruptly. Those lines are treated as a sketch (called the "primal sketch"). Cartoons work because the drawn lines substitute directly for the edges that would be extracted from a real scene.

The use of a computer program to extract edge lines is illustrated in **Chapter 5**. In one commonly used algorithm, a computer program finds the location (to the nearest pixel) where the maximum change in brightness occurs. The sketch extracted by the retina is not quite the same. For one thing, gradual changes in brightness are not as visible as abrupt changes, and the change must be at least several percentage points to be noticed at all. Changes in color are not as precisely located, and some color changes are much more noticeable than others (variations in the green part of the spectrum are noticed least).

Furthermore, people do not interpret the edge line in a consistent way. A simple demonstration can be found in the way we cut out patterns, and there is some indication that there is a sex-correlated behavior involved. Girls cutting cloth to make a garment tend to cut outside the line (better to have seams too wide than too narrow); boys cutting out model airplane parts tend to cut inside the line (so parts will fit together). The same habits carry over to tracing features for computer measurement. A trivial difference, perhaps, but it raises the interesting question, "Is the edge a part of the feature or a part of the surroundings?" In many cases, that depends on whether the feature is dark on a light background (in which case the edge is likely to be seen as part of the feature) or the converse.

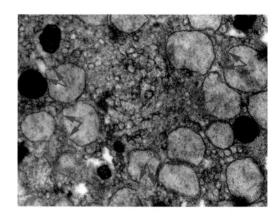

Figure 2.45 TEM (transmission electron microscope) image of stained tissue. The membrane boundaries of the organelles are not visible in some locations (arrows), but human vision "knows" they continue and completes them with simple smooth curves.

In many real images, the boundaries of features are not uniform. Variations in brightness and contrast cause variation in judgment of the location of the feature edge, and hence of its size and shape. In some cases, the boundary disappears in places (**Figure 2.45**). Human vision is not bothered by such gaps (although computer measurement certainly is). We fill in the gaps with simple, smooth curves that may or may not correspond to the actual shape of the feature.

Boundaries are certainly important, but there is evidence that features are represented conceptually not as a collection of boundaries, but as a simplified midline. The pipe-cleaner animals shown in **Figure 2.46** are recognizable because we fill out the bodies from the "skeleton" shown. This is not the actual skeleton of bones, of course, but the one used in computer-based image analysis, a set of midlines sometimes called the medial axis of the object. The topology of the skeleton (the number of branches, ends, and loops) provides critical information for feature recognition by humans and machines.

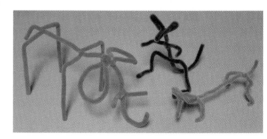

Figure 2.46 Pipe-cleaner animals (elephant, kangaroo, and dachshund) represent solid objects by their skeletons.

Whether the boundaries or the skeletons of features are used for representation, comparisons of the size of features are strongly affected by their shape, position, and brightness. A map of the continental United States illustrates this well (**Figure 2.47**). To compare the sizes of two states, we literally drag the image of one onto the other, in our minds. Since the shapes are different, the fit is imperfect. How the parts that "stick out" are treated depends on their perceived importance. For example,

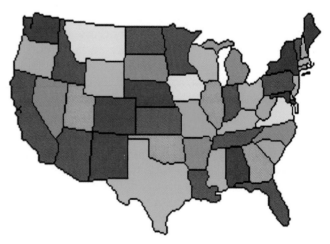

Figure 2.47 The continental United States.

comparing Oklahoma with Missouri is tricky because the panhandle of Oklahoma is pretty skinny and easily overlooked (but Oklahoma is larger than Missouri).

Florida is about the same size as Wisconsin, but they are different colors and far apart, and comparison is very difficult. Colorado has a simple rectangular shape, difficult to compare with Nevada or Oregon, which are not so regular and tend to appear smaller. The greater vertical extent of North Dakota is visually important and leads to the erroneous conclusion that the state is larger than South Dakota. Vertical extent is important in comparing Illinois with Iowa and New York, as well, as are the differences in shape and color (and the fact that New York is far away from Iowa and Illinois).

Visual judgments of size are very error-prone under the best of circumstances, and are easily swayed by seemingly minor factors, several of which have been illustrated in these examples. Another common mistaken judgment of size involves the moon. Most people report that it appears to be larger by one-third to one-half when near the horizon than when high in the sky (**Figure 2.48**), probably because at the horizon there are other structures that the eye can use for comparison. Vertical extent is generally considered more important than horizontal extent (**Figure 2.49**). Features that contrast more with their surroundings are generally considered to be larger than ones with less contrast. Departures from geometrically simple shapes tend to be ignored in judging size.

The context of the scene is also very important. In the discussion of stereoscopic vision and interpretation of the third dimension, it was noted that expectation of constant size is one of the cues used to judge distance. It works the other way, as well. We expect the rules of perspective to apply, so if one feature is higher in the scene than another, and is expected to be resting on the ground, then it is probably farther away, and thus it should appear to be smaller. If it is actually the same size in the image, we would tend to judge it as being larger in actuality. Unfortunately, when viewing images for which the rules of perspective do not apply, this "correction" can lead to the wrong conclusions.

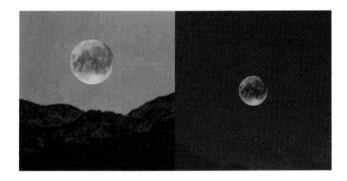

Figure 2.48 Example of the increase in the visual impression of the size of the moon when viewed near the horizon, as compared with the perceived size when the moon is overhead.

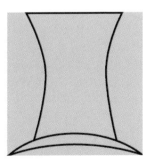

Figure 2.49 The top-hat illusion. In this exaggerated drawing of a top hat, the height appears to be much greater than the width, but in fact they are exactly the same.

Shape (whatever that means)

Shape is extremely important in visual recognition of objects. Even if the size or color of something is changed radically (a miniature pink elephant, perhaps), the shape provides the important information that triggers identification. But what is shape? There are very few common adjectives in English or any other language that really describe shape. We have plenty for size and color, but few for shape. Instead, we describe shape by saying that something is shaped "like an elephant"; in other words, we do not describe the shape at all but simply refer to a representative object and hope that the listener has the same mental image or model that we do, and identifies the same important shape features. The few apparent exceptions to this — adjectives like "round" — actually fall into this same category. Round means "like a circle," and everyone knows what a circle looks like.

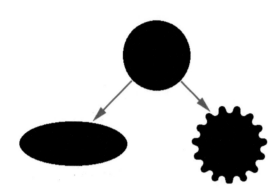

Figure 2.50 The two lower shapes have the same area as the circle but are not circular.

But what does it mean to depart from being round like a circle? There are lots of ways to become less like a circle. **Figure 2.50** shows just two of them: one feature has been stretched horizontally but is still smooth, while the other has remained equiaxial but with a rippled edge. Many other variations with jagged edges, stretching in more or other directions, and so forth, are possible. Which of these features should be considered "rounder?" (several different answers are provided in **Chapter 10**).

When computers measure features in images, there are many mathematical ways that they can describe shape. The most commonly used are simple dimensionless ratios of size measurements, as discussed in **Chapter 10**. One problem with these is that the names used are completely arbitrary and have no familiar (or consistent) meaning. An additional problem with these dimensionless ratios is that they are not unique. It is possible to construct an enormous number of objects whose shapes appear very different to a human but produce the same numerical measure. Still, these shape factors can be very useful for some computer recognition purposes.

It seems that instead of these numerical properties of shape, people rely primarily on two specific kinds of information for shape recognition: fractal dimension and topology. The latter is best illustrated by using a computer processing operation to reduce a shape to its skeleton. The skeleton, discussed in **Chapter 7**, is the midline of the feature, produced by an iterative removal of pixels from the boundary until the only ones left cannot be removed without breaking the feature into pieces. Outlines (edges) and skeletons are simplified object descriptions that are used in some of the classification procedures shown in **Chapter 11**.

Even incomplete delineation of feature skeletons or boundaries is often enough to construct a visual impression (which may or may not be correct). It is this ability to use just a few key features (corners, ends, and branch points) to characterize feature shape that accounts for several common illusions. Kanisza's triangle (**Figure 2.51**) is constructed in the mind by linking together the three well-defined corner points. The linking is always done with smooth, although not necessarily straight, lines.

Once the basic topological form of the object shape has been established, the second property of shape that people seem to instinctively recognize is a measure of the smoothness or irregularity of the boundary. Because so much of the natural world has a geometry that is fractal rather than Euclidean, this takes the form of an ability to detect differences in boundary fractal dimension. The measurement of fractal dimension is discussed in **Chapter 8**, but it must be remembered that even though humans can comparatively rank objects with different boundary irregularities, they do not perform measurements visually.

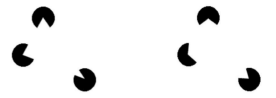

Figure 2.51 *Kanisza's triangle is an illusory region visually formed by linking corner markers with straight lines or gentle curves.*

The most widely accepted method for communicating the information about object shape characteristics that are used for recognition remains showing a picture of the object to another person. For features that are exactly alike, or so nearly alike that the only variations are essentially invisible at the scale of normal viewing, that works fine. Unfortunately, in most of the sciences the objects of interest, whether they are defects in a material, cancerous cells on a slide, or a new species of bug, are not identical. The natural variation is significant, although the clues to recognition (if they are correctly chosen) remain present (although not necessarily visible in every image).

In presenting the "representative image" the scientist attempts to communicate these clues to colleagues. The picture almost always needs an extensive supplement in words (think of Arlo Guthrie's song again, with the "twenty-seven 8 × 10 color glossy pictures with circles and arrows and a paragraph on the back of each one"). But if the viewers are not as familiar with the objects (which is of course the reason for the communication), will they be able to pick out the same features and clues? And does the selected image adequately represent the range of variation in the natural objects? Or correlations between those variations? These dangers are always present in the use of "typical" images, even if the image really does give a fair representation, and in most cases it should probably be admitted that the picture was selected not after analysis showed it to be representative in any statistical sense, but because the picture satisfied some other, unspoken aesthetic criterion (or worse, was the only good quality image that could be obtained). Anecdotal evidence, which is all that a single picture can ever provide, is risky at best and misleading at worst, and should be avoided if it is possible to obtain and present quantitative data. That is another motivation for applying computers to imaging: to obtain enough measurement data for meaningful descriptions.

Context

Recognition of features is often influenced by the context in which they appear. Sometimes this context is supplied by the image itself, but more often it arises from prior knowledge or independent information. In **Figure 2.52**, there are several different representations of the number "five," including ones in languages that we may not know. But once the concept of "fiveness" is accepted, the various representations all become understood. Quite a bit of knowledge and experience that has nothing to do with images is involved in this process, and it happens at higher levels of conscious thought than basic shape recognition. Knowing that pentagons have five sides may help us translate the Greek, or recalling a Cinco de Mayo party may help with the Spanish, and so on.

An interesting insight into this recognition process comes from the study of patients who suffer from synesthesia, a phenomenon in which some kind of cross-wiring in the brain confuses the output from one sense with another. People with synesthesia may report that particular notes played on the piano trigger the sensation of specific tastes, for example. In one of the most common forms of synesthesia, looking at a number produces the sensation of a specific color. For instance, in a printed array of black numbers, the fives may all appear red while the threes are blue (**Figure 2.53**), and the ability to detect and count the features is extremely rapid compared with the need to identify and count the features consciously.

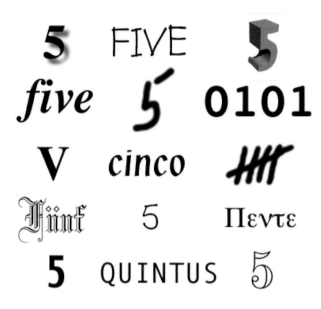

Figure 2.52 Various representations of "five."

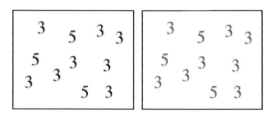

Figure 2.53 Synesthesia may associate specific colors with numbers, so that they "pop out" of an image.

This cross-activation of different sensory pathways in the brain occurs well before the information rises to conscious levels. The alternative representations of "fiveness" shown in **Figure 2.52** do not trigger these colors. Even modest distortions of the printed number, such as unusual or outline fonts, may be enough to prevent it. The study of these types of brain misfunctions is important for an understanding of the processing of sensory information, extraction of abstract concepts, and formation of connections between seemingly separate areas of knowledge that can occur at subconscious and conscious levels. In this instance, it shows that basic shape recognition happens long before the labels, with their semantic content, are applied to features.

It is even possible to have multiple contexts within the same image. This happens particularly when reading words. We tolerate misspellings and sloppy handwriting because there is usually enough redundancy and context to allow the message to be comprehended, even when the image itself is wrong or ambiguous, as shown in the example of **Figure 2.54**.

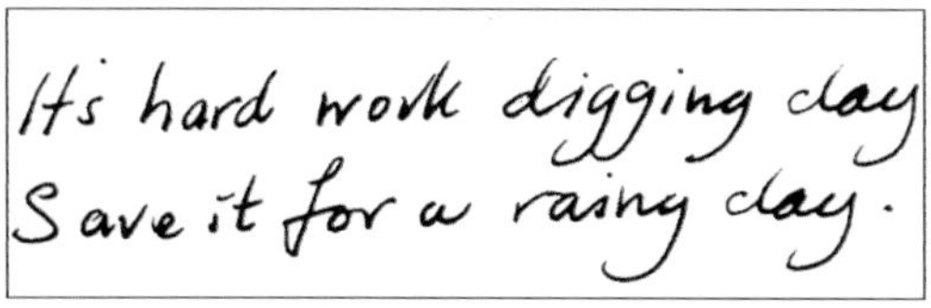

It's hard work digging clay
Save it for a raing clay.

Figure 2.54 The final words in each line are identical in shape, but can be read correctly only because of the context established by the other words.

The importance of context is critical for the correct interpretation of data in scientific images. Our expectations based on prior experience and study, knowledge of how the sample was prepared and how the image was acquired, and even our hopes and fears about how an experiment may turn out can significantly affect visual interpretation and the recognition of features (or failure to recognize them).

Obviously, this works in two different ways. It is important to know enough about the sample and image to correctly interpret it while avoiding the pitfalls that expectation can cause. Some people are better at this than others, and anyone can make the occasional mistake, but fortunately the open nature of scientific publication provides a mechanism for correction.

One frequently encountered problem of context for images arises in microscopy. Sections are typically cut through tissue with a microtome for examination in transmission, or surfaces of opaque materials are prepared by polishing for examination by reflected light (or the equivalent use of the transmission or scanning electron microscope). In all of these cases, the images are inherently two dimensional, but the structure that they represent and sample is three dimensional. It is very difficult for most people to provide a proper context for understanding these images in terms of the three-dimensional structure. Stereology, discussed in **Chapter 9**, provides geometrical relationships that can be used to relate proper measurements on two-dimensional images to three-dimensional structure, but few observers develop sufficient intuition to visually interpret such images correctly.

This seems to be true even after extensive training and developing familiarity with particular three-dimensional structures. Medical doctors rely upon section images from instruments such as magnetic resonance imaging (MRI) and computed X-ray tomography (CAT scans) to study the human body. But it appears from tests and interviews that few of these people have a three-dimensional mental picture of the structure. Instead, they learn to recognize the normal appearance of sections that are almost always taken in a few standard orientations, and to spot deviations from the norm, particularly ones associated with common diseases or other problems.

Arrangements must be made

One thing that people are extremely good at is finding order in an arrangement of objects. Sometimes this quest for simplification finds true and meaningful relationships between objects, and sometimes it does not. Historically, the construction of constellations by playing connect-the-dots among the bright stars in the sky seems to have been carried out by many different cultures (of course, with different results). **Figure 2.55** shows the classical Greek version. Assembling the data needed to construct Stonehenge as a predictor of solstices and eclipses must have taken multiple lifetimes. The Copernican revolution that allowed ellipses to simplify the increasingly complex Ptolemaic circles-and-epicircles model of planetary motion was a quest for this same type of simplification.

Most scientists follow Einstein's dictum that it is important to find the simplest solution that works, but not one that is too simple. The idea is much older than that. William of Occam's "principle of parsimony" is that "one should not increase, beyond what is necessary, the number of entities required to explain anything." Instinctively we all seek the simple answer, sometimes in situations where there is not one to be found. And of course, this applies to the examination of images, also.

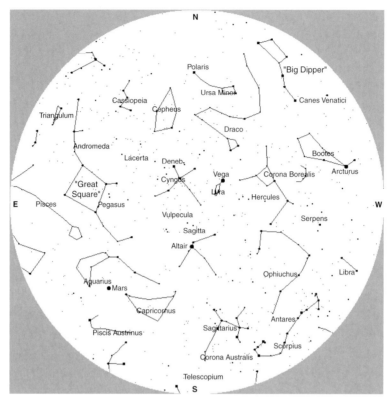

Figure 2.55 *The familiar stellar constellations.*

Finding visual alignments of points in images, or in plots of data, people prefer straight lines or smooth, gradual curves. Linear regression, probably the most widely used (and abused) method of data interpretation, imposes order on a collection of points. Filling in gaps in lines or boundaries is often a useful procedure, but it can lead to mistakes as well. The illusory Kanisza triangles are an example of filling in gaps and connecting points. The process of connecting points and lines is closely related to grouping, which has been discussed before, for instance in the process of forming a number from the colored circles in the color-blindness test images.

Human vision has a built-in directional bias that prefers the vertical, followed by the horizontal, and a strong preference for symmetry. As shown in **Figure 2.56**, that can bias our judgment. It also influences our ability to detect gradients or clustering.

Some processes produce a random distribution of features, like sprinkling salt onto a table. If every feature is completely independent of all the others, a random distribution results. Non-random distributions occur because features either attract or repel each other. Cacti growing in the desert are self-avoiding, because

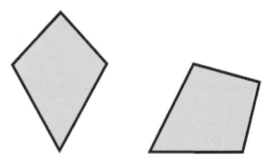

Figure 2.56 *These two shapes are not immediately perceived to be identical. The "kite shape" on the left has a dominant vertical axis of symmetry. The irregular four-sided polygon on the left has a horizontal base.*

each one tries to protect its supply of water and nutrients. Particles floating on a liquid surface may tend to cluster because of surface-tension effects. People are self-avoiding (uniformly spaced) in a marching band, but cluster at parties. In extreme cases, visual observation of clustering or self-avoidance is possible. In most cases, people do not easily see through apparently chaotic distributions to detect these effects, but measurements on digital images (discussed in **Chapter 10**) can frequently provide quantitative characterization.

In general, people do not prefer order. Tests with computer-generated images of apparently random paint droplets showed that completely ordered images were considered boring and not visually stimulating, while completely random ones were considered to be equally uninteresting. When the correlation between size, color, and position obeyed a "pink noise" or fractal relationship, the pictures were most visually interesting to viewers. Interestingly, the same relationships were found in mathematical analyses of several of Jackson Pollock's paintings (**Figure 2.57**).

Apparently, a distribution in which there is just enough hint of order that we must work to find it visually is the most appealing. The implication for noticing (or failing to notice) arrangements of features in scientific images is clear. In addition to arrangements that may be present throughout an image, gradients are often important but are not always easy to detect. The problem is that there can be so many different kinds of gradient. Features can vary in size, shape, orientation, color, density, number, or any combination of these factors, as a function of position. **Chapter 9** illustrates some of the possibilities.

The innate ability that people have for finding order in images is risky. Sometimes we imagine a regularity or order that is not there (e.g., constellations), and sometimes the presence of complexity or superficial disorder hides the real underlying structure. Some orientations are more readily detected than others, and complicated gradients are likely to escape detection unless we know beforehand what to look for. The result is that many real spatial arrangements may be missed, even in two dimensions. Given the additional problems introduced by examining two-dimensional sections through three-dimensional structures, the problem is much worse for three-dimensional spatial arrangements.

Seeing is believing

If human vision is so easily fooled in its interpretation of images, questions can be (and often are) raised about the effects of various image processing procedures that might bias human judgment about the results. This is in part an ethical question, dealing with composites and forgeries that might be intentionally constructed to mislead the observer. That issue is identical to any other case of intentional deception. If someone is willing to invest enough time and skill in creating a forgery, either as an image or other kinds of data, and whether using a computer or not (many excellent forged images have been crafted in the photographic darkroom), it can be done.

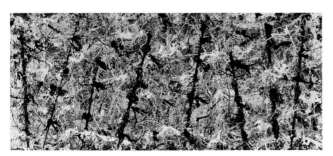

Figure 2.57 Jackson Pollock's Blue Poles #11. *His paintings have been analyzed to determine that they have a fractal structure and a complexity that evolved during his career.*

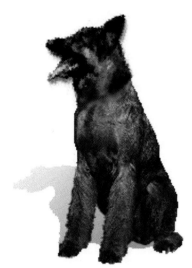

Detecting such forgeries can be very difficult, perhaps impossible in some cases. In the specific case of digital images, the convenience of software tools for cut-and-paste seems to make the task easy, but usually the results are easy to spot. There are plenty of clues that make it possible to detect alterations in images or pasting in parts of one image to another. Some of the obvious ones are shadow lengths and angles that do not match, geometrical inconsistencies, variations in focus, color mismatches, and textures or channel noise that are different (including the way that the noise varies with brightness).

In the example of **Figure 2.58**, the head of a German shepherd has been pasted onto the body of an Irish setter. It is easy to detect the forgery in this case, but it is useful to note the various clues that are present. The first clue is of course the relatively abrupt change in color at the dog's neck. Some color adjustments could have been made to reduce the differences, and the boundary can sometimes be hidden (for instance by putting a collar over it). In this case, some blurring was performed to prevent a sharp line from attracting attention, but the presence of localized blurring and loss of fine detail is itself a clue that something has been done to the image.

Figure 2.58 Example of combining parts of two different images.

A second very common problem with composites is that the lighting on the two parts of the picture is different. The body of the dog is lit from the right side of the picture, while the head is lit from the front. It is also noteworthy that the shadow of the dog does not correspond to the composite, but still has the shape of the original head.

The head image was originally smaller and had to be enlarged and rotated to line up with the body. This resulted in pixelation that does not match the original. The scale of the fine detail is different in the two parts of the image, indicating that they do not belong together. In general, images taken with different cameras and under different lighting conditions have different noise characteristics. The ratio of noise in the red, green, and blue channels and the variation in the noise amplitude with absolute brightness require more effort to measure, but are almost impossible to match when combining images from different sources.

With enough effort (and skill), seamless and virtually undetectable results can be achieved. However, there are few situations in scientific research in which a single image provides conclusive evidence for a result. Creating a family of false images documenting a research study is probably an impractically difficult task, and in any case the hallmark of the scientific method is the ability of an experiment to be duplicated by others, so intentionally forged images are not usually a serious concern.

On the other hand, it is certainly a good idea to keep original images separate from copies that are processed for reproduction, viewing, or measurement, and to keep a careful record of the processing steps so that they can be reported in publications and reproduced as necessary. Some software packages (e.g., Adobe Photoshop CS2) can be configured to do that automatically, saving a history of all processing operations with the image on disk. In some forensic work, this is considered essential.

Of greater concern is the unconsciously introduced bias that can be produced by the selection of the areas that are photographed or the cropping of the photograph to isolate the object(s) of interest. Tabloid newspapers are often faulted for using pictures of celebrities that are taken out of context, but even responsible publications must decide whether the removal of background and surroundings is appropriate or relevant to the story, and it may only be after the fact that such relevance becomes evident.

In the sciences, intentional forgeries are probably rare, and will usually be inconsequential because the scientific method requires that others be able to reproduce and verify results. If a scientist publishes an image without enough information about the procedure, he or she will be criticized. So the information is generally there, and someone else with a comparable skill level and knowledge will serve as a check. That does not mean that every publication has to include such a fine level of detail that anyone, regardless of their ignorance of either the application or the image processing, needs to be able to follow it.

The scientific method of openness and its dependence on confirmation and reproducibility automatically deals with the problem of intentional falsification. It is the unintended errors, which usually have little to do with the image processing and more with the choice of images, choice of specimens, and interpretation of results, that are actually of greater concern. These may involve the human vision system as well, of course, but are usually at heart the result of misunderstanding the experimental background.

An important thing to remember about the image processing techniques discussed and illustrated in this book is that they do not *add* anything to images. Rather, by removing some of the contents of an image, they make it easier to visually access the remaining details, which are presumably relevant and interesting in a particular context. Thus removing or suppressing shading, or noise, or high contrast can reveal the details that were previously hidden. Or increasing local contrast, or converting textural variations to brightness, or substituting one color for another can allow details that were below the threshold of visibility to be seen.

So, in conclusion ...

Human vision is an extremely powerful tool, evolved over millennia to extract from scenes those details that are important to our survival as a species. The processing of visual information combines a hierarchy of highly parallel neural circuits to detect and correlate specific types of detail within images. Many shortcuts that work "most of the time" are used to speed recognition. Studying the failure of these tricks, revealed in various visual illusions, aids in understanding of the underlying processes.

An awareness of the failures and biases of human vision is also important to the scientist who relies on visual examination of images to acquire or interpret data. Visual inspection is a comparative, not a quantitative process, and it is easily biased by the presence of other information in the image. Computer image-analysis methods are available that overcome most of these specific problems, but they provide answers that are only as good as the questions that are asked. In most cases, if the scientist does not visually perceive the features or trends in the raw images, their subsequent measurement will not be undertaken.

There are several classic books that provide a good introduction to human vision without delving too deeply into the fascinating but specialized literature regarding the messy anatomical details of the visual cortex. In particular, see the works by Frisby (1980), Marr (1982), and Rock (1984).

Of course, there is also an extensive literature in many peer-reviewed journals, and in the modern era, no one should neglect to perform a Google search of the Internet, which will locate several sets of course notes on this topic as well as publication reprints and many related sites of varying quality.

3

Printing and Storage

reating hard-copy representations of images, for example to use as illustrations in reports and publications, is important to many users of image processing equipment. It is also usually important to store the images so that they can be retrieved later, for instance to compare with new ones or to transmit to another worker. Both of these activities are necessary because it is rarely possible to reduce an image to a compact verbal description or a series of measurements that will communicate to someone else what we see or believe to be important in the image. In fact, it is often difficult to draw someone else's attention to the particular details or general structure that may be present in an image that we may feel are the significant characteristics present, based on our examination of that image and many more. Faced with the inability to find descriptive words or numbers, we resort to passing a representation of the image on, perhaps with some annotation.

Printing

This book is printed in color, using high-end printing technology not normally available to a single image processing user. That type of printing equipment presents its own set of challenges. But many everyday jobs can be handled very well using quite inexpensive machines; the quality, speed, and cost of both monochrome and color printers are improving rapidly. A typical monochrome (black on white) or color laser printer costs less than $1000 and has become a common accessory to desktop computer systems, particularly serving small networks as found in a typical office or laboratory. These printers are designed primarily to print text and simple graphics such as line drawings. Most can, however, be used to print images as well. Ink-jet printers, which are inexpensive and indeed may be included at modest cost or even free with computer purchases (but which use expensive consumables) are also very capable of printing images. Service bureaus using dye-sublimation or photographic printing methods offer online connection and rapid turnaround. We have come a very long way since computer graphics consisted of printing Christmas posters using Xs and Os on a teletype to represent different gray levels (**Figure 3.1**). In this chapter we examine the technology for printing images that can be used in desktop computer-based image processing systems.

For this purpose it does not matter whether or not the printers use a high-level page description language such as PostScript®, which is used to produce smooth characters and lines at the maximum printer resolution, so long as they allow the computer to transmit to the printer an

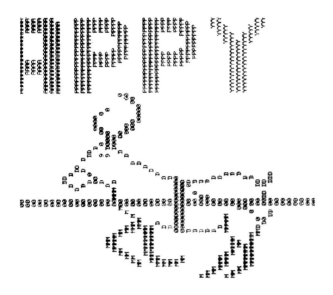

Figure 3.1 Portion of a 1960s-era teletype printout of a Christmas calendar poster.

array of individual pixel brightness values. Most printers that can create any graphics output in addition to simply printing text can be controlled in this way. This means that "daisy wheel" or other formed-character printers (now virtually obsolete) are not useful for imaging. That is how the Snoopy posters were made, by creatively arranging to overprint groups of characters to produce different levels of darkness. But dot-matrix printers using inked ribbons, ink-jet printers, thermal printers, and other devices that form their output as an array of dots on paper *can* be used to print images. The quality of the result is primarily a function of the size and spacing of the dots.

The idea that the juxtaposition of many small dots of a few colors could be visually blended and perceived as continuous-tone colored images was first exploited by artists, notably Georges Seurat, to create a style of pointing known as "pointillism" (**Figure 3.2**). The same principle is now used in cathode-ray tubes (CRT) and liquid crystal displays (LCD), which use pure red, green, and blue to produce an entire spectrum of colors. It is also used for printing, ranging from books like this one to most desktop printers.

A basic level of confusion that often arises in interpreting the specifications of a printer in terms of image quality has to do with "dots per inch" or dpi and "lines per inch" or lpi (sometimes also called pixels per inch for even more confusion). For any of the printers mentioned above, but particularly for laser printers, the specification of dpi resolution is the number of tiny black dots (or whatever color ink or toner is used) that the printer can deposit on paper. Usually, it is the same in both the line (horizontal) and page (vertical) directions on the paper, although some printers have different dpi resolution in the two directions. Normally, the dots are used to form characters and lines. A low number of dpi will cause the characters to look rough and the lines to appear stair-stepped or "aliased." Resolution of 600 to 1200 dpi or more for laser printers is now common, and this level of resolution is capable of producing quite acceptable output for text and line drawings used in reports and correspondence. Ink-jet printers describe the dot size in terms of the volume of liquid ink in each dot, with values of a few picoliters now typical. These dots are small enough to be individually almost invisible, so that the resulting image appears to have continuous tones.

However, the dots placed on the paper by these printers are black, and such printers do not have an adjustable gray scale needed to print images. To create a gray scale for images, it is necessary to use groups of these dots, a technique generally known as halftoning. It is commonly used in newspapers, magazines, and books (including this one), and as we will see, this technique can be used for color as well as monochrome images. The differences in halftone quality between (for instance) a newspaper and a book lie fundamentally in the number of dots per inch that can be placed on the paper and the way they are organized to produce a gray-scale (or color) result.

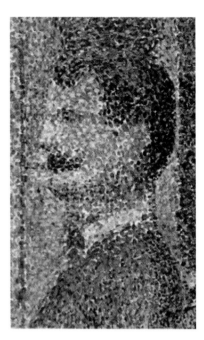

Figure 3.2 Detail from Georges Seurat's La Parade *showing the dots of paint used to create the impression of continuous tones.*

The basis of halftoning lies in the grouping of the individual black dots produced by the printer. A group of (for instance) 16 dots in a 4×4 array can be called a halftone cell. Within the cell, some or all of the dots may actually be printed. Where no dot is printed, the white paper shows through. If the cell is reasonably small, the observer will not see the individual dots but will instead visually average the amount of dark ink and light paper to form a gray scale. In this example, shown in **Figure 3.3**, there are 17 possible levels of gray, ranging from solid black (all dots printed) to solid white (no dots printed).

In a 300-dpi printer, the individual black dots can be placed on the paper with a spacing of 1/300th of an inch in each direction. Grouping these into 4×4 halftone cells would produce $300 \div 4 = 75$ cells per inch. This is close to the resolution of pixels on a typical video display used with an image processing computer (depending on the size of the monitor and the display hardware settings, values from 72 to 90 display pixels per inch are typical). If each pixel corresponds to a halftone cell, then an image can be printed with about the same dimension as it appears on the screen. Each halftone cell uses one of its 17 possible gray levels to represent the gray scale of the pixel. **Figure 3.4** illustrates how these printed cells represent the gray levels in typical anti-aliased text.

Of course, since an original image might typically have 256 gray levels, this seems like a rather poor representation of the brightness information. However, that is not the only or even the most serious limitation. Instant prints from Polaroid® film show only about the same number of distinct gray levels (the film is quite a bit better than the print), and these were considered quite useful for many scientific purposes (for instance, the recording of scanning electron microscope images).

One problem with the halftoning method illustrated above is that the dots and cells are large enough to be visually distinguished by the observer. In a magazine or book, the size of the cells is smaller. The cell size is usually described as a halftone screen or grid: the spacing of the screen in number of lines per inch corresponds to the number of cells per inch discussed above (but be cautious, because sometimes the specification is given as line pairs per inch, since it is a pair of lines, one light and one dark, that composes an element of resolution). A screen with well over 100 lines per inch (often 133 or even as high as 175 lines per inch) is

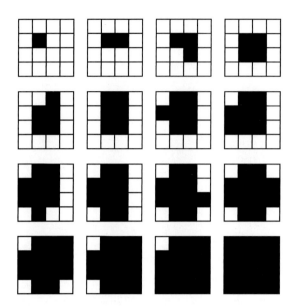

Figure 3.3 Halftone gray scale produced with a 4 × 4-dot cell. Printing dots in all, some, or none of the locations generates 17 different gray values.

used to produce high-quality printed illustrations. Even in a newspaper illustration, a screen of at least 85 lines per inch is typically used. **Figure 3.5** shows several examples of halftone output from a typical laser printer, in which the number of halftone cells is varied to trade off gray-scale vs. lateral resolution. The output from the current generation of desktop laser printers is often adequate for reports, but not for publication. Also, reproduction of such prints is usually difficult and beset by problems such as moiré or interference patterns.

More lines per inch of resolution are desired to preserve the sharpness of features in the image; however, more gray levels must be represented by these more finely spaced cells. That means that the printer (or "imagesetter," as these higher-quality devices that produce films or plates used in offset printing presses are generally called) must be capable of placing a much

Figure 3.4 Representation of a gray-scale display of letters by halftoning.

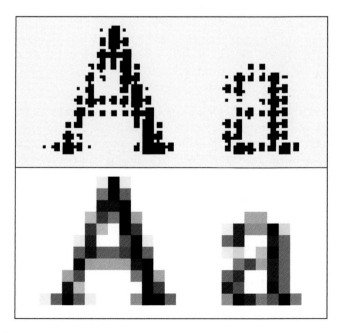

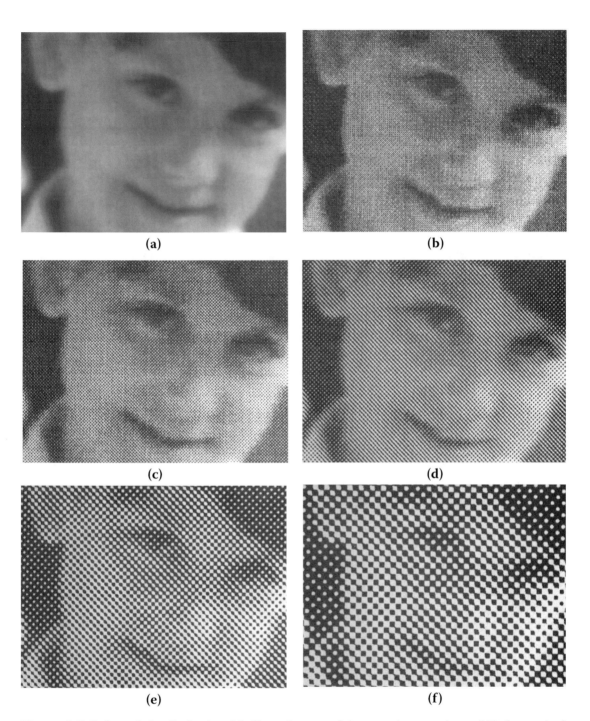

Figure 3.5 *Enlarged detail of printed halftone images of the same image using a 300-dot per inch PostScript laser printer:* ***(a)*** *original image;* ***(b)*** *100 lines per inch;* ***(c)*** *75 lines per inch;* ***(d)*** *50 lines per inch;* ***(e)*** *32 lines per inch;* ***(f)*** *25 lines per inch. Increasing the number of halftone cells improves the lateral resolution at the expense of the number of gray levels that can be shown.*

larger number of very much smaller dots. A gray scale of 65 levels can be formed with an 8 × 8 array of dots in a cell. With a 125-line screen, this would correspond to 8 × 125 = 1000 dpi. This is about the starting point for typeset quality used to print images for commercial purposes. Color (introduced below) imposes additional restrictions that require even higher resolution (smaller dots). Imagesetters used for high-quality printing generally are capable of 2500 to 3000 dots per inch.

An additional difficulty with the halftoning method outlined above arises from the dots themselves. Each of the various printing methods produces dots in a different way. Dot-matrix printers use small pins to press an inked ribbon against the paper. Ink-jet printers produce tiny ink droplets. Some of these printers deposit the ink in a liquid form that penetrates into the paper making slightly fuzzy dots, while in others the ink solidifies and adheres to the paper surface without penetration. The better grades of paper have surface coatings that prevent the ink from spreading or penetrating. Thermal printers, now used primarily in some fax machines, use a pin to pass an electrical current through the coating on a paper. One kind of paper is coated with a white oxide of zinc that is reduced by the current to deposit a dark spot of metal at the location; other thermal papers are based on the chemistry of silver. Laser printers work essentially like a xerographic copier. The light from the laser (or in some versions from a photodiode) falls on a selenium-coated drum and by the photoelectric effect produces a localized electrostatic charge. This in turn picks up carbon particles (the toner or "ink"), which are then transferred to the paper and subsequently heated to remain permanently.

Dots on paper

All of these technologies are limited by the ability to make a small, dark spot on the paper. The size of the carbon particles used as the toner in copier or laser printer cartridges limits the spatial resolution, and special finely ground toner is needed for resolutions of 1200 dpi and higher. The limitation in making higher resolution laser printers is not primarily in the additional memory needed in the printer, nor by the need to focus the light to a smaller spot on the drum, but in the toner particle size. Some systems disperse the toner using liquid carriers to improve the control of toner placement.

Similar restrictions limit the other printing methods. The difficulty of depositing a small but dark ink spot by the impact of a pin onto a ribbon, or the fuzziness of the dot written by thermal printing, have prevented those techniques from advancing to higher resolutions. Ink-jet printers can generate small drops and hence deposit small dots, but the inks tend to spread on the paper. Indeed, the roughness of the paper surface and the need for special coatings (to prevent the inks from soaking into the paper fibers or spreading across the surface or the toner particles from falling off) become critical issues. It is not enough to purchase a high-quality printer; the use of special paper with a proper surface finish for the particular printer is needed to achieve the quality of image printing that the printer technology makes available (Lee and Winslow 1993).

Because the dots produced by printers are generally imperfect and rough-edged, it is hard to control them so that the gray scale produced by the array of dots within the cell is uniform. Most dots are larger than their spacing so that solid black areas can be printed. This is good for printing text characters, which are intended to be solid black. However, it means that the dots overlap some of the white areas in the cell, which darkens the halftone gray scale. **Figure 3.6** shows this for the case of a 6 × 6-dot halftone cell. At the dark end of the scale, adjacent gray levels may be indistinguishable, while at the light end the difference between the first few

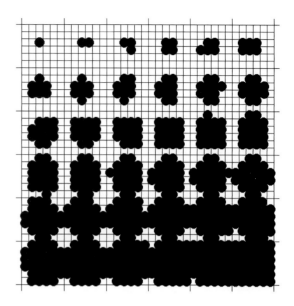

Figure 3.6 A 6 × 6-dot halftone that can produce 37 gray levels. The use of approximately round dots large enough to touch diagonally causes them to overlap and produce darker cells than ideal.

levels may be very great. High-quality printing of images usually tries to avoid pure white and pure black.

For the case of a 4 × 4-dot cell illustrated above using a 300-dpi printer, 17 nominal gray levels, and 75 cells per inch, the darkening or "gain" of the gray scale produces images of poor quality. If the printer resolution is much higher so that finer halftone cells with more steps can be created, it is possible to correct for this tendency to darken the images by constructing a mapping that translates the pixel gray value to a printed gray value that compensates for this effect. These "gamma" curves are applied within the software so that more-or-less equal steps of brightness can be printed on the page. The software drivers that control the flow of information from the computer to the printer handle many chores, including the application of nonlinear corrections for each of the colored inks or toners. Specific correction curves, called ICC (International Color Consortium) curves, must be supplied for each combination of inks and papers used. These can be generated by specific calibration of each system, or curves supplied by the manufacturer may be relied upon. However, note that in the latter case, substituting third-party inks and papers may produce unwanted deviations and poor results.

The human eye does not respond linearly to gray scale, but logarithmically. Consequently, to produce a printed image in which the visual impression of brightness varies linearly with pixel value, a further adjustment of the gamma curve is needed (as shown in **Figure 3.7**) to compress the dark values even more and expand the light ones. Because of these limitations, a printing scale with 65 gray values defined by an 8 × 8-dot halftone cell may be able to show only about half that many shades in the actual printed image.

Halftone grids in a typesetter or imagesetter are not limited by the size or perfection of the dots. Instead of coarse toner particles or contact with an inked ribbon, typesetters use light to expose a photographic emulsion, which is then developed to produce either a film or a print. The size of the silver grains in the film emulsion is far smaller than the effective dot size and the dots can be controlled in both size and shape with great precision. There is still a need for a gamma curve to compensate for the nonlinear response of human vision, however.

If the variation of brightness across an image is gradual and the total number of gray levels is small, a likely consequence is the generation of a visual effect known as banding or posterization. This is illustrated in **Figure 3.8**. The step from one brightness level to the next appears as

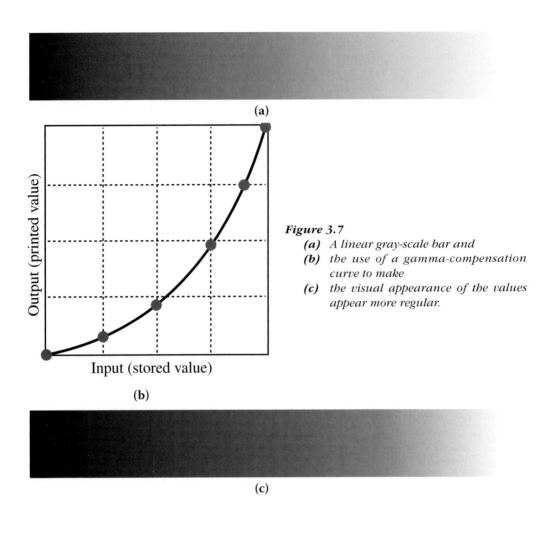

(a)

Output (printed value)

Input (stored value)

(b)

Figure 3.7
   (a) *A linear gray-scale bar and*
   (b) *the use of a gamma-compensation curve to make*
   (c) *the visual appearance of the values appear more regular.*

(c)

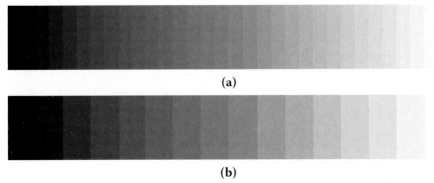

(a)

(b)

Figure 3.8 *A gray-scale bar showing banding when printed with only 32 or 16 gray steps.*

a contour line in the printed image and is visually recognized as a feature in the picture, when in fact it is purely an artifact of the printing process. Banding can be avoided by increasing the number of gray levels used, or in some cases by modifying the way in which the dots within the halftone cell are used to generate the gray scale. Generally, the rule for the maximum number of gray shades available is $1+(dpi/lpi)^2$, where dpi is the printer resolution in dots per inch (e.g., 300 or 600 for a typical laser printer) and lpi is the lines per inch of the halftone screen (e.g., 75 lpi for the example discussed above). This assumes that all of the gray levels can actually be used, subject to the darkening ("dot gain") and gamma effects mentioned above.

In the examples shown in **Figure 3.3** and **Figure 3.4**, an arrangement of dots was used that produced more-or-less round regions of black within a white frame. With a larger dot array in each cell, an even more regular circular pattern can be constructed. The round dot pattern is one of the more commonly used arrangements; however, many others are possible, including lines and crosses (**Figure 3.9**). Each of these produces some visual artifacts that may be useful for artistic effects but generally interfere with viewing the actual image contents. For instance, the diamond pattern used by most PostScript printers as an approximation to round dots causes dot densities less than 50% black to appear quite different from ones that are 50% or more black. The reason for this is that at the 50% point the dots touch from one cell to the next so that the eye perceives a sudden transition from dark dots on a white background to the reverse, even if the individual dots are not visually evident. Of course, all such artifacts degrade the representation of the original gray-scale image.

If the dots within each halftone cell are randomly distributed, fewer visual artifacts are likely. This requires additional computer processing within the printer. Other printers use programs that analyze the neighbor cells (pixels). If cells on one side are dark and on the other side are light, the program may use a pattern of dots that is shifted toward the dark neighbors to produce a smoother edge. This works quite well for generating smooth boundaries for printed text characters and minimizing jagged edges on lines, but it is not clear that it provides any consistent benefit for gray-scale image printing.

Printers of modest dpi resolution cannot produce halftone cells that are small and still represent many gray levels, and visually distracting patterns may appear in images if regular patterns of dots are used within the cells. Hence, another approach used with these printers is to use "dithering" to represent the image. In a simple random dither, each possible position where the printer can place a black dot corresponds to a point in the image whose gray-scale value is examined. If the point is very dark, there is a high probability that the dot should be printed, and vice versa. A random number is generated and compared to the gray scale; if the number is below the gray-scale value for that point (both properly scaled), then the dot is printed on the page.

As shown in **Figure 3.10**, even coarse dithering can produce viewable representation of an image. Many different types of dithering patterns are used, some of them random or pseudorandom and others with various patterned arrangements of the dots. Usually, the particular dither pattern used is determined either by the printer itself or the interface software provided for it. There is a rich literature on the design of dither patterns, but the user of the image-analysis system may not have much control over or choice of the pattern. Dithered images are generally good at showing gradually varying brightness gradients, since human vision responds to an average dot density or spacing. But sharp edges will be blurred, broken up, or displaced because there is no continuous line or boundary printed, and it is difficult to compare the brightness of regions within the image. Dithered printing is usually considered to be a low-end method for producing crude hard copy and not suitable for use in reports or publications.

Figure 3.9 *Printouts of a portion of an image of Saturn (shown in its entirety in* **Chapter 5, Figure 5.26)** *using different dot patterns within the same size halftone cells:*
- *(a)* round;
- *(b)* horizontal line;
- *(c)* diagonal line;
- *(d)* plus;
- *(e)* cross.

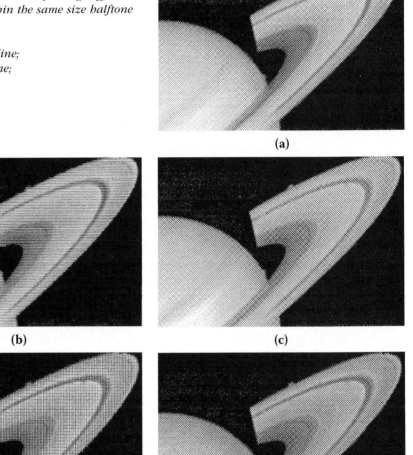

(a)

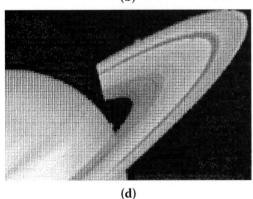

(b)

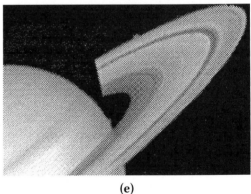

(c)

(d)

(e)

In spite of the limitations discussed above, monochrome image printing using a halftoning method and a printer with 1200-dpi capability is adequate for many kinds of image processing applications, and the resulting images are suitable in quality for reports. Because the printouts cannot be adequately reproduced by office xerographic copiers, it is desirable to make original prints for each copy of the report.

For higher quality work, photographic recording can be used. This process may seem like a step backward, especially when the image may have started out on film in the first place before it was digitized into the computer. But because facilities for handling photographic images, duplicating them, and making halftone screens photographically for printing are well developed, fully understood, and comparatively inexpensive, this is often the most effective solution. Forcing a "high-tech" solution in which images are

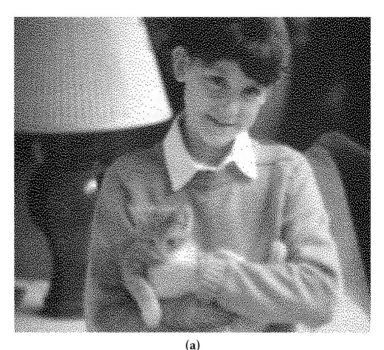

(a)

Figure 3.10 *Two different dither patterns for the "girl" image (shown in **Chapter 1, Figure 1.23**):*
(a) *random dots;*
(b) *patterned dots.*

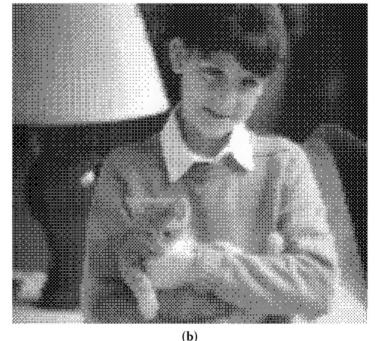

(b)

directly merged into a report within the computer may not be worthwhile in terms of time or cost if only a small number of copies are needed. Mounting photographs on a few pages or inserting them as separate pages is still a quite suitable presentation method. No doubt as printing technology continues to advance, the balance will continue to shift toward direct printing from the computer.

Color printing

Printing color images is considerably more complicated and difficult, but it is increasingly becoming available as a standard computer accessory. The usual method, which you can see by looking at the color images in this book with a magnifier, is to create halftones for each of several different color inks and superimpose them to produce the printed color image. Image-setters typically use four color plates (for cyan, magenta, yellow, and black inks), produced by suitable color-separation software in the computer, for full-color printing. That is not the only possibility, particularly in advertising, where specific additional colors may be introduced to ensure a perfect color match. There are many complexities in the color printing process, however. This section discusses those that are important for most networked or desktop color printers.

Displaying a color image on a computer monitor or television set is accomplished by illuminating red, green, and blue phosphors with the electron beam in the CRT. Large plasma displays and LCDs used for flat-panel monitors, projectors, and notebook computers use a different technology based on colored filters, but also produce red, green, and blue primary colors. There are also large-screen displays (such as used at sporting events) that consist of arrays of discrete lights. Each of these methods generates the colors in different ways, but it is still the visual mixing together of red, green, and blue that produces the full range of colors that can be shown.

This range is called the "gamut" of the device (Stone et al. 1988). In a display that emits red, green, and blue light (RGB), it is possible to generate a large fraction of the total range of colors that the human eye can see. **Figure 3.11** shows the CIE (Commission Internationale de L'Éclairage) color diagram that was introduced in **Chapter 1**, adding the typical color gamut for an RGB display and an ink-jet color printer superimposed on the diagram. One of the features of the CIE diagram is that colors add together along straight lines, so the three phosphor colors define the corners of a triangle that enclose all of the possible color combinations. The missing colors that cannot be generated using these particular phosphors include points near the outside of the diagram, which are the most saturated colors.

As presented in the figure, the concept of gamut applies to the color range that a device can reproduce, but does not address the range of brightness values. This is also an important issue, since (as discussed in **Chapter 2**) human vision is capable of responding to an enormously

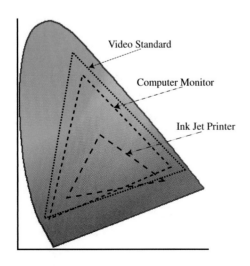

Video Standard

Computer Monitor

Ink Jet Printer

Figure 3.11 *The CIE color diagram discussed in* *Chapter 1,* *with gamuts shown for broadcast television, a typical computer monitor, and a low-end ink-jet printer.*

wide range of brightnesses, much greater than any display (yet alone any hard-copy printout) can reproduce. Cameras, both film and digital, can also record images covering a wider range of brightness values than can be printed out on either photographic dye-based or ink-based printers (Battiato et al. 2003). How, then, can satisfactory representations of scenes with such wide latitude be presented to a human observer?

There is a wide range of literature on the processing of high-dynamic-range images to accomplish this (Debevec and Malik 1997; Durand and Dorsey 2002; Tao and Asari 2005). Most of the techniques rely on maintaining relative brightness differences locally while suppressing them globally, because human vision responds to local changes in brightness but tends to ignore gradual variations. The simplest approach is simply a high-pass filter (which, as discussed in succeeding chapters, suppresses low-frequency changes in the image while keeping or emphasizing high frequencies). Some of these simple methods introduce visible halos around edges, which the more advanced techniques eliminate. Two of the successful techniques are the "retinex" method and homomorphic range compression. The retinex approach is based on the original work in 1963 of Edwin Land (of Polaroid fame). He postulated that human vision depends on spatial comparisons of brightness and color, and his ideas led to many insights into vision that are still the subject of research 40 years later. For a current review, see the January 2004 issue of the *Journal of Electronic Imaging* (Vol. 13, no. 1), which is devoted to "Retinex at 40" and includes a functional implementation of the retinex algorithm for brightness compression using MATLAB® (Funt et al. 2004) as well as numerous other pertinent articles (Ciurea and Funt 2004; Cooper and Baqal 2004; McCann 2004; Rahman et al. 2004; Sobol 2004).

The retinex method operates in the pixel domain and performs comparisons at different scales. The homomorphic method operates instead in Fourier space and is a particularly efficient way to handle the compression of brightness values to fit into a reduced gamut for printing. The procedure is described in **Chapter 6**. As shown in **Figure 3.12**, the result preserves the local contrast while compressing the overall brightness range in the image so that it can be printed. Details emerge from deep shadow areas that were recorded on the original film, while contrast in bright areas is retained.

The concept of gamut applies equally well to other color display and recording devices. However, the gamut is not always as simple in shape as the triangle shown in **Figure 3.11**. For one thing, printing uses subtractive rather than additive color. In terms of the color cube (also introduced in **Chapter 1** and shown in **Figure 3.13**), the blank paper starts off as white, and the addition of cyan, magenta, and yellow inks removes the complementary colors (red, green, and blue, respectively) from the reflected light to produce the possible range of colors. It is common to call these colors CMY (cyan, magenta, yellow) to distinguish them from the additive RGB colors.

The theory of subtractive printing, summarized in **Figure 3.14**, suggests that the mixture of all three colors will produce black (just as with additive RGB color, the summation of all three colors produces white). However, actual printing with CMY inks generally cannot produce a very good black, but instead gives a muddy grayish brown because of impurities in the inks, reflection of light from the surface of the ink (so that it does not pass through all of the ink layers to be absorbed), and difficulty in getting complete coverage of the white paper.

The most common solution is to add a separate, black ink to the printing process. This reduces the need for large amounts of the colored inks, reduces the thickness of ink buildup on the page, and reduces cost. But from the standpoint of image quality, the most important factor is that it allows dark colors to be printed without appearing muddy. The four-color cyan-magenta-

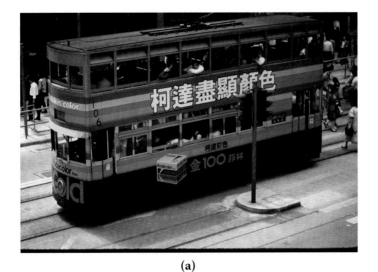

(a)

Figure 3.12 *Homomorphic*
reduction of the brightness
range reveals detail in
shadow areas without
blowing out contrast in the
bright areas:
(a) *original;*
(b) *result.*

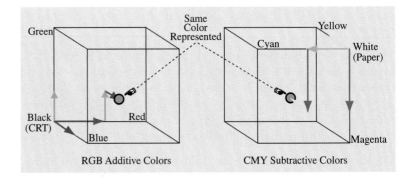

(b)

Figure 3.13 *Comparison*
of RGB (additive) and
CMY (subtractive) color
spaces. The additive color
space adds red, green,
and blue emissive colors
to a black background,
while subtractive color
space removes cyan,
magenta, and yellow
colors from a white
background.

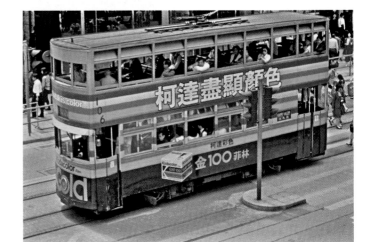

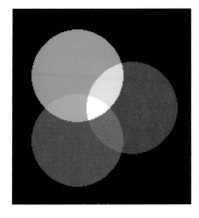
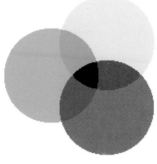

Figure 3.14 Combinations of RGB additive colors on a black background, and CMY subtractive colors on a white background.

yellow-black system (CMYK) uses four halftone screens, one for each ink. However, while converting from RGB colors (or CIE, HSI [hue, saturation, intensity], or any other equivalent color-space coordinate system) to CMY (often called process color) is straightforward, converting to CMYK is not. Rules to calculate how much black to put into various color representations depend on visual response to colors, the kind of paper to be printed, the illumination the print will be viewed with, and even the contents of the images (Sharma 2003).

Algorithms for converting from CMY to CMYK involve specifying levels of undercolor removal (UCR) and gray-component replacement (GCR) that are essentially arbitrary, are little documented, and vary considerably from one software program to another (Agfa 1992). The general approach is to use the value of whichever of the three components (CMY) is darkest to determine an amount of black to be added. For instance, for a color containing 80% cyan, 50% magenta, and 30% yellow, the 30% value would be taken as an index into a built-in calibration curve or lookup table. This might indicate that a 15% value for the black ink should be chosen for gray-component replacement. Then, the amount of the principal color (in this example cyan), or, according to some algorithms, the amounts of all of the colors, would be reduced. It is difficult to design algorithms for these substitutions that do not cause color shifts. Also, the substitutions do not work equally well for printing with different combinations of ink, paper finish, etc.

Color prints are generally not as vivid or saturated as the image appears on the CRT. In addition, the colors depend critically on the paper finish and viewing conditions. Changing the room light will slightly alter the visual appearance of colors on an RGB monitor, but because the monitor is generating its own illumination this is a secondary effect. Since a print is viewed by reflected light, changing the amount of light or the color temperature of room light with a print can completely alter the appearance of the image. The color temperature (a handy way of describing the spectrum of intensity vs. color) of incandescent bulbs, fluorescent bulbs, direct sunlight, or open sky are all quite different. Sunlight is about 5500K, while an incandescent bulb is typically 2900K (warmer, redder), and an overcast sky may be as high as 8000K (colder, bluer). Many computer CRT monitors are close to 6500K.

Human vision can be tricked by combinations of illumination and shadow, inks or other colored coatings, surface finish (smooth or textured in various ways), and even the presence of other adjacent colors in the field of view to change the way we judge colors in an image. These other colors may even lie outside the image itself; consider how a colored mat can change the appearance of an art print. When "true" color prints of an image are required, it is necessary to perform extensive calibrations of a specific printer and monitor so that acceptable fidelity is obtained. This is of great concern in advertising; if you purchase clothing from a mail-order catalog, you expect the colors of the cloth to match the printed photograph, which is no easy task. The process usually works by adjusting the monitor output (with lookup tables in the display hardware) so that the appearance of colors there is tailored to match the ability of a specific printer/paper/ink combination to reproduce them.

For most (but certainly not all) applications of image processing, the purpose of printing in color is to distinguish the variously colored regions present; some inaccuracy in the fidelity of the colors is acceptable. If exact color matching is not necessary in a particular application, then the task becomes much easier, although you will still need to be concerned about the color gamut of the printer, the consistency of colors (to allow comparison of different images or regions), and of course the resolution of the printer. The color gamut is important because colors of increasing saturation in the original image, which can be distinguished on the video display, may become similar in the print image if the saturation exceeds the range of the printer.

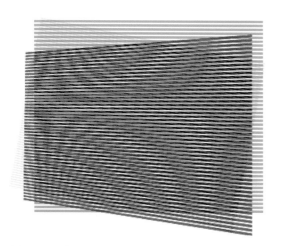

Figure 3.15 Moiré pattern produced by overlaying arrays of color dots.

Producing CMYK halftones (so-called color separations) and superimposing them to produce color prints sounds simple enough, but it harbors many problems that commercial printers must deal with routinely. One is how to superimpose the halftone screens so that they do not produce visual moiré patterns in the image. **Figure 3.15** shows an example of a moiré effect produced by different color patterns. The lines that appear are an artifact of the spacing and alignment of the individual patterns. Traditional offset printing defines "ideal" screen angles for the four CMYK screens as 45° (black), 70° (magenta), 90° (yellow), and 105° (cyan), as shown in **Figure 3.16**. This aligns the colored dots to form small rosettes that together make up the color. **Figure 3.17** shows an example; note that the dots vary in size to control the amount of each color, and that some of the halftone spots may be partly superimposed on each other. Since some inks are partially transparent, this can produce various color biases, depending on the order of printing.

In most printing, the colors are not intended to be superimposed on each other, but printed adjacent to each other, and to allow some white paper to show. Most color printing methods suffer from the fact that as more color is added, the white paper is covered and the appearance becomes darker. This is another reason that high-resolution halftone screens and very small printing dots must be used. Generally, when four halftone grids or color separations are used, the dpi of the printer must be doubled for each color to get a resolution equivalent to that of monochrome printing. In other words, each pixel now requires four interleaved halftone cells, one for each color. Since the dot size for each of the four colors is only one-fourth of the area, printing a solid expanse of one color is not possible, which further reduces the maximum saturation that can be achieved and hence the gamut of the printer.

Most desktop printers do not provide control over the screen angles, and many printers simply use a zero angle for all four screens due to the way the printing mechanism works (for instance, a typical color ink-jet printer). Some page description languages (e.g., PostScript Level

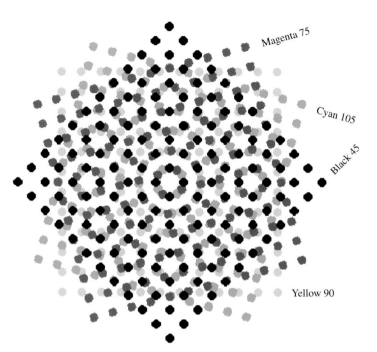

Figure 3.16 *Ideal screen angles for CMYK color printing place the halftone screens at angles of 45° (black), 75° (magenta), 90° (yellow), and 105° (cyan).*

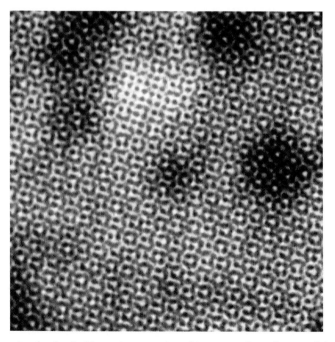

Figure 3.17 *Example of color halftone image printed in an earlier edition of this textbook.*

2) include provision for such control, but only high-end typesetters and imagesetters generally respond to those commands.

All of the problems present in printing monochrome or gray-scale images, such as banding, posterization, limited numbers of intensity levels, and so forth, are also present in producing the color separations. In addition, color printing introduces the additional problems of screen angles and moiré patterns. Finally, alignment and registration of the colors must be considered, since in many printers they are printed one at a time and the paper must be handled in several passes. Some alternative printing methods exist that deposit multiple colors in a single pass, but these have their own problems of allowing inks to dry without mixing.

The printing and registration of colors presents one additional problem in some cases. Consider a region of a uniform color that is a mixture of two or more of the primary printed colors and is adjacent to a region of a different color. At the boundary, the colors must change abruptly from one color to the other. However, the two color screens are not aligned dot for dot, and along the boundary there will be cases in which one of the two left-side color dots may be present close to one of the two right-side color dots. This can give rise to false color lines along boundaries. In graphic arts, such artifacts are usually avoided by trapping to remove the colors at the boundaries in a particular order, or covering up the boundary with a black line. Obviously, such tricks are not available in printing real images, where every pixel may be different.

Printing hardware

The discussion so far of converting the image to CMY or CMYK values and superimposing them as separate halftone screens on the printed page has ignored the physical ways that such color printing is performed (Kang 1997, 1999). Few computer users have ready access to image-setters and offset printing presses with high enough resolution to produce such high-quality results. There is a considerable variation in the quality, cost, and performance of different types of desktop printers. Some of the more common currently available methods include ink-jet, thermal-wax, dye-sublimation, and color laser printers. A comparison of these technologies follows, recognizing that continuous progress in print quality is being made as many vendors compete for their slice of a rapidly growing market. In all of these comparisons, it is important to keep cost in mind. Many of the printers themselves have dropped significantly in price, but the cost of consumables — paper, ink, etc. — keep the overall cost of each copy quite high for several of these devices.

To assist in comparing the various printer types, **Figure 3.18** shows a portion of an image printed using several of the technologies discussed in this section.

Color laser

Color laser printers are the most economical for many applications because they use plain paper and have relatively high speeds. The higher initial cost of the printer is offset by very low cost per copy. They work by separating the image into CMY or CMYK colors and using each image to control the illumination of a separate charged drum that picks up the corresponding color toner and deposits it on the paper. One major design issue with these printers is the difficulty of keeping everything in alignment, so that the paper does not shrink or shift as it goes from one drum through a heater to bake the toner and on to the next drum. The use of a relatively thick paper with a smooth finish helps. In addition, the order in which the toners

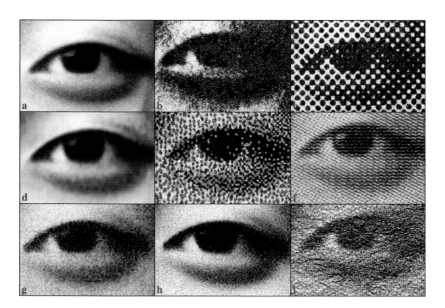

Figure 3.18 Magnified (30×) views of the same image printed using different devices: **(a)** photograph; **(b)** Xerox copy; **(c)** black-and-white laser printer; **(d)** dye-sublimation printer; **(e)** phase-change solid-ink printer; **(f)** color laser printer; **(g)** ink-jet printer in low-resolution mode; **(h)** ink-jet printer in high-resolution mode; **(i)** ink-jet printer using uncoated bond paper. (Courtesy of M. Jurgens, Queens University, Kingston, Ontario.)

must be applied is critical because, with most models presently available, the dots are not really laid down as a set of halftone screens at different angles (as discussed above). Instead, they tend to overlap each other, which makes it difficult to achieve good color saturation or accurate color blending.

Figure 3.19 shows an enlarged example of a color laser printer output. Note that the saturated colors such as red are formed by combining two toner colors (red = blue + magenta) and give good coverage of the white paper, but more subtle colors are not so clear and may appear muddy. In fact, a plot of the gamut (maximum saturation limits for colors) of this type of printer is not too meaningful because the most saturated colors are rather well defined, but the less saturated ones are not and are more difficult to distinguish from each other. Color laser prints are generally a marginal choice for image reproduction, although they may be satisfactory for reports or for computer graphics consisting primarily of saturated colors.

Dye sublimation

Dye-sublimation (or dye-diffusion) printers represent the high end of image quality available in desktop printers. They require special coated paper (or transparency material). The inks or dyes are transferred one at a time from a master color sheet or ribbon to the paper, with a typical resolution of about 300 dpi. A portion of the color ribbon as large as the paper is consumed in making each print, even if only a small amount of the color is needed.

The low resolution value of 300 dpi, as compared with 1200+ dpi for most of the other types of color printers described here, does not indicate the actual print quality because the print is formed in a different way. Rather than assembling tiny printer dots to build up the color, these printers can control the amount of each color more directly. The amount of dye that is transferred from the ribbon to each pixel on the hard copy is controlled by heating the print

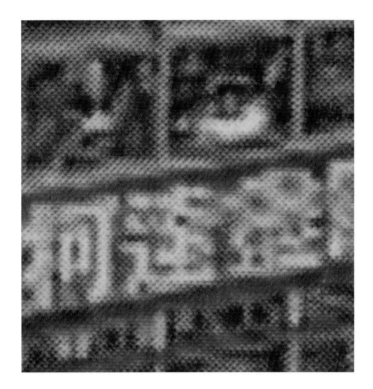

Figure 3.19 Enlarged view of color laser printer output, with areas of fully saturated and unsaturated colors.

head to sublime or vaporize varying amounts of dye. A control to one part in 256 is typical, although the use of a corrective gamma function for each color to balance the colors so that the print appears similar to the screen image (so-called color-matching) may reduce the effective dynamic range for each color to about 1 part in 100. Still, that means that about 1 million (100^3) different color combinations can be deposited at each point in the recorded image.

Dye-sublimation printers do not use a halftone or dither pattern. The dyes diffuse into the polyester coating on the paper and blend to produce continuous color scales. Each of the 300 printed regions per inch on the paper contains a uniform proportioned blend of the three or four dye colors. The lack of any halftone or dither pattern and the blending and spreading of the color dyes within the coating (instead of lying on the surface as inks do) produce an image that is very smooth and pleasing in its appearance. Magnification (**Figure 3.18d**) reveals the continuous tone and the just-visible pixelation pattern.

It is sometimes claimed that these printers are "near photographic" in output quality, but in several important respects that is not true. The saturation is less than that of a good photographic print, so that the color gamut is lower, and the 300-dpi resolution — compounded by the spreading of the dye in the coating — produces much poorer sharpness than a photographic print (which can easily resolve several thousand points per inch). This spreading is somewhat worse along the direction of paper movement than across it, which can cause some distortion in images or make some edges less sharp than others. On the dye-sublimation print, large areas of uniform or gradually varying color will appear quite smooth because there is no dither or halftone to break them up, but edges and lines will appear fuzzy.

In addition to these technical limitations, the relatively high cost of dye-sublimation printers and of their materials has limited their use as dedicated printers for individual imaging systems. At the same time, their rather slow speed (each print requires three or four separate passes with a different color ribbon or a ribbon with alternating color panels) has made them of limited use on networks or for making multiple copies. Still, they have been the preferred choice for making direct hard-copy printouts of images. Several very inexpensive snapshot printers (which produce 4 × 6-in. prints directly from consumer cameras) use this technology. They are even finding use in commercial outlets, where consumers can insert their slides or color negatives into a scanner, select the image and mask it if desired, and then directly print out a hard copy to take home. The glossy finish of the coated paper probably causes many customers to think they have a traditional photographic print, although the effects of temperature, ozone, and humidity on useful life are worse.

Dry ink

Some dry-ink printers (also called phase-change printers, since the ink is melted and transferred to the paper) and thermal-wax printers are used for printing images, although they are best suited to computer graphics because of their bright colors and glossy results. They work well on overhead transparencies, which are fine for producing business graphics presentations, but are not usually an acceptable medium for image processing output. The print head in a thermal-wax printer contains heating elements that melt the wax and transfer the color to the paper. This process is repeated for each color, which may cause alignment problems. In many cases, the dots are too large and the resulting number of shades for each color is too small, and the resolution too poor, to show details well in images. The image appears as flat, shiny plates of ink pressed onto but not into the paper surface (**Figure 3.18e**).

Ink jet

At this time, ink-jet printers are certainly the most widely used devices for producing hard copies of images. The printers are quite inexpensive (although the consumable supplies are not), and the resolution is quite high (many current models offer more than 1200 dpi). However, ink-jet printers are by far the most sensitive to paper quality among all of the technologies discussed here. Quality prints require a paper with both internal sizing and surface coatings to prevent the ink from wicking into the cellulose fibers (**Figure 3.20**), while promoting adhesion and providing a bright white background. Pigments such as $CaCO_3$ or TiO_2 also serve to whiten the paper. Surface coatings such as gelatin or starch are hydrophobic to prevent the ink from spreading, are smoother than the raw cellulose fibers, and can additionally be calendered (passed through a stack of high-pressure rollers during production) to provide an even more uniform surface. Inks must be carefully formulated with very tiny pigment particles (if these are used instead of dyes) to allow small droplets (the current state of the art is 1- to 4-picoliter drops for each tiny printer dot) to be uniformly and consistently transferred to the paper.

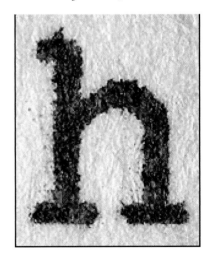

Figure 3.20 Wicking of ink on an uncoated paper.

Longevity of the prints is strongly affected by exposure to ultraviolet light, humidity, temperature, ozone, acidity of the paper, etc. Some manufacturers now offer "archival" quality inks and papers, meaning that the paper has a high pH (usually due to added alkaline buffers to reduce acidity that causes discoloration or physical deterioration of the paper) and a high rag content (fibers other than wood cellulose), and the ink contains pigments that do not break down with exposure to UV radiation. However, it should not be expected that even these prints will survive well for long periods unless storage conditions are carefully controlled. Achieving acceptable lifetimes for computer-printed hard copy continues to present challenges to equipment manufacturers. One of the recent novel developments to improve the lifetime of prints is to "print" an additional layer of transparent material on top of the colored inks to act as a sealant against oxygen and moisture. This also improves the visual appearance of the final prints.

There are two types of inks used in these printers, some containing pigment particles and others containing dyes. The inks containing pigment particles are less affected by paper variables (flatness, surface coatings, etc.) and suffer less environmental degradation by light, moisture, ozone, or other airborne contaminants. Hence, they are often called "archival" inks, although the actual life of prints and the resistance to color shifts during storage still depend upon storage conditions. The pigment particles are not absorbed into the paper or its surface coatings, which makes them more sensitive to smearing or scratching. Dye-based inks, which are more common, dry quickly, and because they are more reflective than pigment-based inks (which produce color mainly by absorbing light) produce brighter colors and a broader range of colors.

To expand the gamut of the printers, and to improve the ability to render subtle shades such as skin tones, many ink-jet printers now use more than the four CMYK inks. In a typical six-color system called CcMmYK, there are two less-saturated cyan and magenta inks available as well. Eight-color systems introduce less-saturated yellow and black inks, and other inks may be used in addition. Algorithms for converting the stored RGB values for each pixel to appropriate blends of multiple inks are complex, proprietary, and highly ad hoc. Many ink-jet printers offer multiple quality levels. The faster settings also consume less ink, producing acceptable draft images with less-saturated colors, while the slower settings are used for final copies.

In light areas of printouts, the individual droplets can be seen (**Figure 3.21a**). Ideally, these would all be perfectly round, identically sized, well-spaced color dots. In practice, droplet uniformity typically deteriorates rapidly as printers age; it is also affected by temperature and, of course, by the absorbency and smoothness of the paper being used. When more color is present and more different ink colors are used, they superimpose on each other and cover more of the paper, producing a darker image (**Figure 3.21b**). As noted previously, this is the opposite behavior to the appearance of the image on the CRT display, where more color produces a brighter pixel.

As mentioned previously, the gamut of a printer is usually described by an outline on a color wheel or CIE diagram of the maximum color saturations achievable, as shown again in

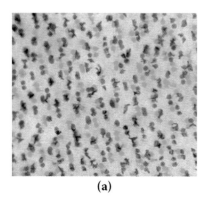

(a)

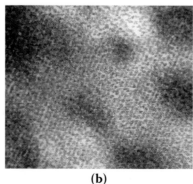

(b)

Figure 3.21 Magnified detail of ink-jet printer output (six-color CcMmYK inks):
(a) light area with well-defined separate dots;
(b) superposition of more colors produces greater saturation but covers more white paper, producing a darker result.

Figure 3.22. The actual situation is much more complicated because saturation varies with brightness, as noted previously. By printing out swatches covering the entire three-dimensional color space, it is possible to construct a more complete representation of a printer's gamut. **Figure 3.23** shows an example, for an Epson six-color ink-jet printer, using the L*a*b* representation of color space described previously. Printers with multiple inks can produce thousands of different hues and modulate colorant density to produce high tonal resolution and subtle difference in color. However, notice that, as with all such gamut plots, there are colors that cannot be represented on the hard copy.

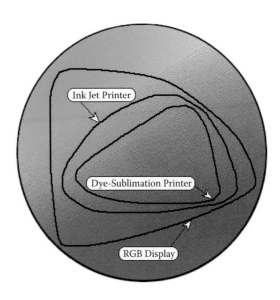

Figure 3.22 Color wheel comparing typical gamuts for ink-jet and dye-sublimation printers.

Ink-jet printers can also be equipped with a selection of gray inks that, when controlled by appropriate software, can do an extremely good job of printing gray-scale images. By selecting different ink densities as well as controlling the placement of tiny drops, a gray scale can be constructed that is very similar to photographic prints and has a very acceptable spatial resolution. Selection of papers with good surface finish is still important.

In summary, ink-jet printers offer hard-copy possibilities that rival (and in some cases surpass) the tonal range and resolution of conventional photographic materials. However, while the initial cost is modest, the per-copy costs are also comparable with photographic prints, and in many cases the longevity is a concern. Properly used, which implies the use of properly calibrated ICC curves specific to the inks and papers used, ink-jet printers are capable of very acceptable results and remain the first choice of many users.

Film recorders

In many cases, especially for color images, printing directly from the computer to paper is expensive and the quality limited. But the image looks good on the computer screen, and it is tempting just to photograph it from there to create slides or prints using conventional film methods. Certainly, this is convenient. I have hundreds of slides that I once used in lectures that were produced in exactly this way. (Today, of course, there are affordable compact projectors that connect directly to laptop computers, allowing for more convenient and higher quality presentations.) I kept a 35-mm camera loaded with slide film on a tripod near my desk. When there was something on the screen that might be useful as a slide, I just moved the camera into position and, with a permanent exposure setting of f8 at 1/2 second (for ASA 100 slide film), snapped the picture. You do need to make sure that there are no reflections of windows or room lights on the monitor. When the roll was finished, I sent it off and got back a box of quite useful slides. I have done this enough times to know that there is no need even to bracket the exposures. The exposure setting of f8 is about optimal for lens sharpness and gives

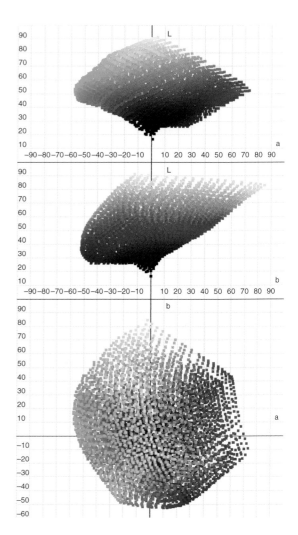

Figure 3.23 *Three-dimensional gamut for a six-color CcMmYK ink-jet printer, displayed as cross sections through L*a*b* color space. (From Rezanaka, I. and Eschbach, R.,* Recent Progress in Ink Jet Technologies, *Society of Imaging Science and Technology, Springfield, VA, 1996. With permission.)*

plenty of depth of field for the slight curvature of the computer monitor, while 1/2 second is long enough to capture enough full raster scans so that no visible line shows where the scan was when the shutter opened or closed.

While these pictures are fine for lecture slides, they are not useful for many other purposes. It is always obvious that they are photographs of the computer screen and not the actual images that have been captured or processed. This is due partly to the fact that they usually include the menu bars, cursor, and other open windows on the screen. It is possible to eliminate those, and many image processing programs have a "photo mode" that displays just the image with the rest of the screen dark.

Unfortunately, there are other clues that reveal how such an image is recorded. It is difficult to align the camera so that it is exactly perpendicular to the center of the screen. This misalignment produces a distortion of the image. In addition, the curvature of the screen causes a pincushion distortion of the image that is hard to overcome, and even with flat-screen displays there tends to be vignetting. Special cameras intended for recording images from computer monitors have hoods to shield against stray light and align the camera lens, and some even incorporate corrective optics to reduce some of the distortions and minimize these problems. Still, other more serious difficulties remain.

Most color displays use an array of red, green, and blue phosphors arranged as triads of round dots. The electron beams are focused onto the phosphors and are further restricted by an aperture screen (shadow mask) that prevents the electrons from straying from one dot to another. The other approach to monitor design, used in the Sony Trinitron®, has a single electron gun, no shadow mask, and the color phosphors arranged in vertical stripes. This design provides brighter images, since more of the screen is covered with phosphor and there is no shadow mask. On the other hand, the colors are less pure and lines or edges are less sharp, depending on their orientation. Varying the intensity of the electron beam controls the relative brightness of the phosphors and thus the resulting color that is perceived by the human observer, who blends the individual dots together. Modern computer displays have color triads with a spacing of about 0.25 mm. Human vision does not resolve these at normal viewing distances, so the colors are visually blended.

The image is made up of a regular pattern of color dots that the film records, perhaps with some systematic distortion due to the screen curvature and camera position. This pattern may be visible when a slide is projected onto a large screen. There is also a temptation to use these films to prepare prints for publication, an application that reveals their major flaw. When the prints are subsequently converted to halftones, the array of dots photographed from the screen interact with the spacing of the halftone screen to produce a moiré pattern that can be quite objectionable.

Film has high resolution, good color saturation and dynamic range, and inexpensive processing, which make it an excellent recording medium. But photographing a color monitor is not the right way to record the image. Dedicated film recorders solve the problems identified here by using a monochrome CRT with a continuous phosphor and a flat face. The continuous phosphor gives a very high resolution with no structure to cause moiré patterns, while the flat face eliminates distortions. With only a single electron beam, sharp focus and uniform intensity can be maintained from center to edges much better than with video displays; the fixed optics also provide sharp focus across the image with no vignetting or distortion.

A motorized filter wheel containing red, green, and blue filters is placed between the CRT and the camera. Software much like that used to drive a printer is used to separate the image into its red, green, and blue components, and these are displayed one at a time on the CRT with the appropriate filter in place. The much higher display resolution allows entire images to be displayed with full pixel resolution, which is not usually possible on the computer monitor (unless you have a very large one). The filter densities are adjusted to balance the film sensitivity, and all three color components are recorded on the same frame of the film. With most recorders, the entire process is automatic, including film transport and compensation for different film speeds and sensitivities (for instance, slide or print film).

The only drawbacks are the exposure time of several seconds and the delay until the film is developed, and of course the cost of the entire unit. The cost varies as a function of resolution (from 2,000 dots horizontally up to as much as 16,000 dots) and the flexibility to handle different sizes and types of film. High-end recorders are used to expose movie film frame by frame to produce movies containing "virtual reality" and rendered computer images (e.g., *Toy Story*), or to restore old classics by removing dirt and making color corrections (e.g., *Snow White*). Recorders that are price-competitive with color printers can be used for routine production of 35-mm slides. Nevertheless, the use of such recorders has not become widespread, and there is still a general preference for printing images directly onto paper.

Another option that can produce photographic prints from computer images is available from a growing number of online services. Photographic labs now offer very inexpensive conversion of uploaded image files to prints or slides. Most return the printed results within days via mail or FedEx. (Wal-Mart lets you pick up the results from your local store in one hour!) For many people, this is a viable alternative to maintaining expensive equipment, but the color fidelity is a variable that is difficult to control. The technicians handling the image files are used to dealing with conventional photographs of real-world scenes, and even then they make color adjustments that are not consistent from lab to lab or from time to time. The color information (such as the color-space description included in Adobe Photoshop®) is often ignored. Faced with scientific or other unfamiliar images, these labs produce results that often introduce color shifts. If you have spent time performing the color calibrations (discussed in **Chapter 1**) to match colors between your camera, display, and printer, it will be frustrating to get results from these labs that are different.

Other presentation tools

In addition to producing hard-copy versions of images to include in reports, another important use of images for publication is their inclusion in Microsoft PowerPoint® and other similar presentation tools. Unfortunately, this also presents several problems to the unwary user.

First, many image-analysis programs display images on the computer monitor with every pixel shown. A "100%" display of a megapixel image is necessary to reveal all of the potentially important detail, but such an image is likely to be larger than the monitor and to require scrolling to view the entire image. Many image-handling programs also record within the image file either the intended output size (in inches) for the entire image or the intended "dpi" (meaning in this instance the number of pixels per inch) with which it is to be printed. These are then used to control the output to the printer so that the proper result is obtained. But when the image is copied from that program and transferred to PowerPoint, that information is likely to be lost. Establishing the proper size of the image on the "slide" can be a problem because, unless a small fragment of the image is used, the image must be reduced in size to fit within the area of the slide, and that means that many of the pixels must be discarded as the image is sampled down to fit the required dimensions. Consequently, many of the details may not be visible in the presentation unless carefully selected regions of interest are chosen.

Second, the color balance and fidelity that was carefully achieved by calibration of the camera, CRT display, and printer (described in **Chapter 1**) resulted in stored ICC curves for those devices. But PowerPoint running under Windows does not use those curves for its slides, so the colors will be different in appearance than they were in the image-analysis program. (This is not a problem on the Macintosh, since ICC curves for the display are part of the operating system and not the responsibility of individual programs.) And unless the projector was also calibrated, it will not match the screen appearance of the images, either.

If images are incorporated in a presentation designed for delivery by HTML (hypertext markup language) documents via the Web, it is also important to remember that Web browsers generally do not respect or use ICC curves or any other form of color control. There are (only) 216 colors that are supposed to be standardized for Web browsers to use, but even for these the appearance on any particular user's monitor is likely to be highly variable. Distributing documents as pdf (Adobe Acrobat®) files is a better choice because it does provide some control over the color information, but you still cannot depend on the calibration of someone else's monitor or printer to view your images.

File storage

People working on a computer-based image-analysis system can save images as disk files. There seems to be no reason to consider these files as being different from any other disk files, which may contain text, drawings, or programs. In one sense this is true: files contain a collection of bytes that can represent any of those things as well as images. But from a practical point of view, there are several reasons for treating image files somewhat differently, because they require somewhat different storage considerations:

1. Image files are usually large. In terms of computer storage, the old adage that a picture is worth a thousand words is clearly a vast understatement. A single video frame (typically stored as 640 × 480 pixels) in monochrome occupies about 300 kB, while one in full color requires about 1 MB. With current digital still-frame cameras having well over 10-megapixel detectors — and with bit depths that require 2 bytes each for red, green, and blue — file sizes can be 60 MB or more. Desktop scanners produce even larger file sizes. A series of images forming a time sequence or a three-dimensional array of voxel data (which can be considered as a series of planes) can be far larger. A 500 × 500 × 500-voxel tomographic reconstruction requires 125 MB, or twice that if the density values for the voxels have a dynamic range that exceeds 256 levels. This means that the storage capacity must be large, preferably open-ended by allowing some kind of removable media, and reasonably fast. It also increases the interest in storage methods that use compression to reduce file size, and it makes it attractive to save reduced-resolution copies of the file (e.g., thumbnails) as rapidly accessible indices.

2. Imaging usually requires saving a large number of files. This reinforces the requirement for large amounts of fast storage, but it also highlights the need for fast access to the stored images. Constructing a database that can access images in a variety of ways, including showing the user small thumbnail representations through the use of keywords and other indexing tools, is an important need that has been recognized by many software producers. Automatically extracting classification data from the image to assist in searching is a more difficult problem.

3. Data management in the era of computers has not yet fully exploited the possibilities of coping with relatively straightforward records that contain text and numbers. The "file cabinet" metaphor is a poor and limited one. Search engines on the Internet compile lists of the words used on trillions of sites so they can produce fast results, but everyone who has used them knows that the process finds many extraneous sites and misses many of interest. Google now offers search-engine capability for an individual's machine, but it does not know as much about the images as the user. The real issue for computerized file storage is access to files and finding documents. The simple act of adding a field that can accommodate an image to a database primarily constructed to hold text entries does not transform the text database into an imaging database. For instance, keeping a picture of each employee in a personnel file may be worthwhile, but it would hardly allow a user to locate employees by knowing what they looked like or by having another photo of them. That would require looking at every image.

One type of database that involves images works in essentially the opposite direction. A geographical information system (GIS) stores multiple images and maps. These record different kinds of information, which is keyed to locations. There may also be text records keyed to those locations. By overlaying and correlating the multiple map representations, it becomes possible to compare the locations of features on one map (e.g., roads or buildings) with those on others (types of soil or vegetation, underground aquifers, etc.). There are important issues to resolve in constructing a GIS, since the various maps and images (including aerial and satellite photos) must be aligned and registered, taking into account their different resolutions. In addition, displaying such rich multidimensional data presents challenges different from those faced in most image databases.

There may be some other factors to consider in designing an optimum system for image storage. For instance, in forensic, medical, and some other applications, it may be important to keep a record of all accesses to the image and of any processing or editing steps that may have been applied. Also, some standardization of storage formats is important if images are to be shared between users or between different systems. Some users may want to archive images essentially forever but rarely access any particular image, while others may make continued and repeated accesses but be willing to discard images after a certain time (or when a project is completed). The data may be intended for access by many users, over a network, or be restricted to a single user. If a set of images is to be distributed widely as a permanent and unalterable resource for reference use, the requirements change again.

There are some beginnings of solutions to most of these problems and indications that many more will be forthcoming. The introduction of the Photo-CD format by Kodak indicates their expectation of considerable consumer usage of this type of storage. It is easy to imagine someone trying to find an old picture of "Aunt Sarah," for example. If the photo is stored as a faded print in an old shoe box, the searcher may have a rough idea of where to look in the attic for the box and then be willing to sort through the contents looking for the picture. But in the era of computer technology, it will seem natural that somehow the computer can find the picture just by being asked for it. Obviously, that is not a trivial task, but many companies are trying to respond to the challenge.

Storage media

Kodak's Photo-CD is an example of one kind of media that is being used for image storage. Actually, we will see below that Photo-CD also defines a storage format, not just the use of CDs (compact disks); it is possible to store images on CDs in other formats as well. Projects as diverse as archaeological digs, medical research, and remote sensing (satellite imagery) have found it convenient and inexpensive to distribute collections of images on CDs or DVDs (digital video disks) as a reference resource. The CD or DVD is just a plastic platter with reflective dots imprinted onto it, physically identical to audio and video disks. The format of the dots on a CD, which mark changes from 1s to 0s rather than the actual bit values, is shown in **Figure 3.24**. The encoding pattern used minimizes the number of pits that are required to store the original data.

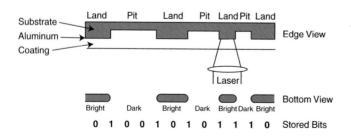

Figure 3.24 Storage format for CD data. Pits and lands in the aluminum layer reflect laser light, with the pits scattering the light and producing a darker reflection. Transitions from bright to dark indicate 1's and places where no transition occurs indicate 0's.

The reflective dots on a CD duplicated in quantity are physically imprinted in a pressing operation and covered by a hard plastic that is quite resistant to damage. This technique lends itself to creating many copies of a disk inexpensively. Current prices for making duplicates from a master are much less than a dollar per copy and continue to decline. Distributing a library of images in this way makes sense, as does distributing software, etc., since practically every modern computer has a reader for these disks and most can also read DVDs.

Data on CDs are written on one single continuous spiral track in blocks of 2048 bytes (plus the block address and some error-detection sums). The entire track is written at one time, which requires the data to be continuously supplied to the write head as the disk spins. The CD format is much more difficult to use as a random-access device for either writing or reading than a conventional computer disk with its multiple circular tracks and fixed sectors, which make locating particular blocks of data much easier.

Pressing CDs from a master creates pits in the plastic substrate that are coated with aluminum and then sealed with a protective plastic layer. The plastic layer not only prevents physical damage, but also prevents oxidation of the aluminum that would reduce its reflectivity. In a CD-R (recordable) disk, the writing is done by a laser whose light is absorbed in a dye layer. The dye decomposes and is deposited on the metal layer, darkens it, and produces the same pattern of reflective and dark regions that the physical lands and pits do in the pressed CD.

CD-R disks are widely used as "write-once" storage devices for archiving files. CD-R drives are inexpensive and can be connected to a computer just like any other disk drive (for instance, using a standard Firewire or USB interface); they are standard equipment on many models. Files are written to a blank disk that costs only a few cents. The writing process is fairly fast; with the 64X drive in the laptop I am writing this on, it takes only minutes to write a full disk. That disk provides storage of more than 600 MB; two such disks will hold this entire book. After it has been written, the CD-R disk can be read in exactly the same drive as a pressed CD-ROM, or used as a master to duplicate the more durable pressed disks in quantity. CD-R disks have become so reliable and inexpensive that many people, myself included, use them instead of floppy disks to transmit even small amounts of data when a physical disk is more suitable than transmission over the Internet.

Rewritable CDs (CD-RW) that use disks of the same size that can be erased and rewritten are slightly more expensive, but share the same problems of slow access speed and lose the advantage of being tamper-proof. Writable but not alterable disks are especially useful in situations (medical and forensic imaging are the most oft-cited examples) in which images must be stored permanently. Such drives are also used for financial records and other applications in which assurances are needed that data cannot be tampered with, either intentionally or accidentally.

DVDs offer a further increase in storage capacity. There are still some uncertainties about the format that will become the standard for DVDs, as manufacturers and content providers line up behind one or another proposal, but this should soon be resolved. In the meantime, DVD-R (DVD read) drives are built into many current computers, even laptops. The entire text and all of the 2000+ illustrations in this book were written onto a DVD-R for backup and for transmission to the publisher.

One of the limitations of the CD and DVD is that, in most cases, this writing operation must be performed in a single session. All of the files to be placed on the disk must be available on the host computer and be written at the same time, so that the disk directory can be created for subsequent reading. In creating the Photo-CD format, Kodak introduced the idea of multiple directories (or multiple sessions) so that a disk could be taken in to the photo finisher to add more images (e.g., another roll of film) to an existing disk. However, not all drives or software that can read CDs are able to access the additional directories, which appear as individual drives rather than one large volume, and there is considerable overhead (about 9 MB) associated with the directories for each additional session.

At present, the most practical use of CDs or DVDs for storing images is to produce entire disks of images or other data for storage or distribution. The images are archival in nature, since users are not able to modify them on the original disk. Reading from CD or DVD drives is generally rather slow. Even the newer drives that operate at 32 times (or more) the speed of the platter used for audio disks have reading speeds an order of magnitude less than a standard magnetic hard disk used in the computer. However, for accessing archival images, that speed may be quite acceptable. The time required to locate the correct disk is the principal impediment.

Magnetic recording

The most common type of hard disks in computers use magnetic storage. The disk platter (of glass or metal) is coated with a thin layer of magnetic material much like that used in audio tapes. Reading and writing are done using a magnetic head that "flies" just above the disk surface, riding on a cushion of air pressure produced by the spinning disk surface, which rotates at speeds from 4,000 to 10,000 rpm. There are exceptions to this method: some drives use a flexible polymer substrate more like simple floppy disks, with the magnetic head in physical contact with the disk coating. Such differences in design affect the long-term durability of the media, the reading and writing speed, the physical density of storage, and the amount of information that can be written onto a single disk. But from the user's point of view, the details of the design technology are secondary considerations.

Removable magnetic storage disks with capacities of several hundred megabytes were fairly common (e.g., the popular "Zip" disk) but are now largely obsoleted by solid-state memory devices (the most common are flash-memory devices that plug into USB ports, with capacities of 4 GB or more at the time of this writing). Removable types of storage are desirable because any conventional hard disk, even one with tens or hundreds of gigabytes of storage, will sooner or later fill up with images (usually sooner). Any system that is intended for serious image-analysis work is going to require some form of removable and hence unlimited storage.

The speed of access of a conventional hard disk is somewhat faster than the removable types and quite a bit faster than accessing data from a CD. Flash memory is also somewhat faster to read or write than a CD, and individual files can be added or removed just like an internal disk drive, but not as quickly. This speed difference makes it attractive to copy files onto a hard disk for access, and to write them to the removable media only when work is at least temporarily complete. With that approach, the hard disk serves as a short-term storage location for work in progress, but the removable media are still used to store images for long-term purposes. The hard disk is also the place where the computer operating system, and all of the various programs including those used for image analysis, are stored.

No consideration needs to be given to floppy disks because of their inability to hold large amounts of data. The typical diskette size of 1.4 MB can usually only hold one or a few images, and sometimes not even that. A single color image obtained from a color scanner with 600-dpi resolution (a relatively low level of performance), taken from an original 8 × 10-in. photograph, would require about 81 MB of storage. Such files are not conveniently stored on floppy disks.

Even a typical video image, requiring about 900 kB, takes up most of one floppy disk. That may be acceptable for giving one image to a colleague, but it is hardly useful for storage of many images, even ignoring the rather slow reading and writing speeds of these drives and the comparative fragility of the disks.

Tape drives are even slower. A single 4-mm tape, the same type of cassette used for digital audio recording, can hold several gigabytes of files, with a drive costing a few hundred dollars. But because access to any particular location on the tape requires rewinding and searching, these devices are really only useful for backing up a random-access hard disk. Saving a collection of images on a tape for archival storage might make sense, however, as it is less expensive than any other form of digital storage except CD-R. Generally, tapes are less robust than disks because they are subject to stretching even in normal use and can easily be damaged by mishandling.

Likewise, magnetic storage is generally less "archival" than optical storage because stray fields or high temperatures can cause accidental erasure. The CD has the best claim to be archival, but this claim applies only to the pressed disks; the CD-R recordable disks claim only a 5- to 10-year life with good storage conditions. Instead of using magnetic tapes and drives simply to back up a large disk drive, it is possible with existing software to treat the tape as though it were a large (and rather slow) disk, that is, to access files randomly. This requires loading into memory a directory identifying where each file is on the tape, which takes memory space. Also, the reading times are not suitable if the files must be accessed very often. But such a medium can be used as a large and inexpensive data storage medium over a network.

One of the most recent developments in storage is network servers with arrays of redundant hard disks (RAID storage) that work in parallel for extremely high speed with error protection. The transmission of large images over Ethernet or WiFi still takes more time than local storage, but the advantages of shifting the responsibilities for maintaining and backing up storage to the IT experts in your organization and the availability of images to all computers on the network makes this an attractive option in many situations.

If your purpose is archival storage of images, then regardless of what medium you select, you should prepare to invest in extra drives and interfaces. It is not likely that any of the current media will be readable by common storage devices in 10 years, so you will need to keep your own spare parts and working systems. The same is true of interfaces and networks: the SCSI and parallel interfaces of a few years ago have been replaced by USB and Firewire now, while Ethernet and WiFi have replaced token ring and AppleTalk®, and all of these may be replaced by other technologies within a few years. It may be difficult to transfer the images to the next generation of computers through different interfaces and networks. If you doubt this, consider the storage media in common use 10 to 20 years ago (8-in. floppy disks, mag-optical disks, Bernoulli and hard-disk cartridges, etc.), none of which can be read with any ease today. Storage media such as punched cards and DECtape, from 20 to 30 years ago, are unreadable except in a few very unusual circumstances because the machines are simply gone or in museums.

Another cost of archival storage is maintaining backup copies at some remote site, with appropriate security and fire protection, and having a routine method of storing regular backups there. It is really not enough simply to back up your hard disk to a tape or CD every Friday and drop the backup off in your safety deposit box on the way home, not if your data are really worth keeping for many years. This is certainly the case for remote sensing tapes (a good example, by the way, of the changing face of storage, as most of the early tapes can be read only on a handful of carefully preserved drives), medical records, and so on. For many kinds of records, and particularly images, photographic film is still the method of choice; it offers decades of storage, takes very little space, and can be accessed with standard equipment.

But for most people, the purpose of storing large numbers of images (certainly hundreds, perhaps thousands, possibly tens of thousands) is not so much for archival preservation as for access. The ability to find a previous image, to compare it with a current one, and to find and measure similarities and differences is an obvious need in many imaging tasks. Choosing a storage technology is not the really difficult part of filling this need. A selection between any of the technologies mentioned above can be based on the trade-offs among cost, frequency and speed of access, and the size of the storage required. The technical challenge lies in finding a particular image after it has been stored.

Databases for images

Saving a large number of images raises the question of how to locate and retrieve any particular image. If the storage uses removable media, the problem is compounded. These problems exist for any large database, for instance one containing personnel or sales records. But some unique problems are involved in searching for images. Database management programs are being introduced with some features intended specifically for images, but much remains to be done in this area. For example, Adobe's Bridge program displays thumbnails of each image and also has searchable metadata ("data about the data," or more specifically, descriptive numeric and textural information that accompanies the actual image), some of which can be specified by the user (such as slide identification, operator, magnification, comments, copyright information, etc.) along with system information such as date and time and image format details. It can also record the full details of all of the image processing operations that are performed on the image, which is important for many applications such as forensics. Measurement programs can automatically add parameter values (such as the number of objects present, measurement results, or color information) to that record, or access it to provide additional searching or classification possibilities. Extending the metadata to include things like the identity of anyone who accesses the file, or to tie in other kinds of data such as reading bar codes from microscope slides, is well within the capability of this approach but has not yet been implemented.

Most database management routines offer the ability to search for entries based on some logical combination of criteria such as keywords or the contents of search fields. For example, it might be useful to search for images recorded between October 1 and 15; from a camera attached to a particular microscope; using transmitted light through a 500-nm color filter; obtained from slide #12345 corresponding to patient ABCDE; etc. It might also be nice to find the images that contain a particular type of feature, for example satellite images of lakes within a certain range of sizes whose infrared signatures indicate that they have a heavy crop of algae.

The first of these tasks can be handled by many existing database searching routines, provided that the classification data have been entered into the appropriate fields for each image. The second task calls for much more intensive computer processing to extract the desired information from each image. It requires close coupling of the image-analysis software with the database management routine. Such a system can be implemented for a specific application (for example, the automatic scanning and screening of Pap-smear slides), but general and flexible solutions are not yet widely available despite considerable efforts.

Searching through multiple fields or lists of keywords is typically specified by using Boolean logic, for instance that the creation date must lie before a certain value AND that either one

OR another particular keyword must be present (and that multiple keywords must occur in close proximity in the text), but that the image must NOT be in color. These types of searches are similar to those used in other kinds of database managers and Internet search engines. A potentially more useful type of search would use fuzzy logic. For instance, looking for features that were "round" and "yellow" does not specify just what criterion is used to judge roundness, nor what range of numeric values are required, nor what combination of color components or range of hue values is sufficiently yellow.

Sometimes described as "query by image content" (QBIC) or "content-based image retrieval" (CBIR), this approach seeks to include visually important criteria such as color, texture, and shape of image objects and regions (Mitra and Acharya 2003; Pentland et al. 1986, 1994; Rui et al. 1999; Yoshitaka and Ichikawa 1999). Depending on the field of use, quite different criteria can be important for searching. For instance, in a medical application the user might want to find "other images that contain a tumor with a texture like this one" (which implies the concept of the object named "tumor," as well as the description of the texture), while in surveillance the target might be "other images that contain objects of similar shape to this airplane." Key issues for such a search include derivation and computation of the attributes of images and objects that provide useful query functionality, and retrieval methods based on similarity as opposed to exact match. Queries can be initiated with one or a few example images ("query by example"), perhaps with subsequent refinement. Effective human interfaces for such query systems are also in development.

In a search by example based on unspecified image contents (color, pattern, feature data, etc.), it is difficult to predict what will be considered significant by the procedure, so that "query by example" is an appealing idea, but it has many pitfalls. Consider the example in **Figure 3.25**: the image at upper left is provided as an example. A few of the responses are shown. But what is the actual intended target? Is the white feature on a pink background important (color is one of the easier things to pick automatically from an image)? If not, the search will have excluded many pictures from consideration. Is the white cockatoo with dark eyes and beak a good match? Not if you want just mammals and not birds. The white kitten is long-haired, like

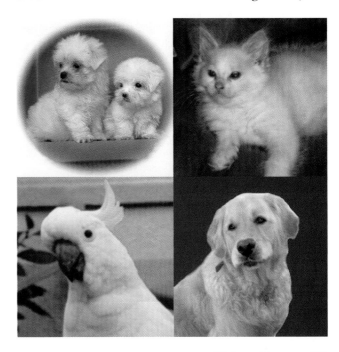

Figure 3.25 *"Query by example" results as discussed in the text.*

the puppies, but the Labrador is a dog rather than a cat. Or maybe it was the round shape of the exterior of the image that mattered, or the presence of two animals. And all of this presupposes that the search was confined to a database of animal pictures to begin with, or we might find automobiles, flowers, and so on, included.

Implementing a search for the example of "round" and "yellow" features would require first measuring a representative sample of features in the images in the database to obtain measures for roundness (perhaps the ratio of shortest to longest dimension, but other shape criteria are discussed in **Chapter 10**) and hue. Some systems also use spatial frequency data to characterize texture. Histograms of frequency vs. value for these parameters would then allow conversion of the adjectives to numbers. For instance, "round" might be taken to mean objects falling within the uppermost 5 to 10% of the range of actual values, and "yellow" the range of hue values bracketing true yellow and enclosing a similar fraction of the observations.

A program that might potentially be shown an example image and then told to search the Internet for similar ones is still far away. Part of the problem is that it is difficult to know beforehand what aspects of an image may later prove to be important. When we search through pictures in a shoebox, they vary widely. This usually allows them to be visually distinguished at a glance, but how will a search program know who Aunt Sarah is? And the meaning of the image content is also obscure except to a human with much additional background knowledge.

For example, **Figure 3.26** shows several images (from a total of more than 600,000!) found on the Internet (each from a different Web site) in a fraction of a second using a search engine

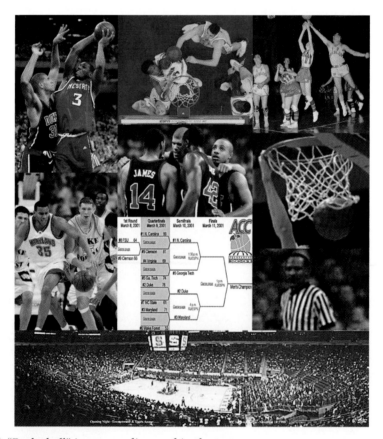

Figure 3.26 *"Basketball" images as discussed in the text.*

with the target "ACC + basketball + tournament + photo." Notice that several of the pictures show several players and the ball, but the uniform colors vary (and one image is not in color). Some do not show the ball, while one shows only the ball and net. Three show neither players nor the ball, but other things that are recognizably connected to basketball (a referee, a tournament bracket chart, and a basketball court). At the present and foreseeable state of the art, showing any one picture to a query-by-example program would not find the others.

An even more difficult scenario is present in many scientific imaging situations. There may be a very large number of quite similar images, such as liver tissue sections with the same colored stain from many patients, or satellite images of populated areas with many buildings, in which visual and machine methods of locating a particular image are hardly useful at all. A very experienced operator may be able to recognize some key features of interest, but not to describe them to the software in a meaningful or exclusive way. In such cases a search based on keywords, dates, patient records, location, etc., may be more appropriate. On the other hand, query-by-content systems have been used successfully for locating paintings and other artwork (Holt and Hartwick 1994) based on the artist's style.

There are several commercial programs that claim to offer some degree of search capabilities for images. By far the best known and most fully documented is the IBM QBIC system, a prototype development kit from IBM Almaden Research with more than 10 years of experience and development (Faloutsos et al. 1994; Flickner et al. 1995; Niblack 1993). It allows a user to query a collection of images based on colors, textures, shapes, locations, and layout. For example, "find an image with a green background and a round red object in the upper left." This and other similar systems first process the images in the files to extract information such as the histogram (for mean and standard deviation of brightness and hue), and to segment the image into homogenous regions for measurement of size and shape, and then search through these signatures for specific numeric values (Marsicoi et al. 1997).

A powerful approach to resolving fuzzy criteria into numeric values ranks all of the observations according to dimension, hue, or some other objective criterion and then uses the rank numbers to decide how well a particular object conforms to the adjective used. If a feature was ranked 10th in roundness and 27th in yellowness out of a few hundred features, it would be considered round and yellow. On the other hand, if it was ranked 79th in one or the other attribute, it would not be. Both of these methods ultimately use numeric values, but judge the results in terms of the actual range of observations encountered in the particular type of application. They do not use traditional "parametric" statistics that try to characterize a population by mean and standard deviation, or other narrow descriptors.

Fuzzy logic offers some powerful tools for classification without requiring the user to decide on numerical limits. However, although fuzzy logic has been enthusiastically applied to control circuits and consumer products, its use in database searching is still rather limited. That, combined with the time needed to measure large numbers of representative images to give meaning to the users' definitions within a particular context, seems to have delayed the use of this approach in image database management. Consequently, most searching is done using specific values (e.g., a creation date after December 1, 2005, rather than "recent") and Boolean matching with user-specified criteria.

Another search strategy uses vectors in n-dimensional parameter space (Kang and Leon 2005). Values for multiple measurement parameters are stored, and for a given target image, the nearest clusters, which have previously been indexed by the database program, are searched for the N closest matches. Each axis (or measurement parameter) can have different weighting applied to determine the n-dimensional distances.

Typically, it is up to the user to establish the criteria, measurement parameters, or other factors such as image metadata (magnification, patient records, date, etc.) that may be interesting for future searches before the database is established and the images are stored away. If the proper fields have not been set up, there is no place to save the values. It is impossible to overstate the importance of designing the proper search fields and lists of keywords or parameters ahead of time, and the difficulty of adding more fields retrospectively. There are no simple guidelines for setting up fields, since each imaging application has unique requirements. Establishing dozens or even hundreds of search fields with large numbers of keywords is a minimum requirement for any image database management routine.

Of course, it is still necessary to fill the search fields with appropriate values and keywords when the image is saved. Some of the fields may be filled automatically with things like date and time, operator name, perhaps some instrument parameters such as magnification or wavelength, location (this could either be latitude and longitude or coordinates on a microscope slide), and so forth. Even patient or sample ID numbers can in principle be logged in automatically; some laboratories are using bar-code labeling and readers to automate this function. Doing this at the time the image is acquired and saved is not too burdensome, but obviously supplying such information retrospectively for a set of images is difficult and error-prone.

However, the really interesting keywords and descriptors still require the human observer to fill in the fields. Recognition and identification of the contents of the image, selection of important characteristics or features while ignoring others, and then choosing the most useful keywords or values to enter in the database is highly dependent on the level of operator skill and familiarity, both with the images and with the program.

Not surprisingly, the entries can vary greatly. Different operators, or the same operator on different days, may produce different classifications. One method that is often helpful in constraining operators' choice of keywords is setting up a glossary of words that the operator can select from a menu, as opposed to free-format entry of descriptive text. The same glossary is later used in selecting logical combinations of search terms.

Values for measurement parameters that are included in the database can usually be obtained from an image-analysis program. In later chapters on image measurement, we will see that automatic counting of features, measurement of their sizes, location, densities, and so forth, can be performed by computer software. But in general this requires a human to determine what it is in the image that should be measured. These programs may or may not be able to pass values directly to the database; in many practical situations, manual retyping of the values into the database is required, offering further opportunities for omissions and errors to creep in.

Even in cases in which the target is pretty well known, such as examining blood-smear slides or scanning the surface of metal for cracks containing a fluorescent dye, there is enough variation in sample preparation, illumination conditions, etc., to require a modest amount of human oversight to prevent errors. And often in those cases the images themselves do not need to be saved, only the numeric measurement results. Saving entire images in a database is most common when the images are *not* all nearly the same, but vary enough to be difficult to describe by a few numbers or keywords.

A very different type of database uses the image as the organizing principle, rather than words or numbers. Numerical or text data in the database is keyed to locations on the images. This approach, mentioned above, is generally called a geographical information system (GIS) and is used particularly when the images are basically maps. Imagine a situation in which a number of aerial and satellite photographs of the same region have been acquired. Some of the images may show visible light information, but perhaps with different resolutions or at different times of day or seasons of the year. Other images may show the region in infrared bands or consist of range images showing elevation. There may also be maps showing roads and buildings, land-use patterns, and the locations of particular kinds of objects (fire hydrants, electrical transformers). Tied to all of this may be other kinds of data, including mail addresses, telephone numbers, and the names of people, for example. Other kinds of information may include temperatures, traffic patterns, crop yields, mineral resources, and so forth.

Organizing this information by location is not a simple task. For one thing, the various images and maps must somehow be brought into registration so that they can be superimposed. The resolution and scales are typically different, and the "depth" of the information is quite variable as well (and certainly consists of much more than a gray-scale value for each pixel). Finding ways to access and present this data so that comparisons can be made between quite disparate kinds of information presents real challenges. Even searching the database is less straightforward than might be imagined.

For instance, selecting coordinates (e.g., latitude and longitude) and then asking for various kinds of information at that location is comparatively straightforward. There are presently computerized maps (distributed on CD) that can be accessed by a laptop computer connected to a GPS (Global Positioning System) receiver that picks up timing signals from the network of satellites to figure out location anywhere on Earth with an accuracy of a few meters. That can obviously be used to bring up the right portion of the map. But if you are driving a car using such a system to navigate, your query may be to "show me the routes to follow to the nearest gas station, or hospital, or to avoid the 5:00 P.M. traffic jam and reach the main highway." Clearly, these questions require access to additional information on streets, traffic lights and timing, and many other things. And that same database can also be accessed by entering a telephone number or zip code. This is current technology; the promise is for much richer databases and more flexible ways to access and display the information.

Browsing and thumbnails

This section started out with the idea that saving images so that they can later be compared with other images is necessary precisely because there is no compact way to describe all of the contents of the image, nor to predict just what characteristics or features of the image may be important later. That suggests that using brief descriptors in a database may not provide a tool adequate to locate particular images later. Consequently, most image databases provide a way for the user to see the image, or at least a low-resolution "thumbnail" representation of it, in addition to whatever logical search criteria may be employed. In spite of the obvious difficulties of visually searching through thumbnail images of many images that share many similarities to locate a particular one of interest, this remains the most widely used approach (Hogan 2005).

Some approaches to image databases write the full image and one or more reduced-resolution copies of the image onto the disk so that they can be quickly loaded when needed. This may include, in addition to the full original copy of the image, a very small version to use as a display thumbnail for browsing, a version with a resolution and color gamut appropriate for the system printer, and perhaps others. Since most of the auxiliary versions of the image are much smaller in storage requirements than the original, keeping the lower resolution copies does not significantly increase the total space required, and it can greatly speed up the process of accessing the images. Kodak's Photo-CD is an example of a storage format that maintains multiple-resolution versions of each image. In some cases it is practical to use a lossy compression technique to save the lower resolution versions of the images to further reduce their storage requirements or to facilitate Internet transmission.

The reason for thumbnails, or some kind of reduced-size representation of the images in the database, is that allowing the user to "browse" through the images by showing many of them on the screen at the same time is often an essential part of the strategy of looking for a particular image. Indeed, one current approach to maintaining an image database provides access from any Web browser, delivering thumbnail views and limited keyword search capabilities simultaneously to many widely distributed viewers via Internet or intranet servers.

The difficulties noted above with keywords and multiple data fields mean that they can rarely be used in a Boolean search to find one particular or unique image. At best, they can isolate a small percentage of the stored images, which can then be presented to the user to make a visual selection. Even highly successful and widely reported search systems like the Automated Fingerprint Identification System (AFIS) rely on skilled human operators to review the 10 to 20 best matches found by the system based on measured values (the minutiae in each fingerprint) to perform conclusive identification.

Current facial-identification software similarly utilizes a set of 20 to 30 dimensional ratios (e.g., the ratio of the distance between the eyes to the distance between the tips of the ears, or the ratio of the distance from nose to upper lip to the distance from eyes to chin, both of which are relatively insensitive to the angle of view of the face) to select a small number of best matches from a database, and then present them to a human operator. The very limited success of these approaches to date is an indication of the difficulty of the task.

Browsing through images is very different from the search strategies that are used for most other kinds of data. It is common on most computer systems, either as part of the system software itself, or as basic utility routines, or as part of applications, to incorporate intelligent search capabilities that can locate files based not only on the values of data fields (e.g., a creation date for the file) or keywords, but also by examining the actual contents of the files. For instance, the word processor being used to write this chapter can search through all of the files on my hard disk for any document containing the phrases "image" and "database" in close proximity to each other, and then show me those files by name and with the phrases displayed in context.

That approach is possible because the files are stored as text. There may be special formatting characters present (and indeed, it is possible to search for those as well: "Find documents containing the word 'large' in Times-Roman italics in at least 14-point type"), but the bulk of the file content is a straightforward ASCII representation of the letters that make up the words and phrases. Searching strategies for text, including ignoring capitalization or requiring an exact match, and allowing for "wild card" characters (e.g., "find documents containing the phrase 'fluorescen# dye'" would find both fluorescent and fluorescence), are widely used. Much effort has gone into the development of efficient search algorithms for locating matches.

A relatively new development in text searches uses natural language rules to interpret the text. This search technique distinguishes among nouns, verbs, and adjectives to extract some meaning from the text. That approach, combined with the use of a thesaurus and dictionary so that words can be substituted, allows specifying target text by entering a few topical sentences, and then having the search engine look for and rank matches. There are also programs that can analyze the vocabulary used in a document, including the combinations of words and grammatical style, to identify the probable author of a document.

How can such techniques be used for images? Certainly there is no way to simply match a specific series of bytes. The image data are typically stored on disk as a sequence of pixel values. For many monochrome images, storage requires 1 byte per pixel, and the values from 0 to 255 represent the gray scale of the data. For images that have greater dynamic range, two bytes per pixel may be needed; some computers store the high byte and then the low byte, and some the reverse. For color, at least 3 bytes per pixel are needed. These can be stored with all three values in some fixed order for each pixel, or the entire row (or even the entire image) can be stored separately for the red, green, and blue values (or some other color-space representation).

There are dozens of different storage formats for images. Few image database management routines support more than a handful of formats, expecting that most users will select a format according to specific needs, or as used by a few particular programs. When images must be imported from some "foreign" format, it is usually possible to translate them using a dedicated program. This is particularly needed when different dedicated computers and programs acquire images from various instruments and then transmit them to a single database for later analysis.

There are a few relatively "standard" formats such as TIFF (tagged image file format) files that are used on several different computer platforms, while others may be unique to a particular type of computer (e.g., PICT on the Macintosh, BMP on the PC) or even proprietary to a particular program (e.g., the PSD format used by Adobe Photoshop). Every camera manufacturer seems to have created its own unique "RAW" format that holds the unmodified, high precsion values read directly from the detector chip, which are subsequently processed in the camera to produce the usual output. The widespread use of a program such as Photoshop can make its format a kind of standard in its own right. Some of the "standards" (TIFF is an excellent example) have so many different options that many programs do not implement all of them. The result is that a TIFF file written by one program may not be correctly read by another program that uses a different subset of the 100 or so options.

Some storage formats include various kinds of header information that describes formats, color tables, and other important data more or less equivalent to the formatting of a text document. Some compress the original data in various ways, and some of the methods do so in a "loss-less" manner that allows the image to be reconstructed exactly, while others accept some losses and approximate some pixel values to reduce the storage requirement.

For instance, the Macintosh PICT format is a lossless method that represents a line of pixels with the same value by listing the value once, and then the number of times it is repeated. For computer graphics, animation, and rendered drawings from drafting programs, this "run-length encoding" (RLE) method is very efficient. It is also used to transmit faxes over telephone lines. But it does not offer much compression for typical real-world images because groups of pixels are not usually uniform.

If compression of the data is present, the computer may be required to read the entire image file and reconstruct the image in memory before anything can be done with it. But even if the data can be scanned directly within the disk file, how can it be searched to locate a particular image based on the contents? There is not generally a specific sequence of pixel values along one line of the image (most images are stored in a raster format, as a series of lines) that is the target. There is not even usually a specific two-dimensional pattern of pixel values. Features in images are more irregular than that, and can occur in unexpected locations, sizes, and orientations.

Statistical averages of the image, as can be summarized in its brightness histogram, most predominant color, etc., may sometimes be useful, but they are rarely computed while searching for a particular image in the database. Instead, if such parameters are considered important, they are determined beforehand, when the image is stored, and written into specific numeric fields in the metadata so that they can be searched using standard logical tests.

There is one approach to data matching that is sometimes applied to this kind of searching. Cross-correlation of a target image with each image in a database is a way to look for images that are similar to the target, in a very particular sense. The use of cross-correlation is discussed and illustrated in **Chapter 6**, because it is usually implemented using Fourier transforms. These can be sped up by using dedicated hardware, but even so it can be quite time consuming to search through a large database for a best match.

One application of this approach is matching surveillance photos to identify targets of possible military interest. For example, cross-correlation of an aerial image of an airport against a database of images of airplanes, each type rotated in many different orientations, will match the type of airplanes and their locations in the image. For more diverse images, or ones containing features that are more variable in their shape, contrast, or color, this method is less suitable.

When images are stored in a database that extends over several physical disks, particularly when removable media are used, many of the images may not be accessible or online when the search is made. The usual solution to this problem is to keep the descriptive keywords and other search fields, plus at least a thumbnail representation of the image, in a file with the main program. This allows rapid searching to find a subset of the images that can be examined visually by the user. Since the program has the location of each image stored in its file, it can then request the user to insert the particular disks to load the actual images. Even with this approach, the search file can be quite large when hundreds or thousands of images are included in the database. The search file can itself require a large (and fast) disk for storage.

On the other hand, there are reasons why the search fields, keywords, thumbnails, and other ancillary information should be stored with the image rather than in a central data file. Such storage makes the file containing the image self-contained, so that it can be copied with all its information intact. It is also possible to maintain a record of who has accessed the image and when, or to keep a detailed record of whatever changes have been made to an image. Such information may be very important in reconstructing the history of processing an image.

Image database programs may also be required to limit access to images, for instance with passwords. A networked file server may allow one group of users to read images from the files, another group to add images to the database, and a third group to process or modify images. Since images are large, moving them across local area networks from a central location to many workstations is a far-from-trivial consideration. This is particularly a concern in medical imaging and remote sensing applications, where a large number of images are to be accessed by a moderate number of users.

Finally, the question for any image searching routine is just how it is to be used. Finding one or several images according to some criteria is usually not the end result but the beginning. How can the image(s) now be loaded into whatever program is to be used for processing or measurement? Some database management programs can act as a filter that is used by any program opening a file. This is convenient for loading images but may not lend itself to adding images to the database. Other management programs can simply locate the images and copy them onto a local disk (and perhaps convert their format or decompress them), so that the user can more easily open them into the desired application.

Lossless coding

There has already been some mention of image compression. This is desired for storage or transmission to reduce the rather large size of most image files, and is quite an active area of study. This section does not review all of the techniques for compression described in the literature (Barni 2006), since most of them are not implemented in standard software packages available for dedicated image processing. Most of the methods fall into just a few categories, and representative examples of each are discussed below.

There are two criteria by which image compression methods can be judged. One is the time needed to accomplish the compression and decompression and the degree of compression achieved. This is particularly important when images are being compressed for "real time" transmission, as in videoconferencing, or perhaps when transmitting large images via the Internet. The second criterion is the degree of preservation of the image. It is this latter area of concern that will be discussed primarily here.

The first and most important distinction between compression methods is whether they are lossless or lossy techniques. A lossless method is one that allows exact reconstruction of all of the individual pixel values, while a lossy method does not. Lossless methods, often referred to as image coding rather than compression, have been around for some time, with much of the original development being directed toward the transmission of images from the space probes. The communication bandwidth provided by these low-power transmitters did not allow sending many images from the remote cameras unless some method was used to reduce the number of bits per pixel.

A simple, early approach was to send just the difference between each pixel and the previous one (sometimes called "delta compression"). Since most areas of the image had little change, this reduced the average magnitude of the numbers, so that instead of requiring (for instance) 8 bits per pixel, fewer bits were needed. This is another way of saying that images are highly correlated. A histogram of the differences between adjacent pixels has a peak near zero and few large values, as shown in **Figure 3.27** and **Figure 3.28** for images that have different histograms of pixel brightness values.

Further approaches to compression used algorithms that examined several preceding pixels, predicted the next value based on some kind of fitting algorithm, and then just stored the

Figure 3.27 Example image ("girl") with its histogram, and the results of compression by calculating differences between each pixel and its left-hand neighbor. The original image has a broad range of pixel brightness values. The histograms of the original and compressed image show that the latter has most values near zero. Contrast of the displayed compression image has been expanded to show pixel differences.

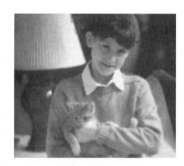

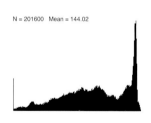

N = 201600   Mean = 144.02

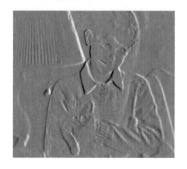

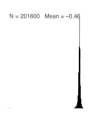

N = 201600   Mean = –0.46

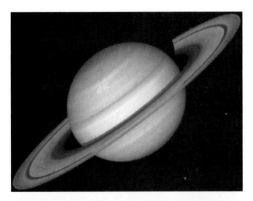
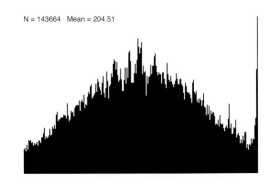
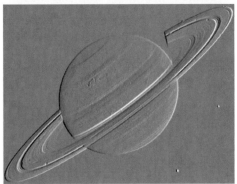
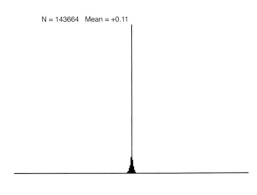

N = 143664   Mean = 204.51

N = 143664   Mean = +0.11

Figure 3.28 Example image ("Saturn") with its histogram, and the results of compression by calculating differences between each pixel and its left-hand neighbor. The original image contains many black pixels. The histograms of the original and compressed image show that the latter has most values near zero. Contrast of the displayed compression image has been expanded to show pixel differences.

difference from that. Advances on those methods use pixels on preceding lines as well, for further improvement in the predicted value and hence reduction in the difference values (Daut et al. 1993). Obviously, a method that looks at preceding lines is suitable for so-called progressive-scan imaging rather than an interlaced scan as used in broadcast television. Most of these compression algorithms were originally designed and utilized with live image sources. If the image has already been stored in memory, then the full array of pixels is available.

An additional refinement codes the differences between a pixel and either its predicted value or its predecessor more efficiently. For instance, in recording each wavelength band in images from the *Landsat* satellite, a 4-bit number is used for most differences, with two values of the 16 possible numbers reserved as flags indicating that a (rare) larger difference value follows, either positive or negative. An average of about 4.3 bits per pixel is needed to store the images, instead of the full 8 bits.

If further optimization is made to allow variable-length codes to be used to represent differences, storage requirements can be further reduced to about 3.5 bits per pixel for the *Landsat* data. One of the most widely used variable-length coding schemes is Huffman coding. This uses the frequency with which different gray values occur in the image in order to assign a code to each value. Shorter codes are used for the more frequently occurring values, and vice versa. This can be done either for the original gray values or for the pixel difference values. Huffman coding is also used for other types of data, including text files. Because some letters are used more than others in English, it is possible to assign shorter codes to some letters (in English, the most frequently used letter is E, followed by T, A, O, I, N, S, H, R, D, L, U). Morse code for letters represents an example of such a variable-length coding for letters (although not an optimal one).

As a simple example of the use of Huffman codes for images, consider an image in which the pixels (or the difference values) can have one of eight brightness values. This would require 3 bits per pixel ($2^3 = 8$) for conventional representation. From a histogram of the image, the frequency of occurrence of each value can be determined and, as an example, might show the following results (**Table 3.1**), in which the various brightness values have been ranked in order of frequency. Huffman coding provides a straightforward way to assign codes from this frequency table, and the code values for this example are shown. Note that each code is unique and no sequence of codes can be mistaken for any other value, which is a characteristic of this type of coding.

Table 3.1. Example of Huffman Codes Assigned to Brightness Values

Brightness Value	Frequency	Huffman Code
4	0.45	1
5	0.21	01
3	0.12	0011
6	0.09	0010
2	0.06	0001
7	0.04	00001
1	0.02	000000
0	0.01	000001

Notice that the most commonly found pixel brightness value requires only a single bit, but some of the less common values require 5 or 6 bits, more than the three that a simple representation would need. Multiplying the frequency of occurrence of each value times the length of the code gives an overall average of

$$0.45 \cdot 1 + 0.21 \cdot 2 + 0.12 \cdot 4 + 0.09 \cdot 4 + 0.06 \cdot 4 + 0.04 \cdot 5 + 0.02 \cdot 6 + 0.01 \cdot 6 = 2.33 \text{ bits/pixel}$$

As the number of values increases, the potential for savings using this type of coding increases.

Using software to perform coding and decoding takes some time, particularly for the more "exotic" methods, but this is more than made up in the decreased transmission time or storage requirements. This is true of all of the coding and compression methods discussed here and is the justification for their use. Information theory sets a lower limit to the size to which an image (or any other file of data) can be reduced, based on the distribution of actual values present. If, for example, an image consists of 256 possible gray levels whose actual frequencies of occurrence (taken from a brightness histogram of the image) are $p_0, p_1, \ldots, p_{255}$, then the entropy of the image is

$$H = -\sum_{i=0}^{255} p_i \cdot \log_2 p_i$$

$$(3.1)$$

Information theory establishes this as a theoretical limit to the number of bits per pixel needed to represent the image, and provides a performance criterion for actual coding methods. If this calculation is applied to the same example with eight gray levels as used above to illustrate Huffman coding, it calculates $H = 2.28$ bits per pixel as a minimum. Huffman coding is not optimal except in the unique case in which the frequencies of occurrence of the various values to be represented are exactly integral powers of $1/2$ ($1/4$, $1/8$, …). But this example indicates that it does offer a useful degree of compression with modest computational needs. Other coding techniques are available that can approach the theoretical limit, but simple methods like Huffman coding are often good enough to be widely used.

Table 3.2 lists the entropy values for a few typical images, which are shown in **Figure 3.29** along with their original brightness histograms and the histograms of difference values between horizontally adjacent pixels. Some of these images have large peaks in their original histograms that indicate there are many pixels with similar brightness values. This affects both the entropy value and, as discussed above, the generation of an optimal Huffman code. Notice the reduction in information density *(H)* as the visual appearance of images becomes simpler and larger areas of uniform brightness are present. Calculating the *H* values for the difference coding of these images reveals a considerable reduction, as shown in **Table 3.2**, averaging about a factor of 2 in additional compression.

Table 3.2. Entropy Values (Bits per Pixel) for Representative Gray-Scale Images Shown in Figure 3.27, Figure 3.28, and Figure 3.29

Image	H (original)	H (difference-coded)
Girl (Figure 3.27)	7.538	3.059
Saturn (Figure 3.28)	4.114	2.019
Bone marrow (Figure 3.29a)	7.780	4.690
Dendrites (Figure 3.29b)	7.415	4.262
Bug (Figure 3.29c)	6.929	3.151
Chromosomes (Figure 3.29d)	5.836	2.968

The entropy definition can be expanded to cover neighbor pairs by summing the joint probabilities of all pairs of two (or more) gray values for neighbors in the same way. This would apply if a coding scheme were used for pairs or larger combinations of pixels, which in theory could compress the image even further.

While it is unusual to apply coding methods to all possible pairs of gray values present, a related coding scheme can be used with images just as it is with text files. This approach scans through the file once looking for any repeating patterns of byte values. In a text file, the letter patterns present in English (or any other human language) are far from random. Some sequences of letters, such as "ing," "tion," "the," and so forth, occur quite often and can be replaced by a single character. In particular cases, common words or even entire phrases may occur often enough to allow such representation.

A dictionary of such terms can be constructed for each document, with segments selected by size and frequency to obtain maximum compression. Both the dictionary itself and the coded document must be stored or transmitted, but for a large document the combination requires much less space than the original. Compression of typical text documents to half of their original size is commonly achieved in this way. For small documents, using a standard dictionary based on other samples of the language may be more economical than constructing a unique dictionary for each file. Dictionary-based methods, known as a "Lempel-Ziv" technique (or

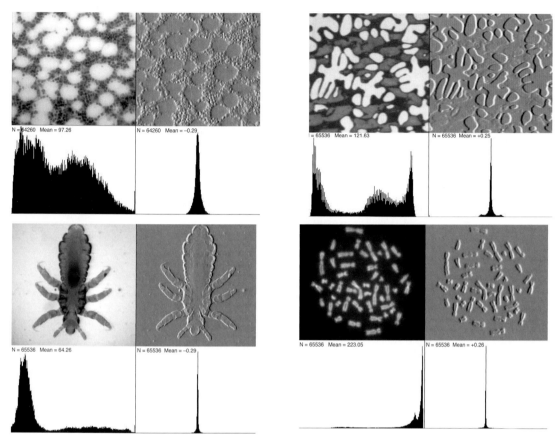

Figure 3.29 *Application of difference compression (autocorrelation) to various test images, with histograms of pixel values. The entropy values are listed in **Table 3.2**.*

one of its variants, such as Lempel-Ziv-Welch, LZW), are commonly used to compress text to reduce file sizes.

Applying the same compression algorithm to images, treating the sequence of bytes just as though they represented ASCII characters, is not so successful (Storer 1992). There are few exactly repeating patterns in most images; even small amounts of random noise cause changes in the pixel values. These noise fluctuations may not be important, and in fact it is easy to argue that much of this "noise" arises in the camera, electronics, and digitization and is not part of the scene itself. But our goal in coding the image is to preserve everything so that it can be reconstructed exactly, and there is no *a priori* reason to discard small fluctuations. Deciding which variations in pixel values represent noise and which represent information is a very difficult task. Because of these fluctuations, whatever their source, few repeating patterns are found, and the compressed image is usually not significantly smaller than the original.

A close cousin of these coding methods is run-length encoding. This was mentioned before as being used in some of the standard file formats. Run-length encoding (RLE) looks for any row of pixel brightness values that repeats exactly, and then replaces it with the value and the number of pixels. For natural gray-scale images, such rows do not occur very often and little compression is achieved. However, for computer graphics, drawings, and animation images, this method can achieve very high compression ratios.

Run-length encoding is particularly appropriate for binary (black and white) images. Fax machines use RLE to send images of pages containing text or images via telephone lines (see **Figure 7.46** in **Chapter 7**). Thresholding is often used (see **Chapter 7**) to reduce images to black and white representations of features and background. Such binary images can be efficiently represented by run-length encoding, and in addition the encoded image is directly useful for performing some measurements on images.

Most of the common image formats used in desktop computers and workstations are lossless representations of images. Some simply record all of the pixel values in some regular order, perhaps with header information that gives the dimensions of the image in pixels, the colors represented by the various values, or other similar information. Some use modest coding schemes such as run-length encoding to speed up the reading and writing process and reduce file size. Some, like TIFF or HDF (hierarchical data format, used for some scientific data files), are actually a collection of possible formats that may or may not include coding and compression, and have within the header a flag that specifies the details of the format in the particular file.

Fortunately, program users rarely need to know the details of the format in use. Either the images have been stored by the same program that will later read them back in, or several programs share one of the more-or-less standard formats, or there is a translation facility from one format to another within the programs or provided by a separate program. Quite a few such translation programs have been developed specifically to cope with the problems of translating image files from one computer platform or program to another.

Reduced color palettes

As part of the storage format for images, many systems try to reduce the number of colors represented within each image. One reason that color images occupy so much storage space is that three color components, usually RGB, are stored for each pixel. In most cases, these occupy 1 byte each, giving 256 possible values for each component. In a few cases, reduction to 32 gray levels ($2^5 = 32$) is used to allow reducing the storage requirements to 2 bytes, but the visual artifacts in these images due to the magnitude of the changes between colors on smoothly varying surfaces may be distracting. In some other cases, more than 8 bits per color component are used, sometimes as many as the 12 bits ($2^{12} = 4096$) that are generally considered to be required to capture all of the dynamic range of color slide film, and this of course represents a further increase in storage requirements.

Some images can be reduced for storage, depending on their ultimate use, by constructing a unique color-coding table. This allows each pixel to have a stored value from 0 to 255 and occupy 1 byte, while the stored value represents an entry in a table of 256 possible colors to be used to display that image. This method may seem to reduce the amount of information in the image drastically, but it corresponds nicely to the way that some computer displays actually work. Instead of a 24-bit display with 8 bits (256 intensity values) for R, G, and B, many low-cost displays use an 8-bit display memory in which each of the possible 256 pixel values is used to select one of 16 million colors (2^{24}). The palette of colors corresponding to each pixel value is stored with the image (it occupies only $3 \times 256 = 768$ bytes) and written to the hardware of the display to control the signals that are output to the CRT or other device. This is sometimes called a lookup table (LUT), since each pixel value is used to "look up" the corresponding display color. Manipulation of the same LUT to produce pseudocolor displays was described in **Chapter 1**.

If the LUT or palette of color values is properly selected, it can produce quite acceptable display quality for visual purposes. Of course, the selection of which 256 colors are to be used to show an entire image (typically containing up to a million pixels) is critical to the success of this method, and various algorithms have been devised to meet the need. The color triplet can be considered (as discussed in **Chapter 1**) as a vector in a three-dimensional space, which may be RGB, HSI, etc. The process of selecting the best palette for the image consists of examining the points in this space that represent the colors of all the pixels in the image, and then finding the clusters of points in a consistent way to allow breaking the space up into boxes. Each box of points of similar color is then represented by a single color in the palette. This process is usually called vector quantization; there are several iterative algorithms that search for optimal results, and all are rather computer-intensive (Braudaway 1987; Gentile et al. 1990; Heckbert 1982; Montagne et al. 2006).

Improvements in both visual quality and speed are obtained by using the YCC (broadcast video, also called YIQ and YUV) space, with the Y (luminance, or brightness) axis given more precision than the two chrominance signals (yellow-blue and red-green), because human vision is more sensitive to changes in brightness than in color. This is the same argument used for reducing the bandwidth used to transmit the color information in television. The scaling of the values is also nonlinear (Balasubramanian et al. 1994), corresponding to the response of the CRT display to changes in signal intensity. In other words, the goal of the color-palette compression is to reproduce the image so that visual observation of the image on a television screen will not show objectionable artifacts such as color banding. And for that goal these methods work well. But if any further quantitative use of the image is intended, the loss of true color information can create obstacles. It can even produce difficulties in printing the images, since the gamut of colors available and the response of the color intensities is different for printing than for CRT displays.

JPEG compression

Much higher compression ratios can often be achieved for images if some loss of the exact pixel values can be tolerated. There is a rich literature discussing the relative merits of different approaches. For instance, the encoding of differences between neighboring pixels can be made lossy and gain more compression simply by placing an upper limit on the values. Since most differences are small, one might represent the small differences exactly but only allow a maximum change of ±7 gray levels. This restriction would reduce the number of bits per pixel from 8 to 4, without any other coding tricks. Larger differences, if they occur, would be spread out over several pixels. Of course, this might distort important edges or boundaries.

Three approaches have become common enough to be implemented in many desktop computers and are fairly representative of the others. The popular JPEG (Joint Photographers Expert Group) standard is widely used in digital cameras and Web-based image delivery. The wavelet transform, which is part of the new JPEG 2000 standard, claims to minimize some of the visually distracting artifacts that can appear in JPEG images. For one thing, it uses much larger blocks — selectable, but typically 1024 × 1024 pixels — for compression, rather than the 8 × 8-pixel blocks used in the original JPEG method, which often produced visible boundaries. Fractal compression has also shown promise and claims to be able to enlarge images by inserting "realistic" detail beyond the resolution limit of the original. Each method will be discussed and examples shown.

The JPEG technique is fairly representative of many of these transform-based compression methods. It uses a discrete cosine transform (DCT) that is quite similar to the Fourier transform method discussed in **Chapter 6**. The JPEG standard is a collaborative effort of the CCITT (International Telegraph and Telephone Consultative Committee) and the ISO (International Standards Organization), and it actually comprises a variety of methods that are not explicitly intended for computer storage; the algorithm deals with a stream of bytes as might be encountered in image transmission.

The JPEG transform consists of several steps:

1. The image is separated into intensity and color channels using the YUV transform (shown in **Chapter 1**) and subdivided into 8 × 8-pixel blocks. If the image is not an exact multiple of 8 pixels in width or height, it is temporarily padded out to that size.
2. Each 8 × 8-pixel block is processed using the discrete cosine transform (DCT). This is closely related to the more familiar Fourier transform, except that all of the values are real instead of complex. The transform produces another 8 × 8 block of values for the frequency components. While the original pixel values are 1 byte = 8 bits (0, …, 255), the transformed data are stored temporarily in 12 bits, giving 11 bits of precision plus a sign bit. Except for the possibility of round-off errors due to this finite representation, the DCT portion of the algorithm does not introduce any loss of data (i.e., the original image can be exactly reconstructed from the transform by an inverse DCT).
3. The 64 coefficients for each block are quantized to a lower precision by dividing by a fixed table of values that gives the least precision for high-frequency terms. Adjusting the "quality" factor in most implementations increases the factors and reduces more terms to low precision or erases them altogether. This is the "lossy" step in the compression. In most cases, more precision is retained for the intensity or luminance than for the color data. This is because, in the intended use of the compression method for human viewing of images, it is generally accepted that more fidelity is needed in image brightness than is needed in color, as mentioned previously.
4. The first of the 64 coefficients for each block is the average brightness or "DC" term. It is represented as a difference from the same term for the preceding block in the image. The blocks are listed in raster-scan order through the image.
5. The remaining 63 coefficients for each block are scanned in a zigzag diagonal order that starts with the lowest frequencies and progresses to the highest. The entire data stream is further compacted by using a Huffman coding as discussed above. This step is loss-free.

The decompression or image reconstruction procedure reverses these steps to produce an image that is similar to the original image. Compression and decompression for the DCT are symmetric (same computational complexity and time requirements). Some other compression methods, such as fractal compression of images and MPEG (Moving Pictures Expert Group) compression of movies, are asymmetric and take much longer to achieve the compression than is needed for decompression during playback.

The loss of high-frequency terms results in some image defects and distortions. Since the loss of precision depends on the magnitude of the values, results are different in the various 8 × 8-pixel blocks in the original image, and the exact nature of the defects will vary from place to place. In general, sharp boundaries, edges, corners, and lines require the highest frequencies to accurately reproduce, and it is these that will show the greatest degradation. The results will depend on exactly where the line or corner lies with respect to the 8 × 8-block boundaries. An

8×8 block of pixels with a uniform gray value would be compressed to a single coefficient that would be accurately encoded, and all of the remaining coefficients would actually be zero so that no loss would occur. Small deviations from this uniform gray might or might not be preserved.

There are several ways in which JPEG, or any other similar approach based on transforms, can be improved. One is to choose the best possible color space in which to represent the image before starting. For instance, Photo-CD (discussed below) uses the CIE color space, while JPEG uses YCC. Second, instead of dividing the image into nonoverlapping tiles, a system using blocks that overlap in both the horizontal and vertical directions can suppress some of the artifacts that appear at block boundaries (Young and Kingsbury 1993). Third, and perhaps most important, the quantization of terms can be made more flexible. Different scaling factors can be used for each color channel or for different colors, for different frequencies, and perhaps different directions, depending on the intended use of the image (for viewing, printing, etc.). These methods can improve the reconstructed image quality at a given level of compression, with no change in reconstruction time. The JPEG 2000 standard, which is widely but not universally now in use, extends the original JPEG method in several ways: images with more than 8 bits per channel are accommodated, the tile size is made variable instead of being fixed at 8×8 pixels, and the wavelet transform is included.

The use of JPEG compression — or indeed any "lossy" compression technique for images — should be restricted to images intended for visual examination and printing, and it should not be used for images intended for measurement and analysis (Russ 1993a). This is true even for relatively high "quality" settings that result in only modest compression. At high compression settings, even visual examination of images can be affected due to aliasing of edges and lines, loss of resolution, and suppression of contrast.

Figure 3.30 shows a real-world image that has been JPEG-compressed by about 30:1 and then reconstructed. The major features are still quite recognizable, but upon closer inspection there are many artifacts present. Besides the blocky appearance, fine details are missing or altered. There has also been a slight shift in the colors present. For measurement purposes, the image fidelity has been seriously compromised. **Figure 3.31** shows a much simpler test image and the results of compression. As the degree of compression is increased, the artifacts become more and more serious until the figure is entirely unrecognizable or unusable.

All of the commonly used compression methods take advantage of the fact that human vision tolerates (and detects) less spatial resolution in the color information than in the brightness. This provides a useful way to detect whether compression has been applied. **Figure 3.32** shows the hue channel from the images from **Figure 3.30**; the uncompressed image has values of hue that vary from pixel to pixel, while the compressed version shows the loss of spatial resolution in the color data.

JPEG compression has been accepted for use in consumer applications and for transmission of images on the Web primarily because most images contain a wealth of redundant information, and human vision and understanding can recognize familiar objects in familiar settings based on only a few clues. For scientific imaging purposes the artifacts introduced by lossy compression are unacceptable. **Figure 3.33** shows an example. The image of the film has been compressed by less than 17:1 and visually appears little changed, but a plot of the average intensity across the film shows that minor peaks have been completely eliminated.

The proprietary Kodak Photo-CD algorithm is also a transform method that shares many of the same advantages and drawbacks as the JPEG method. Because it is intended to work from traditional photographic materials, which have a wide latitude, Photo-CD makes some provision

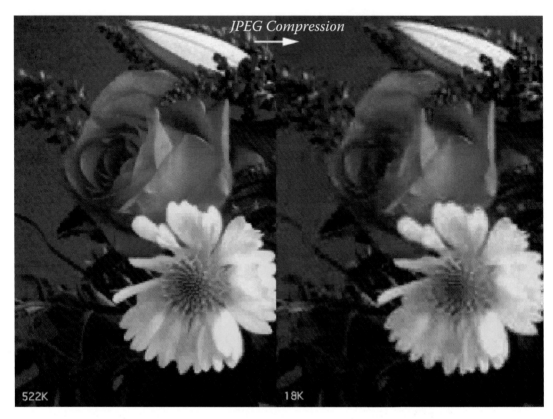

Figure 3.30 Example image ("flowers") and the reconstruction after JPEG compression by a factor of 29:1. Note the differences in highly textured areas at the center of each flower, artifacts along edges of petals, and the discontinuity in the stem at the left.

for the extended range that is often present in such images. Whereas JPEG separates the image first into HSI components, as discussed in **Chapter 1**, Photo-CD uses a modification of the YCC format used for broadcast television, which has one luminance (Y) and two chrominance (C_1 and C_2 or U and V) components (one the red-green balance and the other the yellow-blue balance). However, they cover an extended range in which $Y' = 1.36 \cdot Y$, and the modified C' components are related to RGB by

$$R = Y' + C_2'$$
$$G = Y' - 0.194 \cdot C_1' - 0.509 \cdot C_2' \qquad (3.2)$$
$$B = Y' + C_1'$$

When each of these is mapped to a 256-level (1 byte) value, a nonlinear relationship is used, as shown in **Figure 3.34**. In addition to mapping the film density to the output of a typical CRT display for viewing of the stored image, this method allows recording information beyond the nominal 100% white, which gives visually important highlights to reflections and other features that can be recorded by film, but not by most CCD (charge-coupled device) cameras. However, these differences do not alter the basic similarity of approach, fidelity, and efficiency that Photo-CD shares with JPEG.

Judging the quality of compressed and restored images is not a simple matter. Calculating the statistical differences between the original pixel values and the reconstructed values is often used, but this does not provide a measure that agrees very well with human judgment or with

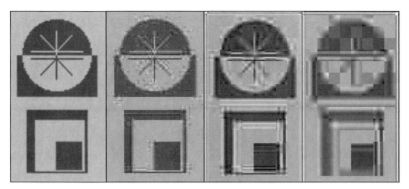

Figure 3.31 *A test pattern and the result of JPEG compression by factors of 3.5:1, 5.8:1, and 7.9:1 (from left to right).*

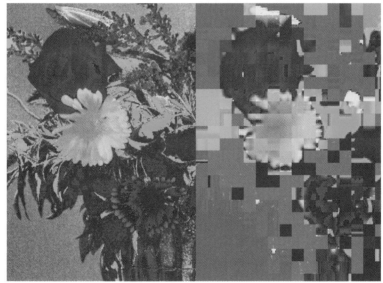

Figure 3.32 *Hue channels from the images in* **Figure 3.30***. The original image (left) has hue values that vary from pixel to pixel, while in the compressed image the hue values are uniform over larger regions.*

the needs of image measurement and analysis. As discussed in **Chapter 2**, human vision responds differently to the same absolute variation between pixels, depending on whether they lie in light or dark areas of the image. Differences are usually more objectionable in the dark areas, because of the logarithmic response of human vision. Differences are also judged as more important in regions that are smooth, or strongly and regularly patterned, than in areas that are perceived as random. Displacing an edge or boundary because of pixel differences is usually considered more detrimental than a similar brightness change in the interior of a feature.

Ranking of image quality by humans is often employed to compare different methods, but even with careful comparisons the results are dependent on lighting conditions, the context of the image and others that have been seen recently, and fatigue. It was the result of extensive human comparisons that led to the selection of the JPEG standard that is now widely implemented. The JPEG method is one of many that rely on first transforming the image from the

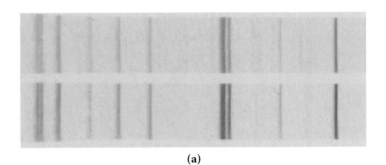

(a)

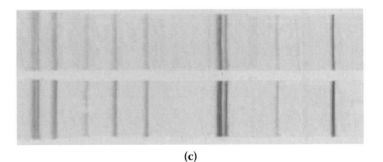

154

036 N = 598 Mean = 49.16 Width = 8

(b)

Figure 3.33 Image of a Debye-Scherer X-ray film before **(a)** and after **(c)** JPEG compression (from 136.3 kB to 8.1 kB). The position and density of the vertical lines provide information about crystallographic structure. A plot of the density profile across the images (images **[b]** and **[d]**, respectively) shows that statistical noise in the spectrum has been removed along with some small peaks, and a new artifact peak introduced, by the compression.

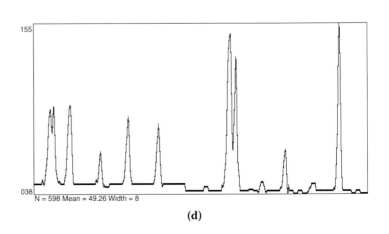

(c)

155

038 N = 598 Mean = 49.26 Width = 8

(d)

familiar spatial domain to another one that separates the information present according to a set of basis functions.

Wavelet compression

The virtue of transforming the image into another space is that it collects the information in a different way. The Fourier method (and its close cousin the DCT used in JPEG compression) separates the information present according to frequency and orientation. If a complete set of these functions is used, it can exactly and completely reconstruct the original image. So using the transform by itself is not a lossy method. But if the complete set of functions is used, the numbers required to specify the magnitude and phase take up just as much storage space as the original image. In

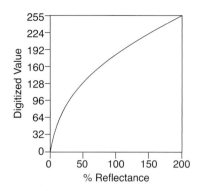

Figure 3.34 Nonlinear encoding of brightness and extended luminance range used in Kodak's Photo-CD format.

fact, usually they take up more because the magnitude and phase values are real numbers, and the original pixel values are likely to have been integers that require less storage space.

There are of course many other sets of basis functions besides the sinusoid functions used in the Fourier approach. Some provide a more efficient representation of the image, in which more of the terms are very small, while some are simply easier to compute. One of the more recently popular methods is the wavelet transform, which offers some computational advantages and can even be obtained optically with lenses and masks (McAulay et al. 1993) or electronically with a filter bank.

The wavelet transform provides a progressive or "pyramidal" encoding of the image at various scales, which is more flexible than conventional windowed approaches like the Fourier transform. The wavelets comprise a normalized set of orthogonal functions on which the image is projected (Chui 1992). The wavelet functions are localized rather than extending indefinitely beyond the image as sinusoids do, so the wavelet transform tends to deal better with the edges of regions and of the image, and its use for compression avoids the "blockiness" or "quilting" sometimes seen in JPEG compression, where the image is subdivided into 8 × 8-pixel blocks before performing a discrete cosine transform.

There are several different wavelet functions commonly used. The simplest is the Haar, which is just a square step, as shown in **Figure 3.35**, that can be shifted across the image and expanded horizontally. Other wavelet functions, such as the Daubechies order-4 wavelet shown, are less obvious but work the same way and may reduce visual artifacts when compression is performed as described below (Welstead 1999). Just as the Fourier summation of sinusoids

Figure 3.35
  Two examples of mother wavelets:
  (a) Haar;
  (b) Daubechies D4.

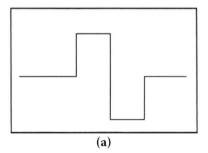

(a)

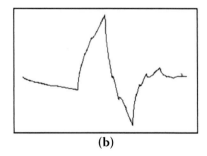

(b)

can be used to reconstruct any arbitrary function, so can the summation of wavelet functions (Daubechies 1992, 1996; Mallat 1989).

To understand the process of the wavelet transform using the Haar functions, consider the following process. First, find the average intensity for the entire image and put this value into a single pixel in the upper left corner of the transform (which will be the same size as the original). Now subdivide the image into quadrants and find the difference between the average values of each quadrant and the global mean. Place these values into a 2 × 2 block of pixels. Similarly, place the difference between each of the two left-hand quadrants and the corresponding right-hand quadrants into one pixel, and then place the vertical differences into one pixel each, as shown in **Figure 3.36**. Repeat this process by subdividing the quadrants, and continue until the individual pixels have been reached.

It is clear that the squares and rectangles in the transform that contain the higher frequency differences (which lie downward and to the right) are much larger and represent much more data than those corresponding to low-frequency information. The subdividing process amounts to working with higher and higher frequencies in the original image, and the reconstruction of the original image can be carried out using selected frequencies. **Figure 3.37** shows the process of reconstruction of the image in **Figure 3.36** by adding back the differences between pixels at progressively smaller steps. The process reconstructs the original image exactly, with-

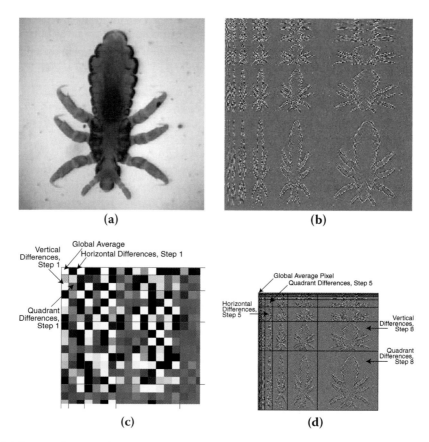

Figure 3.36 *The wavelet transform process applied to an example image ("Bug"). The transform (b) consists of the differences between average values at different scales. These are marked and labeled for the upper left corner of the transform (c) and for the entire transform (d).*

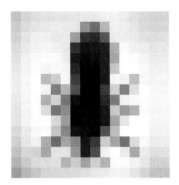
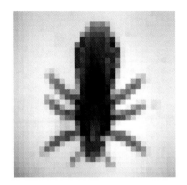
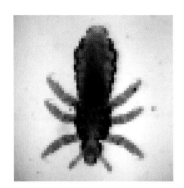

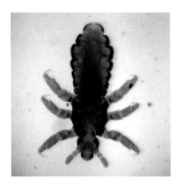

Figure 3.37 Reconstruction (inverse wavelet transform) adds in each higher frequency term successively. In the example, steps 4, 5, 6, and 7 are shown. Step 8 gives back the original image in this case (the dimension, 256 pixels, equals 2^8).

out loss. Applications of this approach to a wide variety of time- and space-dependent signals are taking advantage of its efficiency and compactness. In some cases, analysis of the coefficients can provide information about the image content, just as is commonly done with the Fourier transform.

In principle, all of these transforms take up just as much space as the original, and are loss-free. To achieve compression, the coefficients in the transform are quantized, just as for the JPEG cosine transform. Lossy compression of the image is accomplished by quantizing the magnitudes of the various terms in the transform so that they can be represented with fewer bits and by eliminating those that are very small. This can reduce the amount of space required, but also produces loss in the quality of the reconstructed image and introduces various artifacts.

Filtering selective frequencies using the wavelet transform is accomplished by reducing or eliminating some of the values from corresponding portions of the transform. This is analogous to filtering in Fourier space, discussed in **Chapter 6**.

Figure 3.38 shows the flowers image from **Figure 3.30** after wavelet compression (by a factor of only 6:1). Although the artifacts in the reconstructed image are not visually objectionable, examining the difference between the original and the compressed image reveals many differences in detail, such as color variations and shifts in the location of edges, that would seriously impact quantitative measurements.

The justification for compression is that the loss of particular terms from the transform may not be visible or at least not be objectionable to a human viewer, because the information each term represented was spread throughout the entire image and may have contributed little to any particular feature. This is not always the case. The selection of terms with a small amplitude often means the elimination of high-frequency information from the image, and this may

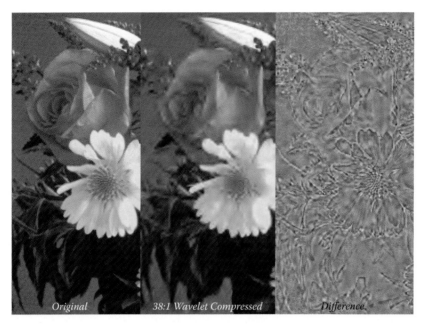

Original   38:1 Wavelet Compressed   Difference

Figure 3.38 *Wavelet transform applied to the "Flowers" image from* **Figure 3.30**. *Subtracting the original from the reconstructed image shows the differences, which are greatest in those areas of the image with more detail.*

be important to define edges and boundaries in particular. Just as the most visually objectionable defect in the JPEG cosine transform is "blocky" artifacts, so the most annoying aspect of the wavelet transform is that details are suppressed more in "busy" parts of the image, making it difficult to predict what details will survive and those that will not.

Compression using lossy methods is often suitable for images to be used in particular applications such as printing, in which the printing device itself may set an upper limit to the fidelity that can be reproduced. It has already been suggested that one use of compression could be to store multiple copies of an image in a database, each with appropriate quality for a specific purpose such as printing or viewing as a thumbnail for searching and recognition. It is also important to determine just how much loss of quality is produced by varying degrees of image compression so that artifacts capable of altering the analysis of reconstructed images are avoided.

Another application in which compression is normally used (wavelet compression, in fact) is fingerprint files, used by law enforcement agencies for identification. The spacing of the friction ridges on fingertips varies only slightly from one individual to another, so the corresponding set of frequencies is preserved while lower frequencies (e.g., due to shading in the image) and higher frequencies (e.g., due to noise or dust) are discarded.

Fractal compression

Barnsley (Barnsley and Hurd 1993) has shown another way to transform an image, using what are often referred to as self-affine distortions of the image (shrinking and displacing copies of the original) as the basis functions. In principle, a complete set of these operations would give a set of parameters as large as the original image. But for many images, a small number of functions are required to reconstruct the original image with acceptable fidelity, providing significant compression. A well-known example of this self-affine image generation is the fern produced by iteratively combining smaller copies of the same basic shape.

The four rules in **Table 3.3** are able to generate a realistic image of a fern. Each rule corresponds to one rotation, displacement, and shrinkage of a subelement of the structure. The rules are applied by starting at any point, selecting one of the rules (with the frequency shown by the probability values, from 1 to 84%), and then moving from the current point to the next point according to the rule. This point is plotted and the procedure iterated to produce the entire figure. The more points, the better the definition of the result, as shown in **Figure 3.39**. The entire fern with 20,000 points shows the self-similarity of the overall shape. As a portion of the image is blown up for examination, more points are required. Finally, the limit of magnification is set by the numerical precision of the values in the computer, as indicated in the figure.

From a mathematical point of view, the four transformations are basis functions or mappings that can be added together in proportion (the p or probability values) to produce the overall object. The same principle has been applied to the compression of photographic images with gray-scale or color pixels, where it is known as the "collage theorem." That there must be such basis functions, or rules for the self-affine distortions, and that they are in principle discoverable is known (Barnsley 1988; Barnsley et al. 1986; Barnsley and Hurd 1993; Barnsley and Sloan 1991; Khadivi 1990). The problem of finding the correct mappings is, however, far from

Table 3.3. Transformations (Basis Functions) for the Fern Image (Figure 3.39)

1	$(p = 0.840)$	$x' = +0.821x + 0.845y + 0.088$
		$y' = +0.030x - 0.028y - 0.176$
2	$(p = 0.075)$	$x' = -0.024x + 0.074y + 0.470$
		$y' = -0.323x - 0.356y - 0.260$
3	$(p = 0.075)$	$x' = +0.076x + 0.204y + 0.494$
		$y' = -0.257x + 0.312y - 0.133$
4	$(p = 0.010)$	$x' = +0.000x + 0.000y + 0.496$
		$y' = +0.000x + 0.172y - 0.091$

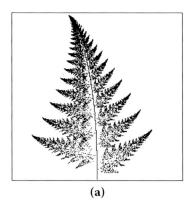

(a)

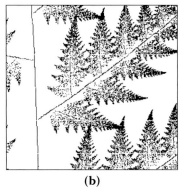

(b)

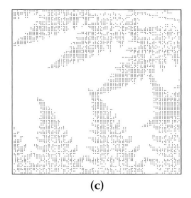

(c)

Figure 3.39 *Image of a fern generated with the four transformation rules shown in* **Table 3.3**. *The structure remains self-similar when expanded, except for the limitation of finite numerical precision in the computer, which rounds off the values in the 100×-expanded image: (a) fern image with 20,000 points; (b) 5× expansion; (c) 100× expansion.*

trivial. Knowing that such functions must exist gives few leads to discovering them. Each mapping consists of a combination of translation, scaling, rotation, and warping. One proprietary method for finding them has been patented (Barnsley and Sloan, U.S. patent no. 5065447). There are formal procedures for performing fractal compression (Fisher et al. 1992; X. Wu et al. 2005), although the results are not necessarily optimal. It has been shown that nonlinear self-affine transforms can also be used and may be more efficient.

This technique is described as "fractal compression" because the reconstruction is carried out iteratively (as shown for the fern) and because it provides ever finer levels of detail. In fact, the method can be continued to produce reconstructed images with detail at a much finer scale than the original used to find the basis functions. Such detail looks very impressive, since the enlarged image never shows flat or smooth areas that indicate loss of resolution. Of course, the detail is not real. It is generated under the assumption that whatever patterns are present at large scale in the image are also present with progressively less amplitude at all finer scales.

Unlike the JPEG and wavelet methods, fractal compression is not symmetrical. The time needed to compress the image is typically much greater than that needed to reconstruct it. Fractal compression also has characteristic artifacts. **Figure 3.40** shows the "Flower" image again, after a 40:1 fractal compression. Subtracting the original from the reconstructed image shows that the colors have been significantly altered, features have been shifted in position, and details inserted that were not present in the original.

Digital movies

There is growing interest in using small computers to produce, edit, and display digital moving pictures. Two emerging standards (or sets of standards) are Apple's QuickTime and Microsoft's Video for Windows. Both of these methods allow the use of various compression techniques, usually called codecs (compressor-decompressor). A codec is a program implementation of one of the compression algorithms such as those described above. In fact, JPEG is one of the methods provided by currently existing codecs available for both QuickTime and Video for Windows. Most of the codecs run in software only, while a few use additional hardware to gain real-time speed. For JPEG, this can be either a digital-signal-processor chip programmed

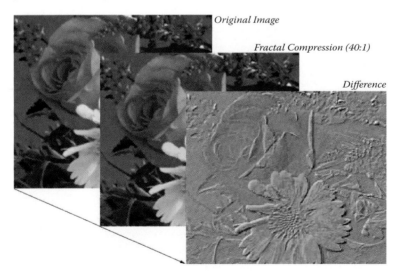

Original Image

Fractal Compression (40:1)

Difference

Figure 3.40 Fractal compression of the "Flowers" image from Figure 3.30. Color changes, shifts in position of features, and insertion of detail are all evident in the difference image.

to execute the discrete cosine transform or a dedicated chip designed specifically for the JPEG algorithm.

However, the JPEG method does not provide as much compression for digital movies as is needed to compress an entire movie onto a single CD-ROM, to broadcast high-definition television (HDTV) images, or to allow digital videoconferencing with images transmitted over relatively low-bandwidth networks because it does not take into account the considerable redundancy of sequential images. In most cases, a series of images on movie film or videotape has large areas of pixels that are not changing at all with time, or are doing so in relatively smooth and continuous ways. It should be possible to compress these, and in fact quite high compression ratios can be tolerated because for such areas the needed quality of the reconstructed image is not high. Human vision tends to ignore portions of images in which nothing interesting is happening and no changes are occurring.

The MPEG standards follow the same approach as JPEG. They are based primarily on the need to compress images to transmit "consumer" video and the forthcoming HDTV, to compress the images enough to permit transmission within the narrow bandwidth used by present television stations, and to fit entire movies onto DVD disks. Of course, for more technical purposes such as tracking features in a sequence of images or for measuring density or color changes as a function of time, different requirements may place different limits on the acceptable quality of reconstruction.

For sequences of images, an additional compression based on similarity between successive frames is employed. MPEG adds several additional steps to reduce the amount of data that must be transmitted. It looks for blocks of similar pixels in successive images, even if they have moved slightly. Only an average of 2 frames per second are normally sent in their entirety. The rest are either encoded as differences from preceding frames or as interpolations between frames. This approach allows overall compression to approach 200:1 with "acceptable" visual appearance.

A typical HDTV proposal presents 1920 × 1080-pixel images at the rate of 30 per second, for a total data rate exceeding 1 gigabit per second. The images use progressive scan (not interlaced), square pixels, and a wider image aspect ratio of 16:9 instead of the 4:3 used in NTSC (National Television Systems Committee) video (and most computer display screens). A typical broadcast TV station has a bandwidth that is 250 times too small. Without examining the debate over HDTV, whose standards are still evolving, we can consider if and how application of these methods may be useful for technical images.

It is important to remember that the criterion for these compression methods is the visual acceptance of the reconstructed image as it is displayed on a television screen. For instance, the MPEG standard, like present broadcast television, encodes the chrominance (color) information with less precision than it does the luminance (brightness) information. This is because tests indicate that human vision of images displayed on a CRT is more tolerant of variations in color than in brightness. The use of images for technical purposes, or even their presentation in other forms such as printed hard copy viewed by reflected light, may not be so forgiving.

The audio compression used in MPEG is used by itself for music recording (the popular MP3 format). The requirement for fidelity is that high frequencies must be preserved well enough so that, for example, overtone sequences allow the listener to distinguish an oboe from a muted trumpet.

Most of the moving-picture compression methods use key frames, which are compressed using the same method as a still picture. Then for every image in the sequence that follows the key frame, the differences from the previous image are determined and compressed. For these difference images, as we have seen above, the magnitude of the values is reduced. Consequently, in performing a further compression of this image by keeping only the "most important" basis functions, the number of terms eliminated can be increased significantly and much higher levels of compression achieved.

Like JPEG, MPEG consists of several options, some of which require more computation but deliver more compression. For instance, motion compensation provides a higher degree of compression because it identifies an overall translation in successive images (for instance, when the camera is slowly panned across a scene) and adjusts for that before comparing locations in one image with the previous frame. The MPEG approach is asymmetric: it requires more computation to compress the original data than to decompress it to reconstruct the images.

One of the consequences of this approach to compression is that it is intended only to go forward in time. From a key frame and then successive differences, you can reconstruct each following image. But you cannot easily go back to reconstruct a previous image except by returning to the nearest preceding key frame and working forward from there. In principle, one key frame at the beginning of each scene in a movie should be enough. In practice, key frames are inserted periodically.

Other compression methods are being developed for sequential images. One is predictive vector quantization, which attempts to locate boundaries in each image, track the motion of those boundaries, and use prediction to generate successive images. Sequences of 8-bit gray-scale images compressed to an average data rate of less than 0.5 bits per pixel have been reported (Hwang et al. 1993; Nicoulin et al. 1993; Wen and Lu 1993; Wu and Gersho 1993). Fractal compression has also been extended to deal with image sequences (Li et al. 1993).

High compression ratios for moving images are appropriate for videoconferencing, where the image quality only has to show who is speaking and perhaps what they are holding. For many consumer applications, in which the final image will be viewed on a screen of only modest resolution (for instance, a cell phone), adequate image quality can be achieved at high compression ratios. Tests with human television viewers have long suggested that it is the quality of the sound that is most important, and significant noise and other defects in the individual images are not objectionable.

However, for most technical applications, the types of artifacts produced by still-image compression are not acceptable, and the additional artifacts introduced as a result of temporal compression make matters worse. The user intending to perform analysis of images from a sequence should certainly begin with no compression at all, and specific compression methods should be accepted only if tests indicate that they are acceptable for the particular purposes for which the images are to be used.

4

Correcting Imaging Defects

This chapter considers a first class of image processing operations, those procedures applied to correct some of the defects in as-acquired images that may be present due to imperfect detectors, limitations of the optics, inadequate or nonuniform illumination, or an undesirable viewpoint. It is important to emphasize that these are corrections that are applied after the image has been digitized and stored, and therefore will be unable to deliver the highest quality result that could have been achieved by optimizing or correcting the acquisition process in the first place.

Of course, acquiring an optimum-quality image is sometimes impractical. If the camera can collect only a small number of photons within a practical period of time or before the scene changes, then the noise present in the image cannot be averaged out by acquiring and adding more photons or video frames, and other noise-reduction means are needed. If the source of illumination cannot be controlled to be perfectly centered and normal to the viewed surface (for instance the sun), or if the surface is curved instead of planar, then the image will have nonuniform illumination that must be corrected afterward. If the viewpoint cannot realistically be adjusted (for instance the path of a space probe or satellite), or if the surface is irregular (as in the case of a metal fracture), then some parts of the scene will be foreshortened; this must be taken into account in comparing sizes or measuring distances.

Even in typical laboratory setups such as light microscopy, keeping the instrument in ideal alignment may be very time-consuming, and achieving adequate stability to collect dim fluorescence images over a long time period can be very difficult, so that it becomes more practical to trade off some of the ultimately achievable image quality for convenience and speed, and to utilize image processing methods to perform these corrections. When the first space-probe pictures were obtained and the need for this type of correction was first appreciated, it required lengthy computations on moderate-sized computers to apply them. It is now possible to implement such corrections on desktop or laptop machines in times measured in seconds, so that they can be practically applied to routine imaging needs.

Contrast expansion

In **Chapter 1** it was noted that the typical digitization process for images produces values from 0 (black) to 255 (white), producing 1-byte (8 bit) values, or for color images 1 byte each for red, green, and blue. If the camera and digitizer have greater precision, the values can have 10, 12, or even more bits of precision and typically occupy 2 bytes each. But while this is the full dynamic range available to the output of the camera sensors, there is no reason to expect that the actual image data will cover the full range. In many situations the recorded image will have a much smaller range of brightness values, which may lie in the middle of the range (intermediate gray values) or toward either the bright or dark end of the range.

The image histogram, a plot of the number of pixels with each possible brightness level, is a valuable tool for examining the contrast in the image. **Figure 4.1** shows an example image in which the histogram covers the full dynamic range and indicates good contrast. There are no pixels that are completely black or white.

If the inherent range of variation in brightness of the image is much smaller than the dynamic range of the camera, subsequent electronics, and digitizer, then the actual range of numbers will be much less than the full range of 0 through 255. **Figure 4.2a** shows an example. The specimen is a thin section through tissue, shown in a bright-field microscope. Illumination in the microscope and light staining of the section produce very little total contrast. The histogram shown next to the image is a plot of the number of pixels at each of the 256 possible brightness levels. The narrow peak and empty regions at the top and bottom of the histogram indicate that many of the possible levels are not used.

Visibility of the structures present can be improved by stretching the contrast so that the values of pixels are reassigned to cover the entire available range. **Figure 4.2b** shows this, as demonstrated by the linear one-to-one mapping. This means that the darkest pixels in the original image are assigned to black, the lightest images are assigned to white, and intermediate gray values in the original image are given new values that are linearly interpolated between black and white. All of the pixels in the original image that had one particular gray value will be assigned the same gray value in the resulting image, but it will be a different value than the one in the original.

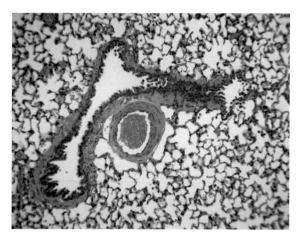

Figure 4.1 Microscope image of a thin slice of tissue, with its brightness histogram. This is an example of good exposure adjustment, since the brightness values cover the entire range without clipping at black or white.

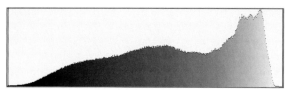

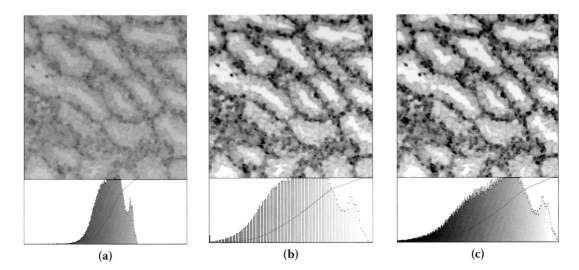

Figure 4.2 (a) *Light-microscope image of stained tissue has very low initial contrast, as shown by its brightness histogram.* **(b)** *Linear expansion of the brightness range by manipulating the display shows a full range of black to white values but causes gaps in the histogram.* **(c)** *Acquiring the image with optimum illumination and camera exposure produces similar contrast but without gaps in the histogram. The red line shows the cumulative or integrated histogram, rising from 0 to 100%.*

This histogram plotted with the image in the figure now shows counts of pixels for gray levels that are spread out across the available brightness scale. However, notice that many of the gray values still show zero values in the histogram, indicating that no pixels have those values. The reassignment of gray values has increased the visual contrast for the pixels present, but it has not increased the ability to discriminate subtle variations in gray scale that were not recorded in the original image. It has also magnified the brightness difference associated with noise in the original image.

Figure 4.2c shows the same field of view recorded to utilize the entire range of the camera and digitizer. This may require adjusting the illumination, camera gain or exposure time, etc., and generally requires trial and error in the settings. The mean brightness of various structures is similar to that shown in **Figure 4.2b**. However, all of the 256 possible gray values are now present in the image, and very small variations in sample density can now be distinguished or measured in the specimen.

This problem is not restricted to bright images. **Figure 4.3a** shows a dark image from a scanning electron microscope (SEM) along with its histogram. The structures on the integrated circuit are revealed when the contrast is stretched out (**Figure 4.3c**), but this also increases the visibility of the noise or random "speckle" variations for pixels that represent the same structure and ideally should be uniform in brightness. The problem of image noise will be dealt with as the next topic in this chapter.

These are rather extreme cases, but it is often not practical to adjust the illumination, camera gain, etc., to exactly fill the available pixel depth (number of gray levels that can be digitized or stored). Furthermore, increasing the brightness range too much can cause pixel values at the dark or light ends of the range to exceed the digitization and storage capacity and to be clipped to the limiting values, which also causes loss of information. **Figure 4.4** shows an example, a micrograph of a cross section through an enamel coating in which the gray-scale range of the bubbles is good, but the polished flat surfaces were brighter than the white limit of the camera

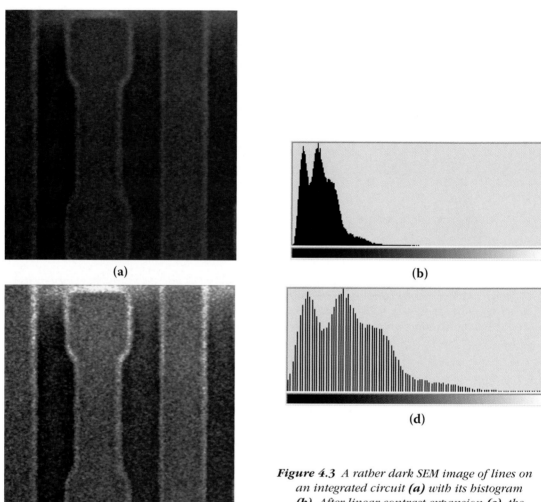

(a)

(b)

(d)

(c)

Figure 4.3 A rather dark SEM image of lines on an integrated circuit (a) with its histogram (b). After linear contrast expansion (c), the features and noise are both more visible, and the histogram (d) shows gaps between values.

and consequently were clipped to a value of 255, losing any detail that might have been present. To avoid such problems, it is common for images to be acquired that do not completely cover the available brightness range.

When contrast expansion is applied to color images, the correct procedure is to convert the image from its stored RGB (red, green, blue) format to L*a*b* or HSI (hue, saturation, intensity) color space, and expand the intensity or luminance scale while leaving the color information unchanged, as shown in **Figure 4.5**. This prevents color shifts that would occur if the individual red, green, and blue histograms were linearly expanded to full scale, as shown in **Figure 4.6**. Such shifts are especially prevalent if the original image consists primarily of just a few colors, or is predominantly of one color.

If these images still have enough different brightness levels to reveal the important features in the specimen, then linear contrast expansion is a useful and acceptable method to increase the viewer's visual discrimination. More important, this expansion may make it possible to more directly compare images acquired with slightly different brightness ranges by adjusting them

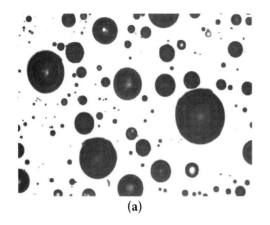

(a)

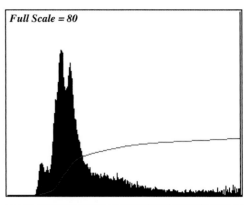

Full Scale = 80

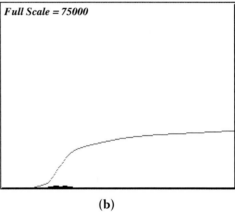

Full Scale = 75000

(b)

*Figure 4.4 Light micrograph of polished section through an enamel coating **(a)**. The histogram **(b)** shows that the majority of the pixels are full white, indicating that they were brighter than the dynamic range and were clipped to 255. It is necessary to expand the vertical scale of the histogram to see the peaks for the pixels with gray values corresponding to the bubbles in the coating. The cumulative histogram rises to only about 30% at the white end of the spectrum, revealing that 70% of the pixels are clipped at white.*

all to the same expanded contrast scale. Of course, this only works if the brightest and darkest classes of features are present in all of the images and fields of view.

Other manipulations of the pixel brightness values can also be performed. These are described as point operations, meaning that the new values assigned depend only on the original pixel value and not on any of its neighbors, and as "one to one," meaning that all pixels that originally had a single gray-scale value are assigned to another single value. However, the process may not be linear. An example would be one that converted brightness to density, which involves a logarithmic relationship. For color images, a transfer function can be used to correct colors for distortion due to the color temperature of the light source, or for atmospheric scattering and absorption in satellite images. These functions can be implemented with either a mathematical function or a lookup table.

Chapter 5 illustrates many of these contrast manipulations to enhance the visibility of structures present in the image.

Noisy images

The linear expansion of contrast shown in the previous examples is often accompanied by an increased visibility for noise (random fluctuations in pixel values) that may be present. Noise is an important defect in images that can take many different forms and arises from various sources.

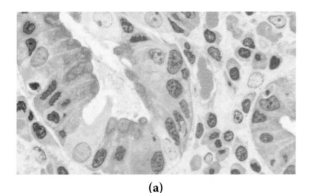

(a)

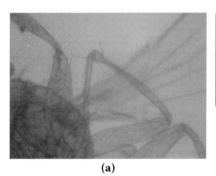

(b)

Figure 4.5
(a) *Light-microscope image of stained tissue, and*
(b) *the result of expanding contrast by converting to HSI space and linearly expanding only the intensity.*

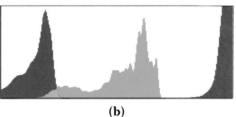

(a)

(b)

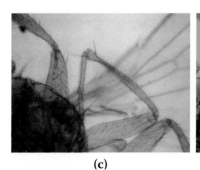

(c)

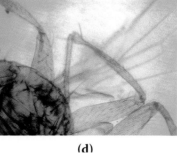

(d)

Figure 4.6
(a) *Light-microscope image of an insect with*
(b) *histograms of the red, green, and blue values.*
(c) *Expanding the intensity while leaving hue and saturation unchanged expands the visible contrast without altering the colors.*
(d) *Expanding the RGB values individually to full range produces color shifts in the image because the proportions of red, green, and blue are changed.*

In **Chapter 1**, **Figure 1.26** illustrated the improvement in image quality (technically, signal-to-noise ratio) by averaging a number of frames. One unavoidable source of noise is counting statistics in the image detector due to a small number of incident particles (photons, electrons, etc.). This is particularly the case for X-ray images from the SEM, in which the ratio of incident electrons to detected X-rays can be from 10^5 to 10^6. In fluorescence light microscopy, the fluoresced-light photons in a narrow wavelength range from a dye or activity probe may also produce very dim images, compounded by the necessity of acquiring a series of very-short-duration images to measure activity as a function of time.

Noisy images may also occur due to instability in the light source or detector during the time required to scan or digitize an image. The pattern of this noise may be quite different from the essentially Gaussian noise due to counting statistics, but it still shows up as a variation in brightness in uniform regions of the scene. One common example is the noise in field-emission SEM images due to the variation in field-emission current at the tip. With a typical time constant of seconds, the electron emission can shift from one atom to another, producing a change of several percent in the beam current. The usual approach to minimize the effects of this fluctuation in the viewed image is to use scan times that are either much shorter or longer than the fluctuation time.

Similar effects can be seen in images acquired using fluorescent lighting, particularly in light boxes used to illuminate film negatives, resulting from an interference or beat frequency between the camera scan and flickering of the fluorescent tube. This flickering is much greater than that of an incandescent bulb, whose thermal inertia smoothes out the variation in light emission due to the alternating current. When the noise has a characteristic that is not random in time and does not exhibit "normal" statistical behavior, it is more difficult to place meaningful numeric descriptors on the amount of noise. However, many of the same techniques can be used, usually with somewhat less efficacy, to reduce the noise. Periodic noise sources, resulting typically from electrical interference or vibration, can be removed using Fourier transform representation of the image, as discussed in **Chapter 6**.

Random noise also arises in the camera chip itself, both due to inherent variations in the sensitivity of each detector and the variations in amplification, losses in the electron transfer process, and random thermal noise. Some of this is a fixed pattern that may or may not be essentially random across the image, and some is random "speckle" noise superimposed on the image data.

Assuming that an image represents the best quality that can practically be obtained, the discussion in this section focuses on ways to suppress noise to improve the ability to visualize and demarcate for measurement the features that are present. The underlying assumptions in all of these methods are that the pixels in the image are much smaller than any of the important details, and that for most of the pixels present, their neighbors represent the same structure. Various averaging and comparison methods can be applied based on these assumptions.

These are very much the same assumptions as those inherent in classical image averaging, in which the assumption is that pixel readings at each location at different times represent the same structure in the viewed scene. This directly justifies averaging or integrating pixel readings over time to reduce random noise. When the signal varies in other ways described above, other methods such as median filtering (discussed below) can be used. These methods are analogous to the spatial comparisons discussed here except that they utilize the time sequence of measurements at each location.

There are important differences between noise reduction by the use of frame averaging to combine many sequential readouts from a camera and the use of a camera that can integrate the charge internally before it is read out. The latter mode is employed in astronomy, fluorescence microscopy, and other applications to very faint images, and is sometimes called "staring" mode, since the camera is simply open to the incident light. The two methods might seem to be equivalent, since both add together the incoming signal over some period of time. However, it is important to understand that there are two quite different sources of noise to be considered.

In a camera used in staring mode, the electrons collected in each transistor on the CCD (charge-coupled device) array include those produced by incoming photons and some from the dark current in the device itself. This current is strongly influenced by thermal noise, which can move electrons around at room temperature. Cooling the chip, either by a few tens of degrees with a Peltier cooler or by hundreds of degrees with liquid nitrogen or even liquid helium, can reduce this thermal noise dramatically. An infrared camera must be cooled more than a visible-light camera because the light photons themselves have less energy, and so the production of a signal electron takes less energy, which means that more dark current would be present at room temperature.

Cameras intended for staring application or long time exposures often specify the operating time needed to half-fill the dynamic range of the chip with dark current. For an inexpensive Peltier-cooled camera, the useful operating time might be several minutes. For a high-quality device used for professional astronomy and cooled to much lower temperatures, it might be tens of hours. Collecting an image in staring mode for that length of time would raise the dark level to a medium gray, and any real signal would be superimposed on that background. Since the production of thermal electrons is a statistical process, not all pixels will have the same background level. Fluctuations in the background thus represent one type of noise in the image that may be dominant for these types of applications to very dim images. In most cases, this source of noise is small compared with the readout noise.

All cameras have some readout noise. In the typical CCD camera, the electrons from each transistor must be transferred many times to be read out as a voltage to the computer. In a CCD camera, more transfers are needed to shift the electrons from one side of the image to the amplifier, and so the resulting noise is greater on one side of the image than on the other. In an interline transfer camera, a separate row of transistors adjacent to each detector is used instead, somewhat reducing the readout noise. Of course, additional sources of noise from the other associated electronics (clock signals, wiring from the camera to the digitizer, pickup of electrical signals from the computer itself, and so forth) may degrade the signal even more. But even if those other sources of noise are minimized by careful design and proper wiring, there is an irreducible amount of noise superimposed on the signal each time the camera image is read out, amplified, and digitized.

This noise is generally random, and hence is as likely to reduce as to increase the brightness of any particular pixel. **Figure 4.7** shows an example of two successive images acquired using a good-quality digital camera and normal lighting. The images look essentially identical except for the motion of the clock hands. However, subtracting one frame from the other (and expanding the contrast as described previously) shows the pixel noise present in the images. With digital cameras, as discussed in **Chapter 1**, the normal procedure is to acquire a single image using an appropriate exposure time and then transfer the digitized values to the computer. However, some camera designs that are not cooled may acquire several shorter exposures and average the results in the computer.

With video cameras, averaging many frames together causes the random noise from readout to partially cancel while the signal continues to add up. The small well size of the transistors on

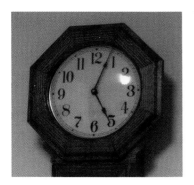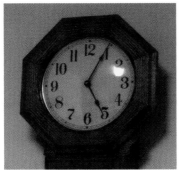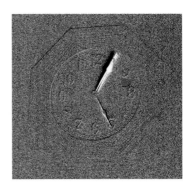

Figure 4.7 Two images of the same view, acquired from a digital camera, and the difference between them (pixels enlarged and contrast expanded to show detail). Except for the differences associated with the motion of the clock hands, the differences are due to random noise in the camera, and are different in the red, green, and blue channels.

the very tiny chip make long exposures impractical The consequence is that frame averaging can reduce the relative magnitude of this source of noise in the image, but cannot eliminate it.

For a very dim image, the optimum situation would be to integrate the signal within the camera chip, but without allowing any single pixel to reach saturation. Then reading the data out once will produce the minimum readout noise and the best image. For a brighter image, or for a camera that can only function at video rates, or one whose detector has a small well size or electron capacity, it may be acceptable to average a sufficient number of successive frames to reduce the pixel variations due to random readout noise. This integration can be done in the frame grabber or in the computer program. The frame grabber is generally restricted by the amount of on-board memory, but it can often collect every frame with no loss of data. The computer program is more flexible, but the time required to add the frames together may result in discarding some of the video frames, so that the total acquisition takes longer (which may not be a problem if the image does not vary with time). Of course, in fluorescence microscopy, bleaching may occur and it may be desirable to collect all of the photons as rapidly as possible, either by frame averaging or, for a very dim image, by using staring mode if the camera is capable of this.

Figure 4.8 shows a comparison of two SEM images taken at different scan rates. The fast-scan image collects few electrons per pixel and so has a high noise level that obscures details in the image. Slowing the scan rate down from 1 sec to 20 sec increases the amount of signal and reduces the noise. The histograms show that the variation of brightness within the uniform region is reduced (the peak is narrowed), which is why the visibility of detail is improved.

Neighborhood averaging

The simplest form of spatial averaging is to add the pixel brightness values in each small region of the image, divide by the number of pixels in the neighborhood, and use the resulting value to construct a new image. **Figure 4.9** shows that this essentially produces an image with a smaller number of pixels. The block size in **Figure 4.9b** is 3 × 3, so that nine pixel values are added. Since the noise in this image is random due to the counting statistics of the small number of photons, the improvement in image quality or signal-to-noise ratio is just the square

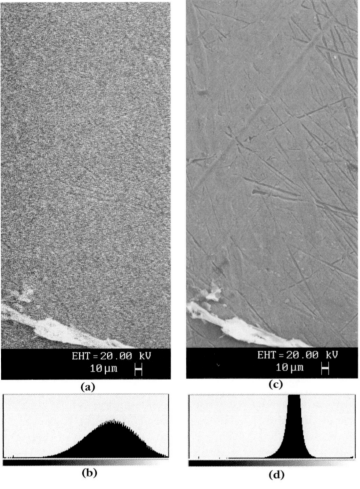

Figure 4.8 SEM images of a scratched metal surface:
(a) 1-sec scan;
(b) histogram of image **a**;
(c) 20-sec scan;
(d) histogram of image **c**.

(a)

(c)

(b)

(d)

root of 9, or a factor of 3. However, the image lateral resolution is seriously impacted, and the small structures in the image can no longer be separately discerned.

The more common way to accomplish neighborhood averaging is to replace each pixel with the average of itself and its neighbors. This is often described as a "kernel" operation, since implementation can be generalized as the sum of the pixel values in the region multiplied by a set of integer weights. The process is also called a "convolution" because it corresponds to a procedure performed in Fourier space (discussed in **Chapter 6**).

$$P^*_{x,y} \frac{\sum\limits_{i,j=-m}^{+m} W_{i,j} \cdot P_{x+i,y+j}}{\sum\limits_{i,j=-m}^{+m} W_{i,j}} \tag{4.1}$$

Equation 4.1 shows the calculation performed over a square of dimension $2m + 1$, which is an odd number. The neighborhood sizes thus range from 3×3, upward to 5×5, 7×7, etc. It is possible to use nonsquare regions; for larger neighborhoods, an approximation of a circle is preferable to a square but somewhat more difficult to implement. The array of weights W for a simple neighbor averaging contains only 1s, and for a 3×3 region could be written as

1	1	1
1	1	1
1	1	1

where we understand the convention that these coefficients are to be multiplied by pixels that surround the central pixel, the total normalized by dividing by the sum of weights (nine in the example), and the value written to the location of the central pixel to form a new image.

As a matter of practicality, since storage space is never unlimited, it is common to write the new image back into the same memory as the original. However, when this is done it is important to use the original pixel values for the summation, and not those new ones that have already been calculated for some of the neighbors. This requires keeping a copy of a few lines of the image during the process.

Neighborhood operations including kernel multiplication are usually applied symmetrically around each pixel. This creates a problem for pixels nearer to the edge of the image than the half-width of the neighborhood. Various approaches are used to deal with this problem, including (a) designing special asymmetrical kernels or rules along edges or in corners, (b) assuming that the image edges are mirrors, so that each line of pixels within the image is duplicated beyond it, (c) extrapolating values from within the image area to the pixels beyond the edge, or (d) assuming that the image wraps around so that the left edge and right edge, and the top and bottom edges, are contiguous. An even simpler approach is sometimes used: the processing is restricted to that portion of the image where no edge conflicts arise. This leaves lines of unprocessed pixels along the edges of the images, equal in width to half the dimension of the neighborhood. None of these approaches is entirely satisfactory, and in general most processing operations sacrifice some pixels from the image edges.

Figure 4.9 shows the effect of smoothing using a 3 × 3-neighborhood average and also a 7 × 7-neighborhood size. The noise reduction is much greater with the larger region, but is accompanied by a significant blurring of the feature edges.

The amount of blurring can be reduced and more control exerted over the neighborhood-averaging procedure by using weight values that are not 1. For example, the values

1	2	1
2	4	2
1	2	1

have several attractive characteristics. First, the central 4 by which the original pixel contents are multiplied is the largest factor, causing the central pixel to dominate the average and reducing blurring. The values of 2 for the four orthogonally touching neighbors and 1 for the four diagonally touching neighbors acknowledge the fact that the diagonal pixels are in fact farther away from the center of the neighborhood (actually by the factor $\sqrt{2}$). Finally, these weights have a total value of 16, which is a power of 2. The use of numbers that are powers of 2 makes it possible to perform multiplications and divisions by bit shifting in the computer, which is very fast.

When the first edition of this book appeared, there was great interest in efficient implementations of image processing operations because computer power was limited. Sets of weight val-

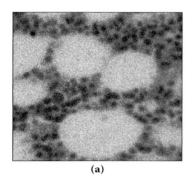
(a)

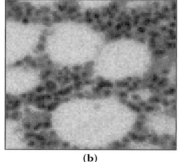
(b)

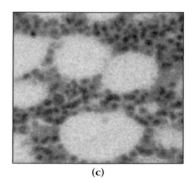
(c)

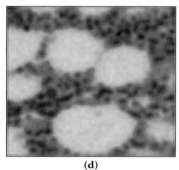
(d)

Figure 4.9 *Smoothing by averaging:*
  (a) *noisy original image (fluorescence light microscopy of bone marrow);*
  (b) *each 3 × 3 block of pixels averaged;*
  (c) *each pixel replaced by the average of itself and its eight neighbors in a 3 × 3 square block;*
  (d) *each pixel replaced by the average of itself and its 48 neighbors in a 7 × 7 square.*

ues commonly used small integers to speed implementation such that the sum of the products would not exceed 32,678 (2^{15}) and so would fit into a single precision integer value. Powers of 2 were favored, and the values were selected with more regard to efficient implementation than to the actual underlying theory. Fortunately, these restrictions are no longer very important. With modern computers, the use of greater precision arithmetic, even floating-point multiplications, is quite fast, and even with the larger multimegapixel images now common, performance speed is adequate for most purposes.

We will see in **Chapter 6**, in the context of processing images in frequency space, that these kernels can be analyzed quite efficiently in that domain to understand their smoothing properties. It turns out from that analysis that one of the very useful "shapes" for a weight kernel is that of a Gaussian. This is a set of weights that approximate the profile of a Gaussian function along any row, column, or diagonal through the center. It is characterized by a standard deviation, expressed in terms of pixel dimensions, and calculated as

$$G(x,y,\sigma) = \frac{1}{2\pi\sigma^2} e^{\left[-\frac{x^2+y^2}{2\sigma^2}\right]}$$

(4.2)

where x and y are the distance in pixels from the center of the kernel. The size of the kernel is generally made large enough that adding another row of terms would insert negligibly small numbers (ideally zeroes) into the array, but of course some zero values will be present anyway in the corners, since they are farther from the central pixel. The standard deviation (σ) for these kernels is the radius (in pixels) containing 68% of the integrated magnitude of the coefficients or, if the kernel is pictured as a three-dimensional (3-D) plot of the integer values, the standard deviation is the volume under the surface. This is a two-dimensional generalization of the usual definition of standard deviation; for a one-dimensional Gaussian distribution, 68% of the area under the curve lies within ±1 σ.

Choosing a set of integers to implement a Gaussian is something of an art, at least for the larger kernels, since the goal is to approximate the smooth analytical curve of the Gaussian. However, the total of the weights must usually be kept smaller than some practical limit to facilitate the computer arithmetic (Russ 1995d). Relaxing that requirement by using double precision integer arithmetic, or floating-point values, allows creating much better results. **Table 4.1** shows several Gaussian kernels with varying standard deviations. The integer values were calculated by scaling the central value to 100 and rounding the smaller values. The kernels thus generated are larger than ones with smaller integers (because small values down to 1% are retained at the edges), which can be important when images with more than 1-byte values are used. For 1-byte values, the kernel size can be reduced somewhat by eliminating these small outer values. Of course, the kernel size increases with the standard deviation as well; the total width of the kernel is about six times the standard deviation.

Table 4.1. Gaussian Kernels with Varying Standard Deviations

σ = **0.5**

2	14	2
14	100	14
2	14	2

σ = **1.0 pixels**

0	0	1	1	1	0	0
0	2	8	14	8	2	0
1	8	37	61	37	8	1
1	14	61	100	61	14	1
1	8	37	61	37	8	1
0	2	8	14	8	2	0
0	0	1	1	1	0	0

σ = **1.5 pixels**

0	0	1	2	3	2	1	0	0
0	2	6	11	14	11	6	2	0
1	6	17	33	41	33	17	6	1
2	11	33	64	80	64	33	11	2
3	14	41	80	100	80	41	14	3
2	11	33	64	80	64	33	11	2
1	6	17	33	41	33	17	6	1
0	2	6	11	14	11	6	2	0
0	0	1	2	3	2	1	0	0

σ = 2.0 pixels

```
0   0   0   0   1   1   1   1   1   0   0   0   0
0   0   1   1   3   4   4   4   3   1   1   0   0
0   1   2   4   8  12  14  12   8   4   2   1   0
0   1   4  11  20  29  32  29  20  11   4   1   0
1   3   8  20  37  54  61  54  37  20   8   3   1
1   4  12  29  54  78  88  78  54  29  12   4   1
1   3   8  20  37  54  61  54  37  20   8   3   1
0   1   4  11  20  29  32  29  20  11   4   1   0
0   1   2   4   8  12  14  12   8   4   2   1   0
0   0   1   1   3   4   4   4   3   1   1   0   0
0   0   0   0   1   1   1   1   1   0   0   0   0
```

σ = 2.5 pixels

```
0   0   0   0   0   0   0   1   1   1   0   0   0   0   0   0   0
0   0   0   0   1   1   1   2   2   2   1   1   1   0   0   0   0
0   0   0   1   2   3   4   5   6   5   4   3   2   1   0   0   0
0   0   1   2   4   7  10  12  14  12  10   7   4   2   1   0   0
0   1   2   4   8  14  20  26  28  26  20  14   8   4   2   1   0
0   1   3   7  14  24  35  45  49  45  35  24  14   7   3   1   0
0   1   4  10  20  35  53  67  73  67  53  35  20  10   4   1   0
1   2   5  12  26  45  67  85  92  85  67  45  26  12   5   2   1
1   2   6  14  28  49  73  92 100  92  73  49  28  14   6   2   1
1   2   5  12  26  45  67  85  92  85  67  45  26  12   5   2   1
0   1   4  10  20  35  53  67  73  67  53  35  20  10   4   1   0
0   1   3   7  14  24  35  45  49  45  35  24  14   7   3   1   0
0   1   2   4   8  14  20  26  28  26  20  14   8   4   2   1   0
0   0   1   2   4   7  10  12  14  12  10   7   4   2   1   0   0
0   0   0   1   2   3   4   5   6   5   4   3   2   1   0   0   0
0   0   0   0   1   1   1   2   2   2   1   1   1   0   0   0   0
0   0   0   0   0   0   0   1   1   1   0   0   0   0   0   0   0
```

σ = 3.0 pixels

0	0	0	0	0	0	1	1	1	1	1	1	1	0	0	0	0	0	0
0	0	0	0	1	1	2	2	3	3	3	2	2	1	1	0	0	0	0
0	0	0	1	2	3	4	5	6	7	6	5	4	3	2	1	0	0	0
0	0	1	2	3	6	8	11	13	14	13	11	8	6	3	2	1	0	0
0	1	2	3	6	10	15	20	24	25	24	20	15	10	6	3	2	1	0
0	1	3	6	10	17	25	33	39	41	39	33	25	17	10	6	3	1	0
1	2	4	8	15	25	37	49	57	61	57	49	37	25	15	8	4	2	1
1	2	5	11	20	33	49	64	76	80	76	64	49	33	20	11	5	2	1
1	3	6	13	24	39	57	76	89	95	89	76	57	39	24	13	6	3	1
1	3	7	14	25	41	61	80	95	100	95	80	61	41	25	14	7	3	1
1	3	6	13	24	39	57	76	89	95	89	76	57	39	24	13	6	3	1
1	2	5	11	20	33	49	64	76	80	76	64	49	33	20	11	5	2	1
1	2	4	8	15	25	37	49	57	61	57	49	37	25	15	8	4	2	1
0	1	3	6	10	17	25	33	39	41	39	33	25	17	10	6	3	1	0
0	1	2	3	6	10	15	20	24	25	24	20	15	10	6	3	2	1	0
0	0	1	2	3	6	8	11	13	14	13	11	8	6	3	2	1	0	0
0	0	0	1	2	3	4	5	6	7	6	5	4	3	2	1	0	0	0
0	0	0	0	1	1	2	2	3	3	3	2	2	1	1	0	0	0	0
0	0	0	0	0	0	1	1	1	1	1	1	1	0	0	0	0	0	0

Figure 4.10 shows a Gaussian kernel plotted as a surface representing the values. Some systems allow entering kernel weights as real numbers, and many systems generate Gaussian kernels as needed when the user enters the standard deviation value.

Because kernel sizes become quite large when the standard deviation of the Gaussian kernel increases, and because the large number of multiplications for each pixel in the image can take a significant amount of time, a strategy that is sometimes used is to approximate a Gaussian smoothing operation by many repetitions of a simple 3 × 3 averaging kernel, which requires only additions rather than multiplications and uses a small neighborhood. As computer speeds have increased, and floating-point arithmetic has become fast due to the incorporation of dedicated arithmetic units, such approximations have become less necessary.

The smoothing operation can be speeded up considerably in the case of Gaussian filters by separating the operation into two simpler ones. Instead of using the entire square array of weights, which for a 15 × 15 kernel would require 225 multiplications and additions, the filter can be separated into a vertical Gaussian blur with a linear array of weights (15 multiplications and additions) followed by a horizontal Gaussian blur (another 15 for a total of 30). **Equation 4.3** is used to calculate the values for the weights, which again can be scaled and rounded as integers.

$$G(x,\sigma) = \frac{1}{\sqrt{2\pi}\cdot\sigma}e^{\left[-\frac{x^2}{2\sigma^2}\right]}$$

(4.3)

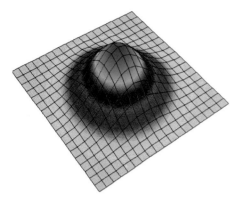

Figure 4.10 Graphical plot of the weight values in a Gaussian smoothing kernel.

The implementation of several types of convolution kernels can be separated in this way, but many cannot, and for the purposes of understanding the algorithms, it is probably better to consider the entire array of weights. In subsequent sections on image processing, we will see other uses for kernels in which the weights are not symmetrical in magnitude and not all positive. The implementation of the kernel will remain the same, except that when negative weights are present, the normalization is usually performed by division by the sum of the positive values only (because in these cases the sum of all the weights is usually zero). For the present, our interest is restricted to smoothing of noise in images.

Figure 4.11 shows the same noisy image as **Figure 4.9**, along with an image of the same region using image averaging to reduce the statistical noise, as illustrated in **Chapter 1**. The figure also shows an enlargement of a portion of the image, in which the individual pixels can be discerned, as an aid to judging the pixel-to-pixel noise variations in uniform regions and the sharpness of boundaries between different structures. Applying smoothing with a Gaussian kernel with a standard deviation of 1.0 pixels to the single-frame noisy image produces the improvement in quality shown in **Figure 4.12**.

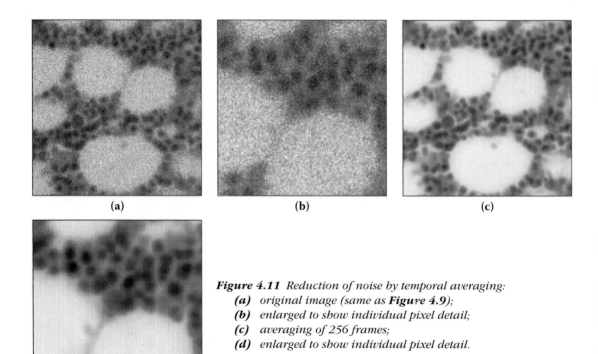

(a)

(b)

(c)

(d)

Figure 4.11 Reduction of noise by temporal averaging:
    *(a) original image (same as **Figure 4.9**);*
    (b) enlarged to show individual pixel detail;
    (c) averaging of 256 frames;
    (d) enlarged to show individual pixel detail.

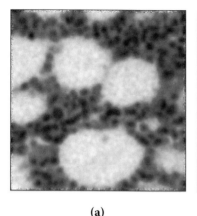 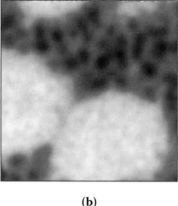

Figure 4.12 Reduction of noise by Gaussian smoothing (compare with Figure 4.11):
(a) application of a Gaussian filter with standard deviation of 1 pixel;
(b) enlarged to show individual pixel detail.

(a)   (b)

This type of averaging can reduce visible noise in the image, but it also blurs edges, displaces boundaries, and reduces contrast. It can even introduce artifacts when two nearby structures are averaged together in a way that creates an apparent feature between them. **Figure 4.13** shows an example in which the lines of the test pattern are blurred by the 11 × 11 averaging window, causing false lines to appear between them.

In our discussion of image enhancement in **Chapter 5**, the use of kernels in which a ring of negative weight values surrounds a positive central peak will be shown. The purpose of this modification is to sharpen edges and avoid some of the blurring that is produced by smoothing out noise. The same method has long been used for the smoothing of one-dimensional signal profiles, such as X-ray diffraction patterns, spectra, or time-varying electronic signals. This is often performed using a Savitsky and Golay (1964) fitting procedure. Tables of coefficients published for this purpose (and intended for efficient application in dedicated computers) are designed to be used just as the weighting coefficients discussed previously, except that they operate in only one dimension. The process is equivalent to performing a least-squares fit of the data points to a polynomial. The smoothed profiles preserve the magnitude of steps while smoothing out noise. **Table 4.2** lists these coefficients for second (quadratic) and fourth (quartic) power polynomials for fits extending over neighborhoods ranging from 5 to 19 points. These profiles are plotted in **Figure 4.14**.

This same method can be extended to two dimensions (Edwards 1982) either by first applying the coefficients in the horizontal direction and then in the vertical direction, or by constructing a full 2-D kernel. **Figure 4.15** shows the application of a 7 × 7 Savitsky and Golay quadratic polynomial to smooth the image from **Figure 4.9**.

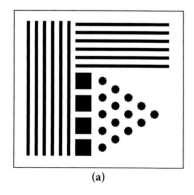 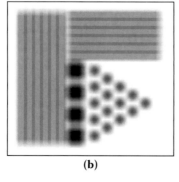

Figure 4.13 Artifacts due to smoothing. Applying an 11 × 11 smoothing kernel to the test pattern in image a produces apparent lines between the original ones, as shown in image **b**.

(a)   (b)

Table 4.2. Savitsky and Golay Fitting Coefficients

5	7	9	Neighborhood Points 11	13	15	17	19
			Quadratic Polynomial Fit				
0	0	0	0	0	0	0	−.0602
0	0	0	0	0	0	−.0650	−.0226
0	0	0	0	0	−.0706	−.0186	.0106
0	0	0	0	−.0769	−.0118	.0217	.0394
0	0	0	−.0839	0	.0380	.0557	.0637
0	0	−.0909	.0210	.0629	.0787	.0836	.0836
0	−.0952	.0606	.1026	.1119	.1104	.1053	.0991
−.0857	.1429	.1688	.1608	.1469	.1330	.1207	.1101
.3429	.2857	.2338	.1958	.1678	.1466	.1300	.1168
.4857	.3333	.2554	.2075	.1748	.1511	.1331	.1190
.3429	.2857	.2338	.1958	.1678	.1466	.1300	.1168
−.0857	.1429	.1688	.1608	.1469	.1330	.1207	.1101
0	−.0952	.0606	.1026	.1119	.1104	.1053	.0991
0	0	−.0909	.0210	.0629	.0787	.0836	.0836
0	0	0	−.0839	0	.0380	.0557	.0637
0	0	0	0	−.0769	−.0118	.0217	.0394
0	0	0	0	0	−.0706	−.0186	.0106
0	0	0	0	0	0	−.0650	−.0226
0	0	0	0	0	0	0	−.0602
			Quartic Polynomial Fit				
0	0	0	0	0	0	.0464	−.0343
0	0	0	0	0	.0464	−.0464	−.0565
0	0	0	0	.0452	−.0619	−.0619	−.0390
0	0	0	.0420	−.0814	−.0636	−.0279	.0024
0	0	.0350	−.1049	−.0658	−.0036	.0322	.0545
0	.0216	−.1282	−.0233	.0452	.0813	.0988	.1063
.25	−.1299	.0699	.1399	.1604	.1624	.1572	.1494
−.5	.3247	.3147	.2797	.2468	.2192	.1965	.1777
1.5	.5671	.4172	.3333	.2785	.2395	.2103	.1875
−.5	.3247	.3147	.2797	.2468	.2192	.1965	.1777
.25	−.1299	.0699	.1399	.1604	.1624	.1572	.1494
0	.0216	−.1282	−.0233	.0452	.0813	.0988	.1063
0	0	.0350	−.1049	−.0658	−.0036	.0322	.0545
0	0	0	.0420	−.0814	−.0636	−.0279	.0024
0	0	0	0	.0452	−.0619	−.0619	−.0390
0	0	0	0	0	.0464	−.0464	−.0565
0	0	0	0	0	0	.0464	−.0343
0	0	0	0	0	0	0	.0458

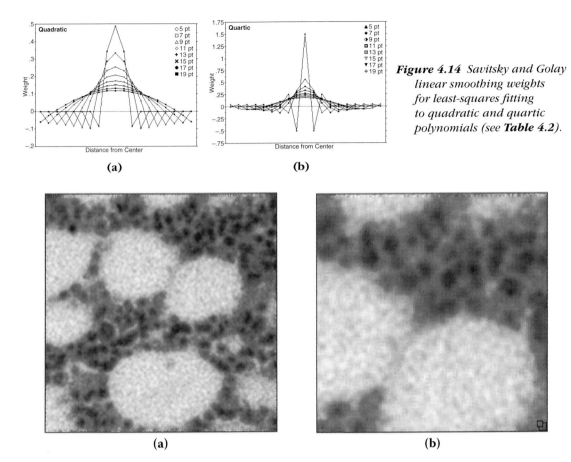

Figure 4.14 *Savitsky and Golay linear smoothing weights for least-squares fitting to quadratic and quartic polynomials (see* **Table 4.2**).

Figure 4.15 *Smoothing with a seven-point-wide quadratic Savitsky and Golay fit:* **(a)** *same image as* **Figure 4.9**, *smoothed;* **(b)** *enlarged to show pixel detail.*

It is interesting to compare the results of this spatial-domain smoothing to that which can be accomplished in the frequency domain. As discussed in **Chapter 6**, multiplication of the frequency transform by a convolution function is equivalent to application of a kernel in the spatial domain. The most common noise-filtering method is to remove high-frequency information, which represents pixel-to-pixel variations associated with random noise. Such removal can be done by setting an aperture on the two-dimensional transform, eliminating higher frequencies, and retransforming. **Figure 4.16** shows the result of applying this technique to the same image as in **Figure 4.9**. A circular low-pass filter with radius = 35 pixels and a 10-pixel-wide cosine edge shape (the importance of these parameters is discussed in **Chapter 6**) was applied. The smoothing is similar to that accomplished in the spatial domain.

As a practical matter, for kernel sizes that are small, or ones that are separable into vertical and horizontal passes like the Gaussian, multiplication and addition of the pixel values in the spatial domain is a faster operation. For kernels that are larger than about 11 × 11 (the limit depends to some extent on the particulars of the individual computer, whether the image can be held entirely in memory or must be accessed from disk, whether multiple processors can be used, etc.), the frequency-domain method will be faster. However, since both procedures are mathematically identical, it is often easier to understand the process based on spatial-domain kernels of weights.

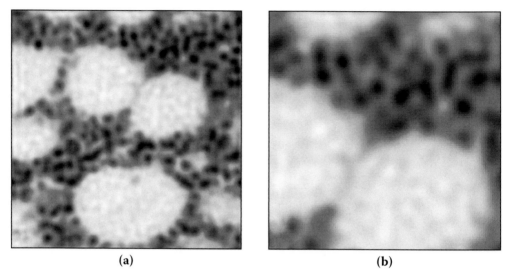

Figure 4.16 *Smoothing in frequency space, using a circular low-pass filter with radius = 35 pixels and a 10-pixel-wide cosine edge shape: (a) application to image in Figure 4.9; (b) enlargement to show pixel detail.*

Neighborhood ranking

Smoothing filters do reduce random noise, but the underlying assumption is that all of the pixels in the neighborhood represent multiple samples of the same value, in other words that they all belong to the same feature. Clearly, at edges and boundaries this is not true, and all of the previously discussed smoothing filters produce some blurring and shifting of edges, which is undesirable. The Gaussian filters produce the least edge blurring for a given amount of noise reduction, but cannot eliminate the blurring altogether.

The use of weighting kernels to average pixels in a neighborhood is a convolution operation, which as illustrated above has a direct counterpart in frequency-space image processing. It is a linear operation that uses all of the pixels in the neighborhood, and in which no information is lost from the original image. There are other processing operations that can be performed in neighborhoods in the spatial domain that also provide noise smoothing. These are not linear and do not utilize or preserve all of the original data.

The most widely used of these methods is based on ranking of the pixels in a neighborhood according to brightness. Then, for example, the median value in this ordered list can be used as the brightness value for the central pixel. As in the case of the kernel operations, this is used to produce a new image, and only the original pixel values are used in the ranking for the neighborhood around each pixel.

The median filter is an excellent rejecter of certain kinds of noise, both random superimposed variations and "shot" or impulse noise in which individual pixels are corrupted or missing from the image. If a pixel is accidentally changed to an extreme value, it will be eliminated from the image and replaced by a "reasonable" value, the median value in the neighborhood. This type of noise can occur in CMOS (complementary metal oxide semiconductor) cameras with "dead" transistors that have no output or "locked" ones that always put out maximum signals, and in interference microscopes for points on a surface with a locally high slope that returns no light.

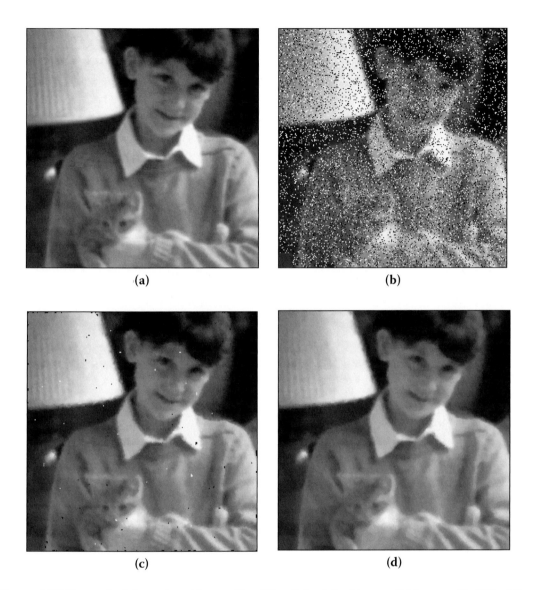

(a)

(b)

(c)

(d)

Figure 4.17 *Removal of shot noise with a median filter: **(a)** original image; **(b)** image with 10% of the pixels randomly selected and set to black, and another 10% randomly selected and set to white; **(c)** application of median filtering to image **b** using a 3 × 3 square region; **(d)** application of median filtering to image **b** using a 5 × 5 octagonal region.*

Figure 4.17 shows an extreme example of this type of noise. In the original image, 10% of the pixels were selected randomly and set to black, and another 10% were set to white. This is a rather extreme amount of noise. However, a median filter is able to remove the noise and replace the bad pixels with reasonable values while causing a minimal distortion or degradation of the image. Two different neighborhoods are used: a 3 × 3 square containing a total of 9 pixels, and a 5 × 5 octagonal (approximately circular) region containing a total of 21 pixels. **Figure 4.18** shows several of the neighborhood regions often used for ranking. Of course, the computational effort required rises quickly with the number of values to be sorted, even using

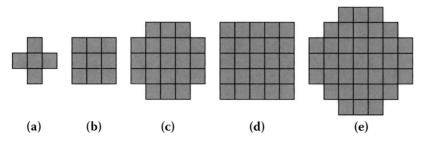

(a)   (b)   (c)   (d)   (e)

Figure 4.18 *Neighborhood patterns used for median filtering:* ***(a)*** *four nearest-neighbor cross;* ***(b)*** *3 × 3 square containing 9 pixels;* ***(c)*** *5 × 5 octagonal region with 21 pixels;* ***(d)*** *5 × 5 square containing 25 pixels;* ***(e)*** *7 × 7 octagonal region containing 37 pixels.*

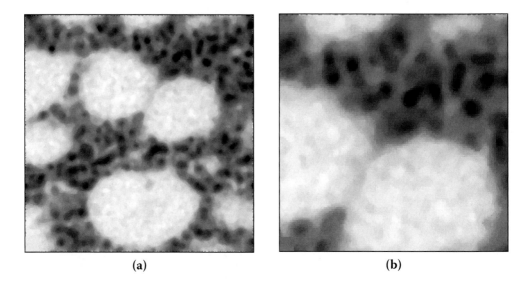

(a)   (b)

Figure 4.19 *Smoothing with a median filter:* ***(a)*** *the same image as in* ***Figure 4.9*** *after application of a 5 × 5 octagonal median filter;* ***(b)*** *enlargement of image to show individual pixels.*

specialized methods that keep partial sets of the pixels ranked separately so that, as the neighborhood is moved across the image, only a few additional pixel comparisons are needed.

Application of a median filter can also be used to reduce the type of random or speckle noise shown before in the context of averaging. **Figure 4.19** shows the same image as in **Figure 4.9**, with a 5 × 5 octagonal median filter applied. There are two principal advantages to the median filter as compared with multiplication by weights. First, the method does not reduce or blur the brightness difference across steps, because the values available are only those present in the neighborhood region, not an average between those values. Second, median filtering does not shift boundaries as averaging may, depending on the relative magnitude of values present in the neighborhood. Overcoming these problems makes the median filter preferred both for visual examination and measurement of images (Huang 1979; Yang and Huang 1981).

Figure 4.20 shows a comparison of uniform averaging, Gaussian filtering, and median filtering applied to a noisy SEM image. The better preservation of edge sharpness by the median filter is apparent. Even with a very large neighborhood (**Figure 4.20e**), the edges do not shift

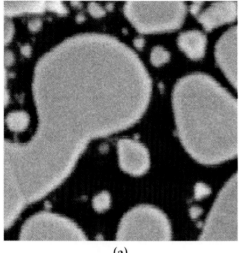

(a)

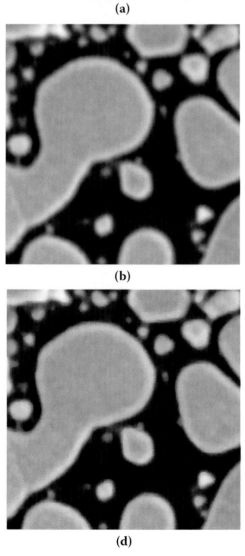

(b)

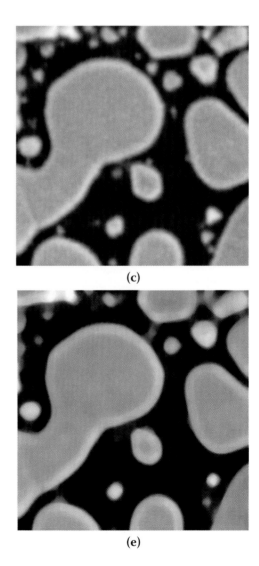

(c)

(d)

(e)

Figure 4.20 Comparison of noise-reduction
techniques (SEM image enlarged to show
pixel detail):
(a) original;
(b) 5 × 5 uniform averaging;
(c) Gaussian filter, standard deviation =
1 pixel;
(d) median filter, 5 × 5 octagonal region;
(e) median filter, radius = 15 pixels.

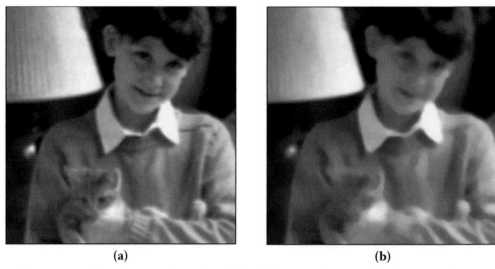

(a)   (b)

Figure 4.21 *Repeated application of a median filter: **(a)** original image; **(b)** after 12 applications (the fine details have been erased and textured regions leveled to a uniform shade of gray, but boundaries have not shifted).*

position, but when the neighborhood radius is larger than the size of any features present, they are eliminated and replaced by values from the surrounding background. This is an essential feature of the median filter, which can sometimes be used to advantage to remove dirt or other small, unwanted features from images. However, for noise-reduction purposes it is usually better (and faster) to repeat the application of a small median than to use a large one.

Because of the minimal degradation to edges from median filtering, it is possible to apply the method repeatedly. **Figure 4.21** shows an example in which a 5 × 5 octagonal median filter was applied 12 times to an image. The fine detail is erased in this process, and large regions take on the same brightness values. However, the edges remain in place and well defined. This type of leveling of brightness due to repetition of median filtering is sometimes described as contouring or posterization (but those terms also have other meanings that will be presented elsewhere).

The concept of a median filter requires a ranking order for the pixels in the neighborhood, which for gray-scale images is simply provided by the pixel value. Color images present a challenge to this idea (Comer and Delp 1999; Heijmans 1994; Sartor and Weeks 2001). Simple application of the ranking operations to the red, green, and blue channels is rarely useful and does not generalize to HSI because hue is an angle that wraps around modulo 360°.

A color median filter can be devised by using as the definition of the median value that pixel whose color coordinates give the smallest sum-of-squares of distances to the other pixels in the neighborhood (Astolo et al. 1990; Oistämö and Neuvo 1990; Russ 1995b). The choice of the color space in which these coordinate distances are measured can also present a problem. As discussed before, HSI space is generally preferred for processing to RGB space, but there is no unique answer to the question of the relative scaling factors of these different spaces, or how to deal with the angular measure of hue values. **Figure 4.22** shows an example of an HSI color median filter used to remove shot noise from an image produced by dead or locked transistors in the camera. The smallest neighborhood shown in **Figure 4.18** was used. Note that the edges and fine lines are retained but single-pixel noise is eliminated.

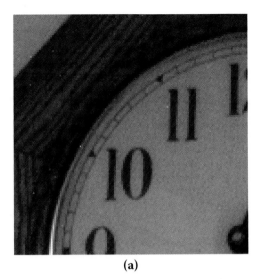
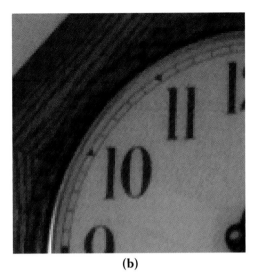

(a)   (b)

Figure 4.22 *Enlarged fragment of a digital camera image with shot noise: (**a**) original; (**b**) color median filter applied.*

The extension of median filtering (or rank-order filtering in general) from a simple ranking of scalar numbers (the gray-scale pixel values) to vectors representing color-space values opens the door to more complex uses of vector ranking. Instead of the vector length, it is possible to construct rankings based on vector angles to remove vectors (colors) that point in atypical directions, or hybrid methods that combine direction and distance (Smolka et al. 2001). Vectors need not be restricted to three dimensions, so it is possible to combine many criteria into a to-

tal measure of pixel similarity. The performance of these methods is bought at the price of computational complexity, but it is possible in some cases to reconstruct images corrupted by up to 70% noise pixels with quite good accuracy.

Sharpening of edges can be accomplished even better with a mode filter (Davies 1988). The mode of the distribution of brightness values in each neighborhood is, by definition, the most likely value. However, for a small neighborhood, the mode is poorly defined. An approximation to this value can be obtained with a truncated-median filter. For any asymmetric distribution, such as would be obtained at most locations near but not precisely straddling an edge, the mode is the highest point, and the median lies closer to the mode than the mean value. This is illustrated in **Figure 4.23**. The truncated-median technique consists of discarding a few extreme values from the neighborhood so that the median value of the remaining pixels is shifted toward the mode. In the example shown in **Figure 4.24**, this is done for a 3 × 3 neighborhood

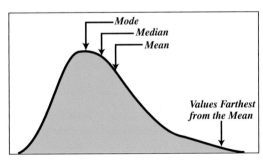

Figure 4.23 *Schematic diagram of an asymmetric histogram distribution of brightness values, showing the relationship between the mode, median, and mean. The truncated-median filter works by discarding the values in the distribution that are farthest from the mean, and then using the median of the remainder as an estimate for the mode. For a symmetrical distribution, values are discarded from both ends, and the median value does not change (it is already equal to the mode).*

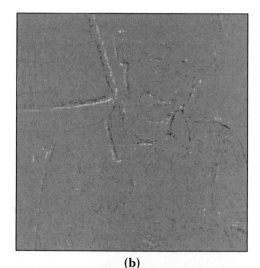

(b)

Figure 4.24 *Application of the truncated median filter to posterize the image from* ***Figure 4.21a:***

- **(a)** one application of the 3 × 3 truncated median;
- **(b)** difference between image **a** and a conventional 3 × 3 median filter, showing the difference in values along edges;
- **(c)** 12 repetitions of the truncated median filter.

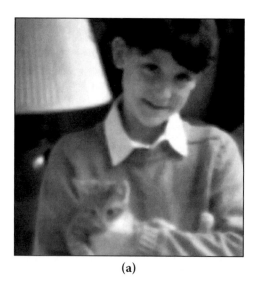

(a)

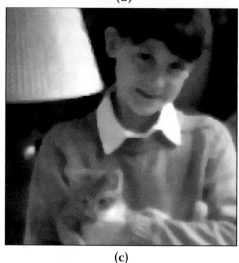

(c)

by skipping the two pixels whose brightness values are most different from the mean, ranking the remaining seven values, and assigning the median to the central pixel.

Another modification to the median filter is used to overcome its tendency to round corners and to erase lines that are narrower than the half-width of the neighborhood. The so-called hybrid median, or corner-preserving median, is actually a three-step ranking operation (Nieminen et al. 1987). In a 3 × 3-pixel neighborhood, pixels can be ranked in two different groups, as shown in **Figure 4.25**. The median values of the 45° neighbors forming an "X" and the 90° neighbors forming a "+" (both groups include the central pixel) are compared with the central pixel, and the median value of that set is then saved as the new pixel value. As shown in **Figure 4.26**, this method preserves lines and corners that are erased or rounded off by the conventional median. In a larger neighborhood, more orientations can be employed; four directions can be used in a 5 × 5 region, producing four values that can be ranked along with the original central pixel value.

The hybrid median can also be extended to color images by using the same approaches for performing the median as described previously. It offers the same advantages of preserving

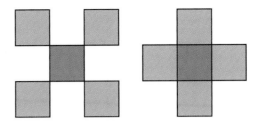

Figure 4.25 Diagram of neighborhood pixels used in the hybrid-median filter. Both groups include the central pixel (color) and are ranked separately. The median of each group, and the central pixel, are then ranked again to select the final median value.

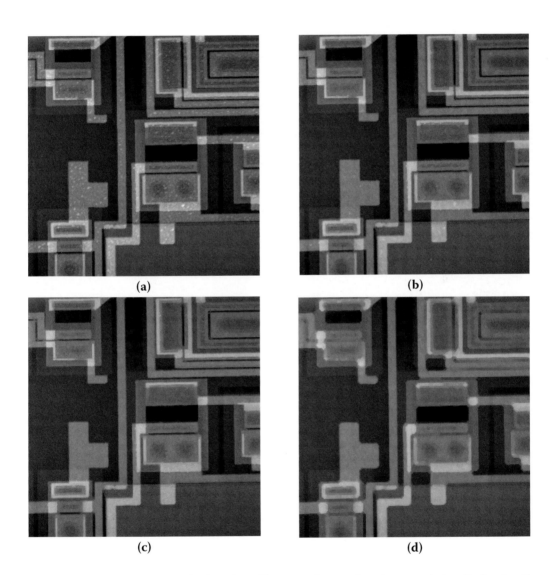

(a)

(b)

(c)

(d)

Figure 4.26 Application of the hybrid-median filter to an image of an integrated circuit, showing the improved retention of lines and corners: *(a)* original image with unwanted surface texture in the deposited metal; *(b)* application of the 5 × 5 hybrid-median filter; *(c)* application of a 9 × 9 hybrid median; *(d)* application of a conventional 5 × 5 median, which removes most of the texture but also rounds corners and fills in lines.

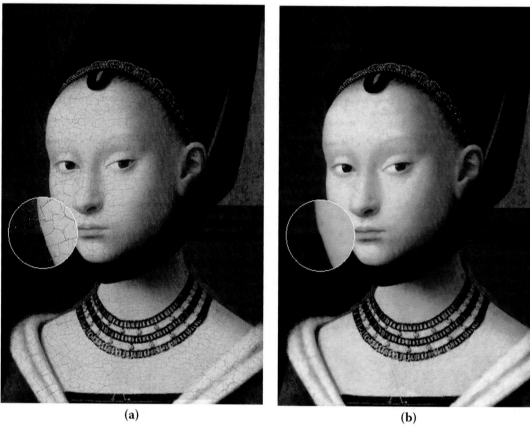

(a)   (b)

Figure 4.27 Portrait of a Lady, *painted in 1470 by Petrus Christus:* **(a)** *present appearance, showing cracks and fading of the colors;* **(b)** *application of a hybrid-median filter to fill in the dark cracks and color compensation to adjust the colors.*

sharp edges and fine lines while reducing random and shot noise. Controlling the size of the neighborhood provides the essential tool for defining the size of the defects to be removed. In the example of **Figure 4.27**, the painting is *Portrait of a Lady*, painted in 1470 by Petrus Christus, a Flemish Renaissance painter (Gemäldegalerie der Staatlichen Museen, Berlin-Dahlem). A smoothing convolution applied to the image would have blended the gray values from the network of fine cracks that have formed in the paint, as well as blurring edges and fine lines. The application of a median filter allows filling in the cracks without blurring edges, much as the pixel noise was removed from the gray-scale images shown previously. The result is a restoration of the appearance of the original painting.

If the hybrid-median filter is applied repeatedly, it can also produce posterization. Because the details of lines and corners are preserved by the hybrid median, the shapes of regions are not smoothed as they are with the conventional median, although the brightness values across steps are still sharpened and posterized.

The fact that the hybrid median involves multiple ranking operations, first within each of the groups of pixels and then to compare those medians with the central pixel, does not impose a computational penalty. Each of the ranking operations is for a much smaller number of values than is used in a square or octagonal region of the same size. For example, a 5-pixel-wide neighborhood contains either 25 (in the square neighborhood) or 21 pixels (in the octagonal neighborhood), which must be ranked in the traditional method. In the hybrid method, each of the groups contains only 9 pixels, and the final comparison involves only five values. Even with the additional logic and manipulation of values, the hybrid method is about as fast as the conventional median.

Posterizing an image, or reducing the number of gray levels so that regions become uniform in gray value and edges between regions become abrupt, falls more into the category of enhancement than correcting defects, but it is mentioned here as a side effect of median filtering. Other methods can produce this effect. One that is related to the median is the extremum filter, which replaces each pixel value with either the minimum or maximum value in the neighborhood, whichever is closer to the mean value. This filter is not edge-preserving and may shift boundaries. When the extremum filter is iterated, it is sometimes called a "toggle" filter (Arce et al. 2000).

Sometimes it is useful to construct a neighborhood that is not round, but has a specific shape based on independent knowledge about the nature of the image. A common defect in video images is the appearance of horizontal lines that indicate variations in signal between the two interlaced fields. A similar defect occurs in atomic force microscope images due to DC (direct current) signal offsets. Movie film often exhibits vertical scratches resulting from wear and tear and rubbing against transport devices. If the direction of the lines or scratches is known, a neighborhood can be constructed to remove it.

Figure 4.28 shows an example of video line noise in a poor-quality surveillance tape. This is a common defect that can arise from dirty recording heads, for example. A median neighbor-

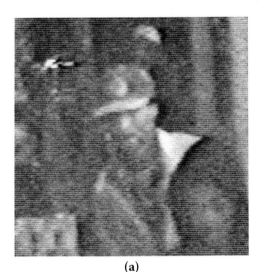

(a)

Figure 4.28
  (a) Surveillance video image with horizontal scan line noise;
  (b) a custom neighborhood to perform median filtering in a vertical direction;
  (c) and the result.

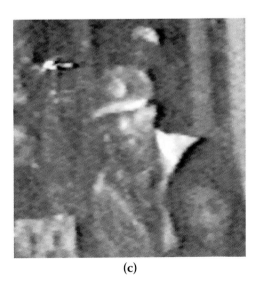

(b)

(c)

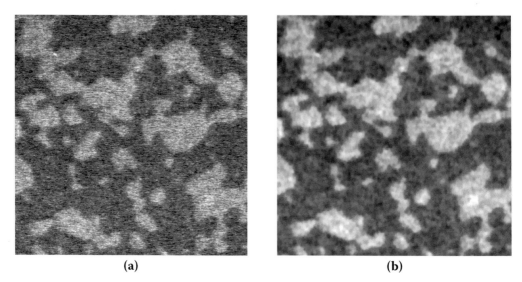

(a)   (b)

*Figure 4.29 Low-voltage SEM image of a thin film, with horizontal streaking **(a)**, and the result of applying a vertical median filter **(b)**.*

hood that is predominantly vertical can eliminate much of the line noise. Similarly, **Figure 4.29** shows horizontal streaks in a low-voltage SEM image in which the scan rate was too high for the amplifier time constant, which blurs information along the scan line direction. Again, a median filter applied in a vertical stripe corrects the problem.

In most simple cases, the neighborhood used in a ranking operation such as a median filter is circular, with a radius selected on the basis of the size of the smallest features to be retained. For computational simplicity, a square neighborhood is sometimes used, which can introduce some directional bias into the results. It is also possible to use an adaptive neighborhood, one that includes pixels based on their value or position. Conditional or adaptive selection starts with a larger neighborhood of candidate pixels, which are then included in the ranking if they meet additional criteria, which can be used in combination. If the number of pixels in the adaptive neighborhood is even rather than odd, so that there is no single median value, several options are available, but the most common is to average the two values in the center of the ranked list. Methods for selecting the pixels in the adaptive neighborhood include:

1. Pixels whose difference from the central pixel is less than some adjustable threshold
2. The N pixels within the larger neighborhood that are closest in value to the central pixel
3. The N pixels within the larger neighborhood that are closest in value to the central pixel and are contiguous to it and to each other (Kober et al. 2001)
4. Weighting the pixels within the neighborhood according to their distance from the central pixel, by entering nearby pixel values more than once into the list to be ranked

At the expense of computational complexity, these methods produce good rejection of impulsive or shot noise (as does the conventional median) and improved rejection of additive random noise while preserving lines and edges. **Figure 4.30** shows an example of the first method listed above.

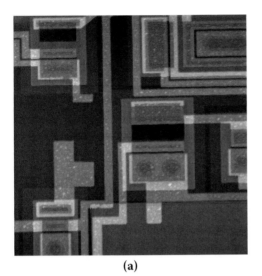 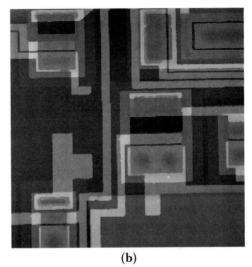

(a)   (b)

*Figure 4.30 Conditional smoothing using an adaptive neighborhood: **(a)** original (same as Figure 4.26a); **(b)** median value of pixels in a 9-pixel-wide circle that are within ±40 gray-level values of the central pixel.*

Other neighborhood noise-reduction methods

A modification to the simple averaging of neighborhood values that attempts to achieve some of the advantages of the median filter is the so-called Olympic filter. The name comes from the system of scoring used in some events in the Olympic games, in which the highest and lowest scores are discarded and the remainder averaged. The same thing is done with the pixel values in the neighborhood. By discarding the extreme values, shot noise is rejected. Then the average of the remaining pixel values is used as the new brightness.

Figure 4.31 shows an application of this method to the image from **Figure 4.9**, which contains random intensity variations or speckle. Because it still causes blurring of edges and still requires sorting of the brightness values, this method is generally inferior to the others discussed and is not often used. **Figure 4.32** shows an application to the shot noise introduced in **Figure 4.17**. The performance is quite poor: the features are blurred and yet the noise is not all removed.

There are other versions of modified or conditional smoothing that omit some of the pixel values in the moving neighborhood from the smoothing operation. The justification is always based on the omitted pixels being different from those that are used, so that they presumably belong to a different region. Most of the techniques take into account both the location of the pixel in the region and the difference in the value from the original central pixel. For example, fitting a function to the pixels can be used to detect a sharp change in the slope and to omit pixels that lie beyond the edge (a technique known as "kriging"). All of these methods make some assumptions about the nature of the image and of the noise present, and the better the assumptions fit the actual image, the better is the result.

One particular instance in which knowledge about the image acquisition is useful for noise reduction applies to digital cameras. As described in **Chapter 1**, the typical camera records separate red, green, and blue signals. Silicon detectors are least sensitive at the blue end of the spectrum, and in addition typical detector designs use fewer blue-filtered transistors than green, resulting in much more speckle noise in the blue channel than in the green. Different

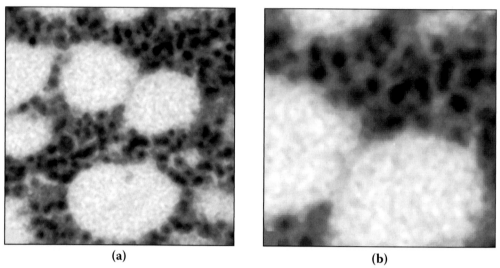

Figure 4.31 *Application of an Olympic filter to Gaussian noise. The four brightest and four darkest pixels in each 5 × 5 neighborhood are ignored, and the remaining 17 averaged to produce a new image: (a) application to the image in* **Figure 4.9**; *(b) enlargement to show pixel detail.*

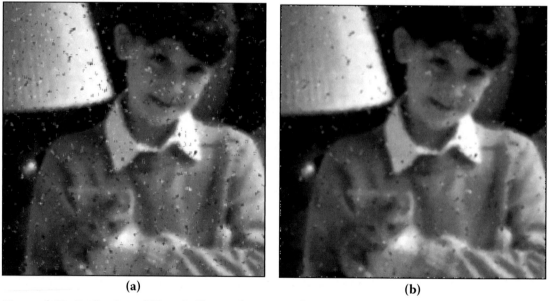

Figure 4.32 *Application of Olympic filter to shot noise. The original image is the same as in* **Figure 4.17b**: *(a) the two brightest and two darkest pixels in each 3 × 3 neighborhood are ignored, and the remaining five averaged; (b) the four brightest and four darkest pixels in each 5 × 5 neighborhood are ignored, and the remaining 17 pixels averaged.*

noise-reduction parameters can therefore be used for the different channels. In **Chapter 5**, the use of principal-components analysis (PCA) is introduced as a way to further separate the noise from the information content of the image so that it can be selectively filtered. In all of these cases, the actual filtering procedures are those that are described in this chapter, either neighborhood-based weighted averaging or rank-based median methods.

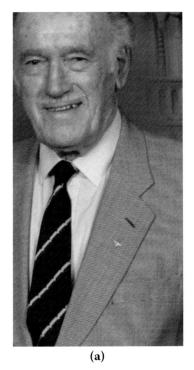

(a)

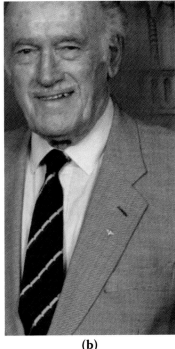

(b)

Figure 4.33 *Removal of moiré interference patterns:*
(a) *original, showing colored fringes on the fabric of the subject's coat;*
(b) *after converting to L*a*b* space and applying Gaussian smoothing to the fringe area in the a and b channels. Because the brightness values are unaltered, the apparent sharpness of the image is not affected.*

Another problem that arises because of the sampling inherent in camera design is color moiré patterns such as shown in **Figure 4.33**. The spacing of the pattern in the cloth of the subject's coat is close to the spacing of the sensors in the detector and at a slight angle, resulting in an interference pattern that typically shifts with slight movements of the subject, and can be very distracting. This type of image defect is commonly seen in television images, for example. Separating the image into L*a*b* channels shows that the interference pattern is almost entirely localized in the two color channels. Smoothing it there using a Gaussian filter corrects the problem, as shown in the figure. Of course, it is impractical to attempt this in real time for television purposes.

There are more complicated combinations of operations that are used for very specific types of images. For instance, synthetic aperture radar (SAR) images contain speckle noise that varies in a known way with the image brightness. To remove the noise, the brightness of each pixel is compared with the average value of a local neighborhood. If it exceeds it by an amount calculated from the average and the standard deviation, then it is replaced by a weighted average value. Using some coefficients determined by experiment, the method is reported (Nathan and Curlander 1990) to perform better at improving signal-to-noise ratio than a simple median filter. This is a good example of a specific processing method based on knowledge of the characteristics of the signal and the noise in a particular situation. In general, any filtering method that chooses between several algorithms or modifies its algorithm based on the actual contents of the image or the neighborhood is called an adaptive filter (Mastin 1985).

Noise is often modeled as a Gaussian additive function, and noise-reduction methods are often tested by adding Gaussian noise to an image, but in fact various noise sources have very widely differing characteristics. Noise that arises from photon or particle counting is generally Poisson, which becomes Gaussian for large numbers. The distribution of exposed grains in film is also approximately Gaussian. The effect of electronic circuitry in cameras and amplifiers can be either additive or multiplicative, and generally affects dark areas differently from bright ones. Noise resulting from light scattering in the atmosphere or from surfaces is generally multiplicative rather than additive. Speckle interferometry encountered in radar imaging is more complex, since it interacts through shifts in phase and polarization. It also tends to have a spatial correlation, which makes it more difficult to model. The removal of speckle by acquiring many short-duration images is used in astronomy, but that is beyond the scope of this text.

Another way of filtering by ranking is to use the maximum and minimum brightness rather than the median. **Figure 4.34** shows the results of a two-step operation. First, the brightest pixel value in each region (a 5 × 5 octagonal neighborhood) was used to replace the original pixel values. Then in a second transformation, the darkest pixel value in each region was selected. This type of combined operation requires two full passes through the image, and during each pass only the previous pixel brightness values are used to derive the new ones.

For reasons that will be discussed in more detail in **Chapter 8**, these types of operations are often described as gray-scale morphological steps, specifically as erosion and dilation, by analogy to the erosion and dilation steps that are performed on binary images. The sequence is also called an opening, again by analogy to operations on binary images. By adjusting the sizes of the neighborhoods (which need not be the same) used in the two separate passes to locate the brightest and then the darkest values, other processing effects are obtained. These are described in **Chapter 5** in the context of image enhancement.

As a method for removing noise, this technique would seem to be the antithesis of a median filter, which discards extreme values. The difference is that this approach makes it possible to selectively remove bright (or dark) noise, whereas the median filter removes both. It may be helpful to visualize the image as a surface for which the brightness represents an elevation. **Figure 4.35** shows a one-dimensional representation of such a situation. In the first pass, the brightest values in each region are used to construct a new profile, which follows the "tops of the trees." In the second pass, the darkest values in each region are used to bring the profile back down to those points that were large enough to survive the first one, giving a new profile

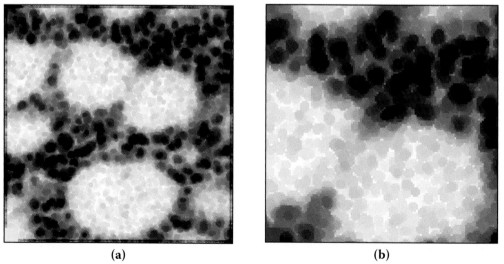

(a)   (b)

*Figure 4.34 Gray-scale opening, or erosion and dilation. Two separate ranking operations are performed on the original image from **Figure 4.9a**. First each pixel value is replaced with the brightest value in the neighborhood (5 × 5 octagonal); then, using this image, each pixel value is replaced by the darkest value in the same size neighborhood: (a) result; (b) enlarged to show pixel detail.*

that ignores the dark noise spikes in the original while retaining the bright features. Applying the same operations in the other order (erosion followed by dilation, called a closing) would have removed bright noise while retaining dark features.

Another method that uses ranking, but in two different size neighborhoods, is useful for locating and removing noise. It is often called a "top-hat" or "rolling-ball" filter. Imagine the brightness values of the pixels to represent the elevation of a surface. A top-hat filter consists of a flat disk that rests on the surface and a central crown of a smaller diameter, as shown in **Figure 4.36**. This filter is centered on each pixel in the image, with the brim "resting" on the surface. Any pixels that "stick up" through the crown of the hat are considered to be noise and are replaced. The replacement value can be either the mean or the median value of the pixels covered by the brim of the hat. (The "rolling ball" name comes from imagining the spots to represent depressions, in which a rolling ball can rest but may or may not be able to touch the bottom of the hole.)

The implementation of this filter uses two neighborhoods, one a round (or approximately round) region corresponding to the inside or crown of the hat, and a second annular neighborhood surrounding it that corresponds to the brim. In each, the maximum (brightest or darkest) value is found. If the difference between the brightest (or darkest) pixel in the interior region and the outside exceeds a threshold (the height of the hat) then the pixel value is replaced with the mean or median of the outside region. As shown in **Figure 4.37**, if the feature fits entirely within the smaller neighborhood (the crown of the hat), it is detected by this operation. If it does not, or if the spacing between features is less than the width of the brim of the hat, then there is no large difference between the inside and outside, and nothing is detected.

The features found using the top-hat or rolling-ball filters can be removed, typically by replacing them with values interpolated from the

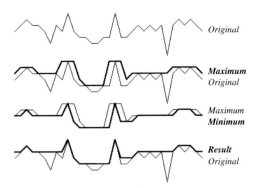

Figure 4.35 *Schematic diagram of the operation of gray-scale erosion and dilation in one dimension, showing (starting from the top): the original profile with result of first (maximum) pass, producing a new profile through brightest points; the second step in which a new profile passes through the darkest (minimum) points in the result from step 1; comparison of the final result with the original profile, showing rejection of noise and dark spikes but retention of bright features.*

Figure 4.36 *Diagram of a top-hat filter. The brim rests on the "surface" that corresponds to the brightness of pixels in the image. Any pixel with a brightness value that is able to rise through the crown of the hat is detected and can be replaced with the mean or median of the outer neighborhood. The inner and outer radius of the brim and the height of the crown are all adjustable parameters.*

brim. An adaptation of this same logic to a trench-shaped neighborhood (a line of pixels forming the inner region, with parallel lines on both sides forming the outer region) can be used to effectively find and remove scratches, provided they have a known direction. This technique is sometimes used to remove scratches when digitizing film, and it is built into the firmware of many scanner models.

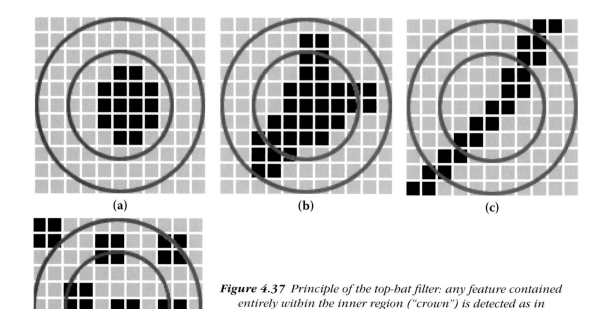

(a)   (b)   (c)

(d)

*Figure 4.37 Principle of the top-hat filter: any feature contained entirely within the inner region ("crown") is detected as in image **a**. Features that are too large for the crown (images **b** and **c**) or are not separated by more than the width of the brim (image **d**) are not.*

Figure 4.38 shows an example. The dust particles on the slide are all smaller than 9 pixels across, so a filter consisting of an inner circle with a radius of 4 pixels and an outer one with a radius of 6 pixels forms the top hat. The dust particles are removed, but since the bug itself is too large to fit inside the inner circle, there is no large difference between the darkest values in the two neighborhoods, and the pixels are not altered.

In the next chapter we will consider the use of this same filter for a different purpose. Instead of removing extreme points as noise or dirt, the same operation can be used to find and keep points of interest that are smaller than the crown of the hat and brighter or darker than the local neighborhood. **Figure 4.38b** also illustrates this function of the top hat. Using the same settings for neighborhood size — but keeping the extreme values and suppressing those that do not have a difference greater than the top-hat threshold — reveals just the dust particles on the slide.

Defect removal, maximum entropy, and maximum likelihood

As shown above, the rolling-ball/top-hat filter can be used to remove small defects by replacing the pixels with a value taken from the surrounding neighborhood. Interpolation is a general tool that can sometimes be used to replace localized defects, either originating in the specimen itself or in the camera (e.g., dirt on the lens). If the defect is large or irregular in shape, smoothing may leave some of the pixel values from the defect remaining in the resulting image, and it may be impractical to use a neighborhood for rank-based filtering that is large enough to encompass it. In many cases, better results can be obtained by filling in the region of the defect using the adjacent values. In the example shown in **Figure 4.39**, a hole in a leaf

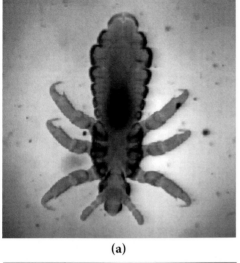

(a)

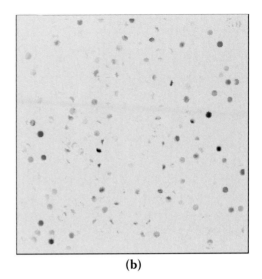

(b)

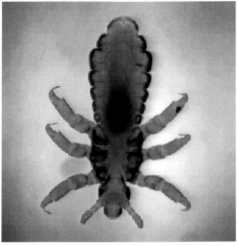

(c)

Figure 4.38 *Operation of the top-hat filter:*
  (a) *original image showing dust particles on the slide containing the insect;*
  (b) *isolation of the dust particles by the top-hat filter, showing the difference in darkness between the values in the crown and brim of the hat;*
  (c) *removal of the dust particles by interpolating values from the brim to replace the darker ones in the crown.*

has been manually circled and the pixels replaced by linear interpolation between the edge pixels. The algorithm is similar in effect to stretching a membrane across an irregular opening with an edge of variable height. The elastic membrane forms a lowest-energy surface. Calculating the pixel values within the region is accomplished in the same way.

Instead of manual outlining, regions can be selected by any of the thresholding techniques discussed in **Chapter 7**. These include specifying a range of brightness or color values that discriminate the defects from their surroundings, or using a region-growing method in which selecting one point in the defect allows the software to include all touching similar pixels. In **Figure 4.40**, this method was used to select the yellow flower. Then the region was enlarged by 2 pixels, and the background interpolated from the edge pixels of the region. This approach can be quite useful for removing manually selected features from images when that is justified by circumstances. It should be noted, however, that it is not proper in the context of scientific imaging to add anything to an image, for instance to replace or cover a feature that has been eliminated. Subtracting the modified image from the original produces an image of just the removed feature, as shown.

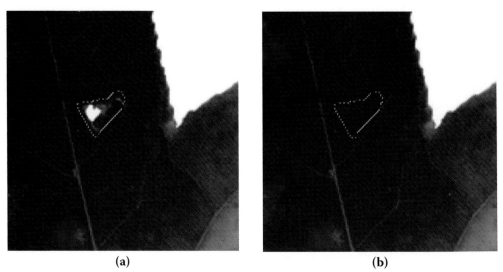

(a)   (b)

Figure 4.39 Defect removal by interpolating from the edges of a region: (a) image of a maple leaf (enlarged) showing a manually drawn region around a hole; (b) interpolation of values from the edge.

Images may contain other defects, such as blur due to motion or out-of-focus optics, in addition to noise. The "inverse filtering" methods described in **Chapter 6** under the topic of deconvolution are quite noise sensitive. When the noise that is present can itself be characterized, it may be possible to use a maximum-entropy approach to remove the artifacts.

Entropy-based methods represent a computer-intensive approach to removing artifacts such as noise or blur from images, based on some foreknowledge about the image contents and some assumptions about the nature of the degradation that is to be removed and of the image that is to be restored (Skilling 1986; Frieden 1988). The conventional description of the method is to imagine an image containing N pixels that has been formed by a total of M photons (where usually $M \gg N$). The number of photons in any single pixel (i.e., the pixel's brightness value) is P_i, where i is the pixel index.

The measured image has normalized pixel brightness values $p_i = P_i / \Sigma P_i$ that only approximate the "true" image that would be collected if there were no artifacts. The p_i values are just the image histogram. The method used to approach this ideal image is to alter pixel brightness values to maximize the entropy in the image, subject to some constraints. The justification for this method is given in terms of statistical probability and Bayes's theorem, and will not be derived here. In some cases this method produces dramatic improvements in image quality.

The "entropy" of the brightness pattern is given in a formal sense by calculating the number of ways that the pattern could have been formed by rearrangement, or $S = M!/P_1!P_2!, ..., P_N!$, where ! indicates factorial. For large values of M, this reduces by Stirling's approximation to the more familiar $S = -\Sigma p_i \log p_i$. This is the same calculation of entropy used in statistical mechanics. In the particular case of taking the log to the base 2, the entropy of the image is the number of bits per pixel needed to represent the image, according to information theory.

The entropy in the image would be minimized in an absolute sense simply by setting the brightness of each pixel to the average brightness and maximized by spreading the values uni-

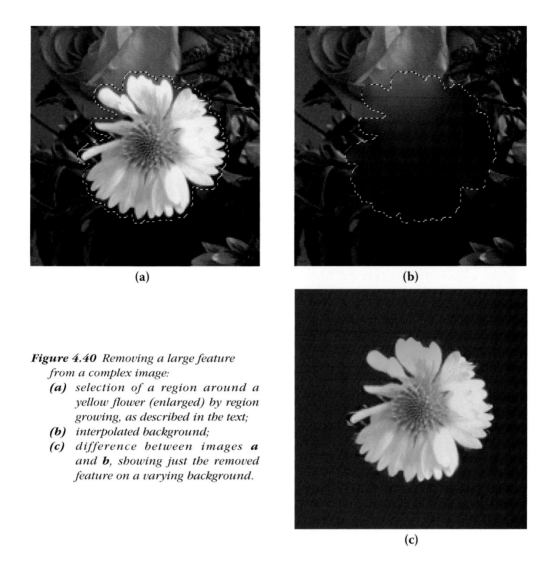

Figure 4.40 *Removing a large feature from a complex image:*
- **(a)** *selection of a region around a yellow flower (enlarged) by region growing, as described in the text;*
- **(b)** *interpolated background;*
- **(c)** *difference between images **a** and **b**, showing just the removed feature on a varying background.*

formly across the entire brightness range. Clearly, neither of these is a "right" solution. It is the application of constraints that produce usable results. The most common constraint for images containing noise is based on a chi-squared statistic, calculated as $\chi^2 = 1/\sigma^2 \Sigma \, (p_i - p_{i'})^2$. In this expression, the p_i values are the original pixel values, the $p_{i'}$ values are the altered brightness values, and σ is the standard deviation of the values. An upper limit can be set on the value of χ^2 allowed in the calculation of a new set of pi' values to maximize the entropy. A typical (but essentially arbitrary) limit for χ^2 is N, the number of pixels in the array.

This constraint is not the only possible choice. A sum of the absolute value of differences, or some other weighting rule, could also be chosen. This is not quite enough information to produce an optimal image, and so other constraints may be added. One is that the totals of the p_i and $p_{i'}$ values must be equal. Bryan and Skilling (1980) also require, for instance, that the distribution of the $p_i - p_{i'}$ values correspond to the expected noise characteristics of the imaging source (e.g., a Poisson or Gaussian distribution for simple counting statistics). And, of course, we must be careful to include such seemingly "obvious" constraints as nonnegativity (no pixel can collect fewer than zero photons). Jaynes (1985) makes the point that there is practically always a significant amount of real knowledge about the image that can be used as constraints but that is assumed to be so obvious that it is ignored.

An iterative solution for the values of $p_{i'}$ produces a new image with the desired smoothness and noise characteristics, which are often improved from the original image. Other formulations of the maximum-entropy approach compare one iteration of the image to the next by calculating not the total entropy, but the cross entropy, $-\Sigma p_i \log(p_i/q_i)$, where q_i is the previous image brightness value for the same pixel or, for a theoretical image, the modeled brightness. In this formulation, the cross entropy is to be minimized. The basic principle remains the same.

Maximum-likelihood reconstruction of an image is another related approach in which the assumption is made that the boundaries between regions should be sharp. In most real images, pixels that straddle any boundary average values from both sides according the exact placement of the edge with respect to the finite size of the pixel. This leads to intermediate brightness or color values that appear to blur the boundary. Reclassifying the pixels to the brightness of one region or the other sharpens the boundaries.

One of the most common statistical approaches to the classification measures the variance of pixels in many subregions of a neighborhood around each pixel, as shown in **Figure 4.41**. Whichever region has the lowest variance is taken to represent the region to which the central pixel should belong, and it is assigned the mean value from that subregion (Kuwahara et al. 1976). **Figure 4.42** shows an application of the method.

When applied to halftoned images that have been digitized with a scanner, this filter can eliminate the halftone patterns, as shown in **Figure 4.43**. Also note that for real objects such as the flowers and leaves shown, in which the edges of objects are naturally shaded, the filter converts the appearance to that of a painting, lithograph, or cartoon.

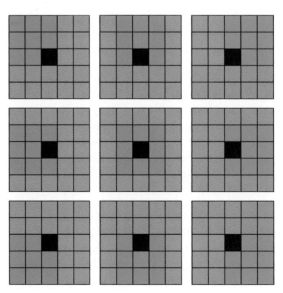

Figure 4.41 *Nine 3 × 3 subregions (green) within a 5 × 5 neighborhood. The Kuwahara filter assigns the mean value of whichever region has the smallest variance to the central pixel (dark).*

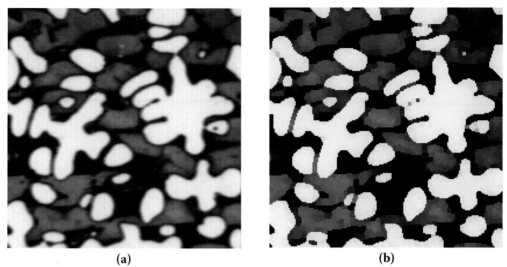

(a)   (b)

Figure 4.42 *Application of a maximum-likelihood filter: **(a)** original image (enlarged to show pixel detail); **(b)** filter applied, resulting in sharp region boundaries.*

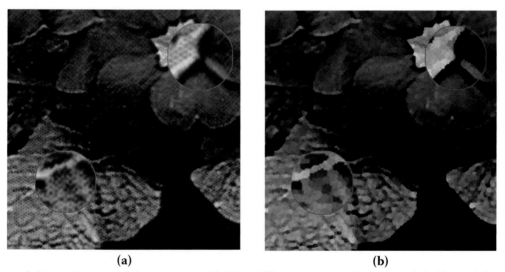

(a)   (b)

Figure 4.43 *Application of the maximum-likelihood filter to a scanned image with halftone: **(a)** original; **(b)** filter applied (regions enlarged to show pixel detail).*

Nonuniform illumination

The most straightforward strategy for image analysis uses the brightness (pixel values) of regions in the image as a means of identification: it is assumed that the same type of feature will have the same brightness (or color, in a color image) wherever it appears in the field of view. If this brightness is different from that of other features, or can be made so by appropriate image processing as discussed in **Chapter 5**, then it can be used to discriminate the features for counting, measurement, or identification. Even if there are a few other types of objects that cannot be distinguished on the basis of brightness or color alone, subsequent measurements may suffice to select the ones of interest.

This approach is not without pitfalls, which are discussed further in **Chapter 7** in conjunction with converting gray-scale images to binary (black and white) images. Other approaches are available, such as region growing or split-and-merge, that do not have such stringent requirements for uniformity of illumination. However, when it can be used, simple brightness thresholding is by far the simplest and fastest method to isolate features in an image, so it is important to consider the problems of shading of images.

When irregular surfaces are viewed, the amount of light scattered to the viewer or camera from each region is a function of the orientation of the surface with respect to the source of light and the viewer, even if the surface material and finish is uniform. In fact, this principle can be used to estimate the surface orientation, using a technique known as shape-from-shading. Human vision seems to apply these rules very easily and rapidly, since we are not generally confused by images of real-world objects.

Most of the images we really want to process are essentially two-dimensional. Whether they come from light or electron microscopes, macroscopic imaging, or satellite images, the variation in surface elevation is usually small compared with the lateral dimensions, giving rise to what is often called "two-and-one-half-D." This is not always the case of course (consider a woven fabric examined in the SEM), but we will treat such problems as exceptions to the general rule and recognize that more elaborate processing may be needed.

Even surfaces of low relief need not be flat, a simple example being the curvature of Earth as viewed from a weather satellite. This will produce a shading across the field of view. So will illumination of a macroscopic or microscopic surface from one side. Even elaborate collections of lights, or ring lights, can only approximate uniform illumination of the scene. Diffusers and umbrellas are useful in studio lighting setups, but in those cases the goal is usually selective rather than uniform illumination.

For transmission microscope imaging, the uniformity of the light source with a condenser lens system can be made quite good, but it is easy for these systems to get out of perfect alignment and produce shading as well. Finally, it was mentioned in **Chapter 1** that lenses or the cameras may cause vignetting, in which the corners of the image are darker than the center because the light is partially absorbed by greater path length in the optics. There may also be effects from the camera sensor itself, such as the influence of nonperpendicular incidence when using wide-angle lenses, which can be corrected by recording a "background" image (this can also be used to remove or reduce the fixed-pattern noise mentioned in **Chapter 1**).

Many of the lighting defects can be minimized by careful setup of the imaging conditions, or if they cannot be eliminated altogether, the defects can be assumed to be constant over some period of time. This assumption allows correction by image processing. In some instances, it is possible to acquire a "background" image in which a uniform reference surface or specimen is inserted in place of the actual samples to be viewed, and the light intensity recorded. This image can then be used to "level" the subsequent images. The process is often called "background subtraction," but in many cases this is a misnomer. If the image-acquisition device is logarithmic with a gamma of 1.0, then subtraction of the background image point by point from each acquired image is correct. If the camera or sensor is linear, then the correct procedure is to divide the acquired image by the background. For other sensor response functions, there is no exactly correct arithmetic method, and the calibrated response must first be determined and applied to convert the measured signal to a linear or logarithmic space.

In the process of subtracting (or dividing) one image by another, some of the dynamic range of the original data will be lost. The greater the variation in background brightness, the greater will be the variation remaining in the image after the leveling process. This loss and the inevitable increase in statistical noise that results from subtracting one signal from another argue that, before resorting to processing methods, all practical steps should be taken first to make illumination uniform and to reduce noise when acquiring the images.

Figure 1.82 in **Chapter 1** showed an example of leveling in which the background illumination function could be acquired separately. This acquisition is most commonly done by removing the specimen from the light path, for instance replacing a microscope slide with a blank one, and storing an image representing the variation. This image can then be used for leveling. **Figure 4.44** shows an example using a copy stand. The base of the stand is painted a flat uniform gray, so removing the object provides an opportunity to record an image of the illumination from the side, and subtracting it effectively levels the original image.

Figure 4.45 shows a situation in which the brightness variation can be extracted directly from the original image. By separating the red, green, and blue channels from the image, it is seen that the green image contains the important detail: the blood vessels in the retina of the eye, which are difficult to view because of the overall brightness variation. The red image has nearly the same variation, so the ratio of the green to red levels the varying background and makes the vessels more uniform in contrast.

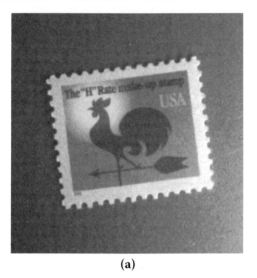

(a)

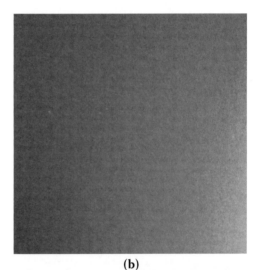

(b)

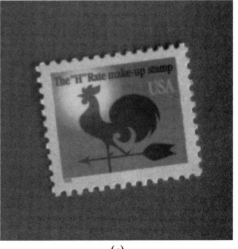

(c)

Figure 4.44 Leveling image brightness by subtracting a measured background:
(a) original image showing sidelighting of an object on a copy stand;
(b) removing the object and recording the background;
(c) subtracting the background point by point produces a uniform result.

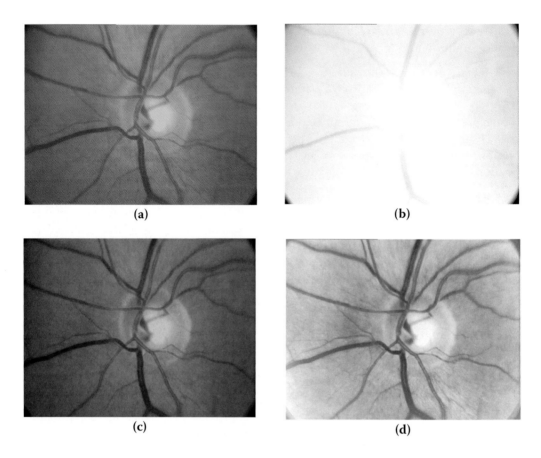

Figure 4.45 *Leveling with a measured background: (a) retina image from an ophthalmoscope, showing shading that makes the capillaries difficult to discern; (b) red channel contains little detail but does show the shading; (c) green channel has most of the contrast in the image; (d) ratio of green to red shows more uniform contrast. (Courtesy of G. Mansoor, University of Connecticut Health Care, Farmington, CT.)*

Another situation in which direct measurement of two images allows dividing to correct for nonuniform brightness arises in the transmission electron microscope. It is common, particularly for inorganic samples in materials science, for the specimens to vary in thickness. Computing the ratio of the conventional bright-field image to the zero-loss electrons isolated by a spectrometer attached to the microscope gives a direct measure of the variation in specimen thickness, which can subsequently be used to quantify concentration and structural measurements.

Fitting a background function

In many cases the background image is not recorded. It may not be practical to remove the specimen, or its presence can be a contributor to the brightness variation. This includes situations in which the specimen thickness varies, which affects the overall absorption of light.

Another case is that in which the surface being examined is tilted or curved, which causes incident light or SEM images to show a varying background. Using the example of **Figure 4.44**, if a background image was not recorded, it may still be possible to generate a background by interpolation.

Rather than the edge-interpolation method shown in **Figure 4.40**, which performs linear interpolation, a polynomial function is used here to define the background brightness. Polynomials are usually a good model for the gradual variation of brightness associated with off-center optics or illumination. Subtracting this function from the entire original image levels the brightness of the object as well as the background, as shown in **Figure 4.46**. This method can be applied whenever representative patches of background (or any structure that should be of the same brightness) can be located to provide adequate coverage of the image area.

By selecting a number of points in the image, a list of brightness values and locations can be acquired. These can then be used to perform least-squares fitting of a function $B(x,y)$ that approximates the background, and the results can be subtracted (or divided) just as a physically acquired background image would be. When the user marks these points, for instance by using

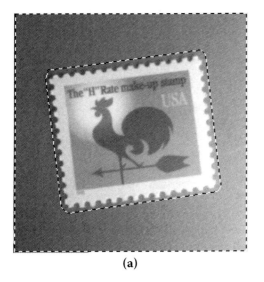

(a)

(b)

Figure 4.46 *Leveling image brightness by interpolation:*
- *(a)* *selecting a background region in* ***Figure 4.44a;***
- *(b)* *smooth polynomial brightness function fit to the background points;*
- *(c)* *leveled result after subtracting the background function from the entire image.*

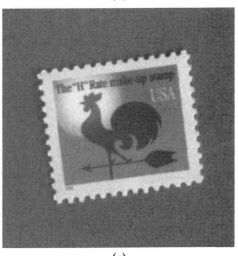

(c)

a pointing device such as a mouse, trackball, or light pen, it is important to select locations that should all have the same brightness and are well distributed across the image. Locating many points in one small region and few or none in other parts of the image requires the function to extrapolate the polynomial, which can introduce significant errors. For a third-order polynomial, the functional form of the fitted background is:

$$B(x,y) = a_0 + a_1 \cdot x + a_2 \cdot y + a_3 \cdot x^2 + a_4 \cdot y^2 + a_5 \cdot xy + a_6 \cdot x^3 + a_7 \cdot x^2 y + a_8 \cdot xy^2 + a_9 \cdot y^3 \qquad (4.4)$$

A second-order polynomial (the first size terms in **Equation 4.4**) has six fitted constants, and so in principle could be fitted with only that number of marked points. A third-order polynomial would have all ten coefficients. However, to get a good fit and diminish sensitivity to minor fluctuations in individual pixels, and to have enough points to sample the entire image area properly, it is usual to require several times this minimum number of points. **Figure 4.47** shows that one effect of leveling is to make the peaks in the image histogram much narrower and better separated, since all of the pixels in the same region have more nearly the same value.

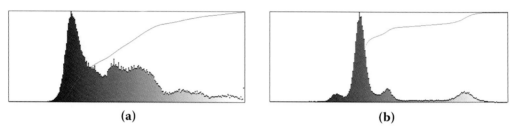

(a)   (b)

Figure 4.47 Effect of leveling on the image histogram: (a) histogram of Figure 4.44a; (b) histogram of Figure 4.46c.

Figure 4.48 shows an example in which the background points can be selected automatically, rather than by a human observer. The SEM image shows particles on a substrate, which because of the geometry of the surface and of the SEM chamber causes a portion of the image to appear darker than the rest. As noted in **Chapter 2**, the human eye is quite tolerant of this kind of gradual brightness variation, and so it is sometimes helpful to apply pseudocolor lookup tables to reveal the shading present in the image. Moving the specimen or changing the magnification alters the pattern of light and dark, in which case it is necessary to perform the correction using the image itself. Fortunately, in many of these situations the variation of background brightness is a smooth and well-behaved function of location and can be approximated by simple functions such as polynomials.

In this instance the particles are brighter than the local background, although the particles near the edges of the image are darker than the background near the center. Using the knowledge that the background consists of the locally dark pixels, and that it should be uniform, the algorithm functions by dividing the image up into many regions (a 9 × 9 grid in the example shown) and finding the darkest pixels in each region. These 81 points are then used to generate the polynomial in **Equation 4.4** and subtract it from the original, which levels the image brightness.

Automatic leveling is easiest when there is a distinct structure or phase present that is well distributed throughout the image area and contains the darkest (or lightest) pixels present. **Figure 4.49** shows an example in which the features (pores) are dark on a light background.

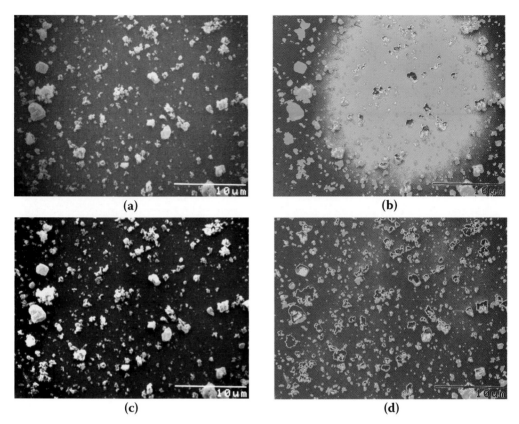

(a) (b)

(c) (d)

Figure 4.48 Leveling image contrast: *(a)* SEM image of particulates on a substrate; *(b)* pseudocolor applied to image *a* to make the shading more visually evident; *(c)* image *b* leveled by polynomial fitting; *(d)* pseudocolor applied to image *c*.

The specimen (a polished ceramic) has an overall variation in brightness due to curvature of the surface. The brightest pixels in each region of the specimen represent the matrix, and so should all be the same. In this example the same grid subdivision of the image was used to select the brightest local values, which are then used to calculate a second-order polynomial (six coefficients) by least-squares. The fitting routine in this case reported a fitting error (root mean square [rms] value) of less than two brightness values out of the total 0 to 255 range for pixels in the image. **Figure 4.49b** shows the calculated brightness using the $B(x,y)$ function, and **Figure 4.49c** shows the result after subtracting the background from the original, pixel by pixel, to level the image. This leveling removes the variation in background brightness and permits setting brightness thresholds to delineate the pores for measurement, as discussed in **Chapter 7**.

This approach to automatic leveling can of course be applied to either a light or a dark background. By simultaneously applying it to both the lightest and darkest pixels in each region of the image, it is possible to stretch the contrast of the image as a function of location, as shown schematically in **Figure 4.50** using a line profile of brightness as an example. This autocontrast method works particularly well when the image loses contrast due to nonuniform illumination or varying sample thickness. **Figure 4.51** shows an example. **Chapter 5** will introduce additional methods that perform adaptive contrast enhancement that varies the adjustments to brightness from one location to another in an image.

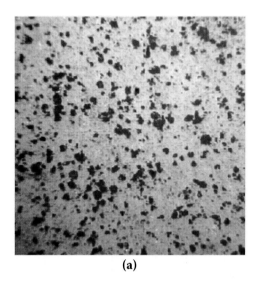

(a)

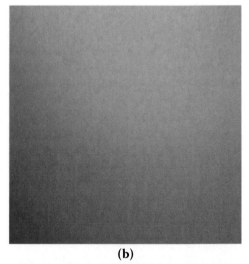

(b)

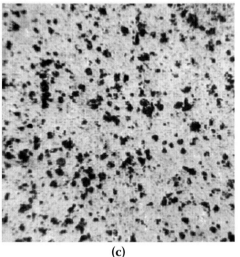

(c)

Figure 4.49 *Automatic leveling of nonuniform illumination:*

(a) *reflection light-microscope image of ceramic specimen, with nonuniform background brightness due to a nonplanar surface;*

(b) *background function calculated as a polynomial fit to the brightest point in each of 81 squares (a 9 × 9 grid);*

(c) *leveled image after subtracting image **b** from image **a**.*

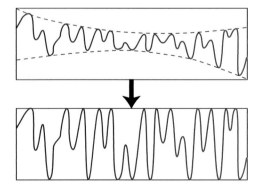

Figure 4.50 *Schematic diagram of automatic contrast adjustment by fitting polynomials to both the brightest and darkest values across an image and stretching the brightness values between those limits.*

Another approach sometimes used to remove gradual variation in overall brightness employs the frequency transforms discussed in **Chapter 6**. It assumes that the background variation in the image is a low-frequency signal that can be separated in frequency space from the higher frequencies that define the features present. If this assumption is justified, and if the frequencies corresponding to the background can be identified, then they can be removed by a simple filter in the frequency-space representation.

Figure 4.52 shows an example of this approach. The brightness variation in the original image is due to off-centered illumination in the microscope. Transforming the image into frequency

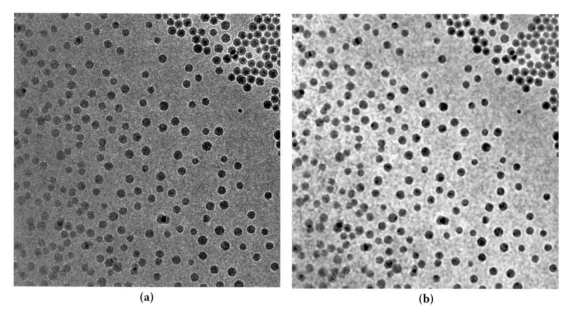

(a)   (b)

Figure 4.51 *TEM image of latex particles:* ***(a)*** *original, with varying contrast due to changing sample thickness;* ***(b)*** *after application of automatic contrast by fitting polynomial functions to light and dark pixel values (after applying a median filter to reduce random pixel noise).*

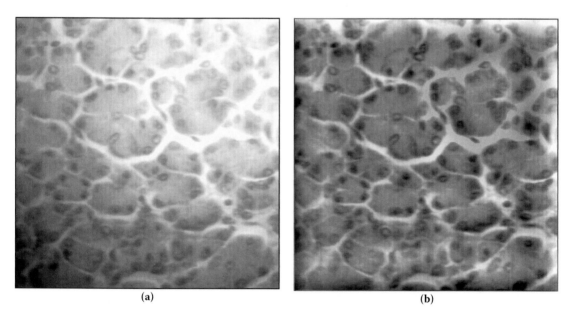

(a)   (b)

Figure 4.52 *Leveling of image brightness and contrast by removal of low-frequency terms in 2-D FFT:* ***(a)*** *original image, showing nonuniform illumination;* ***(b)*** *attempt to level the brightness by reducing the magnitude to zero of the lowest four frequency components. Note that in addition to the variations near the edge, the brightness of similar structures is not constant throughout the image.*

space with a two-dimensional fast Fourier transform (2-D FFT, as discussed in **Chapter 6**), reducing the magnitude of the first four frequency components by filtering the frequency-space image, and then retransforming produces the image shown in the figure.

This method is not entirely successful for this image. The edges of the image show significant variations present because the frequency transform attempts to match the left and right edges and the top and bottom edges. In addition, the brightness of dark and light regions throughout the image that have the same appearance and would be expected to properly have the same brightness show considerable local variations because the brightness variation is a function of the local details, including the actual brightness values, spacing, and the shapes of the features. There are few practical situations in which leveling is satisfactorily performed by this method.

Rank leveling

When the background varies more abruptly than can be fit to simple functions, another approach can be used. This method is especially useful when the surface is irregular, such as details on a fracture surface examined in the SEM or a thin section with a fold viewed in the transmission electron microscope (TEM). The assumption behind this method is that features of interest are limited in size and smaller (at least in one dimension) than the scale of background variations, and that the background is everywhere either lighter than or darker than the local features. Both requirements are often met in practical situations.

Rank neighborhood operations (such as the median filter) were discussed previously in this chapter and are used again in **Chapter 5**. The basic idea behind neighborhood ranking operations is to compare each pixel with its neighbors or combine the pixel values in some small region, usually approximating a circle of adjustable size (**Figure 4.18**). This operation is performed for each pixel in the image, and a new image is produced as a result. In many practical implementations, the new image replaces the original image, with only a temporary requirement for additional storage.

For our present purposes, the neighborhood comparison works as follows: for each pixel, examine the pixels in a 3 × 3 square, a 5 × 5 octagon, or other similar small region. If the background is known to be darker than the features, find the darkest pixel in each neighborhood and replace the value of the original pixel with that darker brightness value. For the case of a background lighter than the features, the brightest pixel in the neighborhood is used instead. These operations are sometimes called gray-scale erosion and dilation, by analogy to the morphological processing applied to binary (black and white) images discussed in **Chapter 7**. The result of applying this operation to the entire image is to shrink the features by the radius of the neighborhood region and to extend the local background brightness values into the area previously covered by features.

Figure 4.53 illustrates this procedure for an image of rice grains on a dark and uneven background. A neighborhood is used here that consists of 21 pixels in an octagonal 5 × 5 pattern centered on each pixel in the image. The darkest pixel value in that region replaces the original central pixel. This operation is repeated for every pixel in the image, always using the original image pixels and not the new ones from application of the procedure to other pixels. After this procedure is complete, the rice grains are reduced in size, as shown in **Figure 4.53b**. Repeating the operation continues to shrink the grains and to extend the background based on the local background brightness.

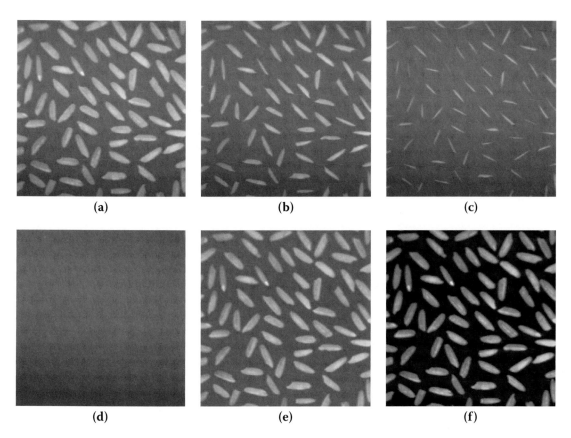

Figure 4.53 *Constructing a background image with a rank operation: **(a)** an image of rice grains with nonuniform illumination; **(b)** each pixel replaced with the darkest neighboring pixel in an octagonal 5 × 5 neighborhood; **(c)** another repetition of the "darkest neighbor" gray-scale dilation operation; **(d)** after four repetitions only the background remains; **(e)** result of subtracting image **d** from image **a**; **(f)** the leveled result with contrast expanded.*

After four repetitions (**Figure 4.53d**), the rice grains have been removed. This removal is possible because the maximum width of any grain is not larger than four times the width of the 5-pixel-wide neighborhood used for the ranking. Knowing how many times to apply this operation depends upon knowing the width (smallest dimension) of the largest features present, or simply watching the progress of the operation and repeating until the features are removed. In some cases, this can be judged from the disappearance of a peak from the image histogram. The background produced by this method has the large-scale variation present in the original image, and subtracting it produces a leveled image (**Figure 4.53f**) that clearly defines the features and allows them to be separated from the background by thresholding. In this particular case, only the darkest values were needed. Usually erosion and dilation are used in combination, as shown in the following examples.

Rank-based methods are particularly suitable for the quite irregular background brightness variations that occur in many natural cases. **Figure 4.54** shows a telescope image of the moon. The uneven illumination produced by the angle of the surface to the sun is one cause of variation, but so is the variation in the albedo of the surface, varying from the mares to the highlands. The background in this case was estimated by applying a gray-scale morphological "closing" operation, which is a sequence of dilation followed by erosion. The first step keeps

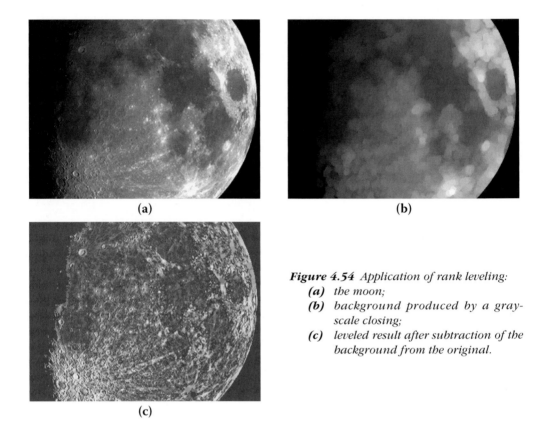

Figure 4.54 *Application of rank leveling:*
- *(a)* *the moon;*
- *(b)* *background produced by a gray-scale closing;*
- *(c)* *leveled result after subtraction of the background from the original.*

the darkest pixel in a 7-pixel-wide octagonal neighborhood (dilation), followed by keeping the brightest values in the same size region (erosion). Subtracting this background from the original makes the markings more visible everywhere on the surface by removing the overall variations.

This method is also useful for examination of particles and other surface decorations on freeze-fractured cell walls in biological specimens, examination of surface roughness on irregular particles or pollen, and other similar problems. In some cases it can be used to enhance the visibility of dislocations in TEM images of materials, which appear as dark lines in different grains whose overall brightness varies due to lattice orientation.

The technique is particularly appropriate for transmission imaging of specimens such as tissue sections in which the density of different organelles produces a background intensity that does not vary in any gradual or consistent pattern, as shown in **Figure 4.55**. The objects of interest are the small gold particles used in this immunogold labeling experiment. Those that lie on cytoplasm are much lighter than those on the darker organelles, and direct thresholding based on brightness is not successful. Applying a gray-scale morphological opening (erosion of the dark features followed by dilation to restore the organelles to their original sizes) produces a background. In this case, the pixel values are a linear measure of the intensity in the TEM, so the background must be divided into the original to produce a leveled result.

Figure 4.56 shows an example in which both leveling techniques are used to complement each other. First a ranked background is created by replacing the dark axons with the locally lighter background, and this is divided into the original image. Then a polynomial fit to the

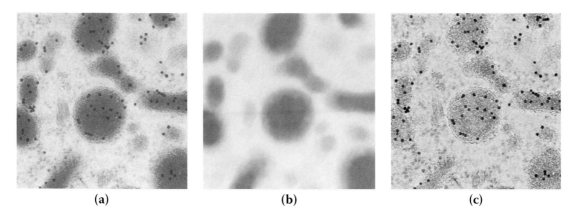

(a)   (b)   (c)

Figure 4.55 Leveling in a transmission image: (a) original TEM image with immunogold particles; (b) background produced by gray-scale opening; (c) leveled result after dividing the background into the original.

brightest and darkest pixel values is used to locally expand the contrast, which helps to reveal even the small dark axon lines.

The ability to level brightness variations by subtracting a background image, whether obtained by measurement, mathematical fitting, or image processing, is not a cost-free process. Subtraction uses up part of the dynamic range, or gray scale, of the image. **Figure 4.57** shows an example. The original image has a shading variation that can be fit rather well by a quadratic function, but this has a range of about half of the total 256 gray levels. After the function has been subtracted, the leveled image does not have enough remaining brightness range to show detail in the dark areas of some features. This clipping can interfere with further analysis of the image.

Color images

Color images sometimes present significant problems for shading correction. A typical example of a situation in which this arises is aerial or satellite imagery, in which the irregularity of the ground or the curvature of the planet surface produces an overall shading. In some cases, this affects only the intensity in the image and leaves the color information unaffected. But depending on the camera response, possible texturing or specular reflection from the surface, atmospheric absorption, and other details of the imaging, it is also possible to find that there are color shifts between different areas in the image.

The same methods used above for gray-scale images can be applied to the intensity channel from a color image. In some instances, the same leveling strategies can be applied to the hue channel, as shown in **Figure 4.58**. This is slightly more complicated than leveling brightness, since the hue values "wrap around" modulo 360°; the simplest solution is to fit the polynomial twice, once with the origin at red and once at cyan, and use whichever gives the better fit. Leveling is practically never useful for application directly to the red, green, and blue channels. When (mis)used in this way, the operations produce color shifts in pixels that alter the image so that it cannot be successfully thresholded, and in most cases does not even "look" right.

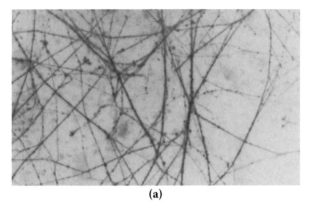

(a)

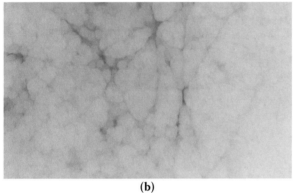

(b)

Figure 4.56 Combined rank and polynomial methods:
(a) *original TEM image of axons;*
(b) *background produced by replacing dark pixels with their brightest neighbors within a five-pixel radius;*
(c) *result of dividing image **a** by image **b**;*
(d) *contrast expanded between automatically fit polynomial limits.*

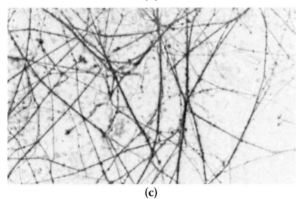

(c)

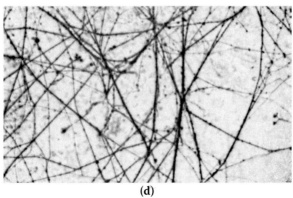

(d)

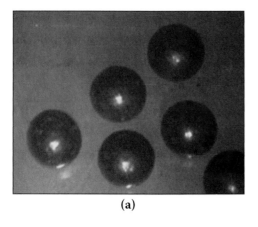

(a)

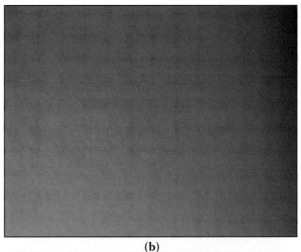

(b)

Figure 4.57 *Effect of leveling on an image with limited gray-scale range:*
(a) *original image;*
(b) *fitted polynomial background;*
(c) *result after subtracting image* ***b*** *from image* ***a****; the background is uniform, but the dark features are not because the original pixels were fully black in the original image.*

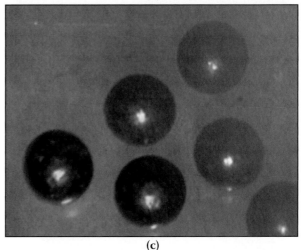

(c)

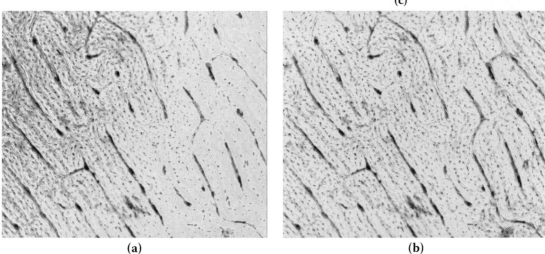

(a)   (b)

Figure 4.58 *Leveling hue:* *(a)* *light micrograph of bone, showing nonuniform color due to misalignment of the bulb in the illuminator;* *(b)* *after polynomial leveling of the hue values.*

Chapter 1 showed an example of another approach. While the various color channels have each been altered by the effects of geometry and other factors, to a first approximation the effect is the same across the spectrum of colors. In that case, it is appropriate to use ratios of one color channel to another to level the effects of nonuniform surface orientation or illumination. Filtering the color image in different wavelengths and then dividing one by another cancels out some of the nonuniformity and produces a leveled image in which similar features located in different areas have the same final appearance.

Figure 4.59 shows an example using a satellite image of the entire Earth. The limb darkening around the edges of the globe is due primarily to viewing angle and secondarily to the effects of atmospheric absorption. Separating the image into separate color channels and obtaining their ratio reveals fine details and levels the overall contrast range. However, this does not produce an image of the globe in which pixels near the limb have their colors "corrected" to be similar to those in the center of the field of view.

The rank-based leveling method can also be applied to color images. In the example of **Figure 4.60**, a red dye has been injected to reveal blood vessels, but the background varies, making the smaller vessels and those at the periphery difficult to detect. Removing the blood

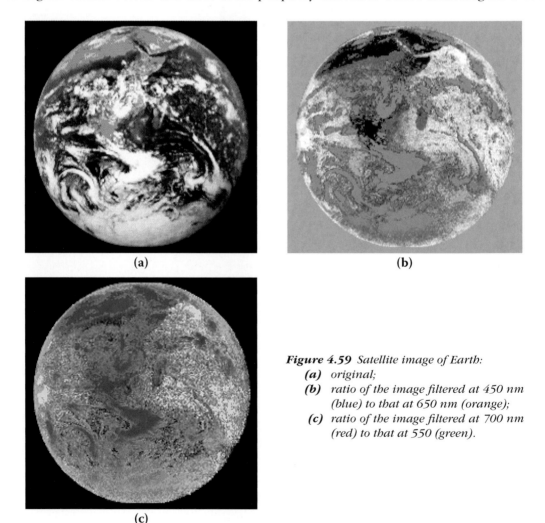

(a)

(b)

(c)

Figure 4.59 *Satellite image of Earth:*
  (a) *original;*
  (b) *ratio of the image filtered at 450 nm (blue) to that at 650 nm (orange);*
  (c) *ratio of the image filtered at 700 nm (red) to that at 550 (green).*

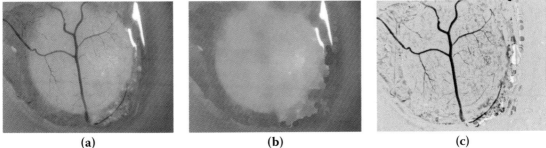

*Figure 4.60 Example of rank leveling in a color image as described in the text: (a) original image; (b) background produced by color opening; (c) result after subtracting image **b** from image **a**. (Courtesy of K. Spencer, The Scripps Research Institute, La Jolla, CA.)*

vessels by replacing each pixel with the color values from its neighbor that is farthest in color space from the selected red color (color erosion), followed by the complementary operation in which each pixel is replaced by its neighbor with the nearest color value (color dilation), produces a background. Subtracting this background image from the original produces optimal contrast for the blood vessels.

Nonplanar views

Computer graphics are often concerned with methods for displaying the surfaces of three-dimensional objects. Some of these methods will be used in **Chapter 13** to display representations of three-dimensional structures obtained from a series of 2-D image slices, or from direct 3-D imaging methods such as tomography.

One particular use of computer graphics that most of us take for granted can be seen each evening on the local news. Most TV stations in the United States have a weather forecast that uses satellite images from a NOAA (National Oceanic and Atmospheric Administration) weather satellite. These pictures show the United States as it appears from latitude 0°, longitude 108° W (the satellite is shifted to 98° W in summertime to get a better view of hurricanes developing in the south Atlantic) at a geosynchronous elevation of about 22,000 miles.

This image shows cloud patterns, and a series of images taken during the day shows movement of storms and other weather systems. In these images, the coastline, Great Lakes, and a few other topographic features are evident, but they may be partially obscured by clouds. Given the average citizen's geographical knowledge, that picture would not help most viewers to recognize their location. So computer graphics are used to superimpose political outlines, such as the state borders, and perhaps other information such as cities or major highways to assist the viewer. Most U.S. TV stations have heavy investments in computer graphics for advertising, news, etc., but they rarely generate these lines themselves, instead obtaining the images with the lines already present from a company that specializes in that niche market.

How are these lines generated? This is not simply a matter of overlaying a conventional map, say a Mercator projection as used in the school classroom, over the satellite image. The curvature of Earth and the foreshortening of the image need to be taken into account. **Figure 4.61** shows a weather satellite image of North America that is clearly foreshortened at the top and also shows noticeable curvature from west to east across the width of the country.

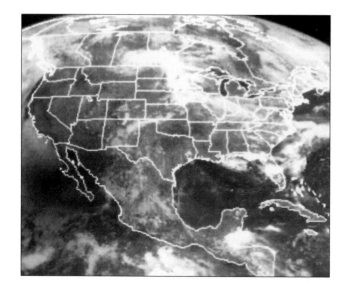

Figure 4.61 GOES-7 image of North America with political boundary lines superimposed. The dark area just west of Baja California is the shadow of the moon during the eclipse of 11 June, 1991. (Courtesy of National Environmental Satellite Data and Information Service, Silver Spring, MD.)

The coordinates, in latitude and longitude, of points on Earth's surface are used to calculate a perspective view of the roughly spherical globe as it is seen from the satellite. Since the viewpoint is constant, this is a one-time calculation, which nevertheless needs to be done for a great many points to construct good outline maps for superposition. The calculation can be visualized as shown in the diagram of **Figure 4.62**.

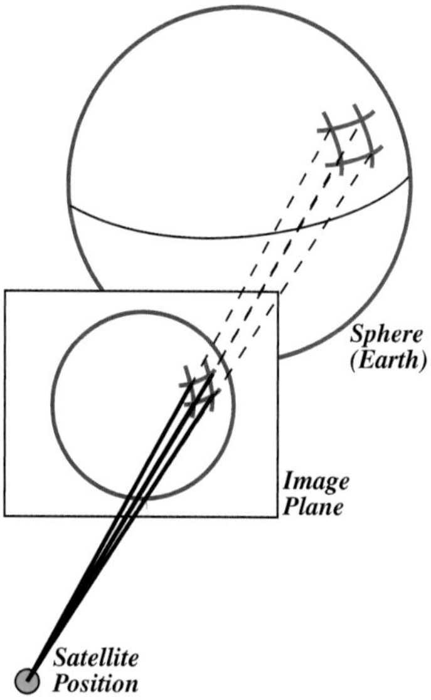

The location of a point on the spherical Earth (specified by its latitude and longitude) is used to determine the intersection of a view line to the satellite with a flat image plane, inserted in front of the sphere. This calculation requires only simple trigonometry, as indicated in **Figure 4.63**. The coordinates of the points in that plane are the location of the point in the viewed image. As shown, a square on the ground is viewed as a skewed trapezoid, and if the square is large enough its sides are noticeably curved.

Sphere (Earth)

Image Plane

Satellite Position

Figure 4.62 Diagram of satellite imaging. As in any perspective geometry, the "flat" image is formed by projecting view lines from the three-dimensional object to the viewpoint and constructing the image from the points at which they intersect the image plane.

Computer graphics

Computer graphics are similarly used to construct perspective drawings of three-dimensional objects so that they can be viewed on the computer screen, for instance in CAD (computer-aided design) programs. The subject goes far beyond our needs here; the interested reader should refer to standard texts such as Foley and Van Dam (1984, 1995) or Hearn and Baker (1986). The display process is the same as that just described, with the addition of perspective control that allows the user to adjust the apparent distance of the camera or viewpoint so as to control the degree of foreshortening that occurs (equivalent to choosing a long or short focal-length lens for a camera; the short focal-length lens produces more distortion in the image).

Ignoring perspective distortion for the moment (i.e., using a telephoto lens), we can represent the translation of a point in three dimensions by matrix multiplication of its x, y, z coordinates by a set of values that describe rotation and translation. This is simpler to examine in more detail in two dimensions, since our main interest here is with two-dimensional images. Con-

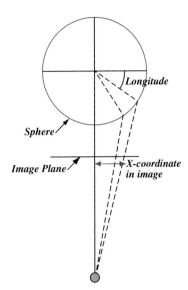

Figure 4.63 Simple trigonometry can be used to calculate the location of points in the image plane from the longitude of the point on Earth and the location of the satellite. This is the view from the North Pole; a similar view from the equator gives the y-coordinate.

sider a point with Cartesian x, y coordinates and how it moves when we shift it or rotate it and the other points in the object with respect to the coordinate system.

From simple geometry we know that a translation of an object simply adds offsets to x and y, to produce

$$x' = x + \Delta x$$
$$y' = y + \Delta y$$

(4.5)

while stretching the object requires multiplicative coefficients, which are not necessarily the same

$$x' = \alpha x$$
$$y' = \beta y$$

(4.6)

and rotation of an object by the angle ϑ introduces an interdependence between the original x and y coordinates of the form

$$x' = x \cos \vartheta - y \sin \vartheta$$
$$y' = x \sin \vartheta + y \cos \vartheta$$

(4.7)

In general, the notation for two-dimensional translations is most commonly written using so-called homogeneous coordinates and matrix notation. The coordinates x, y are combined in a vector along with an arbitrary constant 1 to allow the translation values to be incorporated into the matrix math, producing the result

$$[X'\ Y'\ 1] = [X\ Y\ 1] \cdot \begin{vmatrix} a & b & 0 \\ c & d & 0 \\ e & f & 1 \end{vmatrix}$$

(4.8)

which multiplies out to

$$x' = ax + cy + e$$
$$y' = bx + dy + f$$

(4.9)

By comparing this matrix form to the examples above, we see that the e and f terms are the translational shift values. The a, b, c, d values are the stretching and rotation coefficients. When a series of transformations is combined, including rotation, translation, and stretching, a series of matrices is produced that can be multiplied together. When this happens, for instance to produce rotation about some point other than the origin, or to combine nonuniform stretching with rotation, the individual terms are combined in ways that complicate their simple interpretation. However, only the same six coefficients are needed.

If only these terms are used, we cannot produce curvature or twisting of the objects. By introducing higher-order terms, more complex stretching and twisting of figures is possible. This would produce a more complex equation of the form

$$x' = a_1 + a_2 x + a_3 y + a_4 xy + a_5 x^2 + a_6 y^2 + \ldots \qquad (4.10)$$

and a similar relationship for y'. There is no fundamental reason to limit this polynomial expansion to any particular maximum power except that, as the complexity grows, the number of coefficients needed rises (and the difficulty of obtaining them), and the mathematical precision needed to apply the transformation increases. It is unusual to have terms beyond second power, which can handle most commonly encountered cases of distortion and even approximate the curvature produced by looking at a spherical surface, at least over small ranges of angles.

Of course, some surface mappings are better handled by other functions. The standard Mercator projection of the spherical Earth onto a cylinder (**Figure 4.64**) sends the poles to infinity and greatly magnifies areas at high latitudes. It would require many polynomial terms to approximate it, but since the actual geometry of the mapping is known, it is easy to use the cosecant function that efficiently performs the transformation.

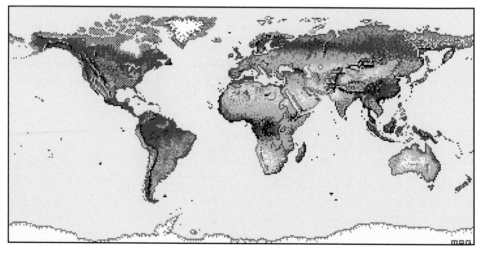

Figure 4.64 *The standard Mercator projection of Earth used in maps projects the points on the sphere onto a cylinder, producing distortion at high latitudes.*

Geometrical distortion

Now we must examine what to do with these mathematical operations. Images are frequently obtained that are not of flat surfaces viewed normally. The example of the satellite image used above is one obvious case. So is viewing surfaces in the SEM, in which the specimen surface is often tilted to increase the contrast in the detected image. If the surface is not flat, different regions may be tilted at arbitrary angles, or continuous curvature may be present. But even with nominally flat but tilted surfaces, the distortion is important if we want to perform any measurements or comparisons within or between images. Many airborne cameras and radars also introduce a predictable distortion (which is therefore correctable) due to the use of a moving or sideways scan pattern, or by imaging a single line onto continuously moving film. In all of these cases, knowing the distortion is the key to correcting it.

This situation does not commonly arise with light microscopy because the depth of field of the optics is so low that surfaces must be flat and normal to the optical axis to remain in focus. There are other imaging technologies, however, that do frequently encounter nonideal surfaces or viewing conditions.

Making maps from aerial or satellite images is one application (Thompson 1966). Of course, there is no perfect projection of a spherical surface onto a flat one, so various approximations and useful conventions are employed. But in each case, there is a known relationship between the coordinates on the globe and those on the map that can be expressed mathematically. But what about the image? If the viewpoint is exactly known, as for the case of the weather satellite, or can be calculated for the moment of exposure, as for the case of a space probe passing by a planet, then the same kind of mathematical relationship can be determined.

This procedure is usually impractical for aerial photographs, as the plane position is not precisely controlled. The alternative is to locate a few reference points in the image whose locations on the globe or the map are known, and then to use these to determine the equations relating position in the image to location on the map. This technique is generally known as image warping or rubber sheeting, and while the equations are the same as those used in computer graphics, the techniques for determining the coefficients are quite different.

We have seen that a pair of equations calculating x', y' coordinates for a transformed view from original coordinates x, y can include constants, linear terms in x and y, plus higher-order terms such as xy, x^2, etc. Adding more terms of higher order makes it possible to introduce more complex distortions in the transformation. If the problem is simply one of rotation, only linear terms are needed, and a constraint on the coefficients can be introduced to preserve angles. In terms of the simple matrix shown in **Equation 4.8**, this would require that the stretching coefficients be equal. That means that only a few constants are needed, and they can be determined by locating a few known reference points and setting up simultaneous equations.

More elaborate stretching to align images with each other or with a map requires correspondingly more terms and more points. In electron microscopy, the great depth of field permits acquiring pictures of samples that are locally flat but oriented at an angle to the point of view, producing distortion that is essentially trapezoidal, as shown in **Figure 4.65**. The portion of the surface that is closest to the lens is magnified more than regions farther away, and distances are foreshortened in the direction of tilt. To measure and compare features on these surfaces, or even to properly apply image processing methods (which generally assume that the neighbor pixels in various directions are at equal distances from the center), it may be necessary to transform this image to correct the distortion. Since the exact tilt angle and working distance may not be known, a method that uses only reference points within the image itself will be needed.

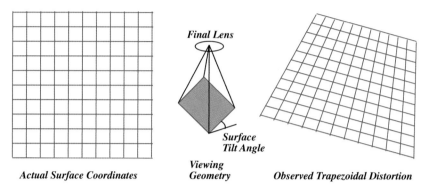

Final Lens

Surface
Tilt Angle

Viewing
Geometry

Actual Surface Coordinates

Observed Trapezoidal Distortion

Figure 4.65 *Trapezoidal distortion commonly encountered in the electron microscope when observing a tilted surface.*

All that is required here is the ability to identify four points whose real x,y coordinates on the surface are known, and whose image coordinates x',y' can be measured. Then the following equations are written

$$x = a_1 + a_2 x' + a_3 y' + a_4 x' y'$$
$$y = b_1 + b_2 x' + b_3 y' + b_4 x' y'$$

(4.11)

for each of the four sets of coordinates. This allows solving for the constants a_i and b_i. Of course, if more points are available, then they can be used to obtain a least-squares solution that minimizes the effect of the inevitable small errors in measurement of coordinates in the image.

By limiting the equation to those terms needed to accomplish the rotation and stretching involved in the trapezoidal distortion that we expect to be present, we minimize the number of points needed for the fit. More than the three terms shown in **Equation 4.11** are required because angles are not preserved in this kind of foreshortening. But using the fewest possible is preferred to a general equation involving many higher-order terms, both in terms of the efficiency of the calculation (number of reference points) and the precision of the coefficients.

Likewise, if we know that the distortion in the image is that produced by viewing a globe, the appropriate sine and cosine terms can be used in the fitting equations. Of course, if we have no independent knowledge about the shape of the surface or the kind of imaging distortion, then other methods such as stereoscopy represent the only practical approach to determining the geometry.

The chief problem that arises with such perspective correction is for features that do not lie on the tilted planar surface, but instead extend in front of or behind it. In the example of **Figure 4.66**, the front of the building is adjusted to show the correct angles and dimensions for the structure, but the light pole that extends out over the street in front appears to be at an angle to the building when in fact it is exactly perpendicular. Notice also that the right side of the building appears to be less sharply focused, which is actually due to the enlargement and interpolation of that portion of the image. Interpolation techniques are discussed below.

Alignment

Another very common situation is the alignment of serial-section images. In some cases there may be no "ground truth" to align with, but only relative alignment between the successive slices. The alignment is performed either by using features within the image that can be rec-

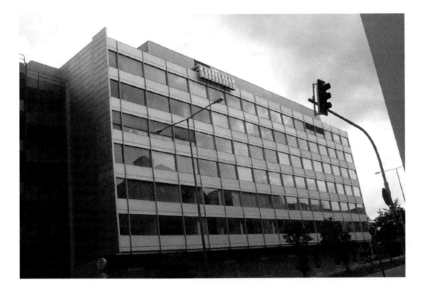

Figure 4.66 Correcting trapezoidal distortion due to a nonperpendicular view.

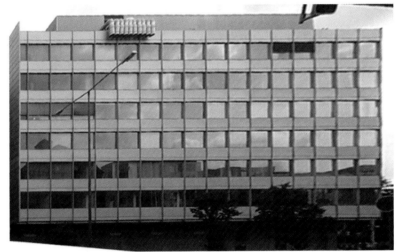

ognized in successive slices, or by introducing fiducial marks such as holes drilled through the specimen block or fibers inserted into it before the sections are cut. The points can be located manually by the user or automatically by the imaging system, although the latter method works best for artificial markings such as holes, and somewhat poorly when trying to use details within the images that match only imperfectly from one section to the next. Relative alignment is discussed in more detail in **Chapter 13**.

Serial sections cut with a microtome from a block of embedded biological material commonly are foreshortened in the cutting direction by 5 to 15% due to compression of the block by the knife. Then they are rotated arbitrarily before they are viewed. Other imaging situations produce sets of images that have different native resolutions and also require scaling as well as rotation and alignment. The result is a need for an alignment equation of the form

$$x = a_1 + a_2 x' + a_3 y' \tag{4.12}$$

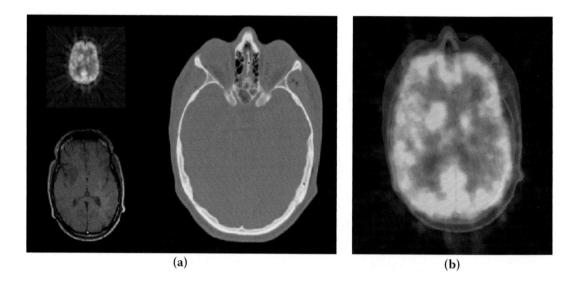

(a)   (b)

*Figure 4.67 Registration of three images — positron-emission tomography (PET), magnetic resonance imaging (MRI), and computed tomography (CT) — with different scales and alignments: **(a)** PET (small), MRI (medium), and CT (large) scans of a human head. The small red, green, and blue dots are the registration points used to determine the stretching and rotation vectors; **(b)** result after registration, with the images displayed in individual color channels.*

with only three constants (and a similar equation for y). Hence, locating three reference points that are common to two sequential images allows one to be rotated and stretched to align with the other. **Figure 4.67** shows a set of images in which three points have been marked as alignment references, and the resulting transformation of the image by stretching and rotating.

This kind of warping can be performed to align images with other images, as in serial-section reconstruction, or to align images along their edges to permit assembling them as a mosaic (Milgram 1975). Alignment of side-by-side sections of a mosaic is often attempted with SEM images but fails because of the trapezoidal distortion discussed previously. The result is that features along the image boundaries do not quite line up, and the mosaic is imperfect. Using rubber sheeting can correct this defect.

Such correction is routinely done for satellite and space-probe pictures. **Figure 4.68** shows an example of a mosaic image constructed from multiple images taken from orbit of the surface of Mars. Boundaries between images are visible because of brightness differences due to variations in illumination or exposure, but the features line up well across the seams. Recently, there has been increased interest in creating mosaics from separate images to generate panoramic views and to overcome the limited resolution (as compared with film) of consumer digital cameras. **Figure 4.69** shows four individual images taken from a single location (by rotating the camera on a tripod) that form a 2 × 2 array with considerable overlap. The wide-angle lens used has produced distortion within each image, and a simple overlapping of the fields does not fit. **Figure 4.70** shows the resulting mosaic that forms a complete image of the building. Note that the images have been distorted to fit together smoothly and that their edges do not form straight lines. This type of mosaic can be very useful for automatically constructing panorama photographs (Brown and Lowe 2003; Brown et al. 2005; Chow et al. 2006; Kim and Hong 2006), but it is rarely useful for measurement purposes.

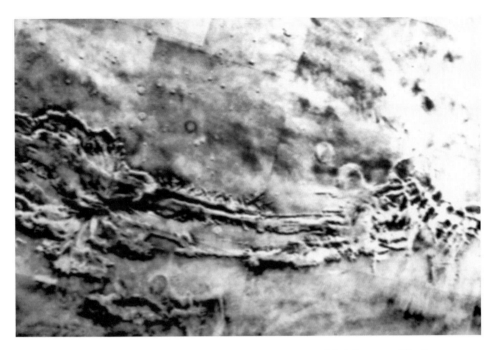

Figure 4.68 *Mosaic image of the Valles Marineris on Mars, assembled from satellite images.*

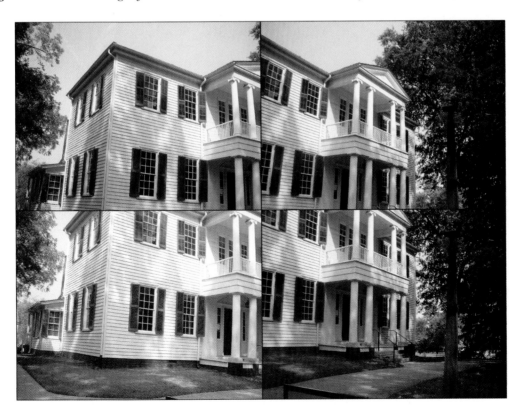

Figure 4.69 *Four images that overlap to provide a 2 × 2 array covering a larger scene. Note the different angles and incompatible lens distortions in each.*

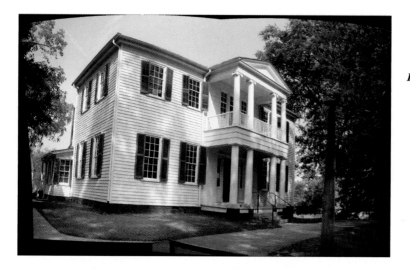

Figure 4.70 The mosaic produced from the images in *Figure 4.69*. *(Mosaic produced using the "autostitch" software from Matthew Brown and David Lowe, University of British Columbia, Vancouver, B.C.)*

For scientific imaging purposes, the use of a microscope stage or other specimen-positioning device that can shift the sample being imaged with reasonable precision while the camera remains fixed would seem to offer the possibility of acquiring images of unlimited size. However, there are more constraints in this situation to assist in the fitting together of the image.

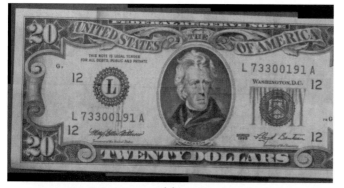

(a)

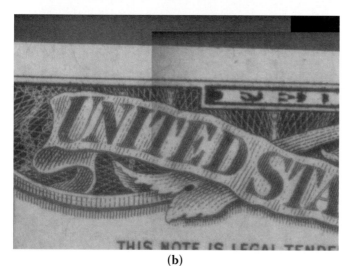

(b)

It is known, for example, that the images can be slightly rotated (the mechanism may have slight wobble or misalignment, and the shifting cannot be counted on to provide exact edge-to-edge alignment), but they cannot be distorted (i.e., straight lines remain straight and angles are unchanged). Hence the process of fitting images together can only shift and rotate the individual image tiles in their entirety.

If the overlap between tiles is between 10 and 20% and if the angular mismatch is no more than a few degrees, then matching each of the tiles together can indeed produce large high-resolution mosaics, as shown in **Figure 4.71**. The matching technique is based on cross-correlation (discussed in **Chapter 6**),

Figure 4.71
  (a) Portion of a large mosaic image assembled from eight individual images, each 1600 × 1200 pixels, from a digital camera, as discussed in the text;
  (b) detail of fit between two image tiles.

and an iterative procedure was used to match all of the tiles together for a best fit. This is particularly effective for images acquired in the atomic force microscope, because the area covered by these devices tends to be rather small, and with the very high spatial resolution it is not feasible to design specimen-shifting hardware that is absolutely precise (Condeco et al. 2000).

Interpolation

When images are being aligned, it is possible to write the equations either in terms of the coordinates in the original image as a function of the geometrically corrected one, or vice versa. In practice it is usually preferable to use the grid of x,y coordinates in the corrected image to calculate for each of the coordinates in the original image, and to perform the calculation in terms of actual pixel addresses.

Unfortunately, these calculated coordinates for the original location will only rarely be integers. This means that the location lies "between" the pixels in the original image. Several methods are used to deal with this problem. The simplest is to truncate the calculated values so that the fractional part of the address is discarded and the pixel lying toward the origin of the coordinate system is used. Slightly better results are obtained by rounding the address values to select the nearest pixel, whose brightness is then copied to the transformed image array. This is called a "nearest neighbor" procedure.

Either method introduces some error in location that can cause distortion of the transformed image. **Figure 4.72** shows examples using a test pattern in which the aliasing or "stair-stepping" of the lines and apparent variations in their width is evident.

When this distortion is unacceptable, another method can be used that requires more calculation. The brightness value for the transformed pixel can be calculated by interpolating between the four pixels surrounding the calculated address. This is called bilinear interpolation, and it is calculated simply from the fractional part of the x and y coordinates. First the interpolation is done in one direction, and then in the other, as indicated in **Figure 4.73**. For a location with coordinates $j+x$, $k+y$ where x and y are the fractional part of the address, the equations for the first interpolation are

$$B_{j+x,k} = (1-x) \cdot B_{j,k} + x \cdot B_{j+1,k}$$

$$B_{j+x,k+1} = (1-x) \cdot B_{j,k+1} + x \cdot B_{j+1,k+1}$$

(4.13)

and then the second interpolation, in the y direction, gives the final value

$$B_{j+x,k+y} = (1-y) \cdot B_{j+x,k} + y \cdot B_{j+x,k+1}$$

(4.14)

Weighted interpolations over larger regions are also used in some cases. One of the most popular is bicubic fitting. Whereas bilinear interpolation uses a 2×2 array of neighboring pixel values to calculate the interpolated value, the cubic method uses a 4×4 array. Using the same notation as the bilinear interpolation in **Equation 4.13** and **Equation 4.14**, the summations now go from $k-1$ to $k+2$ and from $j-1$ to $j+2$. The intermediate values from the horizontal interpolation are

$$B_{j+x,k} = (1/6) \, (B_{j-1,k} \cdot R_1 + B_{j,k} \cdot R_2 + B_{j+1,k} \cdot R_3 + B_{j+2,k} \cdot R_4)$$

(4.15)

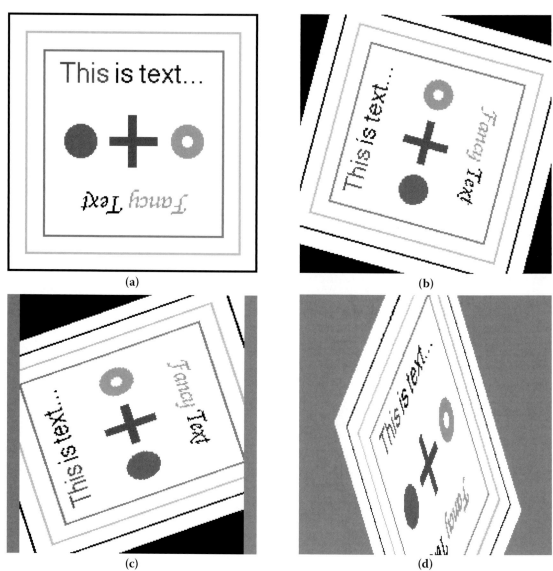

Figure 4.72 *Rotation and stretching of a test image: **(a)** original; **(b)** rotation only, no change in scale; **(c)** rotation and uniform stretching while maintaining angles; **(d)** general rotation and stretching in which angles may vary (but lines remain straight).*

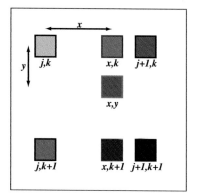

Figure 4.73 *Diagram of pixel interpolation. The brightness values of the neighbors are first interpolated horizontally to determine the brightness values at the locations outlined in red, and then these two values are interpolated vertically to determine the brightness at the target pixel outlined in blue. Interpolation is carried out using the fractional part of the pixel addresses.*

and the interpolation in the vertical direction is

$$B_{j+x,k+y} = (1/6)\,(B_{j+x,k-1}\cdot R_1 + B_{j+x,k}\cdot R_2 + B_{j+x,k+1}\cdot R_3 + B_{j+x,k+2}\cdot R_4) \qquad (4.16)$$

where the weighting factors R_i are calculated from the real part (x or y, respectively) of the address as

$$R_1 = (3 + x)^3 - 4\cdot(2 + x)^3 + 6\cdot(1 + x)^3 - 4\cdot x^3$$
$$R_2 = (2 + x)^3 - 4\cdot(1 + x)^3 + 6\cdot x^3 \qquad (4.17)$$
$$R_3 = (1 + x)^3 - 4\cdot x^3$$
$$R_4 = x^3$$

The bicubic fit is more isotropic than the bilinear method. Interpolation always has the effect of smoothing the image and removing some high-frequency information, but minimizes aliasing or "stair-stepping" along lines and edges. The coefficients in **Equation 4.17** can be varied to produce sharper or smoother results, if desired. Larger neighborhoods are also possible, but these are most often implemented by performing the interpolation in Fourier space (discussed in **Chapter 6**) rather than by directly accessing the neighboring pixels.

Figure 4.74 shows the results of rotating a line (originally a black vertical line one pixel wide) by 17° with no interpolation (selecting the nearest-neighbor pixel value), with bilinear interpolation, and with bicubic interpolation. The aliasing with the nearest-neighbor method is evident. Bilinear interpolation reduces the line contrast more than bicubic, and both assign gray values to adjacent pixels to smooth the appearance of the line.

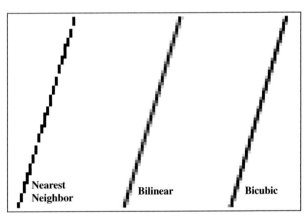

Figure 4.74 Effect of rotating a 1-pixel-wide black line using nearest-neighbor, bilinear, and bicubic interpolation.

The advantage of interpolation is that dimensions are altered as little as possible in the transformation, and boundaries and other lines are not biased or distorted. **Figure 4.75** shows the same examples as **Figure 4.72**, with bilinear interpolation used. Careful examination of the figure shows that the lines appear straight and are not aliased or stair-stepped, because some of the pixels along the sides of the lines have intermediate gray values resulting from the interpolation. In fact, computer graphics programs often use this same method to draw lines and characters in text on CRT displays so that the stair-stepping inherent in drawing lines on a discrete pixel array is avoided. The technique is called anti-aliasing and produces lines whose pixels have gray values according to how close they lie to the mathematical location of the line. This fools the viewer into perceiving a smooth line or character.

Fitting of higher-order polynomials or adaptive spline fits to the pixel intensity values can also be used. This can be particularly useful when enlarging images to reduce the perceived fuzziness that results when sharp edges are spread out by conventional interpolation. **Figure 4.76**

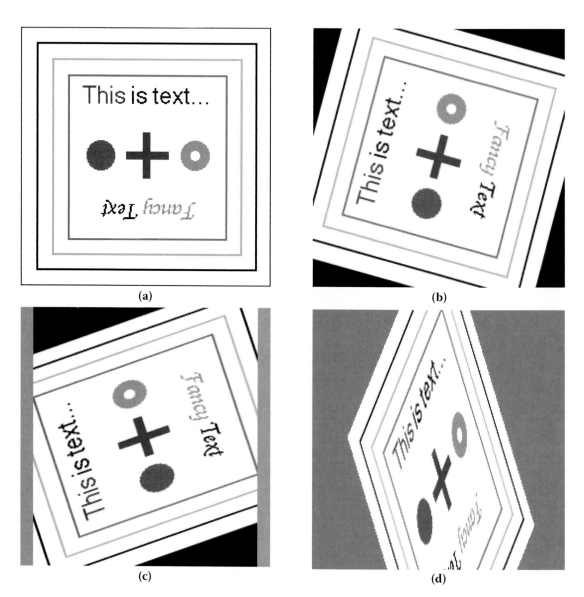

(a)

(b)

(c)

(d)

*Figure 4.75 Same generalized rotation and stretching as in **Figure 4.72**, but with bilinear interpolation. Note the smoothing of the lines and boundaries.*

shows an example (a fragment of the "flowers" image) in which a 4× enlargement has been performed using no interpolation, bilinear interpolation, adaptive spline fitting, or fractal interpolation. The latter inserts false "detail" into the image, while spline fitting maintains the sharpness of edges best.

For image warping, alignment, or enlargement, interpolation has the advantage that dimensions are preserved. However, brightness values are not. With the nearest-pixel method achieved by rounding the pixel addresses, the dimensions are distorted but the brightness values are preserved. Choosing which method is appropriate to a particular imaging task depends primarily on which kind of information is more important and secondarily on the additional computational effort required for the interpolation.

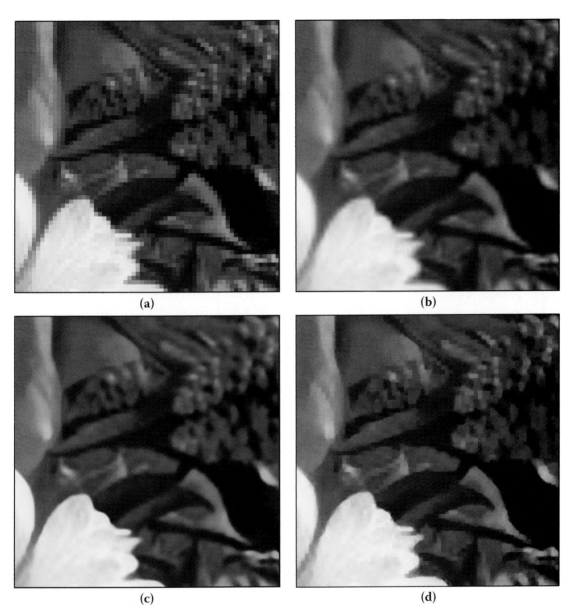

(a)   (b)

(c)   (d)

*Figure 4.76 Enlargement of an image: **(a)** no interpolation (nearest neighbor); **(b)** bilinear interpolation; **(c)** spline fitting; **(d)** fractal interpolation.*

Figure 4.77 illustrates the effect of adding higher-order terms to the warping equations. With quadratic terms, the trapezoidal distortion of a short-focal-length lens or SEM can be corrected. It is also possible to model the distortion of a spherical surface closely over modest distances. With higher-order terms, arbitrary distortion is possible, but this is rarely useful in an image processing situation, since the multiple reference points necessary to determine such a distortion are not likely to be available.

Morphing

Programs that can perform controlled warping according to mathematically defined relationships — or calculate those matrices of values from a set of identified fiducial or reference marks that apply to the entire image — are generally rather specialized. But an entire class of consumer-level programs has become available for performing image morphing based on a net of user-defined control points. The points are generally placed at corresponding locations that are distinctive in the two images. For aligning two faces, for example, points at the tips of the eyes, corners of the mouth, along the hairline and chin line, and so forth, are used as shown in the illustration in **Figure 4.78**.

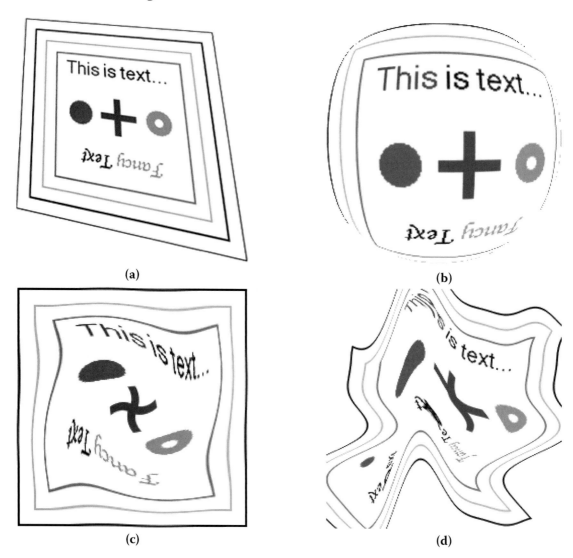

(a)　　　　(b)

(c)　　　　(d)

Figure 4.77 *Some additional examples of image warping using the same original image as* **Figure 4.72:** *(a) quadratic warping showing trapezoidal foreshortening; (b) cubic warping in which lines are curved (approximation here is to a spherical surface); (c) twisting the center of the field while holding the edges fixed (also cubic warping); (d) arbitrary warping in which higher-order and trigonometric terms are required.*

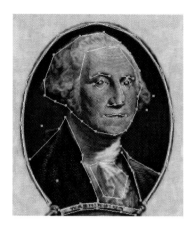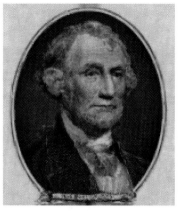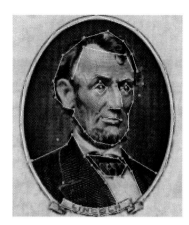

Figure 4.78 *Transformation of George into Abe (pictures from U.S. currency). The corresponding points marked on each original image control the gradual distortion from one to the other. The midpoint frame is plausible as a person and shares feature characteristics with both endpoints. Note that the banner, which is curved in different directions in the two originals, is essentially straight in the composite.*

The program uses the points to form a tessellation of the first image into triangles. (Technically, the choice of which points to use as corners for the triangles is defined by a procedure called a Voronoi tessellation.) Each triangle is uniformly stretched to fit the location of the corner points in the second image. Since the sides of the triangles are uniformly stretched, points along the edges of adjacent triangles are not displaced, although lines may be bent where they cross the boundaries of the triangles. Medical imaging often utilizes this type of morphing, using internal structures as a series of reference points to align patient images with reference standards so that subtle changes can be detected (Rangayyan 2005; Hajnal et al. 2001).

With a triangular mesh and linear stretching of each triangle, lines crossing the boundaries of the triangles would be continuous, but sharply bent. Using spline or cubic equations to control the stretch gives a better appearance by making the curves smooth, but often at the expense of preserving dimensions and thus of making measurements on such images.

The art of using these morphing programs lies primarily in using a sufficient number of control points and their careful placement. The results look quite realistic. This is especially true when a sequence of images is created with progressive motion of the control points from the original to final locations. These morphing "movies" show one image transforming gradually into the second. These effects are used routinely in creating television advertisements. It is not clear whether there are any technical applications requiring image measurement that can be satisfactorily accomplished with these programs, considering the somewhat arbitrary placement of points and the distortion of dimensions and directions.

The ability to use morphing to align images of different objects and produce visually convincing images can be a powerful tool for communicating results to others. This procedure can be useful to show the similarity between two objects, but it is extraordinarily susceptible to misuse, producing apparent matching between different images that are really not the same.

Image Enhancement (Processing in the Spatial Domain)

The preceding chapter discussed methods for correcting or alleviating the principal defects in as-acquired images. There is a fuzzy area between simply correcting these defects and going beyond to enhance the images. Enhancement is the subject of this chapter. Methods are available that increase the visibility of one portion, aspect, or component of an image, generally by suppressing others, whose visibility is diminished. In this regard, image processing is a bit like word processing or food processing. It is possible to rearrange things to make a product that is more pleasing or interpretable, but the total amount of data does not change. In the case of images, this generally means that the number of bytes (or pixels) is not reduced.

In contrast to image processing, most image-analysis procedures attempt to extract only the "important" information from the image. An example would be to identify and count features in an image, reducing the amount of data from perhaps a million bytes to a few dozen, or even a single "Yes" or "No" answer in some quality control, medical, or forensic applications.

Image enhancement can be performed for several reasons. One is simply to make the image easier to visually examine and interpret. Many of the procedures described here are based to some degree on the response or the requirements of the human visual system. Some are purely *ad hoc* methods that have been found over time to be useful. Others are based on the physics of image generation (e.g., light interaction with subjects) or the operation of optical components and image detectors (e.g., removing distortion or correcting for the response of solid-state cameras). The latter are not necessarily more complicated to apply. For example, Sharma (2005) demonstrates a calculation — based on the passage of light through a document and its reflection from print on both surfaces — that is used to separate the two images and remove "show through" in a scanned document. Other reasons for image enhancement are to facilitate printing of images or to allow automatic methods to perform measurements, as will be the subject of later chapters.

Image processing for purposes of enhancement can be performed in either the spatial domain (the array of pixels that compose our conventional representation of the image) or other domains, such as the Fourier domain discussed in **Chapter 6**. In the spatial domain, pixel values can be modified according to rules that depend on the original pixel value (local or point processes). In addition, pixel values can be combined with or compared with others in their immediate neighborhood in a variety of ways. Examples of each of these approaches were presented in **Chapter 4**, which showed how brightness values could be replaced to expand image contrast or how to smooth noise by kernel averaging or median filtering. The techniques used in this chapter employ the same basic classes of tools to perform further enhancements.

It is worth noting here that two-dimensional (2-D) images typically consist of a very large number of pixels, from about a quarter million to several million. Even a point process that simply modifies the value of each pixel according to its previous content requires that the computer address each pixel location. For a neighborhood process, each pixel must be addressed many times, and the processing speed slows down accordingly. Fast processors and high-speed memory access (and a lot of memory) are essential requirements for this type of work. Some machines use dedicated hardware —shift registers and array processors, boards with dedicated memory and custom addressing circuits, or multiple processors with special programming — to permit near-real-time processing of images when that is economically justified. As CPU speeds have increased, the need for special hardware has diminished. With more memory, entire images can be accessed rapidly without the need to bring in pieces, one at a time, from disk storage.

As desktop computer power has increased, the implementation of increasingly complex algorithms for image enhancement has become practical. Many of these algorithms are not new, dating from decades ago and often developed in conjunction with the need to process images from satellites and space probes, but until recently they had only been performed using large computers or special-purpose systems. Most can now be satisfactorily applied to images routinely, using personal computers.

This chapter does not address the implementation methods that can speed up various processing operations, but it is significant to understand that such coding "tricks" were very important 20 and even 10 years ago, as a way to make computer image processing practical. With the development of faster computers, larger data buffers, and smarter compilers, these concerns have faded. In today's computing environment, which facilitates the implementation of increasingly complex algorithms, it is generally more important that the programmer attempt to write clear and well-documented code than to squeeze out tiny performance increments at the cost of producing specialized routines that cannot be easily transferred from one platform to another. There is also greater impetus to implement algorithms exactly and with all appropriate precision rather than to accept compromises and approximations.

Contrast manipulation

Chapter 4 showed examples of expanding the contrast of a dim image by reassigning pixel brightness levels. In most systems, this can be done almost instantaneously by writing a table of values into the display hardware. This lookup table (LUT) substitutes a display brightness value for each stored value and thus does not require actually modifying any of the values stored in memory for the image. Linearly expanding the contrast range by assigning the darkest pixel value to black, the brightest value to white, and each of the others to linearly interpolated shades of gray makes good use of the display and enhances the visibility of features in the image.

It was also shown, in **Chapter 1**, that the same LUT approach can be used with colors by assigning a triplet of red, green, and blue values to each stored gray-scale value. This pseudo-color also increases the visible difference between similar pixels; sometimes it is an aid to the user who wishes to see or show small or gradual changes in image brightness.

A typical computer display can show 2^8 or 256 different shades of gray, and can produce colors with the same 2^8 brightness values for each of the red, green, and blue components to produce a total of 2^{24} or 16 million different colors. This is often described as "true color," since the gamut of colors that can be displayed is adequate to reproduce most natural scenes. It does not imply, of course, that the colors displayed are photometrically accurate or identical to the original color in the displayed scene. Indeed, that kind of accuracy is very difficult and requires special hardware and calibration. If the original image has more than 256 brightness values (is more than 8 bits deep) in each color channel, some type of lookup table is required even to display it on the screen.

More important, the 16 million different colors that such a system is capable of displaying, and even the 256 shades of gray, are far more than the human eye can distinguish. Under good viewing conditions, we can typically see only a few tens of different gray levels and a few hundreds of distinguishable colors. That means that the display hardware of the image processing system is not being used very well to communicate the image information to the user. If many of the pixels in the image are quite bright, for example, they cannot be distinguished. If there are also some dark pixels present, we cannot simply expand the contrast. Instead, a more complicated relationship between stored and displayed values is needed.

In general, the manipulation of pixel brightness is described in terms of a transfer function relating the stored brightness value for each pixel to a displayed value. If this relationship is one-to-one, then for each stored value there will be a corresponding and unique (although not necessarily visually discernible) displayed value. In some cases, it is advantageous to use transfer functions that are not one to one: several stored values are displayed with the same brightness value, so that other stored values can be spread further apart to increase their visual difference.

Figure 5.1 shows an image (the surface of dried paint, viewed in the scanning electron microscope [SEM]) in which the 256 distinct pixel brightness values cannot all be discerned on the computer display cathode-ray tube (CRT); the printed version of the image is necessarily much worse. As discussed in **Chapter 3**, the number of distinct printed gray levels in a halftone image is determined by the variation in dot size of the printer. The imagesetter used for this book is capable of much higher resolution and more gray levels than a typical office laser printer, but not as many as a CRT or a photograph.

For comparison purposes, a good-quality photographic print can reproduce 20 to 40 gray levels (the negative can do much better). An instant print such as the Polaroid film commonly used with laboratory microscopes can show 10 to 15. However, both have much higher spatial resolution, and so the images appear sharper to the eye.

Even so, looking at the original image in **Figure 5.1**, the viewer cannot see the detail in the bright and dark regions of the image, even on the video screen (and certainly not on the print). Modifying the LUT can increase the visibility in one region or the other, or in both dark and bright regions, provided something else is given up in exchange. **Figure 5.1** shows several modifications to the original image produced simply by manipulating the transfer function and the LUT by creating a new relationship between stored and displayed brightness. Some of these modifications are useful in that they reveal additional detail, while others were adjusted purely for visual effect.

Note some of the imaging possibilities. A nonlinear relationship can expand one portion of the gray-scale range while compressing another. In photographic processing and also in analog display electronics, this is called varying the gamma (the slope of the exposure-density curve). Using a computer, however, we can create transfer functions that are far more complicated, nonlinear, and arbitrary than can be achieved in the darkroom.

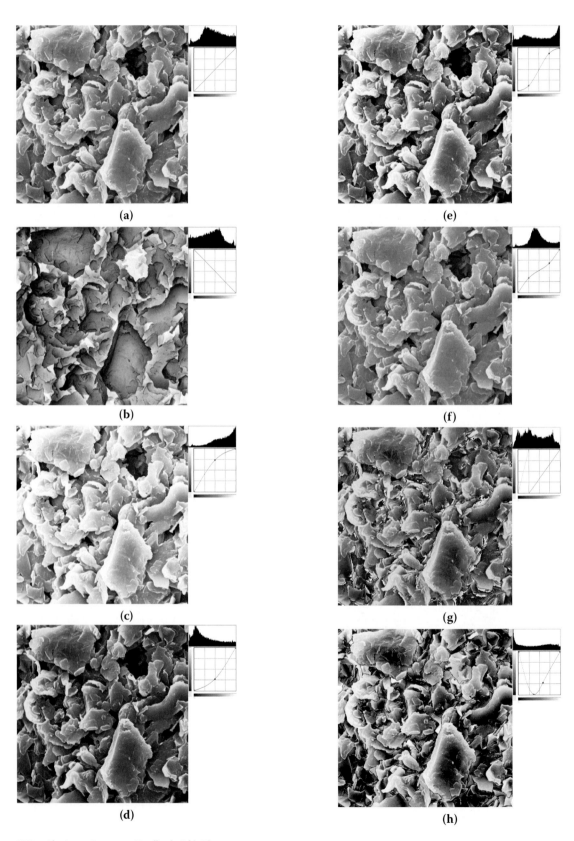

*Figure 5.1 (See facing page.) An original image with a full range of brightness values, and several examples of arbitrary display transfer functions that expand or alter the contrast in various parts of the range. The plot with each image shows the stored pixel brightness values on the horizontal axis and the displayed brightness on the vertical axis. The histogram of each resulting image is also shown. **(a)** The original image has a transfer function that is the identity function, so that actual stored brightnesses are displayed; **(b)** inverted (negative) image; **(c)** increasing gamma brightens middle grays and shows increased detail in shadows; **(d)** reducing gamma darkens middle grays and shows increased detail in bright areas; **(e)** increased contrast; **(f)** decreased contrast; **(g)** banded or wraparound; **(h)** solarization.*

Reversing all of the contrast range produces the equivalent of a photographic negative, which sometimes improves the visibility of details. **Figure 5.2** illustrates this with an example of an X-ray image; these are commonly examined using negatives. Reversing only a portion of the brightness range produces a visually strange effect, called solarization by photographers, that can also be used to show detail in both shadowed and saturated areas (**Figure 5.1h**).

Increasing the slope of the transfer function so that it "wraps around" produces an image (**Figure 5.1g**) in which several quite different stored brightness values can have the same display brightness. If the overall organization of the image is familiar to the viewer, this contouring may not be too disruptive, and it can increase the visibility for small differences. However, as with the use of pseudocolor, this kind of treatment is easily overdone and can confuse rather than enhance most images.

Certainly, experimentally modifying the transfer function until the image "looks good" and best shows those features of most interest to the viewer provides an ultimately flexible tool. The technique increases the visibility of some image details but hides others, according to the judgment of the operator. Of course, the same can be said of manipulating image contrast in darkroom printing. In most cases, it is desirable to have more reproducible and meaningful transfer functions available that can be applied equally to a series of images, so that proper comparison is possible.

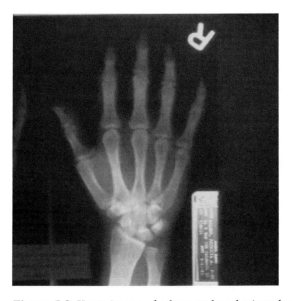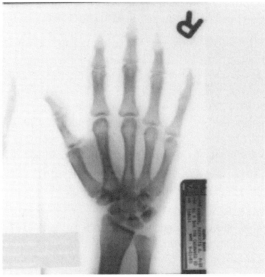

Figure 5.2 X-ray image of a human hand, viewed as a positive and a negative.

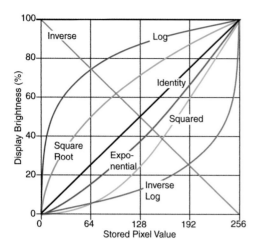

The most common kinds of transfer functions are curves of displayed vs. stored brightness following simple mathematical relationships such as logarithmic or power-law curves. An increased gamma curve (**Figure 5.1c**) compresses the displayed brightnesses at the bright end of the scale while expanding those at the dark end. This kind of relationship can also convert an image from a camera with a linear response to the more common logarithmic response. A reduced gamma curve (**Figure 5.1d**) does the opposite.

Figure 5.3 *Examples of display transfer functions.*

Figure 5.3 illustrates some of the more commonly used arithmetic functions that are applied to modify image brightness values. Any of these functions can be used in addition to contrast expansion if the image did not originally cover the full range from black to white, which stretches the original scale to the full range of the display. Curves or tables of values for these transfer functions can be precalculated and stored so that they can be loaded quickly to modify the display LUT. Many systems allow quite a few different tables to be kept on hand for use when an image requires it, just as a series of color LUTs may be available on disk for pseudocolor displays.

Histogram equalization

In addition to standard mathematical functions, it is sometimes advantageous to construct a transfer function for a specific image. Unlike the arbitrary functions shown above, however, we desire a specific algorithm that gives reproducible and (hopefully) optimal results. The most popular of these methods is called histogram equalization (Stark and Fitzgerald 1996). To understand it, we must begin with the image brightness histogram.

Figure 5.4 shows an example using the same original image as **Figure 5.1a**. The conventional histogram plot shows the number of pixels in the image having each of the 256 possible values of stored brightness. Peaks in the histogram correspond to the more common brightness values, which often correspond to particular structures that are present. Valleys indicate brightness values that are less common in the image. The data can also be plotted as a cumulative curve (shown in red in **Figure 5.4a**), which is simply the integral or summation of the values. If this curve is used as the display transfer function, the result (**Figure 5.4b**) is a display in which all of the available 256 brightness values are equally used. The histogram of this processed image (**Figure 5.4c**) shows this uniform distribution and a linear cumulative plot. This procedure is called histogram equalization.

Generally, images have unique brightness histograms. Even images of different areas of the same sample or scene, in which the various structures present have consistent brightness levels wherever they occur, will have different histograms, depending on the area covered by each structure. Changing the overall illumination or camera settings will shift the peaks in the histogram. In addition, most real images exhibit some variation in brightness within features (e.g., from the edge to the center) or in different regions.

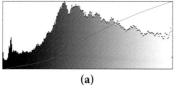

(a)

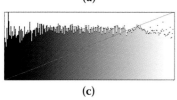

(c)

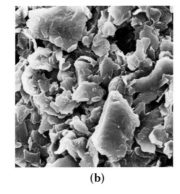

(b)

Figure 5.4 Histogram equalization: **(a)** *histogram of the original image in* **Figure 5.1a** *with the cumulative total shown in red;* **(b)** *application of the equalization function to the image;* **(c)** *histogram after processing, showing a uniform distribution of values and a linear cumulative plot.*

From the standpoint of efficiently using the available gray levels on the display, some gray-scale values are underutilized. It might be better to spread out the displayed gray levels in the peak areas selectively, compressing them in the valleys so that the same number of pixels in the display show each of the possible brightness levels. Histogram equalization accomplishes this redistribution by reassigning the brightness values of pixels based on the image histogram. Individual pixels retain their brightness order (that is, they remain brighter or darker than other pixels), but the values are shifted, so that an equal number of pixels have each possible brightness value. In many cases, this spreads out the values in regions where different regions meet, showing detail in areas with a high brightness gradient.

An image having a few regions in which the pixels have very similar brightness values presents a histogram with peaks. The sizes of these peaks give the relative area of the different phase regions and are useful for image analysis. Performing a histogram equalization on the image spreads the peaks out while compressing other parts of the histogram by assigning the same, or very close, brightness values to those pixels that are few in number and have intermediate brightnesses. This equalization makes it possible to see minor variations within regions that appeared nearly uniform in the original image.

The process is quite simple. For each brightness level j in the original image (and its histogram), the new assigned value k is calculated as

$$k = \sum_{i=0}^{j} N_i / T$$

(5.1)

where the sum counts the number of pixels in the image (by integrating the histogram) with brightness equal to or less than j, and T is the total number of pixels (or the total area of the histogram).

Figure 5.5 shows an example of an image with significant peaks and valleys. The original metallographic specimen has three phase regions with dark, intermediate, and light-gray values. Histogram equalization spreads out the values in the peaks, making the differences between pixels great enough to be visible. This shows the shading within the bright phase regions, indiscernible in the original image. Because the original image did not cover the full black-to-white range, and contained only 8 bits of data, the resulting histogram (**Figure 5.5d**) shows numerous gaps, even though the cumulative plot shows that the general distribution of values is uniform. In addition, some pixels that originally had different values are now assigned the same value.

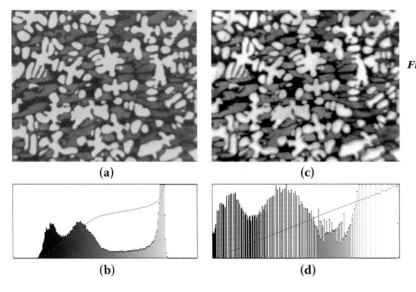

Figure 5.5 *Histogram equalization applied to an 8-bit gray-scale image:*
(a) original image;
(b) histogram showing peaks and valleys and incomplete coverage of the brightness range;
(c) after equalization;
(d) resulting histogram.

For a color image, it is possible to show three histograms corresponding to the three color axes or channels. As shown in **Figure 5.6**, this can be done equally well for RGB (red, green, blue), HSI (hue, saturation, intensity), or YUV (Y = luminance, U and V = red-green and yellow-blue chrominance) color coordinates. These sets of histograms are incomplete, however, in that they do not show the combinations of values that are associated in the same pixels. A three-dimensional histogram, in which points in the histogram have coordinates that correspond to the color values and show the number of pixels with each possible combination of values, is illustrated in **Figure 5.7**. Dark values indicate a large number of pixels with a particular combination of components. The projections of the three-dimensional histogram onto each of the two-dimensional faces of the cube are shown. This approach will be used again in **Chapter 7** in the context of selecting color combinations for thresholding and in **Chapter 10** for measuring the colocalization of intensity in different color channels (e.g., different fluorescent dyes).

Performing histogram equalization on the individual color channels produces unfortunate and often bizarre results, because the proportions of the various colors are altered differently in different regions of the image. The correct procedure is to work in HSI or L*a*b* space, leaving the color information unchanged and processing just the brightness or luminance values. As shown in **Figure 5.8**, this can produce substantial improvements in the visibility of details, particularly for images with a very large range of brightness values.

Equalization is just one example of histogram shaping. Other predetermined shapes, including ones that try to equalize the values in terms of human brightness perception, are also used (Frei 1977). **Figure 5.9** compares several different functions, all of which are most easily understood by the shape of the cumulative histogram. In all cases, the reassignment of some pixel brightness values opens up gaps in the histogram and combines some values so that pixels initially different in brightness are given the same value. One of the arguments for using higher-bit-depth images is that their brightness values can be manipulated without creating gaps in a 256-value histogram or creating visible contouring or posterization of the resulting image.

Any of these histogram-manipulation procedures — whether simple linear stretching, application of a predetermined mathematical transfer function, or histogram equalization — need not be performed on an entire image. Enhancing a portion of the original image, rather than the

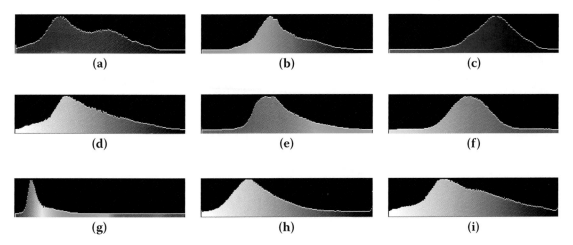

Figure 5.6 *Histograms of individual planes in a color image (the image, a microscope thin section of pancreas, is shown as **Figure 1.51** in **Chapter 1**: **(a)** red; **(b)** green; **(c)** blue; **(d)** luminance (Y); **(e)** chrominance (U); **(f)** chrominance (V); **(g)** hue; **(h)** saturation; **(i)** intensity*

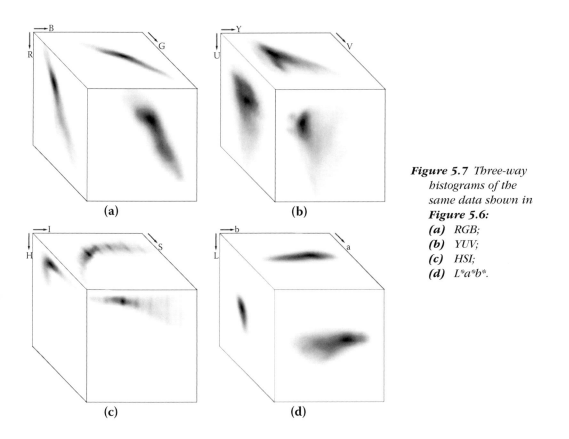

Figure 5.7 *Three-way histograms of the same data shown in* **Figure 5.6:** **(a)** *RGB;* **(b)** *YUV;* **(c)** *HSI;* **(d)** *L*a*b*.*

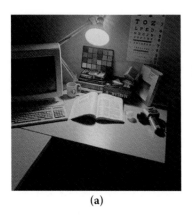 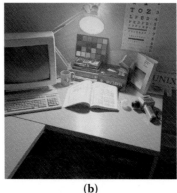

(a) (b)

Figure 5.8 *Histogram equalization applied to the brightness channel of a color image:*
(a) *original;*
(b) *processed result.*
(From Reinhard, E. et al., ACM Trans. Graphics *21(3): 267–276. [2002] With permission.)*

entire area, is also useful in many situations. This is particularly true when large regions of the image correspond to different types of structures or scenes and are generally brighter or darker than the rest of the image. When portions of an image can be selected, either manually or by some algorithm based on the variation in the brightness or contents, a selective equalization can be used to bring out local detail.

Figure 5.10 shows regions of the same test image used previously, with several regions separately selected and modified. Two of these regions are arbitrary rectangular and elliptical shapes, drawn by hand. In many cases, this kind of manual selection is the most straightforward way to specify a region. The other areas follow the outlines of the structure itself, either particles or holes, which can be isolated from the rest of the image because locally the boundary is sharp. Methods for locating boundary edges are discussed later in this chapter. Each of the regions was processed based solely on the histogram of the pixels within it, producing greater local contrast and increased detail visibility. When these operations are applied to only a portion of the entire image, it is necessary to actually modify the contents of the stored image to alter the display rather than simply adjusting the display LUT.

Histogram modification of regions within an image can dramatically improve the local visibility of details, but it usually alters the relationship between brightness and structure. In most cases, it is desirable for the brightness level of pixels associated with a particular type of feature in the image to be the same, wherever in the field of view it may occur. This allows rapid classification of the features for counting or measurement, whether it is done by a human or by the computer. Local modification of the gray-scale relationship voids this assumption, making the display brightness of features dependent on other features that happen to be nearby or in the selected region.

Histogram modification assigns the same new gray value to each pixel having a given original gray value, everywhere in the region. The result is that regions often have very noticeable and abrupt boundaries, which may or may not follow feature boundaries in the original image. Another approach performs the adjustment in a region around each pixel in the image, with the result applied separately to each individual pixel based on its surrounding neighborhood. This is normally done by specifying a neighborhood size (typically round or square). All of the pixels in that region are counted into a histogram, but after the adjustment procedure, the new value is applied only to the central pixel. This process is then repeated for each pixel in the image, always using the original brightness values to construct each region histogram.

Figure 5.11 shows an example in which local histogram equalization has been applied to every pixel in the image. A round neighborhood with a radius of 6 pixels was centered on each

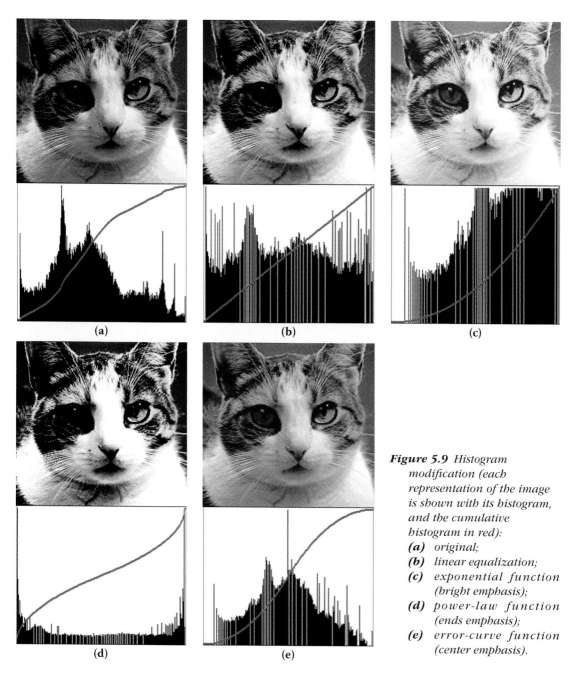

Figure 5.9 *Histogram modification (each representation of the image is shown with its histogram, and the cumulative histogram in red):*
(a) original;
(b) linear equalization;
(c) exponential function (bright emphasis);
(d) power-law function (ends emphasis);
(e) error-curve function (center emphasis).

pixel in the image, and the histogram of the 137 pixels within the neighborhood was used to perform the equalization. However, the new pixel value is kept only for the central pixel, which is then used to construct a new image. Some programs implement local equalization using a square neighborhood, which is slightly easier computationally but is less isotropic. The actual calculation is quite simple, since for each pixel the equalized brightness value is just the number of darker pixels in the neighborhood. Since the neighborhood contains 137 pixels, the procedure produces an image in which the maximum number of distinct brightness values is 137, instead of the original 256, but this is still more than can be visually distinguished

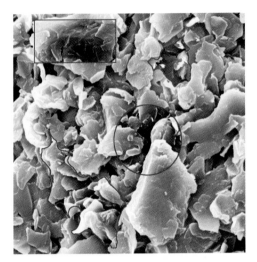

Figure 5.10 Selective contrast enhancement by histogram modification can be performed in any designated region of an image. In this example, several regions have been selected (outlined in red for visibility) and histogram equalization performed within each one separately.

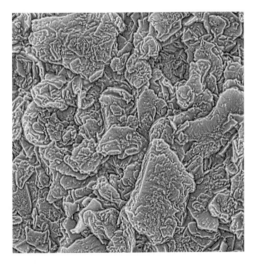

Figure 5.11 Local equalization applied to the same image as in Figure 5.1a. The local detail is enhanced while large-scale contrast is suppressed.

in the display. Even for a small neighborhood (for instance, a 5-pixel-wide circle contains 21 pixels), the number of gray values is generally enough for visual examination.

As is evident in the example, the process of local equalization makes pixels that were slightly — even imperceptibly — brighter than their surroundings brighter still, and vice versa. This enhances contrast near edges, revealing details in both light and dark regions. However, it can be seen in the example that in nominally uniform regions, this can produce artificial contrast variations that magnify the visibility of noise artifacts in the image. In general, it is important to remove or reduce noise, as discussed in **Chapter 4**, before performing enhancement operations.

The example image also shows that the result of local equalization is to reduce the overall or large-scale contrast in the image. The bright particle surfaces and dark holes are all reduced to an average gray, which hides much of the overall shape of the structure. Sometimes this reduction is not desirable, and can be offset by adding back a percentage of the original image to the processed result. In other cases, as shown in **Figure 5.12**, the large-scale changes in brightness are merely confusing and best eliminated.

Changing the size of the neighborhood used in local processing offers some control over the process, as shown in the figure. As long as the neighborhood is large enough to encompass the scale of the texture present and yet small enough to suppress the long-range variations in brightness, the results are usually satisfactory (Z. Q. Wu et al. 2005). Other modifications that are more effective (and generally combined under the term "adaptive" processing) are to weight the pixels according to how close they are to the center of the neighborhood, or according to how similar they are in brightness to the central pixel, or to include in the neighborhood only pixels "similar" to the central one. Histogram equalization is the most widely used local processing method, and since equalization is performed by constructing a histogram of the pixels and finding the midpoint of that histogram, the weighting is accomplished by assigning values greater or less than 1 to the pixels for use in summing up the histogram.

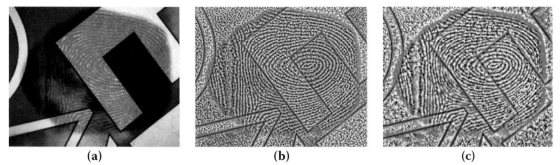

Figure 5.12 *The effect of neighborhood size:* **(a)** *the original image shows a fingerprint on a magazine cover, which is difficult to visually distinguish on the dark and light printed regions;* **(b)** *a neighborhood with a radius of 2 pixels contains 21 pixels;* **(c)** *a radius of 7 pixels contains 177 pixels. Both results suppress the contrast from the background and make the friction ridge markings in the fingerprint evident.*

Another local equalization technique that enhances the visibility of detail is variance equalization. This also uses a moving neighborhood in which a calculation is performed that modifies only the central pixel. The statistical variance of the pixels in the region is calculated and compared with that for the entire image, and the pixel values are adjusted up or down to match the local variance to the global. The result is again to increase the contrast in uniform areas, as shown in **Figure 5.13**. The surface indentations and scratches on the coin are much more visible after processing, particularly when the surface geometry is reconstructed with the enhanced contrast applied to the rendered surface.

When it is used with color images, local or adaptive equalization is properly applied only to the intensity data. The image is converted from its original RGB format in which it is stored internally to an HSI or L*a*b* space; the intensity values are then modified and combined with the original hue and saturation values so that new RGB values can be calculated to permit display of the result. This preserves the color information, which would be seriously altered if the red, green, and blue channels were equalized directly, as shown in **Figure 5.14** (Buzuloiu et al. 2001).

Laplacian

Local, or neighborhood, equalization of image contrast produces an increase in local contrast at boundaries, as shown in **Figure 5.15**. This has the effect of making edges easier for the viewer to see, consequently making the image appear sharper (although, in this example, the increased noise visibility within the uniform grains offsets this improvement). There are several other approaches to edge enhancement that are less sensitive — to overall brightness levels, noise, and the type or scale of detail present — than the equalization discussed above.

The first set of operations uses neighborhoods with multiplicative kernels identical in principle to those used in **Chapter 4** for noise smoothing. In the section on smoothing, kernels were written as an array of integers. For example,

$$
\begin{array}{ccc}
1 & 2 & 1 \\
2 & 4 & 2 \\
1 & 2 & 1
\end{array}
$$

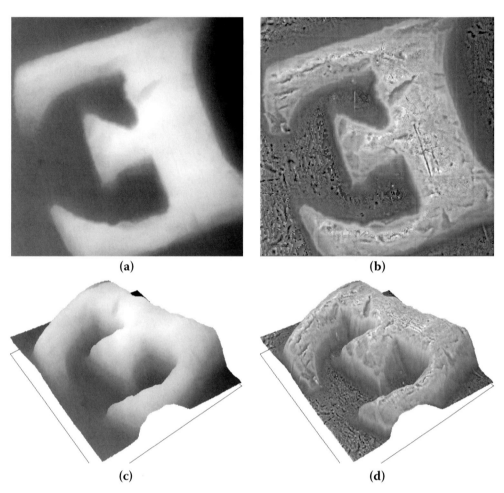

Figure 5.13 *Local enhancement applied to a surface image: **(a)** original (raised letter on a coin); **(b)** local variance equalization applied; **(c)** rendered surface with the original image contrast; **(d)** rendered surface with the equalized result applied to show the surface detail.*

This 3 × 3 kernel is understood to mean that the central pixel brightness value is multiplied by 4, the values of the four touching neighbors to the sides and above and below are multiplied by 2, and the four diagonally touching neighbors by 1. The total value is added up and then divided by 16 (the sum of the nine weights) to produce a new brightness value for the pixel. Other arrays of weights were also shown, some involving much larger arrays than this simple 3 × 3. For smoothing, all of the kernels were symmetrical about the center (at least, they approximated symmetry within the constraints of a square-pixel grid and integer values) and had only positive weight values.

A very simple kernel that is still roughly symmetrical, but does not have exclusively positive values, is the classic 3 × 3 Laplacian operator

$$
\begin{array}{ccc}
-1 & -1 & -1 \\
-1 & +8 & -1 \\
-1 & -1 & -1
\end{array}
$$

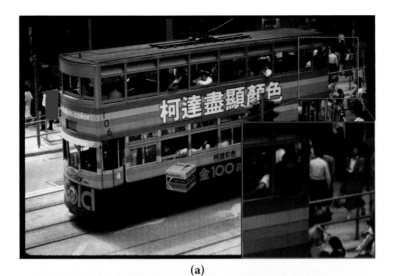

(a)

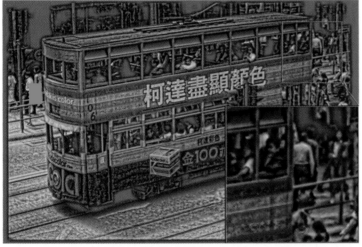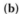

(b)

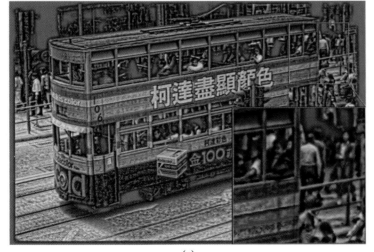

(c)

Figure 5.14 *Color photograph:*
(a) original;
(b) adaptive equalization of the individual red, green, and blue channels;
*(c) adaptive equalization of intensity, leaving hue and saturation unchanged. Note the increased visibility of figures and detail in shadow areas, and the false color variations present in image **b**.*
(Courtesy of Eastman Kodak Co.)

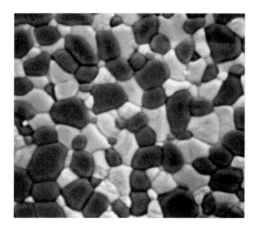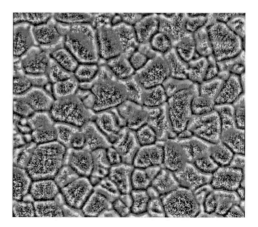

Figure 5.15 Local equalization of a two-phase material (alumina-zirconia). Note the increased contrast at boundaries, and the noise artifacts within the grains.

This subtracts the brightness values of each of the eight neighboring pixels from eight times the central pixel. Consequently, in a region of the image that is uniform in brightness or has a uniform gradient of brightness, the result of applying this kernel is to reduce the gray level to zero. When a discontinuity is present within the neighborhood in the form of a point, line, or edge, the result of the Laplacian is a nonzero value. It can be either positive or negative, depending on where the central point lies with respect to edge, etc.

To display the result when both positive and negative pixel values can arise, it is common to add a medium gray value (128 for the case of an image in which gray values are represented with a range from 0 to 255) so that the zero points are middle gray and the brighter and darker values produced by the Laplacian can be seen. Some systems instead plot the absolute value of the result, but this tends to produce double lines along edges that are confusing both to the viewer and to subsequent processing and measurement operations.

As the name of the Laplacian operator implies, it is an approximation to the linear second derivative of brightness B in directions x and y

$$\nabla^2 B \equiv \frac{\partial^2 B}{\partial x^2} + \frac{\partial^2 B}{\partial y^2}$$

(5.2)

which is invariant to rotation, and hence insensitive to the direction in which the discontinuity runs. This highlights the points, lines, and edges in the image and suppresses uniform and smoothly varying regions, with the result shown in **Figure 5.16**. By itself, this Laplacian image is not very easy to understand. Adding the Laplacian enhancement of the edges from the original image restores the overall gray-scale variation, which the human viewer can comfortably interpret. It also sharpens the image by locally increasing the contrast at discontinuities, as shown in the figure. This can be done simply by changing the weights in the kernel (and eliminating the offset of 128), so that it becomes

−1	−1	−1
−1	+9	−1
−1	−1	−1

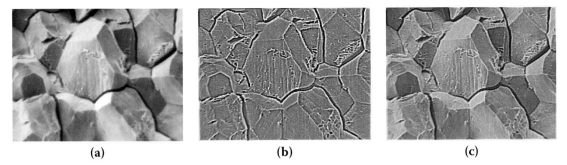

Figure 5.16 *Enhancement of contrast at edges, lines, and points using a Laplacian:* **(a)** *original SEM image of ceramic fracture;* **(b)** *application of Laplacian operator;* **(c)** *addition of the Laplacian to the original image.*

This kernel is often described as a sharpening operator because of the increased image contrast that it produces at edges. Justification for the procedure can be found in two different explanations. First, consider blur in an image to be modeled by a diffusion process in which brightness spreads out across the image, which would obey the partial differential equation

$$\frac{\partial f}{\partial t} = k\nabla^2 f \tag{5.3}$$

where the blur function is $f(x,y,t)$ and t is time. If this is expanded into a Taylor series around time τ, we can express the unblurred image as

$$B(x,y) = f(x,y,\tau) - \tau\frac{\partial f}{\partial t} + \frac{\tau^2}{2}\frac{\partial^2 f}{\partial t^2} - \cdots \tag{5.4}$$

If the higher-order terms are ignored, this is just

$$B = f - k\tau\nabla^2 f \tag{5.5}$$

In other words, the unblurred image B can be restored by combining the Laplacian (times a constant) with the blurred image. While the modeling of image blur as a diffusion process is at best approximate and the scaling constant is unknown or arbitrary, this at least gives some plausibility to the approach.

At least equally important is the simple fact that the processed image "looks good." As pointed out in **Chapter 2**, the human visual system itself concentrates on edges and ignores uniform regions (Hildreth 1983; Marr 1982; Marr and Hildreth 1980). This capability is hardwired into our retinas. Connected directly to the rods and cones of the retina are two layers of processing neurons that perform an operation very similar to the Laplacian. The horizontal cells in the second layer average together the signals from several neighboring sensors in the first layer, and the bipolar cells in the third layer combine that signal with the original sensor output. This is called local inhibition and helps us to extract boundaries and edges. It also accounts for some of the visual illusions shown previously.

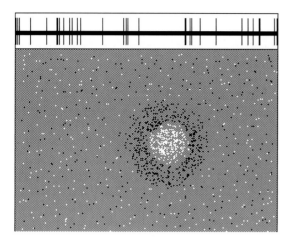

Figure 5.17 Experimental results plotting the output from a single retinal ganglion in the optic nerve as targets consisting of small white or black circles are moved slowly across the visual field. The central cluster of white dots shows a positive response to the white circle, and there is a reduction in pulses when the white target lies in the field of a neighboring receptor. The dark target gives a complementary result.

Inhibition is a process that takes place within the eye itself. Connections between the neurons within the retina suppress the output from one region according to its neighbors. Inhibition is useful for edge detection, but it also affects our visual comparisons of size and orientation. **Figure 5.17** shows a typical result from an experiment in which the output from a single retinal ganglion in the optic nerve (shown as a time sequence across the top) is plotted as a small white target is slowly moved across the visual field. The cluster of white dots shows the location of the corresponding receptor on the retina. Notice the zone around the receptor that is very poor in white dots. Light shining on neighboring receptors inhibits the output from the central receptor. Presenting a dark spot in the visual field produces additional output from the receptor when it lies within the zone of inhibition, and suppresses output when it lies on the receptor. Selecting different ganglia will map other receptor cells, including those that surround the one shown. Each cell inhibits output from its neighbors.

To observe the effect of the simple 3 × 3 sharpening kernel illustrated above, **Figure 5.18** shows an image fragment (enlarged to show individual pixels) and the actual pixel values (shown as integers in the usual 0 to 255 range) before and after the filter is applied. The effect of the filter is to make the pixels on the dark side of an edge darker still and those on the bright side brighter still, thus increasing the edge contrast. A modification of this technique can be used to restrict the edge enhancement to just the brighter or darker side, which may improve the visual appearance of the result, as shown in **Figure 5.19**, depending on whether the local region is dark or light. Also notice in this example that the filter is applied only to the intensity channel of the image, leaving color information unchanged. As for all image processing operations, this is important because operating on the original red, green, and blue channels produces variations in the proportions of the values that alter the colors and seriously degrade the visual appearance of the processed image. **Figure 5.20** illustrates this difference.

Another way to describe the operation of the Laplacian is as a high-pass filter. In **Chapter 6**, image processing in the Fourier domain is discussed in terms of the high- and low-frequency components of the image brightness. A low-pass filter, such as the smoothing kernels discussed in **Chapter 4**, removes or suppresses the high-frequency variability associated with random noise, which can cause nearby pixels to vary in brightness. Conversely, a high-pass filter allows these high frequencies to remain (pass through the filter) while removing the low frequencies corresponding to the gradual overall variation in brightness.

As with smoothing kernels, there are many different sets of integers and different-size kernels that can be used to apply a Laplacian to an image. The simplest just uses the four immediately touching pixels that share a side with the central pixel.

$$
\begin{array}{ccc}
 & -1 & \\
-1 & +4 & -1 \\
 & -1 & \\
\end{array}
$$

One problem with the small kernels shown above is that the differences are strictly local, comparing the central pixel with its immediate neighbors. The most common type of noise consists of random variations between adjacent pixels, even within homogeneous regions of an image, and so it will be made more visible by this approach.

A somewhat more general method for enhancing the visibility of details and edges is the unsharp mask. The name "unsharp mask" may seem odd for a technique that makes images appear visually sharper. It comes from the origins of the method, which has traditionally been applied in the photographic darkroom. **Figure 1.29** in **Chapter 1** illustrates the steps. First, a contact print is made from the original negative onto film, at 1:1 magnification but slightly out of focus or blurred. After the film is developed, a new print is made with the two negatives sandwiched together. The light areas on the original negative are covered by dark areas on the printed negative, allowing little light to come through. Only regions where the slightly out-of-focus negative does not match the original are printed. This is somewhat similar to the Laplacian, which subtracts a smoothed (out of focus) image from the original to suppress gradual changes and pass high frequencies or edges, but it allows the blurring to extend over a greater (and adjustable) distance.

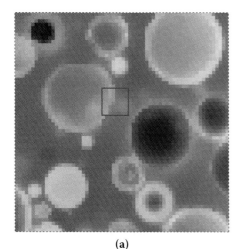

(a)

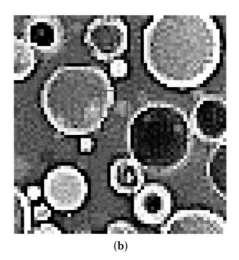

(b)

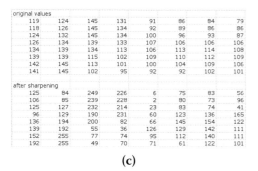

original values							
119	124	145	131	91	86	84	79
118	126	145	134	92	89	86	86
124	132	145	134	100	96	93	87
126	134	139	133	107	106	106	106
134	139	134	113	106	113	114	108
139	139	115	102	109	110	112	109
142	145	113	101	100	104	109	106
141	145	102	95	92	92	102	101

after sharpening							
125	84	249	226	6	75	83	56
106	85	239	228	2	80	73	96
125	127	232	214	23	83	74	41
96	129	190	231	60	123	136	165
136	194	200	82	66	145	154	122
139	192	55	36	126	129	142	111
152	255	77	74	95	112	140	111
192	255	49	70	71	61	122	101

(c)

Figure 5.18 *Operation of the 3 × 3 sharpening filter:*
(a) fragment of an original image (an epoxy containing bubbles);
(b) image after application of the filter, showing edges delineated by bright and dark borders;
(c) pixel values from the region outlined in red.

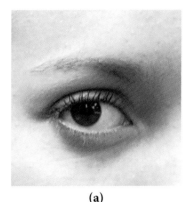

(a)

Figure 5.19 *Allowing only dark or light edge enhancement:*
   (a) *original image (detail);*
   (b) *dark border only;*
   (c) *light border only;*
   (d) *both light and dark borders.*

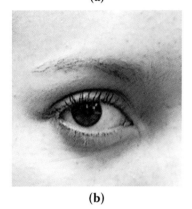

(b)

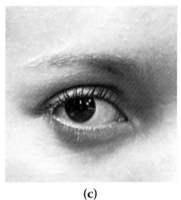

(c)

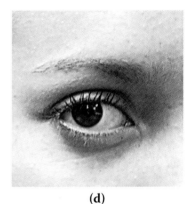

(d)

Computer implementation of the unsharp mask typically applies a Gaussian blur to one copy of the image, which is then subtracted from the original. Just as for the Laplacian, the result usually is added back to the original to provide emphasis to the edges and detail while retaining some of the overall image contrast. Applying the unsharp mask operator increases the visibility of fine detail while suppressing overall variations in brightness. **Figure 5.21** shows an example using the same X-ray image from **Figure 5.2**. In the original image, the bones in the fingers are thinner and hence not as dense as those in the wrist, and the written label is hardly visible. The processed image makes these more readily visible.

Closely related to unsharp masking, in fact the most general form of this technique, is the subtraction of one smoothed version of the image from another having a different degree of smoothing. This is called the "difference-of-Gaussians" (DoG) method and is believed (Marr 1982) to be similar to the way the human visual system locates boundaries and other features. The DoG method is practically identical in shape to another function that is also used, the Laplacian of a Gaussian, or LoG. (This edge extractor is also sometimes called a Marr-Hildreth operator.)

The DoG technique is superior to the unsharp mask in its ability to suppress random pixel noise variations in the image. Smoothing the image using a Gaussian kernel with an appropriate but small standard deviation suppresses high-frequency noise, while the second Gaussian smooth (with a larger standard deviation, usually two to five times greater than first one) removes both the noise and important edges, lines, and detail. The difference between the two images then keeps only those structures (lines, points, etc.) that are in the intermediate size range between the two operators. Rather than being a high-pass filter, the DoG is more properly described as a band-pass filter that allows a selected range of frequencies or spacings to be kept.

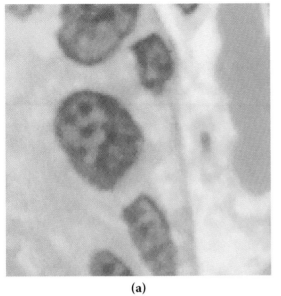

(a)

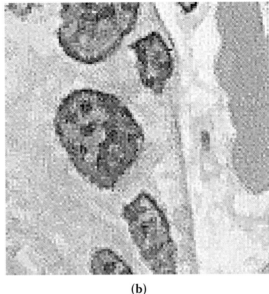

(b)

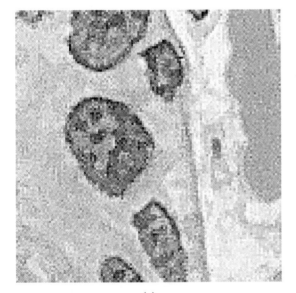

(c)

Figure 5.20 *Effect of color space on processing:*
- *(a) original image (enlarged fragment of a microscope image of stained tissue);*
- *(b) image after processing intensity channel but not hue or saturation, showing an increase in noise visibility as well as edge sharpness;*
- *(c) image after processing RGB channels, showing an increase in noise visibility and the introduction of new, random colors for individual pixels*

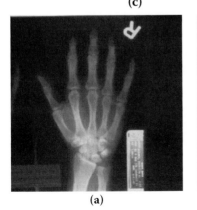

(a)

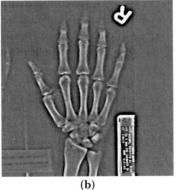

(b)

Figure 5.21 *Application of an unsharp mask to an X-ray image of a human hand:*
- *(a) original;*
- *(b) processed.*

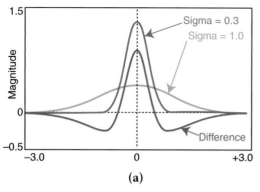

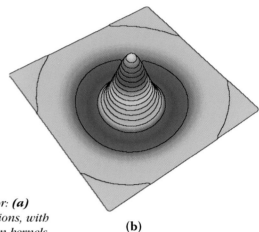

(a)

(b)

Figure 5.22 *The difference-of-Gaussian (DoG) operator:* **(a)** *two Gaussian curves with different standard deviations, with their difference;* **(b)** *difference between two Gaussian kernels, plotted as an isometric view. The "moat" of values around the central peak contains negative values.*

A plot of two Gaussian curves with different standard deviations, and their difference, is shown in **Figure 5.22**; the difference is similar to a cross section of the Laplacian when both standard deviations are small, and to the unsharp mask when the smaller one is negligible. Because of the shape of these kernels when they are plotted as isometric views, they are sometimes described as a Mexican hat or sombrero filter; this name is usually reserved for kernels with more than one positive-weighted pixel at the center. **Figure 5.23** shows a comparison of the application of a simple 3 × 3 Laplacian-based sharpening filter, an unsharp mask, and a DoG filter to a noisy SEM image.

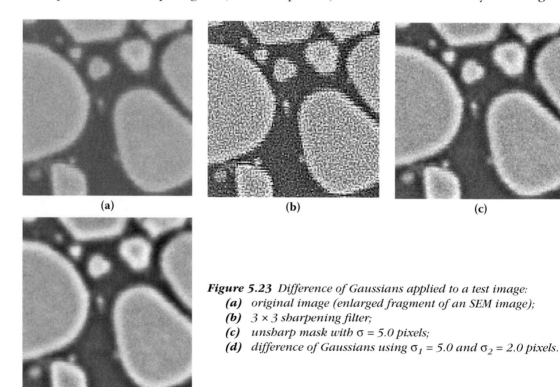

(a)

(b)

(c)

(d)

Figure 5.23 *Difference of Gaussians applied to a test image:*
    (a) *original image (enlarged fragment of an SEM image);*
    (b) *3 × 3 sharpening filter;*
    (c) *unsharp mask with* σ = 5.0 *pixels;*
    (d) *difference of Gaussians using* σ_1 = 5.0 *and* σ_2 = 2.0 *pixels.*

Historically, kernels used for convolution have been relatively small and have used integer weights to make the arithmetic as fast as possible. Constructing a kernel such that the negative values (a) have the same total as the positive ones (to avoid shifting the overall brightness), (b) are reasonably isotropic (so that feature and edge orientations are equally enhanced regardless of their directionality), and (c) actually conform to the shape of Gaussian curves or to the difference of Gaussians is at best an art form. Earlier editions of this book included a few examples. Fortunately, with the advent of faster computers capable of floating-point arithmetic, this need not be an issue. The appropriate filters can be constructed as needed, interactively, while observing the resulting enhancement of the image. The same option shown previously of applying the effect selectively to the bright or dark sides of a step can be added. And of course the operation of the filter in a hue-saturation-intensity (HSI) or L*a*b* space, rather than RGB, is assumed.

Derivatives

The Laplacian, unsharp mask, and DoG filters are good for general-purpose visual enhancement, but not the best tool to use in all cases. One situation that arises involves images in which the detail has a single, known orientation. Examples include chromatography preparations in which proteins are spread along lanes in an electrical field (**Figure 5.24**) or tree-ring patterns from drill cores (**Figure 5.25**). Applying a first derivative to such an image, in the direction of important variation, enhances the visibility of small steps and other details, as shown in the figures. Of course, for an image with digitized finite pixels, a continuous derivative cannot be performed. Instead, the difference value between adjacent pixels can be calculated as a finite derivative. This difference is somewhat noisy, but averaging in the direction perpendicular to the derivative can smooth the result, as shown in the examples.

Typical kernels used for a directional first derivative are:

1	0	−1	or	0	1	0	−1	0
2	0	−2		0	2	0	−2	0
1	0	−1		0	4	0	−4	0
				0	2	0	−2	0
				0	1	0	−1	0

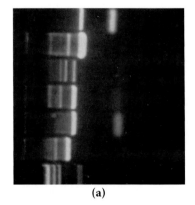

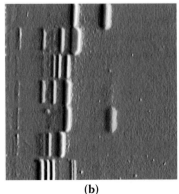

Figure 5.24 Image of a protein-separation gel:
(a) original;
(b) horizontal derivative using a 3 × 3 kernel.

(a) (b)

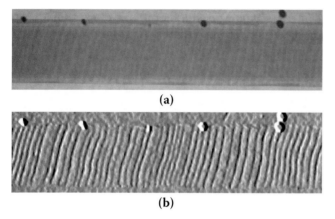

(a)

(b)

Figure 5.25 Image of tree rings in a drill core:
(a) original;
(b) horizontal derivative using a 3 × 3 kernel.

Note that the original central pixel's value does not enter into the calculation at all. Instead, the differences are formed between neighbors to the left and right. Obviously, this pattern can be rotated to other directions, such as

2	1	0	or	1	2	1
1	0	−1		0	0	0
0	−1	−2		−1	−2	−1

Of course, other kernel values can be devised that will also produce derivatives. As the kernel size increases, the number of different possible directions increases. Because this is fundamentally a one-dimensional derivative, it is possible to directly use the coefficients of Savitsky and Golay (1964), which were originally published for use with such one-dimensional data as spectrograms or other strip-chart recorder output. These coefficients, like the smoothing weights shown in **Chapter 4**, are equivalent to a least-squares fitting of a high-order polynomial to the data. In this case, however, the first derivative of the polynomial is evaluated at the central point. Second-degree (quadratic) and fourth-degree (quartic) polynomials are shown in **Table 5.1** and **Table 5.2**, respectively.

Adjusting the orientation of the derivative to be perpendicular to the predominant structure in an image can produce useful results, as shown in **Figure 5.26**. However, note that while this so-called "embossing" effect enhances the visibility of the cloud patterns and a portion of the rings in this picture of Saturn, it effectively hides the details where they are oriented parallel to the derivative direction, whereas the Laplacian-based sharpening highlights the details regardless of orientation.

The ability to hide detail that has a particular orientation is, in fact, a useful attribute that can sometimes be exploited to reveal other information in an image. **Figure 5.27** and **Figure 5.28** illustrate the possibilities.

Finding edges

As shown above, the Laplacian, which is a second derivative, is not an ideal tool for demarcating edges (Berzins 1984; Heath et al. 1997). In most cases, boundaries or edges of features or

Table 5.1. Coefficients for First-Derivative Quadratic Fit

Neighborhood Points

No.	5	7	9	11	13	15	17	19	21	23	25
−12											−.0092
−11										−.0109	−.0085
−10									−.0130	−.0099	−.0077
−9								−.0158	−.0117	−.0089	−.0069
−8							−.0196	−.0140	−.0104	−.0079	−.0062
−7						−.0250	−.0172	−.0123	−.0091	−.0069	−.0054
−6					−.0330	−.0214	−.0147	−.0105	−.0078	−.0059	−.0046
−5				−.0455	−.0275	−.0179	−.0123	−.0088	−.0065	−.0049	−.0038
−4			−.0667	−.0364	−.0220	−.0143	−.0098	−.0070	−.0052	−.0040	−.0031
−3		−.1071	−.0500	−.0273	−.0165	−.0107	−.0074	−.0053	−.0039	−.0030	−.0023
−2	−.2000	−.0714	−.0333	−.0182	−.0110	−.0071	−.0049	−.0035	−.0026	−.0020	−.0015
−1	−.1000	−.0357	−.0250	−.0091	−.0055	−.0036	−.0025	−.0018	−.0013	−.0010	−.0008
0	0	0	0	0	0	0	0	0	0	0	0
+1	+.1000	+.0357	+.0250	+.0091	+.0055	+.0036	+.0025	+.0018	+.0013	+.0010	+.0008
+2	+.2000	+.0714	+.0333	+.0182	+.0110	+.0071	+.0049	+.0035	+.0026	+.0020	+.0015
+3		+.1071	+.0500	+.0273	+.0165	+.0107	+.0074	+.0053	+.0039	+.0030	+.0023
+4			+.0667	+.0364	+.0220	+.0143	+.0098	+.0070	+.0052	+.0040	+.0031
+5				+.0455	+.0275	+.0179	+.0123	+.0088	+.0065	+.0049	+.0038
+6					+.0330	+.0214	+.0147	+.0105	+.0078	+.0059	+.0046
+7						+.0250	+.0172	+.0123	+.0091	+.0069	+.0054
+8							+.0196	+.0140	+.0104	+.0079	+.0062
+9								+.0158	+.0117	+.0089	+.0069
+10									+.0130	+.0099	+.0077
+11										+.0109	+.0085
+12											+.0092

regions appear at least locally as a step in brightness, sometimes spread over several pixels. The Laplacian gives a larger response to a line than to a step, and to a point than to a line. In an image that contains noise, which is typically present as points varying in brightness due to counting statistics, detector characteristics, etc., the Laplacian will show such points more strongly than the edges or boundaries that are of interest. Also, directional first derivatives only highlight edges in a direction perpendicular to their orientation. Using one-dimensional derivatives to extract one-dimensional data from two-dimensional images is a relatively specialized operation that does not address the needs of most real pictures.

Extending the same principles used in the directional derivative to locating boundaries with arbitrary orientations in two-dimensional images is one of the most common of all image enhancement operations. The problem, of course, is finding a method that is insensitive to the (local) orientation of the edge. One of the earliest approaches to this task was the Roberts'

Table 5.2. Coefficients for First-Derivative Quartic Fit

					Neighborhood Points						
No.	5	7	9	11	13	15	17	19	21	23	25
−12											+.0174
−11										+.0200	+.0048
−10									+.0231	+.0041	−.0048
−9								+.0271	+.0028	−.0077	−.0118
−8							+.0322	−.0003	−.0119	−.0159	−.0165
−7						+.0387	−.0042	−.0182	−.0215	−.0209	−.0190
−6					+.0472	−.0123	−.0276	−.0292	−.0267	−.0231	−.0197
−5				+.0583	−.0275	−.0423	−.0400	−.0340	−.0280	−.0230	−.0189
−4			+.0724	−.0571	−.0657	−.0549	−.0431	−.0335	−.0262	−.0208	−.0166
−3		+.0873	−.1195	−.1033	−.0748	−.0534	−.0388	−.0320	−.0219	−.0170	−.0134
−2	+.0833	−.2659	−.1625	−.0977	−.0620	−.0414	−.0289	−.0210	−.0157	−.0120	−.0094
−1	−.6667	−.2302	−.1061	−.0575	−.0346	−.0225	−.0154	−.0110	−.0081	−.0062	−.0048
0	0	0	0	0	0	0	0	0	0	0	0
+1	+.6667	+.2302	+.1061	+.0575	+.0346	+.0225	+.0154	+.0110	+.0081	+.0062	+.0048
+2	−.0833	+.2659	+.1625	+.0977	+.0620	+.0414	+.0289	+.0210	+.0157	+.0120	+.0094
+3		−.0873	+.1195	+.1033	+.0748	+.0534	+.0388	+.0320	+.0219	+.0170	+.0134
+4			−.0724	+.0571	+.0657	+.0549	+.0431	+.0335	+.0262	+.0208	+.0166
+5				−.0583	+.0275	+.0423	+.0400	+.0340	+.0280	+.0230	+.0189
+6					−.0472	+.0123	+.0276	+.0292	+.0267	+.0231	+.0197
+7						−.0387	+.0042	+.0182	+.0215	+.0209	+.0190
+8							−.0322	+.0003	+.0119	+.0159	+.0165
+9								−.0271	−.0028	+.0077	+.0118
+10									−.0231	−.0041	+.0048
+11										−.0200	−.0048
+12											−.0174

Cross operator (Roberts 1965). It uses the same difference technique shown previously for the one-dimensional case, but with two-pixel differences at right angles to each other, as diagrammed in **Figure 5.29**. These two differences represent a finite approximation of the derivative of brightness. Two-directional derivatives can be combined to obtain a magnitude value that is insensitive to the orientation of the edge by squaring, adding, and taking the square root of the total.

This method has the same problems as the difference method used in one dimension. Noise in the image is magnified by the single-pixel differences. Also, the result is shifted by half a pixel in both the x and y directions. In addition, the result is not invariant with respect to edge orientation. As a practical matter, the computers in common use when this model was first proposed were not very fast, nor were they equipped with separate floating-point math co-processors. This made the square root of the sum of the squares impractical to calculate. Two

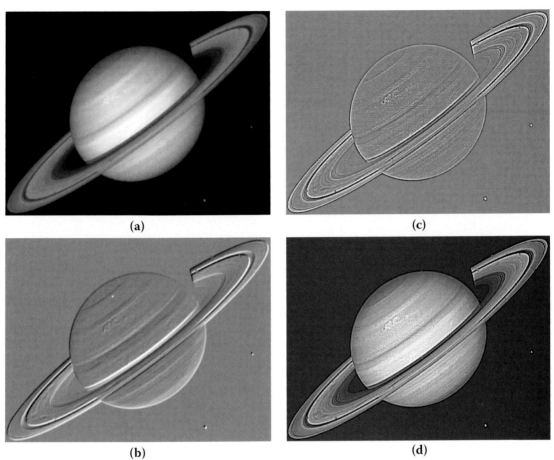

(a)

(c)

(b)

(d)

Figure 5.26 *Comparison of a directional derivative with the Laplacian operator: **(a)** original; **(b)** derivative from the upper left applied; **(c)** nondirectional Laplacian kernel applied; **(d)** result after adding images **c** and **a**.*

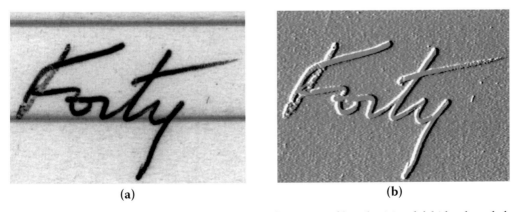

(a)

(b)

Figure 5.27 *Applying a horizontal derivative to this image of handwriting **(a)** hides the ruled lines on the paper **(b)**.*

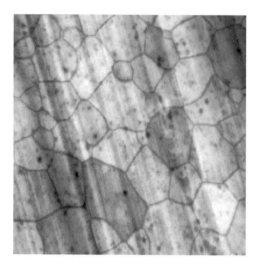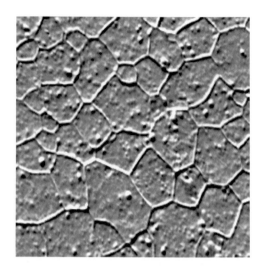

Figure 5.28 Applying a derivative parallel to the rolling marks on this aluminum foil suppresses them and makes the grain structure of the metal more accessible.

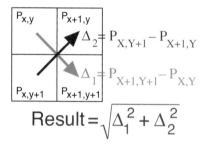

Figure 5.29 Diagram of Roberts' Cross operator. Two differences in directions at right angles to each other are combined to determine the gradient.

alternatives were used: adding the absolute values of the two directional differences, or comparing the two absolute values of the differences and keeping the larger one. Both of these methods make the result quite sensitive to direction. In addition, even if the square root method is used, the magnitude of the result will vary because the pixel spacing is not the same in all directions, and edges in the vertical and horizontal directions spread the change in brightness over more pixels than edges in the diagonal directions. In the comparison sequence shown later in this chapter (in **Figure 5.32b**), the Roberts' Cross image uses the square root of the sum of squares of the differences. Even so, the image is characterized by varying sensitivity with respect to edge orientation, as well as a high noise sensitivity.

Just as for the example of the horizontal derivative, the use of a larger kernel offers reduced sensitivity to noise by averaging several pixels and eliminating image shift. In fact, the derivative kernels shown previously, or other similar patterns using different sets of integers, are widely used. Some common examples of these coefficients are shown in **Table 5.3**.

It actually makes little difference which of these patterns of values is used, as long as the magnitude of the result does not exceed the storage capacity of the computer being used. If this is limited to a single byte per pixel, the limits would be values between –127 and +128, since the result of this operation can be either negative or positive. If large steps in brightness are present, this can result in the clipping of the calculated values, so that major boundaries are broadened or distorted to see smaller ones. The alternative is to employ automatic scaling, using the maximum and minimum values in the derivative image to set the white and dark values. To avoid loss of precision, this requires two passes through the image: one to perform the calculations and find the extreme values and another to actually compute the values and scale

Table 5.3. Several Examples of Directional Derivative Filter Weights

A			B			C			D		
+1	0	-1	+1	0	-1	+1	-1	-1	+5	-3	-3
+1	0	-1	+2	0	-2	+2	+1	-1	+5	0	-3
+1	0	-1	+1	0	-1	+1	-1	-1	+5	-3	-3
+1	+1	0	+2	+1	0	+2	+1	-1	+5	+5	-3
+1	0	-1	+1	0	-1	+1	+1	-1	+5	0	-3
0	-1	-1	0	-1	-2	-1	-1	-1	-3	-3	-3
+1	+1	+1	+1	+2	+1	+1	+2	+1	+5	+5	+5
0	0	0	0	0	0	-1	+1	-1	-3	0	-3
-1	-1	-1	-1	-2	-1	-1	-1	-1	-3	-3	-3

and so forth, for eight rotations.

the results for storage, or one to perform the calculations and temporarily store intermediate results with full precision and another to rescale the values to fit the range for pixel values.

As for the Roberts' Cross method, if the derivatives in two orthogonal directions are computed, they can be combined as the square root of the sums of their squares to obtain a result independent of orientation. This is just the normal method for combining two vectors, one in the horizontal and one in the vertical direction, to get the length of the vector that represents the local gradient of the brightness change.

$$\text{Magnitude} = \sqrt{\left(\frac{\partial B}{\partial x}\right)^2 + \left(\frac{\partial B}{\partial y}\right)^2}$$

(5.6)

This is the Sobel (1970) method. It is one of the most commonly used techniques, even though it requires a modest amount of computation to perform correctly. (As for the Roberts' Cross, some early computer programs attempted to compensate for hardware limitations by adding or comparing the two values, instead of squaring, adding, and taking the square root.)

With appropriate hardware, such as a shift register or array processor, the Sobel operation can be performed in essentially real time. This usually means 1/30th of a second per image, so that conventional video images can be processed and viewed. It often means viewing one frame while the following one is digitized, but in the case of the Sobel, it is even possible to view the image live, delayed only by two video scan lines. Two lines of data can be buffered and used to calculate the horizontal and vertical derivative values using the 3 × 3 kernels shown previously. Specialized hardware to perform this real-time edge enhancement is used in some military applications, making it possible to locate edges in images for tracking, alignment of hardware in midair refueling, and other purposes.

At the other extreme, some general-purpose image-analysis systems that do not have hardware for fast math operations approximate the Sobel by using a series of operations. First, two derivative images are formed, one using a horizontal and one a vertical orientation of the kernel.

Then each of these is modified using a LUT to replace the value of each pixel with its square. The two resulting images are added together, and another LUT is used to convert each pixel value to its square root. No multiplication or square roots are needed. However, if this method is applied in a typical system with 8 bits per pixel, the loss of precision is severe, reducing the final image to no more than 4 bits (16 gray levels) of useful information.

A more practical way to avoid the mathematical operations needed to calculate the square root of the sum of squares needed by the Sobel is the Kirsch (1971) operator. This method applies each of the eight orientations of the derivative kernel and keeps the maximum value. It requires only integer multiplication and comparisons. For many images, the results for the magnitude of edges are very similar to the Sobel. In the example of **Figure 5.30** vertical and horizontal derivatives of the image, and the maximum derivative values in each of eight directions, are shown.

Figure 5.31 and **Figure 5.32** illustrate the formation of the Sobel edge-finding image and compare it with the Laplacian, Roberts' Cross, and Kirsch operators. The example image contains many continuous edges running in all directions around the holes in the carbon film, as well as some straight edges at various orientations along the asbestos fibers. The Laplacian image is quite noisy, and the Roberts' Cross does not show all of the edges equally well. The individual vertical and horizontal derivatives are shown with the zero value shifted to an intermediate gray, so that both the negative and positive values can be seen. The absolute values are also shown. Combining the two directional derivatives by a sum, or maximum operator, produces quite noisy and incomplete boundary enhancement. The square root of the sum of squares produces a good image, with little noise and continuous edge markings. The result from the Kirsch operator is visually similar to the Sobel for this image.

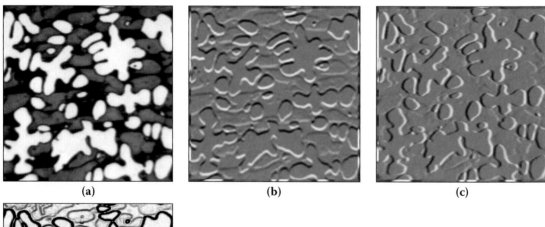

(a) (b) (c)

Figure 5.30
  (a) *A metallographic image with*
  (b and c) *two directional derivatives, and*
  (d) *the Kirsch image produced by keeping the maximum value from each direction.*

(d)

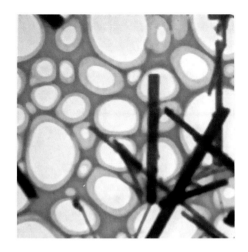

Figure 5.31 Original image (asbestos fibers on a holey carbon film, imaged in a TEM). This image is the basis for the processing shown in Figure 5.32.

In addition to the magnitude of the Sobel operator, it is also possible to calculate a direction value (Lineberry 1982) for the gradient vector at each pixel as

$$\text{Direction} = \text{Arc Tan}\left(\frac{\partial B/\partial y}{\partial B/\partial x}\right)$$

(5.7)

Figure 5.33 shows the vector results from applying the Sobel operator to the image of **Figure 5.31**. The magnitude and direction are encoded, but the vector field is too sparse to show any image details. If the calculation is used to assign a value to each pixel for the gradient direction, the values can be scaled to the gray scale of the image. If typical pixel values from 0 to 255 are used to represent angles from 0 to 359°, each step in gray scale corresponds to about 1.4° in vector orientation.

Figure 5.34 shows only the direction information for the image in **Figure 5.31**, using gray values to represent the angles. The progression of values around each more-or-less circular hole is evident. The use of a pseudocolor scale for this display is particularly suitable, since a rainbow of hues can show the progression without the arbitrary discontinuity required by the gray scale (in this example, at an angle of 0°). Unfortunately, the pixels within relatively homogeneous areas of the features also have colors assigned, because at every point there is some direction to the gradient, and these colors tend to overwhelm the visual impression of the image. A solution is to combine the magnitude of the gradient with the direction, as shown in **Figure 5.35**. This is the image from **Figure 5.30**, processed to show the magnitude and the direction of the Sobel edge gradient, the latter in color. These two images are then combined so that the intensity of the color is proportional to the magnitude of the gradient. The result clearly shows the orientation of boundaries.

Another way to improve the resulting image is to show the direction information only for those pixels that also have a strong magnitude for the brightness gradient. In **Figure 5.36** this is done by using the magnitude image as a mask, selecting (by thresholding, as discussed in **Chapter 7**) the 40% of the pixels with the largest gradient magnitude, and showing the direction only for those pixels. This is particularly suitable for selecting pixels to be counted as a function of color (direction) for analysis purposes.

Figure 5.36 also shows a histogram plot of the preferred orientation in the image. This kind of plot is particularly common for interpreting the orientation of lines, such as dislocations in metals and the traces of faults in geographic maps. In **Figure 5.37**, the orientation of the collagen fibers is measured using this same technique. The plot shows that they are not isotropically oriented, with about twice as many pixels showing an orientation of about 70°. Further examples of measurement using this tool will be discussed below, as will the use of the direction image to reveal image texture or to select regions of the image based on the texture or its orientation.

When the oriented features do not fill the image, but are either isolated fibers or edges of features, they can be selected for measurement by using the Sobel magnitude image. Thresholding this image to select only the points whose gradient vector is large, and then applying

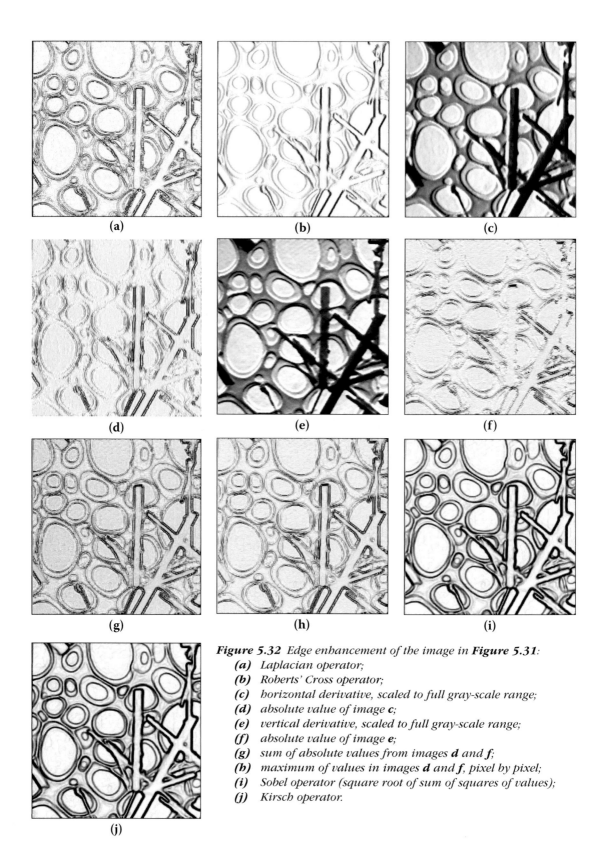

Figure 5.32 Edge enhancement of the image in *Figure 5.31*:
- *(a)* Laplacian operator;
- *(b)* Roberts' Cross operator;
- *(c)* horizontal derivative, scaled to full gray-scale range;
- *(d)* absolute value of image *c*;
- *(e)* vertical derivative, scaled to full gray-scale range;
- *(f)* absolute value of image *e*;
- *(g)* sum of absolute values from images *d* and *f*;
- *(h)* maximum of values in images *d* and *f*, pixel by pixel;
- *(i)* Sobel operator (square root of sum of squares of values);
- *(j)* Kirsch operator.

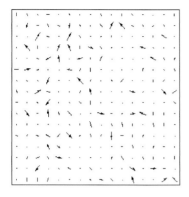

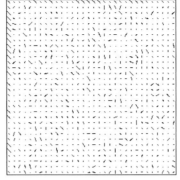

Figure 5.33 *Applying a Sobel operator to the image in* *Figure 5.31*. *Each vector has the direction and magnitude given by the operator, but even the fine vector field is too sparse to show image details.*

Figure 5.34 *Gray-scale representation of direction of the Sobel operator for the image in* *Figure 5.31*.

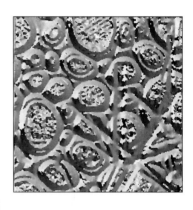

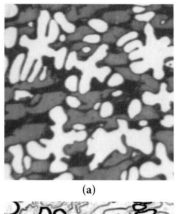

(a)

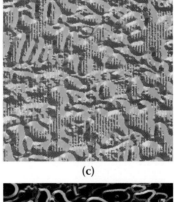

(c)

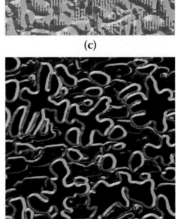

(b)

(d)

Figure 5.35 *Combining the magnitude and direction information from the Sobel gradient operator:*
(a) *original gray-scale image (from* *Figure 5.30);*
(b) *Sobel gradient magnitude;*
(c) *Sobel direction (color-coded);*
(d) *combining magnitude (as intensity) and direction (as hue).*

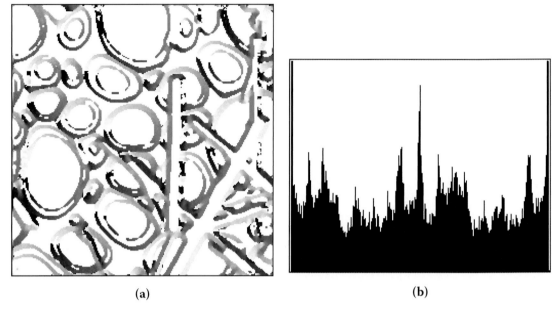

(a)   (b)

Figure 5.36 *Uses of the edge-orientation image in* **Figure 5.34***: (a) masking only those pixels whose edge magnitude is large (the 40% of the pixels with the greatest magnitude); (b) histogram of orientation values in which the horizontal axis of the histogram (255 brightness values) represents the angular range 0 to 360°.*

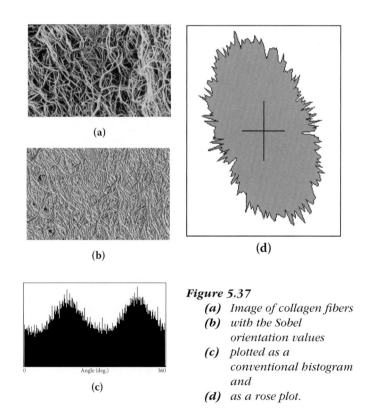

(a)

(b)

(d)

0   Angle (deg.)   360

(c)

Figure 5.37

    (a)   *Image of collagen fibers*
    (b)   *with the Sobel orientation values*
    (c)   *plotted as a conventional histogram and*
    (d)   *as a rose plot.*

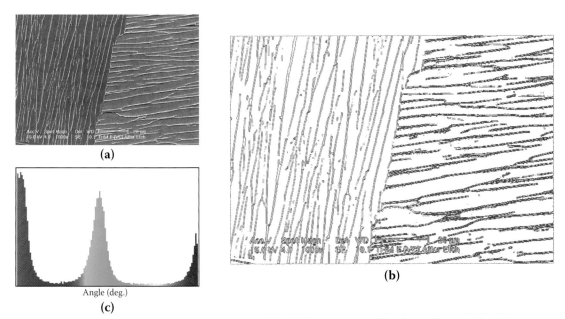

(a)

(b)

(c)

Angle (deg.)

Figure 5.38 *Lamellar structure in a titanium alloy: **(a)** SEM image; **(b)** edges color-coded with orientation and selected by magnitude of the Sobel gradient; **(c)** histogram of orientations from 0 to 180°. (Courtesy of H. Fraser, Ohio State University, Columbus.)*

the resulting binary image as a selection mask to eliminate pixels that are not of interest for orientation measurement, produces a result as shown in **Figure 5.38**.

Orientation determination using the angle calculated from the Sobel derivatives is not a perfectly isotropic or unbiased measure of boundary orientations because of the effects of the square-pixel grid and the limited number of points sampled. With a larger kernel of values, weights can be assigned to better correspond to how far away the pixels are from the center. With a 5- or 7-pixel-wide neighborhood, a more smoothly varying and isotropically uniform result can be obtained, and the effect of random noise in the image is minimized, although the line breadth becomes greater, as shown in **Figure 5.39**.

The use of an edge-enhancing operator to modify images is useful in many situations. We have already seen examples of sharpening using the Laplacian to increase the contrast at edges and make images appear sharper to the viewer. Gradient or edge-finding methods also do this,

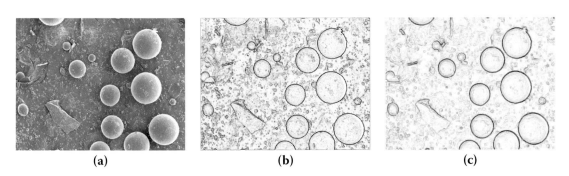

(a)   (b)   (c)

Figure 5.39 *Effect of neighborhood size on edge delineation: **(a)** original (SEM image of spherical particles); **(b)** 3-pixel-wide neighborhood; **(c)** 7-pixel-wide neighborhood.*

but they also modify the image so that its interpretation becomes somewhat different. Since this contrast increase is selective, it responds to local information in the image in a way that manipulating the brightness histogram cannot.

Performing derivative operations using kernels can be considered as a template-matching or convolution process. The pattern of weights in the kernel is a template that gives the maximum response when it matches the pattern of brightness values in the pixels of the image. The number of different kernels used for derivative calculations indicates that there is no single best definition of what constitutes a boundary. Also, it might be helpful at the same time to look for other patterns that are not representative of an edge.

These ideas are combined in the Frei and Chen (1977) algorithm, which applies a set of kernels to each point in the image. Each kernel extracts one kind of behavior in the image, only a few of which are indicative of the presence of an edge. For a 3 × 3-neighborhood region, the corresponding kernels, which are described as orthogonal or independent basis functions, are shown in Table 5.4.

Table 5.4 Kernels for a 3 × 3 Neighborhood Region

Kernel 0

1	1	1
1	1	1
1	1	1

Kernel 4

$\sqrt{2}$	-1	0
-1	0	1
0	1	$-\sqrt{2}$

Kernel 1

-1	$-\sqrt{2}$	-1
0	0	0
1	$\sqrt{2}$	1

Kernel 5

0	1	0
-1	0	1
0	-1	0

Kernel 2

-1	0	1
$-\sqrt{2}$	0	$\sqrt{2}$
-1	0	1

Kernel 6

-1	0	1
0	0	0
1	0	-1

Kernel 3

0	-1	$\sqrt{2}$
1	0	-1
$-\sqrt{2}$	1	0

Kernel 7

1	-2	1
-2	4	-2
1	-2	1

Kernel 8

-2	1	-2
1	4	1
-2	1	-2

Only kernels 1 and 2 are considered to indicate the presence of an edge. The results of applying each kernel to each pixel are therefore summed to produce a ratio of the results using kernels 1 and 2 to those for the other kernels. The cosine of the square root of this ratio is the vector projection of the information from the neighborhood in the direction of "edgeness," and this is assigned to the pixel location in the derived image.

The advantage, compared with more conventional edge detectors such as the Sobel, is sensitivity to a configuration of relative pixel values independent of the magnitude of the brightness, which can vary from place to place in the image. **Figure 5.40b** shows an example of the Frei and Chen operator, which can be compared with several other techniques.

All of the preceding edge-finding methods produce lines along edges that are broad, and only approximately locate the actual boundary. The Canny filter (Canny 1986; Olsson 1993) attempts to locate the edge to the most probable single-pixel location. It is based on finding the zero crossing of the derivative of the brightness. As shown in **Figure 5.40c**, this is attractive from the standpoint of locating the edge, but tends in many cases to break the line up into discontinuous pieces.

Figure 5.41 shows an example using a different method. The specimen is a polished aluminum metal examined in a light microscope The individual grains exhibit different brightnesses because their crystallographic lattices are randomly oriented in space so that the etching procedure used darkens some grains more than others. It is the grain boundaries that are usually important in studying metal structures, since the configuration of grain boundaries, the result of prior heat treatment and processing, controls many mechanical properties.

The human visual process detects the grain boundaries using its sensitivity to boundaries and edges. Most image-analysis systems use a gradient operation, such as a Sobel, to enhance the boundaries prior to measuring them. In the example in **Figure 5.41**, a statistical method has been employed instead. This is still a local neighborhood operation, but does not use a kernel of weights. The variance operator calculates the sum of squares of the brightness differences for the neighborhood of pixels surrounding each pixel in the original image (in the example, a circular neighborhood with a radius of 2.5 pixels). The variance value is small in uniform regions of the image and becomes large whenever a step is present. In this example, the dark lines (large magnitudes of the variance) are further processed by thinning to obtain the single-pixel lines that are superimposed on the original image. This thinning or ridge-finding method is discussed further below.

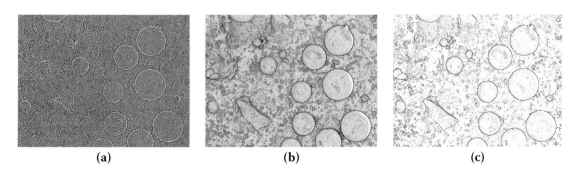

(a) (b) (c)

Figure 5.40 *Several neighborhood operators applied to the image from* ***Figure 5.39a****: (a) Laplacian; (b) Frei and Chen edge detector; (c) Canny edge detector.*

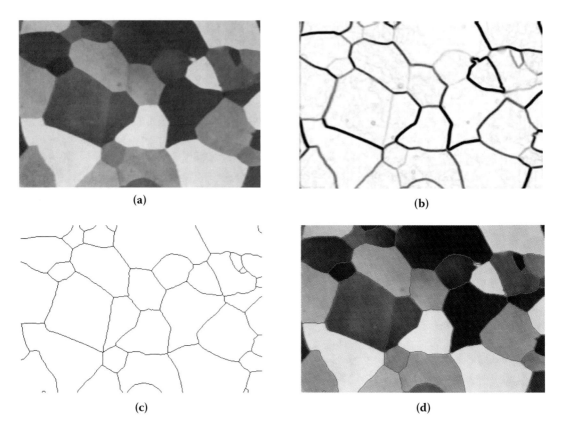

(a)

(b)

(c)

(d)

Figure 5.41 *Delineating boundaries between grains: (a) aluminum metal, polished and etched to show different grains (contrast arises from different crystallographic orientation of each grain, so that some boundaries have less contrast than others); (b) variance edge-finding algorithm applied to image **a**; (c) skeletonization (ridge finding) applied to image **b** (points not on a ridge are suppressed); (d) grain boundaries, produced by thresholding and skeletonization of the boundaries to a single line of pixels, shown superimposed on the original image.*

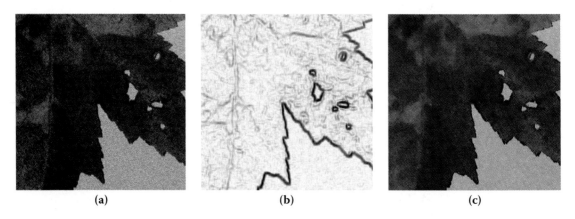

(a)

(b)

(c)

Figure 5.42 *Use of edge detection to control image processing: (a) original image fragment showing pixel noise; (b) edge image (Sobel operator), which is used as a mask; (c) result of smoothing the regions away from edges and sharpening the regions along the edge.*

There are several reasons for the interest in edge-finding operators. One is that the locations of the boundaries are useful for various measurement operations. A second is that the edges form a "primal sketch" of the scene, which can be useful for high-level software used in robotics that tries to "understand" a scene in terms of the geometry of the objects present. But an additional purpose is to facilitate further image processing. Image-sharpening operations, described previously, work by increasing the contrast at edges. But they also tend to increase the visibility of random noise in areas of the image away from the edge. By using a mask based on the result of an edge-locating operator to restrict the regions where the sharpening operator is applied, and conversely applying some smoothing in regions away from edges to reduce noise, the overall appearance of images can be improved (Kim and Allebach 2005; Kotera and Wang 2005).

This "trick" for improving the visual appearance of noisy images by sharpening just the edge detail has been popular for some time with digital photographers using programs like Photoshop that make it easy to limit the application of filters to arbitrary regions of an image. The mask, or alpha channel, uses the pixel value (0 to 255) to control the amount of application of the various filters. **Figure 5.42** shows an example. This is another example of an adaptive processing method that varies the application of filters (in this case, selects between several possibilities), depending on the local neighborhood around each pixel (Greenberg and Kogan 2005).

Rank operations

The neighborhood operations discussed in the preceding section use arithmetic operations (multiplication, addition) to combine the values of various pixels. Another class of operators that also use neighborhoods instead performs comparisons and ranking. Several of these operations are analogous to the previously described methods, but they use ranking rather than arithmetic.

In **Chapter 4**, the median filter was introduced. This sorts the pixels in a region into brightness order, finds the median value, and replaces the central pixel with that value. Used to remove noise from images, this operation eliminates extreme values from the image. Rank operations also include the maximum and minimum operators, which find the brightest or darkest pixels in each neighborhood and place that value into the central pixel. By loose analogy to the erosion and dilation operations on binary images, which are discussed in **Chapter 8**, these are sometimes called gray-scale erosion and dilation (Heijmans 1991). One effect of such ranking operations was demonstrated in **Chapter 4**, in the context of removing features from an image to produce a background for leveling.

Rank operators can be used to produce an edge-enhancement filter conceptually similar in some ways to a Sobel filter. The horizontal "derivative" is calculated as the difference between the median value of the right-hand column of pixels and that of the left-hand column in the neighborhood. A vertical derivative is obtained in the same way, and the edge strength is then computed as the square root of the sum of squares. This does not perform well on diagonal lines, so two more differences are calculated in the diagonal directions to determine another square root value, and the greater of the two is used. The method requires more computation than a traditional Sobel and does not generally produce superior results.

An even simpler rank-based filter uses the difference between the brightest and darkest pixel in the neighborhood, called the range operator. As shown in **Figure 5.43**, this difference is small within uniform regions and increases at edges and steps. It shares some similarities with the variance operator but generally does not perform as well. One of the important vari-

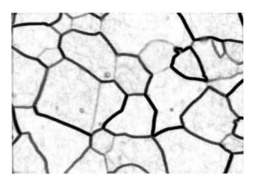

Figure 5.43 *Range operator applied to the image from* *Figure 5.41a*, *showing the difference between the brightest and darkest pixels in a circular neighborhood of radius 2.5 pixels.*

ables in the use of a rank operator is the size of the neighborhood. Generally, shapes that are squares (for convenience of computation) or approximations to a circle (to minimize directional effects) are used. As the size of the neighborhood is increased, however, the computational effort in performing the ranking increases rapidly. Also, these ranking operations cannot be easily programmed into specialized hardware, such as array processors.

Several uses of rank operators are appropriate for image enhancement and the selection of one portion of the information present in an image. For example, the top-hat operator (Bright and Steel 1986) was described in **Chapter 4** as a way to find and remove bright or dark noise. If we assume that the goal of the operator is to find dark points, then the algorithm compares the minimum brightness value in a small central region with the minimum brightness value in a surrounding annulus. If the difference between these two values exceeds some arbitrary threshold, then the value of the central pixel is retained. Otherwise it is removed. The logic can be inverted to find bright points.

The top-hat filter is basically a point or feature finder. The size of the feature is defined by the smaller of the two neighborhood regions, which can be as small as a single pixel in some cases. The larger region defines the local background, which the points of interest must exceed in brightness. The top-hat filter uses an inner and outer neighborhood, so it has some resemblance to a Laplacian or DoG operator. However, unlike the Laplacian, which subtracts the average value of the surrounding background from the central point, the top-hat method finds the extreme brightness in the larger surrounding region (the "brim" of the hat) and subtracts that from the extreme point in the interior region. If the difference exceeds some arbitrary threshold (the "height" of the hat's crown), then the central pixel is kept.

Figure 5.44 shows a case in which the small (and quite uniformly sized) dark features are gold particles in Golgi-stained muscle tissue. In this example, simply thresholding the dark particles does not work because other parts of the image are just as dark. A linear filter method (convolution) such as unsharp masking, accomplished in the example by subtracting the average value (using a Gaussian smoothing filter with a standard deviation of 0.6 pixels) from the original, produces an image in which the particles are quite visible to a human viewer but are still not distinguishable by thresholding. The top-hat filter isolates most of the particles (excluding a few that touch each other).

The top-hat filter is an example of a suppression operator. It removes pixels from the image if they do not meet some criteria of being "interesting" and leaves just those pixels that do. Another operator of this type, which locates lines rather than points, is variously known as ridge-finding or gray-scale skeletonization (by analogy to skeletonization of binary images, discussed in **Chapter 8**). We have already seen a number of edge-finding and gradient operators that produce bright or dark lines along boundaries. These lines are often wider than a single pixel, and it may be desirable to reduce them to a minimum width (Bertrand et al. 1997).

The ridge-finding algorithm suppresses pixels (by reducing their value to zero) if they are not part of the center ridge of the line. When the method is applied to any of the edge-finding gradient operations, it tends to reduce the image to a sketch, much like the Canny filter.

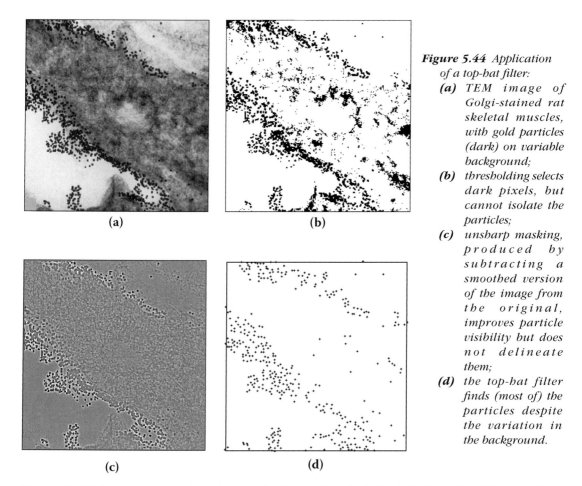

(a)   (b)

Figure 5.44 Application of a top-hat filter:
(a) *TEM image of Golgi-stained rat skeletal muscles, with gold particles (dark) on variable background;*
(b) *thresholding selects dark pixels, but cannot isolate the particles;*
(c) *unsharp masking, produced by subtracting a smoothed version of the image from the original, improves particle visibility but does not delineate them;*
(d) *the top-hat filter finds (most of) the particles despite the variation in the background.*

(c)   (d)

Figure 5.45 shows an example using a color image in which the Sobel gradient filter was first applied to the individual red, green, and blue channels, followed by ridge-finding.

Many structures (e.g., cells or grains) are best characterized by a continuous network, or tessellation, of boundaries. **Figure 5.46a** shows an example, a ceramic containing grains of two different compositions (the dark grains are alumina and the light ones zirconia). The grains are easily distinguishable by the viewer, but it is the grain boundaries that are important for measurement to characterize the structure, not just the boundaries between light and dark grains, but also those between light and light or dark and dark grains.

Figure 5.46 compares the application of various edge-finding operators to this image (all performed on a 3 × 3-neighborhood region). In this case, the variance produces the best boundary demarcation while minimizing extraneous marks due to the texture within the grains. Thresholding this image (as discussed in **Chapter 7**) and processing the binary image (as discussed in **Chapter 8**) to thin the lines to single-pixel width produces an image of only the boundaries, as shown in **Figure 5.47**. It is then possible to use the brightness of the pixels in the original image to classify each grain as either α or β. Images of only those boundaries lying between α and α, β and β, or α and β can then be obtained (and measured, as discussed in later chapters). It is also possible to count the number of neighbors around each grain and use a color or gray scale to code them, as shown in **Figure 5.48**. This goes beyond the usual scope of image processing, however, and into the realm of image measurement and analysis, which is taken up in **Chapter 10**.

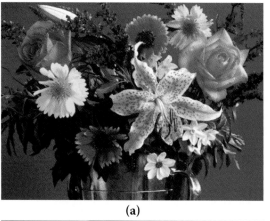

(a)

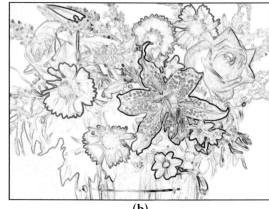

(b)

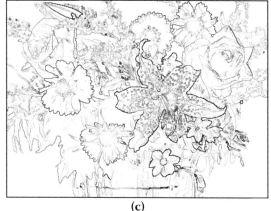

(c)

Figure 5.45 Thinning or ridge finding applied to a color image:
(a) original;
(b) Sobel gradient filter applied to the RGB channels;
(c) each color channel thinned by a ridge-finding suppression filter.

A range image, such as those from the atomic force microscope (AFM), the interference microscope, or from radar imaging, assigns each pixel a brightness value representing elevation. Rank operations are particularly well suited to such images and can often be used to locate boundaries. **Figure 5.49** shows an example, an AFM image of the topography of a deposited coating. Performing a gray-scale erosion (replacing each pixel with the brightest pixel in a 5-pixel-wide neighborhood) and subtracting from the original produces a set of lines along the boundaries. The tessellation of lines is useful for counting and measuring the individual structures in the coating.

For range images (particularly radar images used in surveillance), searching for a target pattern can be accomplished using a special class of adaptive operators. A top-hat filter of the right size and shape can be used for the task, but better performance can be achieved by adjusting the parameters of size and especially height according to the local pixel values (Verly and Delanoy 1993). For example, the threshold difference in brightness between the inner and outer regions could be made a percentage of the brightness rather than a fixed value. In principle, the more knowledge available about the characteristics of the target and of the imaging equipment, the better is the adaptive filter that can be made to find the features and separate them from background. In practice, these approaches seem to be little used and are perhaps too specific for general applications.

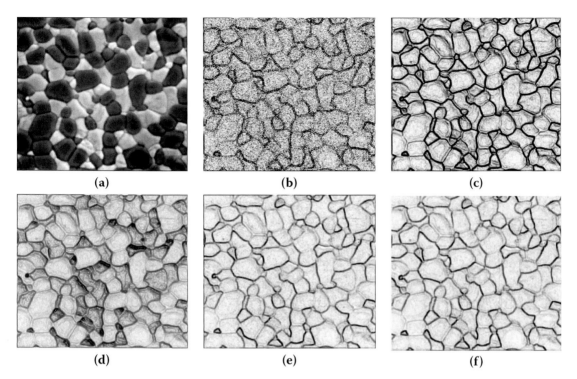

(a)   **(b)**   **(c)**

                (d)   **(e)**   **(f)**

Figure 5.46 *Locating boundaries: **(a)** original SEM image of thermally etched alumina-zirconia multiphase ceramic (the two phases are easily distinguished by brightness, but the boundaries between two light or two dark regions are not); **(b)** absolute value of the Laplacian; **(c)** Sobel gradient operator; **(d)** Frei and Chen edge operator; **(e)** variance operator; **(f)** range operator. (Courtesy of Dr. K. B. Alexander, Oak Ridge National Labs, Oak Ridge, TN.)*

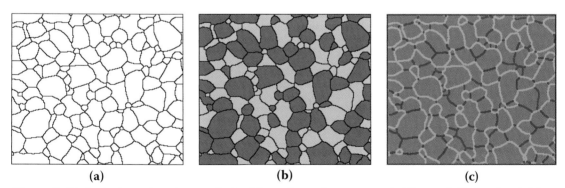

                (a)   **(b)**   **(c)**

Figure 5.47 *Grain-boundary images derived from the variance image in **Figure 5.46e** by thresholding and skeletonization: **(a)** boundaries between the grains; **(b)** grains coded to show phase identification: yellow = light (zirconia) grains, magenta = dark (alumina) grains; **(c)** boundaries color-coded by type: red = boundaries between two dark (alumina) grains, making up 16.2% of the total, blue = boundaries between two light (zirconia) grains, making up 15.2% of the total, green = boundaries between a light and dark grain, making up 68.6% of the total boundary.*

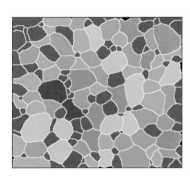

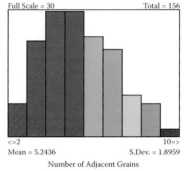

Figure 5.48 *The grains from Figure 5.47 color-coded to show the number of neighbors touching each, and a plot of the frequency of each number of neighbors. Further analysis shows that both the size and the number-of-neighbor plots are different for the two different phases.*

Full Scale = 30   Total = 156
<=2   10=>
Mean = 5.2436   S.Dev. = 1.8959
Number of Adjacent Grains

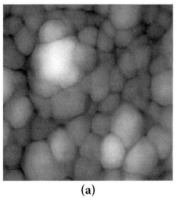

(a)

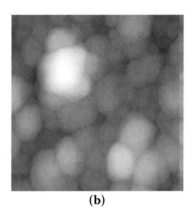

(b)

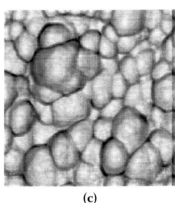

(c)

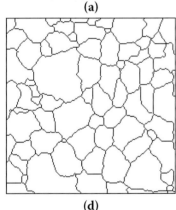

(d)

Figure 5.49 *AFM image of a deposited coating, showing a series of gently rounded bumps:*
(a) the original range image (gray scale proportional to elevation);
(b) use of a rank filter to replace each pixel with its brightest neighbor;
*(c) difference between images **b** and **c**, showing boundary delineation;*
*(d) thresholding and skeletonizing of image **c** to get boundary lines.*

Texture

Many images contain regions characterized not so much by a unique value of brightness or color, but by a variation in brightness that is often called texture. This is a somewhat loosely defined term that refers to the local variation in brightness from one pixel to the next or within a small region. If the brightness is interpreted as elevation in a representation of the image as a surface, then the texture is a measure of the surface roughness, another term with multiple meanings and measures.

Rank operations are one tool that can be used to detect this texture in images. The simplest of the texture operators is simply the range or difference between maximum and minimum brightness values in the neighborhood. For a flat or uniform region, the range is small. Larger values of the range correspond to surfaces with a larger roughness. The size of the neighborhood region must be large enough to include dark and light pixels, which generally means being larger than any small uniform details that may be present.

Figure 5.50 shows an example in which the original image has a histogram with a single broad peak and no ability to distinguish the visually smooth and textured regions based on brightness. The range image (using a 5-pixel-wide circular neighborhood) produces different brightness values that allow thresholding. The smooth regions (the curds in this microscope image of cheese) produce a low range value, while the highly textured protein produces a larger range value. The overall shading of the image is also removed by the filter. A second texture-extraction method, also shown in the figure, is the calculation of the statistical variance of the pixel values in a moving neighborhood (a 5-pixel-wide circular neighborhood), which

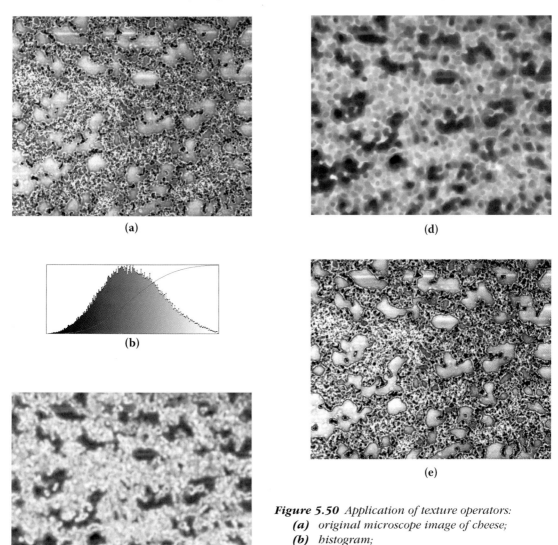

(a)

(d)

(b)

(c)

(e)

Figure 5.50 *Application of texture operators:*
(a) original microscope image of cheese;
(b) histogram;
(c) range operator applied;
(d) variance operator applied;
(e) region outlines from thresholding image ***d*** *superimposed on the original.*

can also distinguish the regions in this image. Note that both the range and variance operators were also used above with a smaller neighborhood size to locate edges.

Satellite images are often appropriate for characterization by texture operators. Various categories of land use (crops, construction, etc.) produce distinctive textures in these images that humans can recognize. Therefore, methods have been sought that duplicate this capability in software algorithms. In a classic paper on the subject, Haralick listed 14 such texture operators that utilize the pixels within a region and their brightness differences (Haralick et al. 1973; Haralick 1979; Weszka et al. 1976). The region used was not a neighborhood around each pixel; rather, the region comprised all of the pixels within a contiguous block delineated by some boundary or other identifying criterion such as brightness, etc. A table was constructed with the number of adjacent pixel pairs within the region as a function of their brightnesses. This pixel table was then used to calculate the texture parameters.

In **Equation 5.8** below, the array $P(i,j)$ contains the number of nearest-neighbor pixel pairs (in 90° directions only) whose brightnesses are i and j. R is a renormalizing constant equal to the total number of pixel pairs in the image or any rectangular portion used for the calculation. In principle, this can be extended to pixel pairs that are separated by a distance d and to pairs aligned in the 45° direction (whose separation distance is greater than the pixels in the 90° directions). The summations are carried out for all pixel pairs in the region. Haralick applied this to rectangular regions, but it is equally applicable to pixels within irregular outlines.

The first parameter shown is a measure of homogeneity using a second moment. Since the terms are squared, a few large differences will contribute more than many small ones. The second parameter is a difference moment, which is a measure of the contrast in the image. The third is a measure of the linear dependency of brightness in the image, obtained by correlation.

$$f_1 = \sum_{i=1}^{N} \sum_{j=1}^{N} \left(\frac{P(i,j)}{R} \right)^2$$

$$f_2 = \sum_{n=0}^{N-1} n^2 \left\{ \sum_{|i-j|=n} \left(\frac{P(i,j)}{R} \right) \right\}$$

$$f_3 = \frac{\sum_{i=1}^{N} \sum_{j=1}^{N} [i \cdot j \cdot P(i,j)/R] - \mu_x \cdot \mu_y}{\sigma_x \cdot \sigma_y}$$

(5.8)

In these expressions, N is the number of gray levels, and μ and σ are the mean and standard deviation, respectively, of the distributions of brightness values accumulated in the x and y directions. Additional parameters describe the variance, entropy, and information measure of the brightness value correlations. Haralick has shown that when applied to large rectangular areas in satellite photos, these parameters can distinguish water from grassland, different sandstones from each other, and woodland from marsh or urban regions, as well as the planting patterns for different crops.

When calculated within a small moving neighborhood centered on each pixel, the same calculated values can be scaled to create a derived image in which brightness differences represent textural variations. Applications in medical imaging (Zizzari 2004), microscopy, remote sensing, and others make use of these tools. In any given instance, it sometimes requires experimentation with several texture operators to find the one that gives the best separation between the features of interest and their surroundings, although the chosen operator may not apply the same logic as the human vision system does to perform the same discrimination. **Figure 5.51** illustrates the use of the Haralick angular second moment operator (f_2 above) applied in a moving neighborhood centered on each pixel to calculate a texture value, which is then assigned to the pixel. The figure also shows the entropy calculated in a circular neighborhood (radius = 3 pixels).

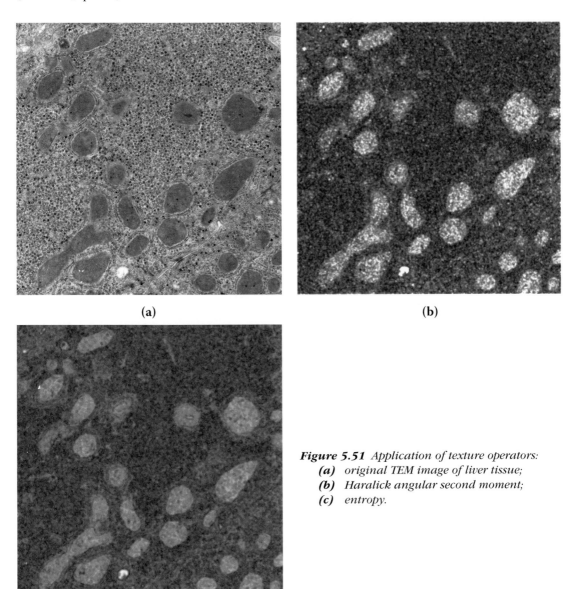

(a)

(b)

(c)

Figure 5.51 Application of texture operators:
  (a) original TEM image of liver tissue;
  (b) Haralick angular second moment;
  (c) entropy.

Fractal analysis

The characterization of surface roughness by a fractal dimension has been applied to fracture surfaces, wear and erosion, corrosion, etc. (Fahmy et al. 1991; Mandelbrot et al. 1984; Mecholsky and Passoja 1985; Mecholsky et al. 1986, 1989; Srinivasan et al. 1990; Underwood and Banerji 1986). It has also been shown (Peleg et al. 1984; Pentland 1983) that the brightness pattern in images of fractal surfaces is also mathematically a fractal and that this also holds for SEM images (Russ 1990a). A particularly efficient method for computing the fractal dimension of surfaces from elevation images is the Hurst coefficient, or rescaled range analysis (Feder 1988; Hurst et al. 1965; Russ 1990c). This procedure plots, on log-log axes, the greatest difference in brightness (or elevation, etc.) between points along a linear traverse of the image or surface as a function of the search distance. When the range is scaled by dividing by the standard deviation of the data, the slope of the resulting line is directly related to the fractal dimension of the profile.

Performing such an operation at the pixel level is interesting because it can permit local classification that can be of use for image segmentation. Processing an image so that each pixel value is converted to a new brightness scale indicating local roughness (in the sense of a Hurst coefficient) permits segmentation by simple brightness thresholding. It uses two-dimensional information on the brightness variation, compared with the one-dimensional comparison used in measuring brightness profiles.

Application of the operator proceeds by examining the pixels in the neighborhood around each pixel in the original image, out to a maximum radius typically in the range of 4 to 7 pixels (a total neighborhood diameter of 15 pixels, counting the central one). The brightest and darkest pixel values in each of the distance classes are found and their difference used to construct a Hurst plot. Performing a least-squares fit of the slope of the log (brightness difference) vs. log (distance) relationship characterizes the slope and intercept of the texture, and either value can be selected and scaled to fit the brightness range of the display. The procedure is time consuming compared with simple neighborhood operations such as smoothing, etc., but it is still well within the capability of typical desktop computer systems. **Figure 5.52** and **Figure 5.53** illustrate the results.

Implementation notes

Many of the techniques discussed in this chapter and in **Chapter 4** are neighborhood operators that access pixels in a small area around each central pixel, perform some calculation or comparison with those values, and then derive a new value for the central pixel. In all cases, this new value is used to produce a new image, and it is the original values of pixels that are used in the neighborhood around the next pixel as the operation is repeated throughout the image.

Most image-analysis systems, particularly those operating in desktop computers, have limited memory (particularly when the large size of images is considered). Creating a new image for every image processing operation is an

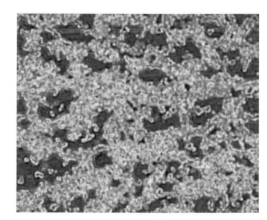

Figure 5.52 *Fractal texture operator applied to the image from **Figure 5.50a**. The intercept of the plot for pixels within a radius of 4 pixels is used to set the gray-scale value for each pixel.*

inefficient use of this limited resource. Consequently, the strategy generally used is to perform the operation "in place," i.e., to process one image and replace it with the result.

This requires only enough temporary memory to hold a few lines of the image. The operations are generally performed left to right along each scan line and top to bottom through the image. Duplicating the line that is being modified, and keeping copies of the preceding lines whose pixels are used, allows the new (modified) values to be written back to the original image memory. The number of lines is simply $(n + 1)/2$, where n is the neighborhood dimension (e.g., 3×3, 5×5, etc.). Usually, the time required to duplicate a line from the image is small, and by shuffling through a series of pointers, it is only necessary to copy each line once when the moving process reaches it, and then reuse the array for subsequent vertical positions.

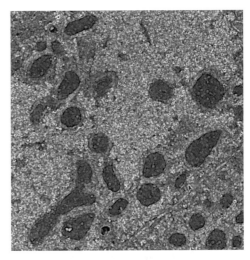

Figure 5.53 Fractal texture operator applied to the image from *Figure 5.51a*. The slope of the plot for pixels within a radius of 6 pixels is used to set the gray-scale value for each pixel.

Some of the previously described image processing methods create two or more intermediate results. For example, the Roberts' Cross or Sobel filters apply two directional derivatives whose magnitudes are subsequently combined. It is possible to do this pixel by pixel, so that no additional storage is required. However, in some implementations, particularly those that can be efficiently programmed into an array processor (which acts on an entire line through the image at one time), it is faster to obtain the intermediate results for each operator applied to each line and then combine them for the whole line. This requires only a small amount of additional storage for the intermediate results.

Another consideration in implementing neighborhood operations is how to best treat pixels near the edges of the image. The possibilities include having special neighborhood rules near edges to sort through a smaller set of pixels, duplicating rows of pixels at edges (i.e., assuming each edge is a mirror), extrapolating values beyond the edge, or using wraparound addressing (i.e., assuming that the left and right edges and the top and bottom edges of the image are contiguous). None of these methods is universally optimum.

Image math

The image processing operations discussed so far in this chapter operate on one image and produce a modified result that can be stored in the same image memory. Another class of operations uses two images to produce a new image (which may replace one of the originals). These operations are usually described as image arithmetic, since operators such as addition, subtraction, division, and multiplication are included. They are performed pixel by pixel, so that the sum of two images simply contains pixels whose brightness values are the sums of the corresponding pixels in the original images. There are also additional operators that, for example, compare two images to keep the brighter (or darker) pixel, obtain the absolute difference, or base the comparison on neighborhood values (for instance, keeping the pixel with the greater local variance as a means of combining images with different focus settings, or adding pixels in proportion to mean neighborhood values to blend images taken with different exposures). Other two-image operations, such as Boolean OR/AND logic, are generally applied to binary images; these will be discussed in that context in **Chapter 8**.

Actually, image addition has already been used in a method described previously. In **Chapter 4**, the averaging of images to reduce noise was discussed. The addition operation is straightforward, but a decision is required about how to deal with the result. If two 8-bit images (with brightness values from 0 to 255 at each pixel) are added together, the resulting value can range from 0 to 510. This exceeds the capacity of the image memory if single-byte integers are used. One possibility is simply to divide the result by 2, obtaining a resulting image that is correctly scaled to the 0 to 255 range. This is what is usually applied in image averaging, in which the *N* images added together produce a total, which is then divided by *N* to rescale the data.

Another possibility is to find the largest and smallest actual values in the sum image and then dynamically rescale the result to this maximum and minimum, so that each pixel is assigned a new value B = range × [(sum − minimum)/(maximum − minimum)], where range is the capacity of the image memory, typically 255. This is superior to performing the division by 2 and then subsequently performing a linear expansion of contrast, as discussed in **Chapter 4**, because the precision of the resulting values is higher. When the integer division by 2 is performed, fractional values are truncated and some information may be lost.

On the other hand, when dynamic ranging or automatic scaling is performed, it becomes more difficult to perform direct comparison of images after processing, since the brightness scales may not be the same. In addition, autoscaling takes longer, since two complete passes through the image are required: one to determine the maximum and minimum and one to apply the autoscaling calculation. Many of the images printed in this book have been autoscaled to maximize printed contrast. In most cases this operation has been performed as part of the processing operation to maintain precision.

Adding images together superimposes information and can, in some cases, be useful in creating composites that help to communicate complex spatial relationships. We have already seen that adding the Laplacian or a derivative image to the original can help provide some spatial guidelines to interpret the information from the filter. Usually, this kind of addition is handled directly in the processing by changing the central value of the kernel. For the Laplacian, this modification is called a sharpening filter, as noted previously.

Subtracting images

Image subtraction is widely used and is more interesting than the addition operation. In **Chapter 4**, subtraction was used to level images by removing background. This chapter has already mentioned uses of subtraction, such as that employed in unsharp masking, where the smoothed image is subtracted, pixel by pixel, from the original. In such an operation, the possible range of values for images whose initial range is 0 to 255 becomes −255 to +255. The data can be rescaled to fit into a single byte, replacing the original image, by dividing by 2 and adding 128, or the same previously described autoscaling method for addition can be employed. The same advantages and penalties for fixed and flexible scaling are encountered.

In some cases, the absolute difference may be preferred to simple subtraction of a background. **Figure 5.54** shows a phase-contrast image of cells on a slide. Images such as this, in which features have pronounced bright and dark shadows on opposite sides, are very difficult to measure because there are different criteria to define an edge on the two sides, and the edges on the top and bottom are not revealed at all but are inferred by the viewer. Using a large

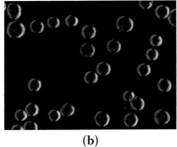
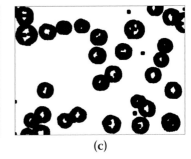

(a) (b) (c)

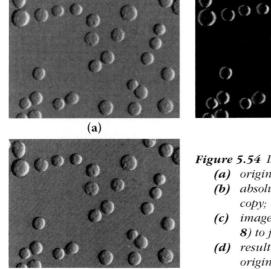

Figure 5.54 Isolating features in a phase contrast image:
- **(a)** original image;
- **(b)** absolute difference between original and a median-filtered copy;
- **(c)** image **b** thresholded and dilated (as discussed in **Chapter 8**) to join left and right shadows;
- **(d)** resulting boundaries after erosion, superimposed on the original image.

(d)

median filter to remove the shadows produces a "background" image without the features. The absolute difference between this and the original shows both shadows as bright. Thresholding this image produces two disconnected arcs, but dilation of the binary image (discussed in **Chapter 8**) merges the two sides. After filling and eroding this back to the original size, the outlines of the cells are adequately delineated for useful measurement.

Subtraction is primarily a way to discover differences between images. **Figure 5.55** shows two images of coins and their difference. The parts of the picture that are essentially unchanged in the two images cancel out and appear as a uniform medium gray except for minor variations due to the precision of digitization, changes in illumination, etc. The coin that has been moved between the two image acquisitions is clearly shown. The dark image shows where the feature was; the bright one shows where it has gone.

Subtracting one image from another effectively removes from the difference image all features that do not change while highlighting those that do. If the lighting and geometry of view is consistent, the only differences in pixel values where no changes occur are statistical variations in the brightness due to camera or electronic noise. The bright and dark images show features that have been removed from or added to the field of view, respectively.

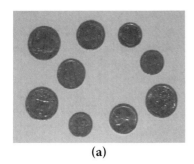
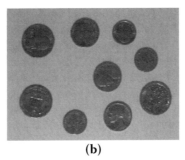
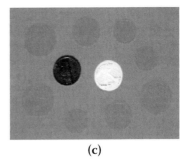

(a) (b) (c)

Figure 5.55 Showing image differences by subtraction: **(a)** original image; **(b)** image after moving one coin, **(c)** difference image after pixel by pixel subtraction.

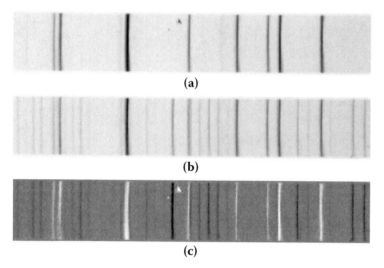

(a)

(b)

(c)

Figure 5.56 Image subtraction to enhance the visibility of details:

(a and b) scanned images of films from a Debye Scherer X-ray camera, taken with similar compounds;

(c) the difference between image *b* and image *a* showing the low intensity lines present in one film due to the presence of trace compounds in the sample.

Even in the presence of some noise, subtraction of two images can be an effective way to identify small differences that might otherwise escape notice. **Figure 5.56** shows an example. The image shows two films from a Debye-Scherer X-ray camera. The vertical lines show the exposure of the film by X-rays that were diffracted from a tiny sample, with each line corresponding to reflection from one plane of atoms in the structure of the material. Comparing the films from these similar samples shows that most of the lines are similar in position and intensity, demonstrating that the two samples are in fact quite similar in composition. The presence of trace quantities of impurities is revealed by additional faint lines in the image. Subtraction of one set of lines from the second increases the relative amount of noise, but it also reveals the presence of lines from the trace compounds as well as the difference in intensity of the lines that match. These can then be measured and used for identification.

A major use of image subtraction is quality control. A master image is acquired and stored that shows the correct placement of parts on circuit boards (**Figure 5.57**), the alignment of labels on packaging, etc. When the image is subtracted from a series of images acquired from subsequent objects, the differences are strongly highlighted, revealing errors in production.

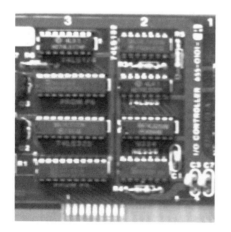 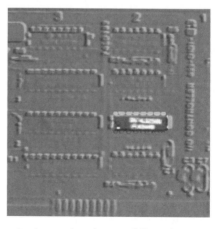

Figure 5.57 Difference images for quality control. A master image is subtracted from images of each subsequent part. In this example, the missing chip in a printed circuit board is evident in the difference image.

This subtraction is often carried out at video frame rates using dedicated hardware. Since it is unrealistic to expect parts to be exactly aligned, a tolerance can be specified by the area of bright and dark (mismatched) pixels present after the subtraction.

The same technique is used in reconnaissance photos to watch for the appearance or disappearance of targets in a complex scene. Image warping, as discussed in **Chapter 4**, may be required to align images taken from different points of view before the subtraction can be performed. A similar method is used in astronomy. "Blinking" images taken of the same area of the sky at different times is the traditional way to search for moving planets or asteroids. This technique alternately presents each image to a human viewer, who notices the apparent motion of the point of light that is different in the two images while ignoring the stationary stars. Some applications of computer searching based on subtraction have been used, but for dim objects in the presence of background noise, this has not proved to be as sensitive as a human observer.

In the example shown in **Figure 4.7** of **Chapter 4**, two images were acquired a little more than 1 minute apart. The difference between the two clearly shows the motion of the minute hand. The very small motion of the hour hand is also shown, which would be much too small to be noticed by viewing the images side by side.

Object motion can be measured using subtraction if the features are large enough and if the sequential images are acquired fast enough so that they overlap in successive frames. In this case, the subtraction shows a bright area of mismatch that can be measured. The length of the unmatched region divided by the elapsed time gives the velocity; direction can be determined by the orientation of the region. This technique is used at microscopic scales to track the motion of cells on slides in response to chemical cues and at macroscopic scales in animal studies to track motion within a cage or pen. (In the latter case, applying unique color tags to each animal makes it easier to keep track of individuals.)

At the other extreme, subtraction is used to track ice floes in the North Atlantic from satellite photos. For motion between two successive images that is too great for this method, it may be possible to identify the same objects in successive images based on size, shape, etc., and thus track motion. Or, one can assume that where paths cross, the points causing the least deviation of the path give the correct match (**Figure 5.58**). However, the direct subtraction technique is much simpler and more direct.

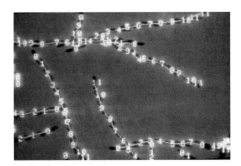

Multiplication and division

Image multiplication is perhaps the least used of the mathematics modes, but it is generally included for the sake of completeness in systems offering the other arithmetic operations. Multiplication can be used to superimpose one image on another, for example to add texture to a surface (often called "bump mapping"). Similar multiplicative superimposition can be used to add fluorescence or other emission images to a reflection or transmission image.

Figure 5.58 *Analysis of motion of multiple objects. Where the paths of the swimming microorganisms cross, they are sorted out by assuming that the path continues in a nearly straight direction. (From Gualtieri, P. and Coltelli, P., J. Computer Assisted Microsc. 3. 15–22. With permission.)*

One of the difficulties with multiplication is the extreme range of values that can be generated. With 8-bit images whose pixels can have a range between 0 and 255, the possible products can range from 0 to more than 65,000. This is a 2-byte product, only the high byte of which can be stored back into the same image memory unless automatic scaling is used. The values in the resulting image can suffer a significant loss of precision.

The magnitude of the numbers also creates problems with division. First, division by 0 must be avoided. This is usually done by adding 1 to all brightness values, so that the values are interpreted as 1 to 256 instead of 0 to 255. Then it is necessary to multiply each pixel in the numerator by some factor that produces quotients covering the 0 to 255 range while maintaining some useful precision for the ends of the range. Automatic scaling is particularly useful for these situations, but it cannot be used in applications requiring comparison of results with each other or with a calibration curve.

An example of division in which automatic scaling is useful is the removal of background (as discussed in **Chapter 4**) when linear detectors or cameras are used. An example of division when absolute values are required is the calculation of ratios of brightness from two or more *Landsat* bands (an example is shown in **Chapter 1**) or two or more filter images when examining fluorescent probes in a light microscope. In fluorescence microscopy, the time variation of emitted light intensity is normalized by alternately collecting images through two or more filters at different wavelengths above and below the line of interest, and then calibrating the ratio against the activity of the element(s) of interest. In satellite imagery, ratios of intensities (particularly from the Landsat Thematic Mapper satellite: band 4 = 0.5 to 0.6 µm, band 5 = 0.6 to 0.7 µm, band 6 = 0.7 to 0.8 µm, and band 7 = 0.8 to 1.1 µm) are used for terrain classification and the identification of some rock types. The thermal inertia of different rock formations can also be determined by ratioing images obtained at different local times of day, as the formations heat or cool.

As an example of mineral identification, silicates exhibit a wavelength shift in the absorption band with composition. Granites, diorites, gabbros, and olivine peridots have progressively decreasing silicon content. The absorption band shifts to progressively longer wavelengths in the 8- to 12-µm thermal infrared band as the bond-stretching vibrations between Si and O atoms in the silicate lattice change. The Landsat Thermal Infrared Multispectral Mapper satellite records six bands of image data in this range that are combined and normalized to locate the absorption band and identify rock formations. Carbonate rocks (dolomite and limestone) have a similar absorption response in the 6- to 8-µm range. At radar wavelengths, different surface roughnesses produce variations in reflected intensity in the Ka, X, and L bands, and these can be combined in the same ways to perform measurements and distinguish the coarseness of sands, gravels, cobbles, and boulders (Sabins 1987).

In the same way, bands of 0.55 to 0.68 µm (visible red) and 0.72 to 1.10 µm (reflected infrared) from multispectral satellite imagery are used to recognize vegetation. The first band records the chlorophyll absorption, and the second gives the reflection from the cell structure of the leaves. The ratio $(B_2 - B_1)/(B_2 + B_1)$ eliminates variations due to differences in solar elevation (illumination angle) and is used to measure the distribution of vegetation in images. Typically, this approach also combines data from successive scans to obtain the spectral vegetation index as a function of time. Other ratios have been used to image and to measure chlorophyll concentrations due to phytoplankton in the ocean (Sabins 1987). **Figure 5.59** shows a simplified approximation of this method using the ratio of near-infrared to blue wavelengths to isolate vegetation in satellite imagery.

Ratios are also used in astronomical images. **Figure 5.60** shows infrared images of the star-forming region in NGC-2024. Infrared light penetrates the dust that blocks much of the visible light. Ratios or differences of the different wavelength images show details in the dust and enhance the visibility of the young stars. This can be a useful supplement to the combination of channels for direct color viewing.

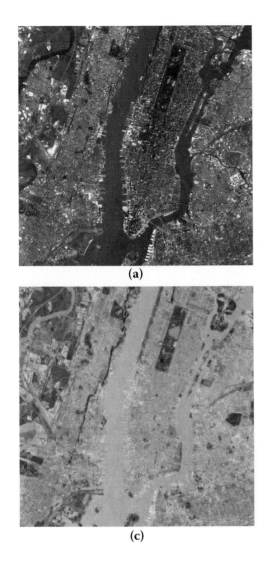

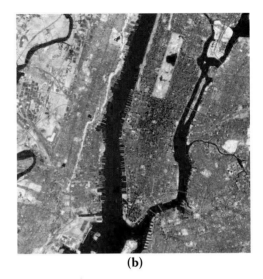

(a)

(b)

(c)

Figure 5.59 Landsat thematic mapper images of New York City:
- *(a)* Band 1 (visible blue);
- *(b)* Band 4 (near infrared);
- *(c)* ratio of Band 4 to Band 1 (showing vegetation areas).

Principal components analysis

When multiband images are acquired — whether the various visible and infrared channels detected in remote sensing or just the red, green, and blue channels of a typical digital camera — there is no reason to expect that any individual band will contain the most significant representation of the structure in the subject. This is particularly true when the individual channels contain other information, such as the various signals that can be acquired by an AFM or the multiple elements that can be detected by their X-ray emission in the SEM.

Principal components analysis (PCA) of multivariate data sets is a standard statistical method that was developed in the first half of the 20th century. An $N \times N$ (the number of channels) matrix is set up holding all of the covariance values between the channels. The eigenvectors of the matrix are the principal-components axes. This provides researchers with a method for transforming their source-data axes into a set of orthogonal principal axes. If each pixel's value is used as a coordinate to plot its location in the color space, the principal axis is fitted through the data so that it fits the greatest dispersion of values; then the second axis is orthogonal to it and fits the greatest remaining dispersion, and so on. For a three-channel image, transforming to a principal

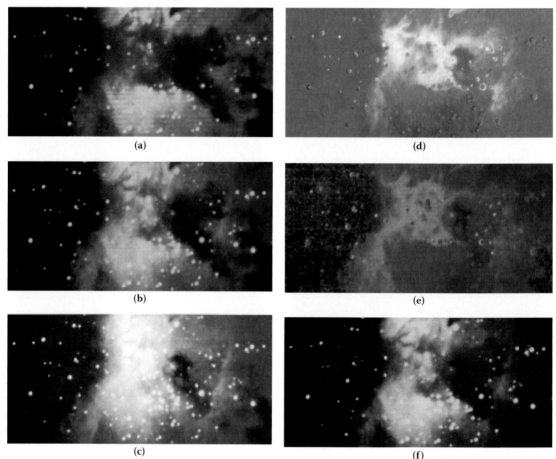

(a)   (d)

(b)   (e)

(c)   (f)

Figure 5.60 *Combining views of NGC-2024 to show star forming regions and dust. **(a)** 1.2 μm infrared image; **(b)** 1.6 μm infrared image; **(c)** 2.2 μm infrared image; **(d)** 2.2 μm image minus 1.6 μm image; **(e)** 1.6 μm image divided by 1.2 μm image; **(f)** the original three channels combined as RGB color channels.*

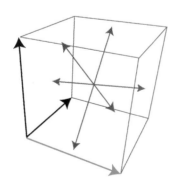

Figure 5.61 *Illustration of principal components axes (orange) within an RGB color space.*

components space (**Figure 5.61**) creates three new channels in which the first (most significant) contains the most structural contrast and information. The principle is the same when more channels are present, but the graph is harder to draw.

The rank for each axis in the principal set represents the significance of that axis as defined by the variance in the data along that axis. Thus, the first principal axis is the one with the greatest amount of scatter in the data and consequently the greatest amount of contrast and information, while the last principal axis represents the least amount of information. This technique is particularly useful for extracting the maximum contrast and structural information from a set of images, as well as finding correlations between the source variables and determining if any are degenerate or redundant in their contribution. Except for remote-sensing applications, the technique has not been widely applied to the field of imaging (Neal and Russ 2004).

Noise and image artifacts (including those from JPEG compression) are typically relegated to the least significant channel(s). Processing the least significant channel before transforming back to RGB can be used to remove image noise, as shown in **Figure 5.62**. In this example, a very noisy image from a consumer-grade pocket digital camera, taken by available dim light (but with brightly lit windows), shows considerable pixel noise. A conventional approach to such an image would be to apply noise reduction primarily to the blue channel, which typically contains more noise than the others, or to use a color median filter, as described in the previous chapter. A markedly superior result was obtained by transforming to principal components and applying a median filter to the least significant channel, then retransforming to RGB. In some instances, this method is also capable of removing JPEG artifacts and the residual pattern of the color filters (e.g., a Bayer pattern) used on the chip before color interpolation. This is, of course, a specialized technique that is rather time consuming for routine application.

It is often useful to examine the information that PCA produces about the source channels. X-ray maps produced by an SEM provide an example. Typically, more than three elements are of interest, both in terms of their distribution and their colocalization, since this gives information about the compounds or phases present. Further, while we can pick many combinations of three elements to display as RGB channels, we would like to be able to delineate all of the phase boundaries in a single image. By definition, the principal-components transform provides a way to do both of these things. **Figure 1.31** and **Figure 1.32** of **Chapter 1** showed

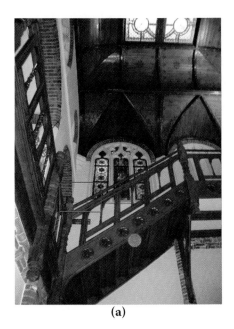

(a)

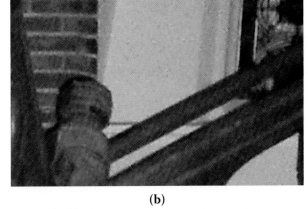

(b)

(c)

Figure 5.62 Noise reduction in PCA space:
- *(a)* original image with outline showing detail region;
- *(b)* detail of original noisy image;
- *(c)* after processing as described in text.

9 SEM X-ray maps, presented three at a time in the red, green, and blue channels of different images. The original individual channels are reproduced here as **Figure 5.63**. As explained previously, it is not possible to display more than three channels in unique colors. This limitation arises from the fact that human vision has three kinds of cones, and so displays use three kinds of phosphors (red, green, and blue); you cannot assign another color (e.g., yellow) to a fourth element because yellow will appear wherever the red and green elements are colocated. Principal-components analysis produces much more useful images by combining the basic elements to show structural and phase locations. **Figure 5.64** combines the three most significant channels to show the phase distribution. This was done by placing those three channels into the L*, a*, and b* channels of a color image, producing unique colors for each combination of elements.

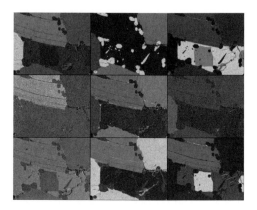

Figure 5.63 Nine individual elemental SEM X-ray maps from a Mica specimen (in order, Al, Ca, Fe, K, Mg, Na, O, Si, Ti).

The analysis of the principal-components data starts with the covariance matrix generated by the transform. The matrix in **Table 5.5** shows the result for the nine elements in these X-ray maps. Each row shows the significance of the principal channel (second column) and the contributions of each source channel to that principal vector. Notice that the three most significant channels, which were used to generate **Figure 5.65**, account for more than 83% of the information in the nine original images. The components of the source channels are a function of the phase composition. This numerical data can be visualized using colocalization plots. Plotting nine-dimensional space is difficult, but the projection of this space onto any pair of axes shows

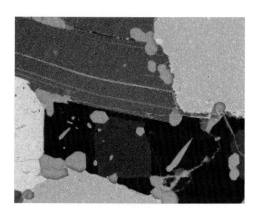

*Figure 5.64 Combining the three most significant channels from the nine channels in **Figure 5.63** to produce a color display showing the phase distribution (compare to **Figure 1.32** in **Chapter 1**).*

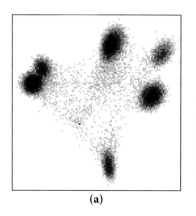

(a)

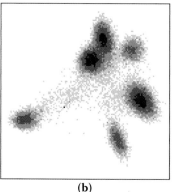

(b)

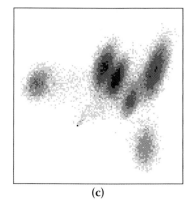

(c)

*Figure 5.65 Selected colocalization plots for the PCA results: **(a)** Channel 1 vs. Channel 2; **(b)** Channel 2 vs. Channel 3; **(c)** Channel 2 vs. Channel 5.*

Table 5.5. Principal Components Analysis of Mica Images for Nine Elements

Original Channel

PCA Channel	Significance (%)	Al	Ca	Fe	K	Mg	Na	O	Si	Ti
1	49.46	0.2355	0.2220	−0.6026	0.0382	0.2542	0.1113	−0.0576	0.6330	−0.2228
2	20.92	0.3970	−0.6890	0.0469	0.4005	0.1582	0.0778	0.2075	0.1687	0.3202
3	12.86	0.0696	−0.1735	0.5571	-0.2819	0.0398	0.0488	0.2768	0.3730	−0.5963
4	7.08	−0.3950	−0.1648	0.0958	−0.5195	0.2579	−0.0264	−0.1497	0.4030	0.5346
5	4.77	−0.5419	0.0872	0.1360	0.5372	0.5940	−0.1062	0.0736	0.0025	−0.1489
6	2.21	0.1996	0.6134	0.3236	0.1417	−0.0364	0.1429	0.4673	0.1924	0.4267
7	1.33	−0.1258	0.0303	0.2784	0.4181	−0.4934	−0.0253	−0.5417	0.4388	0.0271
8	0.79	0.4676	0.1694	0.3360	−0.0694	0.4913	0.1527	−0.5807	−0.1812	0.0144
9	0.57	−0.2411	−0.0733	−0.0388	0.0236	−0.0572	0.9606	−0.0116	−0.0829	−0.0366

the frequency with which various combinations of those values occur as a gray-scale intensity. Dark clusters of points correspond to regions in the original image with characteristic values of the original data. The six clusters shown in the colocalization plots in **Figure 5.65** represent the phases present in the sample. These correspond to the six various colored regions in **Figure 5.64**.

There are many other common applications for which multispectral images are useful. For biological samples, the use of different excitation wavelengths for various stains and dyes produces multiple source channels suitable for PCA. In addition, many of the most effective stains do not produce as much color contrast as desired for visualization or for subsequent thresholding and measurement. To make effective use of PCA techniques, the selection of specimen preparation and imaging techniques should be broadened to include as wide a variety of stains, wavelengths, bright and darkfield illumination, and other conditions as possible. The principal-components transform will, by definition, maximize contrast in the most significant channels.

Even with conventional RGB images, use of the principal components to maximize contrast can make processing and measuring samples with difficult or complex staining more tractable. In **Figure 5.66**, the original image shows a stained intestinal tissue sample. The brown background is a common effect of many stains, but this makes thresholding the structure difficult, since brown contains red, green, and blue. Applying a principal-components transform to the image produces an increase in contrast, as shown in the figure. Assigning the resulting channels to red, green, and blue produces a color image in which the boundaries of the cells are distinct from the background and the internal structure of the cell is distinct, making thresholding an easier task. Compare this result with **Figure 1.52** in **Chapter 1**, where the hue values of the pixels were used to construct an image.

One of the most difficult problems in measurement of stained tissue arises when the stain produces only subtle differences in saturation or brightness and very little color variation. Transforming to another color space, such as L*a*b* or HSI, does not produce enough contrast or variation to threshold the different structures. Even visualization is difficult. By using a principal-components transform and assigning the most significant channels to the red, green, and blue channels for display (**Figure 5.67**), the structure is revealed clearly and measurements can be made.

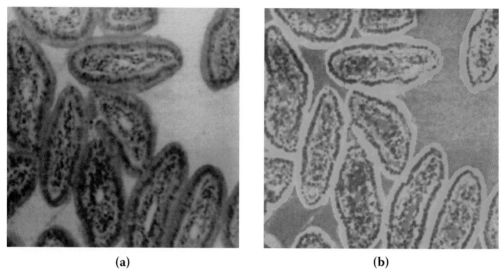

(a)   (b)

Figure 5.66 Maximizing contrast using PCA: (a) original (light micrograph of stained mouse intestine); (b) principal components channels displayed as RGB.

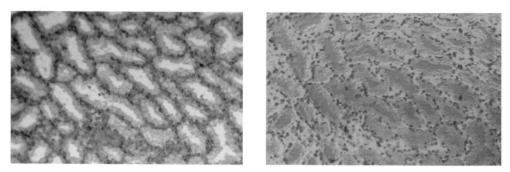

Figure 5.67 Maximizing contrast using PCA: (a) original (light micrograph of stained tissue); (b) principal components channels displayed as RGB.

Other image combinations

Image math also includes the logical comparison of pixel values. For instance, two (or more) images can be combined by keeping the brighter (or darker) of the corresponding pixels at each location. One example arises in polarized light microscopy, as shown in **Figure 5.68**. The use of polarizer and analyzer with specimens such as mineral thin sections produces images in which some grains are colored and others dark, a function of analyzer rotation. Combining images from several orientations and keeping just the brightest value for each pixel produces an image that shows all of the grains. The same technique can be used with transmission electron microscope (TEM) images of thin metal foils, where it is applied to combine images in which some grains are darkened due to electron diffraction effects, or to remove dark contours that result from bending of the foil. Macroscopic images of rough objects with lighting from several sides can be similarly combined.

The same logic is used to build up a confocal scanning light microscope (CSLM) image with great depth of field. Normal light-microscope images have limited depth of field because of the high numerical aperture of the lenses. In the CSLM, the scanning light beam and aperture on

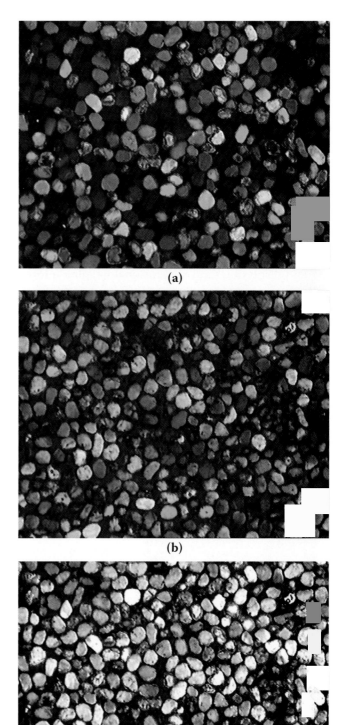

(a)

(b)

(c)

Figure 5.68

(a, b) Thin section of sandstone viewed by polarized light:

(c) different orientations of the analyzer; maximum-brightness image from six rotations.

the detector reduce this depth of field even more by eliminating light scattered from any point except the single point illuminated in the plane of focus.

A single, two-dimensional image is formed by scanning the light over the sample (or, equivalently, by moving the sample itself with the light beam stationary). For a specimen with an irregular surface, this image is very dark, except at locations where the surface lies in the plane of focus. By moving the specimen vertically, many such planar images can be acquired. However, at each pixel location, the brightest value of light reflectance occurs at the in-focus point. Consequently, the images from many focal depths can be combined by keeping only the brightest value at each pixel location to form an image with an unlimited depth of field. **Figure 5.69** shows an example.

An additional effect can be produced by shifting each image slightly before performing the comparison and superposition. **Figure 5.70** shows an example. The 26 individual images, four of which are shown, are combined in this way to produce a perspective view of the surface. (This image was also shown in **Chapter 1**, **Figure 1.60**, as an example of one mode of collecting and displaying three-dimensional imaging information.)

Extended-focus image can also be produced with conventional optics. If a series of images is captured with planes of focus that cover the range of depth of the specimen, they can be combined by keeping at each pixel location the value from whichever image in the series is in best focus. **Figure 5.71** shows a simple example in which two images are used. It would be possible in this example to cut and paste to combine the in-focus regions of the two images, which are well separated, but in general we prefer to have an algorithmic way to select the best focus at each location in the series.

There are several ways to make this selection, all of which are local adaptations of the same algorithms used for automatic focusing of optics (discussed in **Chapter 1**) and typically look for maxima in the image contrast or some selection of high-frequency information as the criterion for focus (Boyde 2004; Forster et al. 2004). One rapid method that generally works well is to go through all of the images in the sequence, at each pixel location, using a small neighborhood to calculate the local variance in brightness. This statistical value rises sharply when the image is in focus, and allows selecting the pixel value that should be kept to build up an extended-focus image, as shown in **Figure 5.72**.

This procedure is easily adapted to use with the light microscope, which has fixed lenses and shifts the distance of the specimen from the objective lens to focus the image. That provides a series of images that are aligned and at the same magnification. With

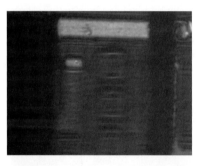

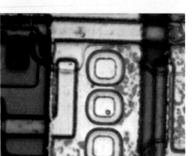

Figure 5.69 Combining CSLM images by keeping the brightest value at each pixel location. Images a shows one individual focal-plane image from a series of 25 on an integrated circuit. Only the portion of the surface that is in focus is bright. Since the in-focus point is brightest, combining all of the individual planes produces a result that shows the entire surface in focus.

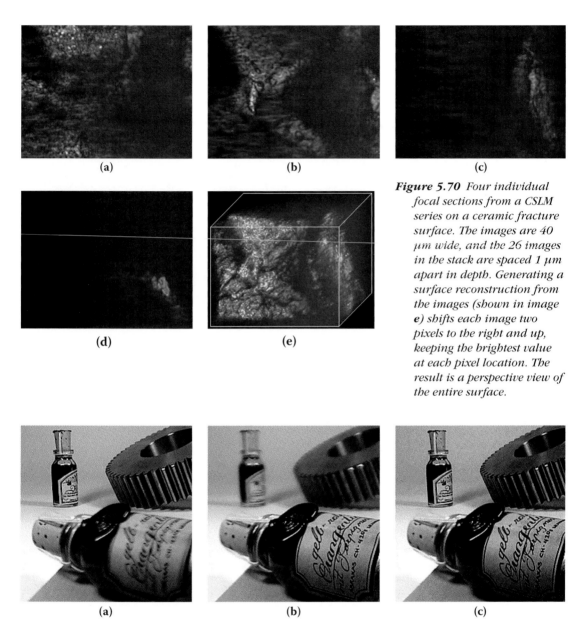

Figure 5.70 *Four individual focal sections from a CSLM series on a ceramic fracture surface. The images are 40 μm wide, and the 26 images in the stack are spaced 1 μm apart in depth. Generating a surface reconstruction from the images (shown in image e) shifts each image two pixels to the right and up, keeping the brightest value at each pixel location. The result is a perspective view of the entire surface.*

(a)　　　(b)　　　(c)

(d)　　　(e)

(a)　　　(b)　　　(c)

Figure 5.71 *Merging two images to obtain extended depth of field: (a, b) original images; (c) combined result.*

macroscopic imaging it is more difficult to acquire a proper sequence. The camera-to-subject geometry must be tightly controlled, and it is not proper to focus each image by adjusting the lens optics (which also changes the magnification). Instead, with a telephoto lens, the camera must be moved toward or away from the subject. However, when these conditions are met, it is possible to obtain depth of field limited only by the camera lens physically striking the subject, as shown in **Figure 5.73**.

Another situation that calls for merging multiple images of the same scene or subject arises with extreme levels of brightness. Depending on the well size of the camera sensor and the bit

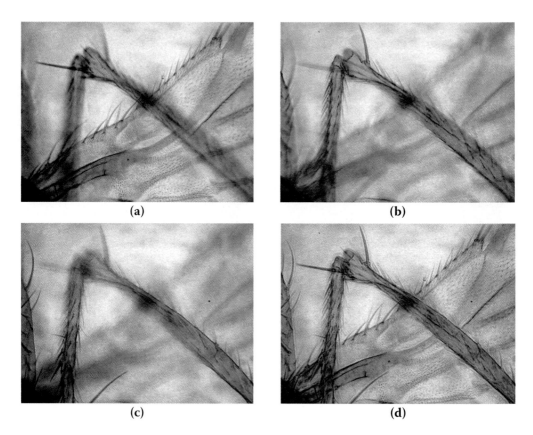

(a)   (b)

(c)   (d)

Figure 5.72 *Extended focus with microscope images:* (*a,b,c*) *individual focal planes showing a fly's wing and leg;* (*d*) *merged result using the maximum of local variance to select pixel values from each plane.*

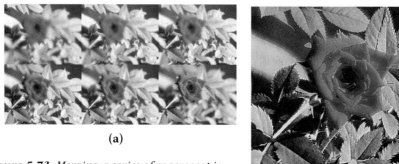

(a)

Figure 5.73 *Merging a series of macroscopic images to obtain extended depth of field:*
(*a*) *sequence of images obtained by shifting camera distance to subject;*
(*b*) *merged result.*

(b)

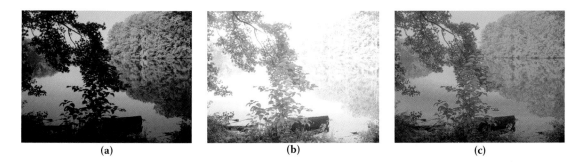

Figure 5.74 *Merging two images with different exposures: **(a, b)** originals; **(c)** merged result*

depth of the digitization, it may not be possible to capture the entire range of brightness in a scene in a single image. Film cameras are also limited in the maximum range of brightness that can be recorded. If the scene is static, acquiring two or more images with different exposure times may offer a solution. In the example of **Figure 5.74**, two such images are combined by examining the average brightness in a small neighborhood around each pixel location and then calculating a weighted average of the individual scenes so that values that are clipped to black or white are ignored, local contrast is maintained, and the overall scene appearance is preserved. This makes it possible to see detail in both the shadow area (which is completely black in one image) and in the bright areas (which are completely white or "blown out" in the other).

A further, but somewhat different problem arises with images that have a high range of contrast. Whether these are obtained by merging multiple images or by using a camera that can accommodate a high dynamic range, it can be difficult to display or print such images because of the limitations of the output devices. This limitation is more severe for hard-copy printing than for CRT and liquid-crystal displays (LCD), but neither can adequately handle the range of brightnesses that a human viewer can visually interpret in a scene. This has generated interest in finding ways to compress the overall brightness range of an image in such a way that local contrast is preserved and detail remains visible, as discussed and illustrated in **Chapter 3**.

Processing Images in Frequency Space

What frequency space is all about

It is unusual to pick up a book on image analysis without finding at least a portion of it devoted to a discussion of Fourier transforms (see especially Gonzalez and Wintz 1987; Jain 1989; Pratt 1991). In part, this is due to the utility of working in frequency space to perform certain image measurement and processing operations. Many of these same operations can be performed in the original (spatial or pixel domain) image only with significantly greater computational effort. Another reason for the lengthy sections on these methods is that the authors frequently come from a background in electrical engineering and signal processing and so are familiar with the mathematics and the use of these methods for other types of signals, particularly the one-dimensional (time varying) electrical signals that make up much of our modern electronics.

However, the typical image analyst interested in applying computer methods to images for purposes of enhancement or measurement may not be comfortable with the pages of mathematics (and intimidating notation) used in these discussions. Furthermore, he or she may not have the fortitude to relate these concepts to the operation of a dedicated image-analysis computer. Unable to see the connection between the topics discussed and the typical image problems encountered in real life, the potential user might therefore find it easier to skip the subject. This is a loss, because the use of frequency-space methods can offer benefits in many real-life applications, and it is not essential to deal deeply with the mathematics to arrive at a practical working knowledge of these techniques.

The Fourier transform and other frequency-space transforms are applied to two-dimensional images for many different reasons. Some of these have little to do with the purposes of enhancing visibility and selection of features or structures of interest for measurement. For instance, some of these transform methods are used as a means of image compression to reduce the amount of data in the original image for greater efficiency in transmittal or storage. In this type of application, it is necessary to reconstruct the image (bring it back from the frequency to the spatial domain) for viewing. It is desirable to be able to accomplish both the forward and reverse transform rapidly and with a minimum loss of image quality. Image quality is a somewhat elusive concept that certainly includes the alteration of brightness levels and color values, definition and location of feature boundaries, and introduction or removal of fine-scale texture in the image. Generally, the greater the degree of compression, the greater the loss of image fidelity, as shown in **Chapter 3**.

Speed is usually a less important concern to image measurement applications, since the acquisition and subsequent analysis of the images are likely to require some time anyway, but the computational advances (both in hardware and software or algorithms) made to accommodate the requirements of the data compression application help to shorten the time for some other processing operations as well. On the other hand, the amount of image degradation that can be tolerated by most visual uses of the compressed and restored images is far greater than is usually acceptable for image-analysis purposes. Consequently, the amount of image compression that can be achieved with minimal loss of fidelity is rather small.

Since in most cases the transmission of an image from the point of acquisition to the computer used for analysis is not a major concern, we will ignore this entire subject here and assume that the transform retains all of the data, even if this means that there is no compression at all. Indeed, most of these methods are free from any data loss. The transform encodes the image information completely and it can be exactly reconstructed, at least to within the arithmetic precision of the computer being used (which is generally better than the precision of the original image sensor or analog-to-digital converter).

Although there are many different types of image transforms that can be used, the best known (at least, the one with the most recognizable name) is the Fourier transform. This is due in part to the availability of a powerful, efficient algorithm for computing it, known as the fast Fourier transform (FFT) (Bracewell 1989; Cooley and Tukey 1965), which is described below. Although some programs actually perform the computation using the fast Hartley transform (FHT) (Bracewell 1984, 1986; Hartley 1942; Reeves 1990), the frequency space images are usually presented in the same form that the Fourier method would yield. For the sake of explanation, it is easiest to describe the better-known method.

The usual approach to developing the mathematical background of the Fourier transform begins with a one-dimensional waveform and then expands to two dimensions (an image). In principle, this can also be extended to three dimensions or more, although it becomes more difficult to visualize or display. Three-dimensional transforms between the spatial domain (now a volume image constructed of voxels instead of pixels) and the three-dimensional frequency space are used, for example, in some tomographic reconstructions.

The mathematical development that follows has been kept as brief as possible, but if you suffer from "integral-o-phobia," then it is permitted to skip this section and go on to the examples and discussion, returning here only when (and if) a deeper understanding is desired.

The Fourier transform

Using a fairly standard nomenclature and symbology, begin with a function $f(x)$, where x is a real variable representing either time or distance in one direction across an image. It is common to refer to this function as the spatial- or time-domain function and the transform F introduced below as the frequency-space function. The function f is a continuous and well-behaved function. Do not be disturbed by the fact that, in a digitized image, the values of x are not continuous but discrete (based on pixel spacing) and that the possible brightness values are quantized as well. These values are considered to sample the real or analog image that exists outside the computer.

Fourier's theorem states that it is possible to form any one-dimensional function $f(x)$ as a summation of a series of sine and cosine terms of increasing frequency. The Fourier transform of the function $f(x)$ is written $F(u)$ and describes the amount of each frequency term that must be added together to make $f(x)$. It can be written as

$$F(u) = \int_{-\infty}^{+\infty} f(x)e^{-2\pi iux}dx$$

(6.1)

where i is (as usual) $\sqrt{-1}$. The use of the exponential notation relies on the mathematical identity (Euler's formula)

$$e^{-2\pi iux} = \cos(2\pi ux) - i\sin(2\pi ux)$$

(6.2)

One of the very important characteristics of this transform is that, given $F(u)$, it is possible to recover the spatial-domain function $f(x)$ in the same way.

$$f(x) = \int_{-\infty}^{+\infty} F(u)e^{2\pi iux}du$$

(6.3)

These two equations together comprise the forward and reverse Fourier transform. The function $f(x)$ is generally a real function, such as a time-varying voltage or a spatially varying image brightness. However, the transform function $F(u)$ is generally complex, the sum of a real part R and an imaginary part I.

$$F(u) = R(u) + iI(u)$$

(6.4)

It is usually more convenient to express this in polar rather than Cartesian form

$$F(u) = |F(u)| \cdot e^{i\varphi(u)}$$

(6.5)

where $|F|$ is called the magnitude and φ is called the phase. The square of the magnitude $|F(u)|^2$ is commonly referred to as the power spectrum, or spectral density, of $f(x)$.

The integrals from minus to plus infinity can in practice be reduced to a summation of terms of increasing frequency, limited by the finite spacing of the sampled points in the image. The discrete Fourier transform is written as

$$F(u) = \frac{1}{N}\sum_{x=0}^{N-1} f(x) \cdot e^{-i2\pi ux/N}$$

(6.6)

where N depends on the number of sampled points along the function $f(x)$, which are assumed to be uniformly spaced. Again, the reverse transform is similar (but not identical; note the absence of the $1/N$ term and the change in sign for the exponent).

$$f(x) = \sum_{u=0}^{N-1} F(u) \cdot e^{i2\pi ux/N}$$

(6.7)

The values of u from 0 to $N-1$ represent the discrete frequency components added together to construct the function $f(x)$. As in the continuous case, $F(u)$ is complex and can be written as real and imaginary components or as magnitude and phase components.

The summation is normally performed over terms up to one-half the dimension of the image (in pixels), since it requires a minimum of two pixel brightness values to define the highest frequency present. This limit is described as the Nyquist frequency. Because the summation has half as many terms as the width of the original image, but with each term having a real and imaginary part, the total number of numeric values produced by the Fourier transform is the same as the number of pixels in the original image width (or the number of samples of a time-varying function), so there is no compression. Since the original pixel values are usually small integers (e.g., 1 byte for an 8-bit gray-scale image), while the values produced by the Fourier transform are floating-point numbers (and double-precision numbers in the best implementations), this actually represents an expansion in the storage requirements for the data.

In both the continuous and the discrete cases, a direct extension from one-dimensional functions to two- (or three-) dimensional ones can be made by substituting $f(x,y)$ for $f(x)$ and $F(u,v)$ for $F(u)$, and then performing the summation or integration over two (or three) variables instead of one. Since the dimensions x,y,z are orthogonal, so are the u,v,w dimensions. This means that the transformation can be performed separately in each direction. For a two-dimensional image, for example, it is possible to perform a one-dimensional transform on each horizontal line of the image, producing an intermediate result with complex values for each point. Then a second series of one-dimensional transforms can be performed on each vertical column, finally producing the desired two-dimensional transform.

The program fragment listed below shows how to compute the FFT of a function. It is written in Fortran, but can be translated into any other language (you may have to define a type to hold the complex numbers). Upon input to the subroutine, F is the array of values to be transformed (usually the imaginary part of these complex numbers will be 0) and LN is the power of 2 (up to 10 for the maximum 1024 in this implementation). The transform is returned in the same array F. The first loop reorders the input data; the second performs the successive doubling that is the heart of the FFT method; and the final loop normalizes the results.

```
SUBROUTINE FFT(F,LN)
COMPLEX F(1024),U,W,T,CMPLX
PI=3.14159265
N=2**LN
NV2=N/2
NM1=N-1
J=1
DO 3 I=1,NM1
        IF (I.GE.J) GOTO 1
        T=F(J)
```

```
                F(J)=F(I)
                F(I)=T
1               K=NV2
2               IF (K.GE.J) GOTO 3
                J=J-K
                K=K/2
                GOTO 2
3               J=J+K
        DO 5 L=1,LN
                LE=2**L
                LE1=LE/2
                U=(1.0,0.0)
                W=CMPLX(COS(PI/LE1),-SIN(PI/LE1))
                DO 5 J=1,LE1
                        DO 4 I=J,N,LE
                                IP=I+LE1
                                T=F(IP)*U
                                F(IP)=F(I)-T
4                               F(I)=F(I)+T
5                       U=U*W
        DO 6 I=1MN
6               F(I)=F(I)/FLOAT(N)
        RETURN
        END
```

Applying this one-dimensional transform to each row and then each column of a two-dimensional image is not the fastest way to perform the calculation, but it is by far the simplest and is actually used in many programs. A somewhat faster approach, known as a butterfly because it uses various sets of pairs of pixel values throughout the two-dimensional image, produces identical results (Johnson and Jain 1981). Storing an array of W values as predetermined constants can also provide a slight increase in speed. Many software math libraries include highly optimized FFT routines. Some of these allow for array sizes that are not an exact power of 2.

The resulting transform of the original image into frequency space has complex values at each pixel. This is difficult to display in any readily interpretable way. In most cases, the display is based on only the magnitude of the value, ignoring the phase. If the square of the magnitude is used, this is referred to as the image's power spectrum, since different frequencies are represented at different distances from the origin, different directions represent different orientations in the original image, and the power at each location shows how much of that frequency and orientation is present in the image. This display is particularly useful for isolating periodic structures or noise, which is discussed below. However, the power spectrum by itself cannot be used to restore the original image. The phase information is also needed, although it is rarely displayed and is usually difficult to interpret visually. Because the magnitude or power values usually cover a very large numeric range, most systems display the logarithm of the value instead, and that is the convention used here.

Fourier transforms of real functions

A common illustration in introductory-level math textbooks on the Fourier transform (which usually deal only with the one-dimensional case) is the quality of the fit to an arbitrary, but simple, function by the sum of a finite series of terms in the Fourier expansion. **Figure 6.1** shows the familiar case of a step function, illustrating the ability to add up a series of sine waves to produce the desired step. The coefficients in the Fourier series are the magnitudes of each increasing frequency needed to produce the fit. **Figure 6.2a** shows the result of adding together the first 4, 10, and 25 terms. Obviously, the greater the number of terms included, the better the fit (especially at the sharp edge). **Figure 6.2b** shows the same comparison for a ramp function. One of the important characteristics of the Fourier transform is that the first few terms include much of the information, and adding more terms progressively improves the quality of the fit.

Notice in both of these cases that the function is actually assumed to be repetitive or cyclical. The fit goes on past the right and left ends of the interval as though the function were end-lessly repeated in both directions. This is also the case in two dimensions; the image in the spatial domain is effectively one tile in an endlessly repeating pattern. If the right and left edges or the top and bottom edges of the image are different, this can produce very noticeable effects in the resulting transform. One solution is to embed the image in a larger one consisting

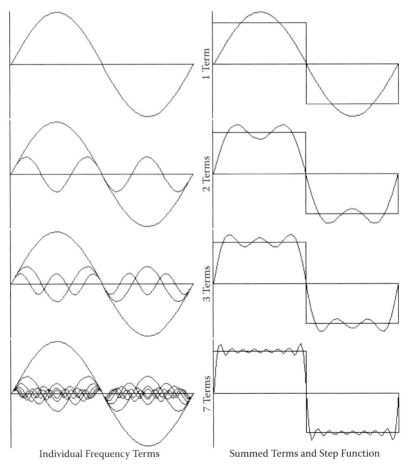

Individual Frequency Terms   Summed Terms and Step Function

Figure 6.1 *Summation of Fourier frequency terms to fit a simple step function.*

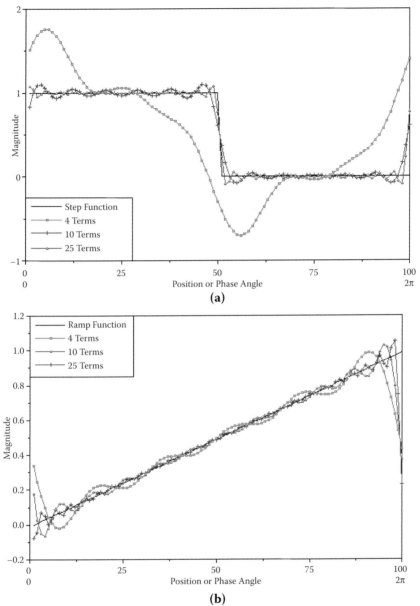

Figure 6.2 *Match between a step function **(a)** and a ramp function **(b)** and the first 4, 10, and 25 Fourier terms.*

of either zeroes or the average brightness value of the pixels. This "padding" allows applying the FFT procedure to images whose dimensions are not an exact power of 2 (64, 128, 256, 512, 1024, …) but makes the image up to twice as large in each direction, requiring four times as much storage and calculation. It is useful particularly when correlation is performed between images of different sizes, as discussed below.

The magnitudes of the Fourier coefficients from the transforms shown in **Figure 6.2** are plotted as amplitude vs. frequency (**Figure 6.3**). Notice that the step function consists only of odd terms, while the magnitudes for the ramp-function transform decrease smoothly, but for

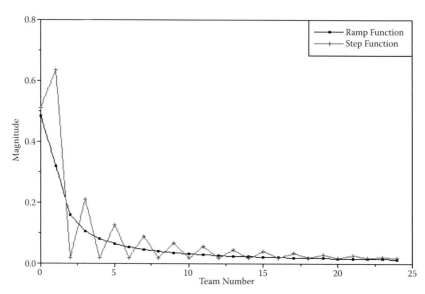

Figure 6.3 *Magnitude of the first 25 Fourier terms fit to the step and ramp in **Figure 6.2**.*

both functions the first few terms (the low frequencies) are large and the higher-order terms (the high frequencies) have smaller values. Rather than the magnitudes, it is somewhat more common to plot the power spectrum of the transform, and to plot it as a symmetric function extending to both sides of the origin (zero frequency, or the mean image brightness value. As noted above, the power is simply the square of the magnitude. Because the range of values can be very large, the power spectrum is usually plotted with a logarithmic or other compressed vertical scale to show the smaller terms usually present at high frequencies along with the lower-frequency terms.

Figure 6.4 reiterates the duality of the Fourier-transform process. The spatial and frequency domains show the information in very different ways, but the information is the same. Of course, the plot of amplitude or power in the frequency transform does not show the important phase information, but we understand that the values are actually complex. Shifting the spatial-domain image does not alter the amplitude values, but it does change the phase values for each sinusoidal component.

It is important to recall, in examining these transforms, that the axes represent frequency. The low-frequency terms provide the overall shape of the function, while the high-frequency terms are needed to sharpen edges and provide fine detail. The second point to be kept in mind is that these terms are independent of each other. (This is equivalent to the statement that the basis functions — the sinusoidal waves — are orthogonal.) Performing the transform to determine coefficients to higher and higher frequencies does not change the previous ones, and selecting any particular range of terms to reconstruct the function will do so to the greatest accuracy possible with those frequencies.

Proceeding to two dimensions, **Figure 6.5** shows four images of perfectly sinusoidal variations in brightness. The first three vary in spacing (frequency) and orientation; the fourth is the superposition of all three. For each, the two-dimensional frequency transform is particularly simple. Each of the pure tones has a transform consisting of a single point (identifying the frequency and orientation). Because of the redundancy of the plotting coordinates, the point is

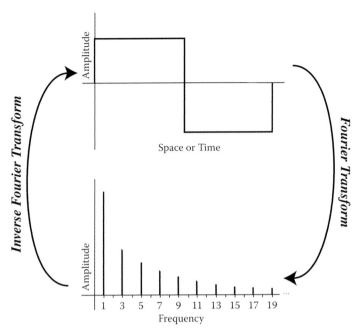

Figure 6.4 *Role of the forward and inverse transform and the spatial- and frequency-domain representations of a step function.*

shown in two symmetrical locations around the origin, which by convention lies at the center of the power-spectrum plot.

Two-dimensional power spectra are easiest to describe using polar coordinates. The frequency increases with radius ρ, and the orientation depends on the angle θ. **Figure 6.6** shows two images with the same shape in different orientations. The frequency transforms rotate with the feature. The power-spectrum display shows three lines of values that correspond to the series of sinusoids needed to specify each of the edges of the original (spatial domain) triangle.

It is common to display the two-dimensional transform with the frequencies plotted from the center of the image, which is consequently redundant. (The top and bottom or left and right halves are simply duplicates, with rotational symmetry about the origin.) In some cases, this

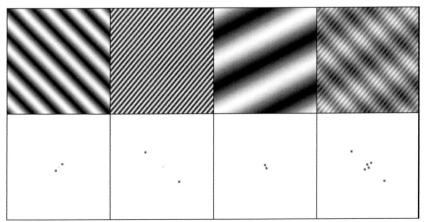

Figure 6.5 *Three sinusoidal patterns, their frequency transforms, and their sum.*

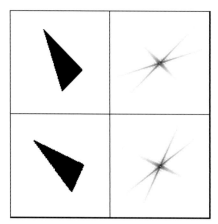

Figure 6.6 Rotation of a spatial-domain image (left) and the corresponding rotation of the frequency transform (right).

image is shifted so that the origin is at the corners of the image and the highest frequencies are in the center. One format can be converted to the other by swapping quadrants of the display. For the purposes of image processing (removing or selecting specific frequencies, etc.), the display with the origin centered is simplest to use and has been adopted here.

The power spectrum of the low-frequency (largest spacing) sinusoid has a point close to the origin, and the higher-frequency sinusoids have points farther away and in directions that identify the orientation of the lines. The value at the origin is called the DC level and simply represents the average brightness of the original image. The superposition of the three sinusoids in **Figure 6.5** produces an image whose frequency transform is simply the sum of the three individual transforms. This principle of additivity will be important for much of the discussion below. Subtracting the information from a location in the frequency transform is equivalent to removing the corresponding information from every part of the spatial-domain image.

Figure 6.7 shows a two-dimensional step consisting of a rectangle. The two-dimensional frequency transform of this image produces the same series of diminishing peaks in the x- and y-axis directions as the one-dimensional step function. The darkness of each point in the power-spectrum display represents the log of the square of the amplitude of the corresponding frequency. Limiting the reconstruction to only the central (low frequency) terms produces the reconstructions shown. Just as for the one-dimensional case, this limits the sharpness of the edge of the step and produces some ringing (oscillations near the edge) in the overall shape. The line profiles through the image show the same shape as previously discussed for the one-dimensional case.

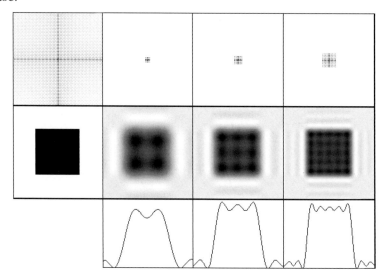

Figure 6.7 A two-dimensional step function and its frequency transform (left), and reconstructions with different numbers of terms (shown as a portion of the frequency transform). The bottom row shows horizontal line profiles through the center of the reconstructed spatial image.

Frequencies and orientations

It is helpful to develop a little familiarity with the power-spectrum display of the frequency-space transform of the image using simple images. In **Figure 6.8a**, the lines can be represented by a single peak because their brightness profile is perfectly sinusoidal; thus only a single frequency is present. If the line profile is different, for example more like a square wave than a sinusoid, more terms are needed to represent the shape, and consequently more peaks appear in the power spectrum at increasing frequencies. **Figure 6.8b** shows an example in which the frequency transform consists of a series of peaks at multiples of the lowest frequency, in the same orientation (perpendicular to the line angle).

In **Figure 6.8c**, the lines have the aliasing common in computer displays (and in halftone printing technology), in which the lines at a shallow angle on the display are constructed from a series of steps corresponding to the rows of display pixels. This further complicates the frequency transform, which now has additional peaks representing the horizontal and vertical steps in the image that correspond to the aliasing, in addition to the main line of peaks seen in the figure.

It is possible to select only the peaks along the main row and eliminate the others with a mask or filter, as will be discussed below. After all, the frequency-domain image can be modified just like any other image. If this is done and only the peaks in the main row are used for the inverse transformation (back to the spatial domain), the aliasing of the lines is removed. In fact, that is how the images in **Figure 6.8a** and **Figure 6.8b** were produced. This will lead naturally to the subject of filtering (discussed in a later section), or removing unwanted information from spatial-domain images by operating on the frequency transform. For example, it offers one practical technique to remove aliasing from lines and make them visually smooth.

The idealized examples shown in the preceding tutorial show that any periodic structure in the original spatial-domain image will be represented by a peak in the power-spectrum image at a radius corresponding to the spacing and a direction corresponding to the orientation. In a real image, which typically consists of mostly nonperiodic information, any such peaks will be superimposed on a broad and sometimes noisy background. However, finding the peaks is generally much easier than finding the original periodic structure. Also, measuring the peak locations accurately is much easier and more accurate than trying to extract the same information from the original image, because all of the occurrences are effectively averaged together in the frequency domain.

Figure 6.9 shows an example of this kind of peak location measurement. The spatial-domain image is a high-resolution TEM (transmission electron microscope) image of the lattice structure in pure silicon. The regular spacing of the bright spots represents the atomic structure of the lattice. Measuring all of the individual spacings of the spots would be very time consuming and not particularly accurate. The frequency-domain representation of this image shows the periodicity clearly. The series of peaks indicates that the variation of brightness is not a simple sine wave, but contains many higher harmonics. The first-order peak gives the basic atomic spacing (and orientation), which can be measured by interpolating the peak position to a fraction of a pixel width, corresponding to an accuracy for the atom spacing of a few parts in ten thousand. The spacing of the features that produce the point in the power spectrum is simply the width of the image (e.g., 256 pixels in the example, times whatever calibration applies) divided by the distance in pixels from the origin to the center of the peak in the power spectrum.

The figure also shows several other characteristic features found in many FFT power-spectrum displays. The dark vertical and horizontal lines correspond to the sequence of terms

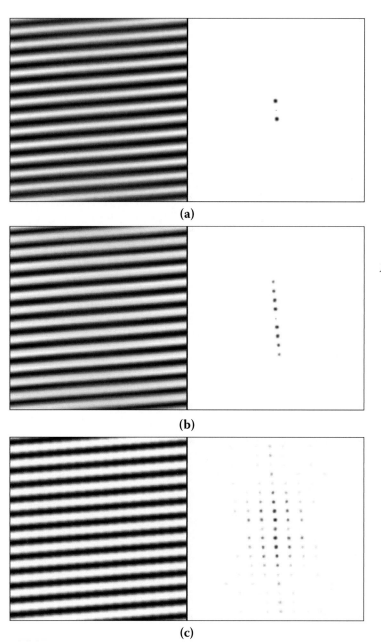

Figure 6.8 *A set of lines (left) and their frequency transform (right):* *(a)* *sinusoidal lines;* *(b)* *with a nonsinusoidal brightness profile;* *(c)* *the lines from image **b** with aliasing.*

needed because the left and right edges and the top and bottom edges of the image do not match. Recall that the mathematics of the Fourier transform assume that the functions being transformed are continuous, so that the image is repeated to the left and right and above and below the original. Also, notice that the power-spectrum display has a darker vertical band of values (larger amplitudes) in the center, with a rather abrupt drop in magnitude beyond about one-third of the radius. That is an indication that there is no information at high frequencies in the horizontal dimension, and reveals the limited resolution of the camera used to record the original image. As noted in **Chapter 1**, many cameras record images with more pixels than they can actually resolve, and as will be shown below, the Fourier transform can be used to measure actual image resolution.

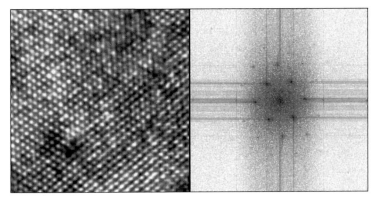

Figure 6.9 *High-resolution TEM image of atomic lattice in silicon (left), with the frequency transform (right). (Courtesy of Dr. S. Chevacharoenkul, Microelectronics Center of North Carolina, Research Triangle.)*

To the electron microscopist, the power-spectrum image of the frequency-domain transform looks just like an electron diffraction pattern, which in fact it is. The use of microscope optics to form the diffraction pattern is an analog method of computing the frequency-domain representation. This can be done with any image by setting up suitable optics. While it is a fast way to obtain the frequency-domain representation, this method has two serious drawbacks for use in image processing.

First, the phase information is lost when the diffraction pattern is recorded, so it is not possible to reconstruct the spatial-domain image from a photograph of the diffraction pattern. (Recording the entire diffraction pattern including the phase information results in a hologram, from which the original image *can* be reconstructed.) It is possible to perform the reconstruction from the diffraction pattern in the microscope by using suitable lenses (indeed, that is how the microscope functions), so in principle it is possible to insert the various masks and filters discussed below. However, making these masks and filters is difficult and exacting work that must usually be performed individually for each of the images to be enhanced. Consequently, it is much easier (and more controllable) to use a computer to perform the transform and to apply any desired masks.

It is also easier to perform measurements on the frequency-domain representation using the computer. Locating the centers of peaks by curve fitting would require recording the diffraction pattern (typically with film, which may introduce nonlinearities or saturation over the extremely wide dynamic range of many patterns), followed by digitization to obtain numerical values. Considering the speed with which a spatial-domain image can be recorded, the frequency transform calculated, and interactive or automatic measurement performed, the computer is generally the tool of choice. This analysis is made easier by the ability to manipulate the display contrast so that both brighter and dimmer spots can be seen, and to use image processing tools such as background leveling and a top-hat filter to isolate the peaks of interest.

When spots from a periodic structure are superimposed on a general background, the total power in the spots expressed as a fraction of the total power in the entire frequency transform gives a useful quantitative measure of the degree of periodicity in the structure. This can also be used to compare different periodicities (different spacings or orientations) by comparing summations of values in the power spectrum. For electron diffraction patterns, this is a function of the atomic density of various planes and the atomic scattering cross sections.

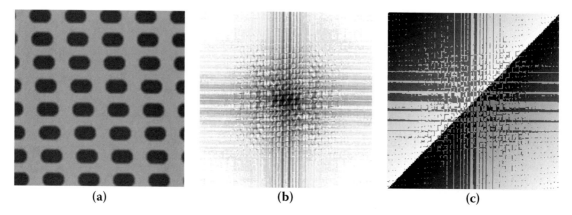

(a)   (b)   (c)

Figure 6.10 *Test image consisting of a regular pattern (a) with its frequency-transform power spectrum (b) and phase values (c).*

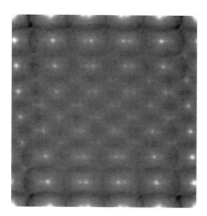

Figure 6.11 *Retransformation of Figure 6.10 with all phase information set to zero.*

While the display of the power spectrum corresponds to a diffraction pattern and is the most familiar presentation of frequency-space information, it must not be forgotten that the phase information is also needed to reconstruct the original image. **Figure 6.10** shows a test image, consisting of a regular pattern of spots, and its corresponding power spectrum and phase values. If the phase information is erased (all phases set to zero), the reconstruction (**Figure 6.11**) shows some of the same periodicity, but the objects are no longer recognizable. The various sine waves have been shifted in phase, so that the feature boundaries are not reconstructed.

The assumption that the image is one repetition of an endless sequence is also important. Most real images do not have perfectly matching left and right or top and bottom edges. This produces a large step function at the edge, which is more apparent if the image is shifted by an arbitrary offset (**Figure 6.12**). As noted previously, this does not alter the power-spectrum image, although the phase image is shifted. The discontinuity requires high-frequency terms to fit, and since the edges are precisely horizontal and vertical, the power-spectrum display shows vertical and horizontal lines superimposed on the rest of the data, which are visible in **Figure 6.10b**. For the test pattern, the result of eliminating these lines from the original frequency transform and then retransforming is shown in **Figure 6.13**. The central portion of the image is unaffected, but at the edges the discontinuity is no longer sharp because the many frequencies needed to create the step functions at the edges are missing. The pattern from each side has been reproduced crossing over to the other side of the boundary, superimposed on the correct data.

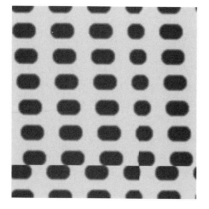

Figure 6.12 *The test image of Figure 6.10 with an arbitrary spatial shift, showing the discontinuities at the image boundaries.*

Preferred orientation

Figure 6.14 shows another example of a periodic structure, only much less perfect and larger in scale than the lattice images above. The specimen is a thin film of magnetic material viewed in polarized light. The stripes are oppositely oriented magnetic domains in the material that are used to store information in the film. The frequency transform of this image clearly shows the width and spacing of the domains. Instead of a single peak, there are arcs that show the variation in orientation of the stripes, which is evident in the original image but difficult to quantify.

The length of the arcs and the variation of brightness (power) with angle along them can be easily measured to characterize the preferred orientation in the structure. Even for structures that are not perfectly periodic, the integrated power as a function of angle can be used to measure the preferred orientation. This is identical to the results of autocorrelation operations carried out in the spatial domain, in which a binary image is shifted and combined with itself in all possible displacements to obtain a matrix of fractional values, but it is much faster to perform with the frequency-domain representation. Also, this makes it easier to deal with gray-scale values.

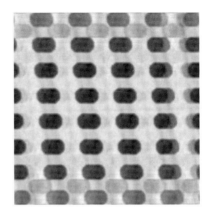

Figure 6.13 Retransformation of *Figure 6.10* with the central cross (horizontal and vertical lines) reduced to zero magnitude, so that the left and right edges of the image, and the top and bottom edges, are forced to match.

Reconstructing periodic structures that are not perfectly aligned can be performed by selecting the entire arc in the frequency transform. **Figure 6.15** illustrates this with a virus particle. The TEM image of the negatively stained virus hints at the internal helical structure, but does not show it clearly. In the frequency transform, the periodic spacing and the variation in direction is evident. The spacing can be determined (2.41 nm) by measuring the distance from the center to the arc, and the helix angle determined from the length of the arc. Retransforming only these arcs shows the periodicity, but this is not limited spatially to the virus particle. Using the spatial-domain image as a mask (as discussed in **Chapter 8**) makes the internal helical pattern evident.

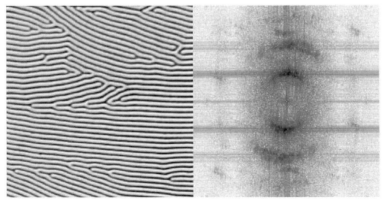

Figure 6.14 Polarized light image of magnetic domains in thin film material (left), with the frequency transform (right).

One particular type of preferred orientation in images, which arises not from the specimen but rather from the imaging system itself, is astigmatism. This is a particular problem with electron microscopes because of the operating principles of electromagnetic lenses. Even skilled operators devote considerable time to making adjustments to minimize astigmatism, and it is often very difficult to recognize it in images in order to correct it. Astigmatism results in the defocusing of the image and a consequent loss of sharpness in one direction, sometimes

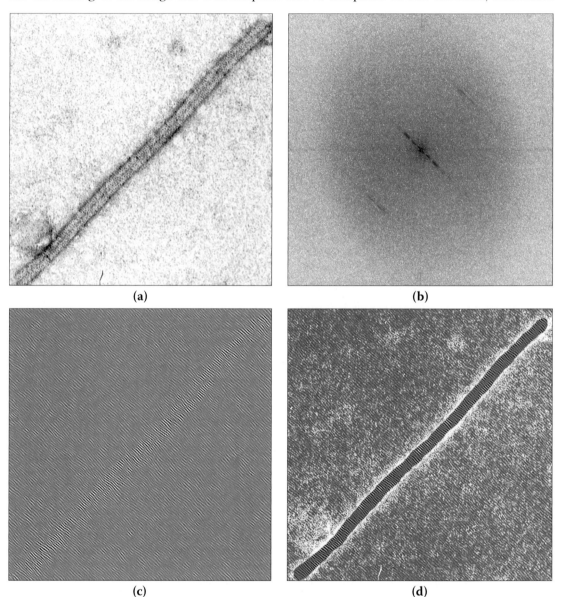

(a)   (b)

(c)   (d)

Figure 6.15 *TEM image of a virus: (a) original image, in which the internal helical structure is difficult to discern; (b) frequency transform of image a, in which the regular repeating structure of the virus and its angular variation in orientation is evident; (c) retransformation of just the peaks in the frequency transform, in which the periodic lines are not limited to the virus; (d) using the virus particle as a mask, the helical pattern becomes evident. (Courtesy of Dr. R. L. Grayson, Virginia Polytechnic Institute, Blacksburg, VA.)*

with an improvement in the perpendicular direction. This becomes immediately evident in the frequency transform, since the decrease in brightness or power falls off radially (at higher frequencies) and the asymmetry can be noted.

Figure 6.16 shows an example. The specimen is a cross section with three layers. The bottom is crystalline silicon, above which is a layer of amorphous (noncrystalline) silicon, followed by a layer of glue used to mount the sample for thinning and microscopy. The glue is difficult to distinguish by eye from the amorphous silicon. Frequency transforms for the three regions are shown. The regular structure in the pattern from the crystalline silicon gives the expected diffraction pattern. While the two regions above do not show individual peaks from periodic structures, they are not the same. The amorphous silicon has short-range order in the atomic spacings based on strong covalent bonding, but this local order is not visible to the human observer because of its chaotic overall pattern. This shows up in the frequency transform as a white cross in the dark ring, indicating that in the 45° directions there is a characteristic distance and direction to the next atom. This pattern is absent in the glue region, where there is no such structure.

In both regions, the dark circular pattern from the amorphous structure is not a perfect circle, but an ellipse. This indicates astigmatism. Adjusting the microscope optics to produce a uniform circle will correct the astigmatism and provide uniform resolution in all directions in the original image. It is much easier to observe the effects of small changes in the frequency-space display than in the spatial-domain image.

The frequency transform of an image can be used to optimize focus and astigmatism. When an image is in focus, the high-frequency information is maximized to sharply define the edges. This provides a convenient test for sharpest focus. **Figure 6.17** shows a light-microscope image that is in focus. The line profiles of the power spectrum in both the vertical and horizontal directions show a more gradual drop-off at high frequencies than **Figure 6.18**, which is the same image out of focus. In **Chapter 1**, methods for automatic focusing of optics were described that functioned by maximizing the high-frequency content of the image. This is

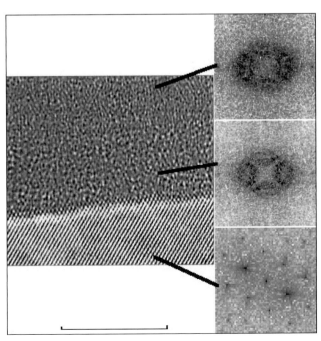

Figure 6.16 TEM image of cross section
of crystalline and amorphous silicon,
and glue, with frequency transforms
of each region shown at right.
(Courtesy of Dr. S. Chevacharoenkul,
Microelectronics Center of North
Carolina, Research Triangle.)

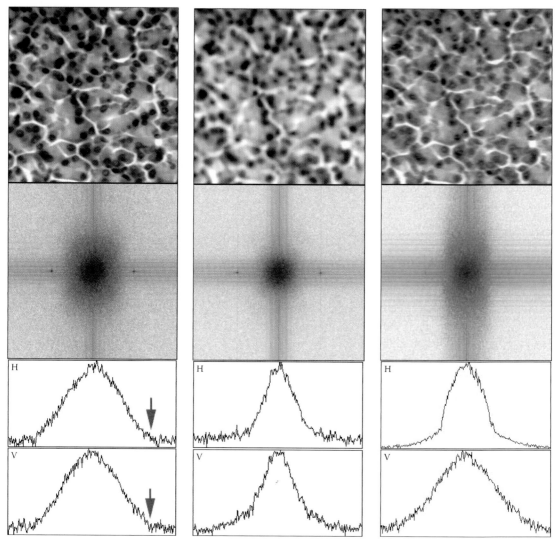

Figure 6.17 *Out-of-focus image with its power spectrum and horizontal and vertical line profiles, showing presence of high-frequency information as compared with Figure 6.18. Red arrows indicate actual resolution limit, as discussed in text.*

Figure 6.18 *Out-of-focus image with its power spectrum and horizontal and vertical line profiles, showing loss of high-frequency information as compared with Figure 6.17.*

Figure 6.19 *Astigmatic image produced by misaligning lens, with its power spectrum and horizontal and vertical line profiles showing different high-frequency components.*

easily visualized using the Fourier-transform power spectrum. When astigmatism is present (**Figure 6.19**), the power spectrum is asymmetric, as shown by the profiles.

Profiles of the power spectrum also provide a convenient tool for measuring the actual resolution of images to characterize various types of cameras and acquisition devices, as discussed in **Chapter 1**. Most image-acquisition procedures store an image that has somewhat more pixels than the actual resolution. As shown by the red arrows in **Figure 6.17**, the power spectrum shows a definite break in slope. This indicates the frequency at which the real information in the image ends; only noise is present at higher frequencies (smaller spacings).

Figure 6.20 shows a test pattern of radial lines recorded with a video camera. Due to the finite spacing of detectors in the video camera used, as well as limitations in electronics bandwidth that eliminate the very high frequencies required to resolve small details, these lines are incompletely resolved where they are close together. **Figure 6.21** shows the two-dimensional Fourier-transform power spectrum of this image. The power spectrum is plotted as a surface in **Figure 6.22** to emphasize the drop-off in magnitude, which is different in the horizontal and vertical directions. As is common in

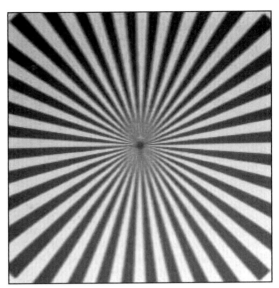

Figure 6.20 *Test pattern image used for Figures 6.21, 6.22, 6.23 and 6.37.*

video, the resolution along each scan line is poorer than the vertical resolution. **Figure 6.23** shows the complete set of data using color. One image shows the real and imaginary components of the transform and the other the magnitude and phase, encoded in different color channels. While technically complete, these displays are rarely used because the phase information is confusing to the viewer.

In the power spectrum, it is evident that there is a well-defined boundary, different in the x and y directions, beyond which the magnitude drops abruptly. This corresponds to the image resolution, which is different in the horizontal and vertical directions. In many cases, it is not so obvious where the physical source of resolution limitation lies. It can arise from the finite spacing of detectors in the camera or from various electronic effects in the amplification and digitization process. However, the Fourier-transform power spectrum will still show the limit, permitting the resolution of any imaging system to be ascertained.

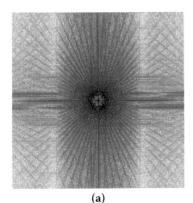

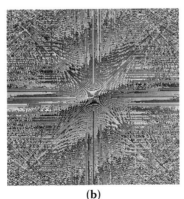

Figure 6.21 *Fourier transform of the test image in Figure 6.20:*
(a) *power-spectrum magnitude;*
(b) *phase (angles from 0 to 180° displayed as gray-scale values from black to white).*

(a)

(b)

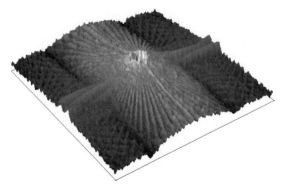

Figure 6.22 *The power spectrum from*
Figure 6.21 *presented as an isometric view.*

Texture and fractals

Besides the peaks in the power spectrum resulting from periodic structures that may be present and the ultimate limitation at high frequencies due to finite image resolution, it may seem as though there is only a noisy background containing little useful information. This is far from true. Many images represent the brightness of light scattered from surfaces, or other data such as surface elevation. In these images, the roughness or texture of the surface is revealed and can be measured from the power spectrum.

The concept of a fractal surface dimension will not be explained here in detail, but is discussed in **Chapter 14**. Surfaces that are fractal have an area that is mathematically undefined. It is greater than the projected area covered by the irregular surface and increases as the measurement scale becomes finer. The fractal dimension can be determined from the slope of a line on a log-log plot of measured area vs. the size of the measuring tool. Many naturally occurring surfaces resulting from wear, erosion, agglomeration of particles, or fracture are observed to have this character. It has also been shown that images of these surfaces, whether produced by the scattering of diffuse light or the production of secondary electrons in an SEM (scanning electron microscope), are also fractal. That is, the variation of brightness with position obeys the same mathematical relationship. The fractal dimension is an extremely powerful and compact representation of the surface roughness, which can often be related to the history of the surface and the properties that result.

Measuring surface fractals directly is rarely practical, although it can be done physically by determining the number of molecules of various gases that can adhere to the surface as a function of their size. One common imaging approach is to reduce the dimensionality and measure the fractal dimension of a boundary line produced by intersecting the surface with a sampling plane. This can be produced by either cross-sectioning or by polishing down into the surface to produce islands. In either case, the rougher the surface, the more irregular is the line. In the case of polishing parallel to the surface to produce islands, the perimeter line also has a fractal dimension (the slope of a log-log plot relating the measured line length and the length of the measurement tool), which is just 1.0 less than that of the surface.

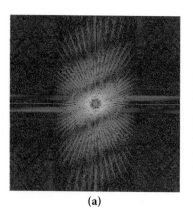

(a)

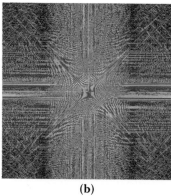

(b)

Figure 6.23 *Color representations of the Fourier transform from* **Figure 6.21**:
(a) *YUV image in which U = real, V = imaginary;*
(b) *RGB image in which intensity = magnitude, hue = phase.*

For a fractal surface, the power spectrum shows the superposition of sinusoids of all frequencies and orientations that have a specific shape: the magnitudes of the coefficients in a Fourier transform of a fractal curve decrease exponentially with the log of frequency, while the phases of the terms are randomized. This can be understood qualitatively, since by definition a fractal curve is self-similar and has detail extending to ever-finer scales (or higher frequencies). This also implies that the proportion of amplitudes of higher-frequency terms must be self-similar. An exponential curve satisfies this criterion.

Plotting the log of the amplitude (or the power spectrum, which is the square of the amplitude) versus the logarithm of frequency produces a straight-line plot, which is easily analyzed. There is a simple relationship between the fractal dimension of a profile and the exponential decrease in magnitude of the terms in a Fourier expansion, as had been predicted by Feder (1988). This correlation makes it practical to use the radial decrease of magnitude in a two-dimensional Fourier-transform image as a measure of roughness and the directional variation of that decrease as a measure of orientation (Mitchell and Bonnell 1990; Russ 1990b, 1994).

Figure 6.24 shows a range image (brightness represents elevation) for a fractal surface, with its Fourier-transform power spectrum. Plotting log (amplitude) vs. log (frequency) as shown in **Figure 6.25** produces a straight line, and a plot of the histogram of the phase values shows a uniform random distribution, which confirms the fractal geometry of the surface. The slope of the plot gives the dimension of the surface (which must lie between 2.0 for a Euclidean surface and 2.999… for one so irregular that it effectively fills three-dimensional space) as Fractal Dimension = (6 + slope)/2, or about 2.2 for the example shown. This is an isotropic surface produced by shot blasting a metal, so the slope is the same in all directions.

Figure 6.26 shows another surface, this produced by machining, with tool marks oriented in a specific direction. Similar analysis of this surface shows (**Figure 6.27**) that while it is still fractal (with average dimension about 2.25), it is not isotropic. There are actually two ways to depart from isotropy: one is changing the slope of the log (amplitude) vs. log (frequency) plot, and the other is its intercept, as a function of direction. **Chapter 14** discusses fractal surface geometry in more detail (see also Russ 1994, 2001b).

Measuring the two-dimensional Fourier transform is more efficient than measuring many individual brightness profiles in the original image. It also allows any periodic structures that may be present to be ignored, since these show up as discrete points in the frequency-transform image and can be skipped in determining the overall exponential decrease in the magnitude values. In other words, it is possible to look beyond the periodic structures or noise (e.g., arising from electronic components) in the images and still characterize the underlying chaotic but self-similar nature of the surface.

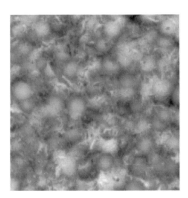 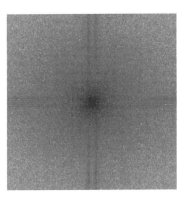

Figure 6.24 Range image of a shot-blasted metal surface, with its Fourier-transform power spectrum.

Isolating periodic noise

It was noted previously (and shown in **Figure 6.5** for a simple case) that the frequency transform has a property of separability and additivity. Adding together the transforms of two original images or functions produces the same result as the transform of the sum of the originals. This idea opens the way to using subtraction to remove unwanted parts of images. It is most commonly used to remove periodic noise, which can be introduced by the devices used to record or transmit images, or by some kinds of environmental interference (such as illumination or vibration). We will see some examples below. If the frequencies associated with the noise can be determined (often possible directly from the Fourier transform), then setting the amplitude of those terms to zero will leave only the desired remaining parts of the information. This can then be inverse-transformed back to the spatial domain to produce a noise-free image.

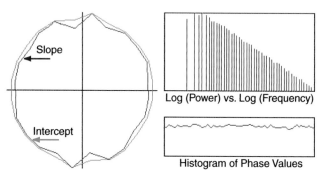

Figure 6.25 Analysis of the Fourier-transform data showing the isotropic fractal nature of the surface in *Figure 6.24*.

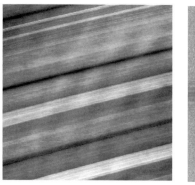

Figure 6.26 Range image of a machined metal surface, with its Fourier-transform power spectrum.

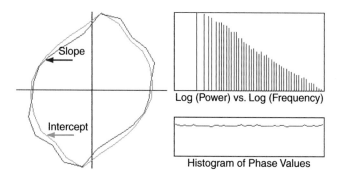

Figure 6.27 Analysis of the Fourier-transform data showing the anisotropic fractal nature of the surface in *Figure 6.26*.

The same method of removing selected frequencies can be used for a more basic type of filtering as well. **Figure 6.28** shows an image with its Fourier-transform power spectrum. There are no evident "spikes" or noise peaks, just the usual gradual reduction in the amplitude of higher frequencies. Keeping the low frequencies and removing the high frequencies can be accomplished by zeroing the amplitude of all sinusoids above a selected frequency. The red circle in **Figure 6.28b** was used to perform this "low pass" filtering operation (i.e., passing or keeping the low frequencies), to produce the result in **Figure 6.28c**. Conversely, keeping the high frequencies and removing the low frequencies (a high-pass filter) produces the result in **Figure 6.28d**.

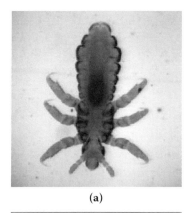
(a)

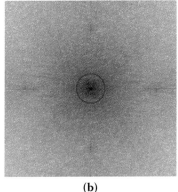
(b)

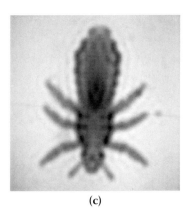
(c)

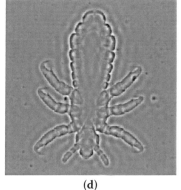
(d)

Figure 6.28 Frequency filtering using the Fourier transform:
  (a) original image;
  (b) power spectrum with a circular-frequency cutoff;
  (c) retransforming just the low frequencies inside the circle (a low-pass filter);
  (d) retransforming just the high frequencies outside the circle (a high-pass filter).

Except for the ringing around boundaries (discussed below), the results are exactly the same as those for Gaussian smoothing and Laplacian sharpening, shown in the two preceding chapters. In fact, it can be shown mathematically that the operations are exactly the same whether performed in the frequency domain or in the pixel domain.

In this illustration of filtering, portions of the Fourier-transform image were selected based on frequency, which is why these filters are generally called low-pass and high-pass filters. Usually, selecting arbitrary regions of the frequency domain for reconstruction produces "ringing" artifacts, unless some care is taken to shape the edges of the filter region to attenuate the data smoothly. This can be seen in the one-dimensional example of the step function in **Figure 6.1** and the corresponding two-dimensional example of **Figure 6.7**. If only the first few terms are used, then in addition to not modeling the steepness of the step, the reconstruction has oscillations near the edge, which are generally described as ringing.

It is necessary to shape the edge of the filter to prevent ringing at sharp discontinuities. This behavior is well known in one-dimensional filtering (used in digital signal processing, for example). Several different shapes are commonly used. Over a specified width (usually given in pixels, but of course ultimately specified in terms of frequency or direction), the filter magnitude can be reduced from maximum to minimum using a weighting function. The simplest function is linear interpolation (also called a Parzen window function). Better results can be obtained using a parabolic or cosine function (also called Welch and Hanning window functions, respectively, in this context). The most elaborate filter shapes do not drop to the zero or minimum value, but extend a very long tail beyond the cutoff point. One such shape is a Gaussian. **Figure 6.29** shows several of these shapes.

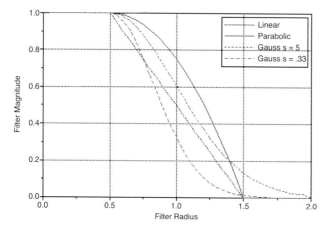

Figure 6.29 *Some common filter edge profiles.*

Another filter shape often used in these applications is a Butterworth filter, whose magnitude can be written as

$$H = 1 / \left[1 + C \left(\frac{R}{R_0} \right)^{2n} \right]$$

(6.8)

where R is the distance from the center of the filter (usually the center of the power-spectrum image, or zero-frequency point), and R_0 is the nominal filter cutoff value. The constant C is often set equal to 1.0 or to 0.414; the value defines the magnitude of the filter at the point where $R = R_0$ as either 50% or $1/\sqrt{2}$. The integer n is the order of the filter; its most common values are 1 or 2. **Figure 6.30** shows comparison profiles of several Butterworth low-pass filters (those that attenuate high frequencies). The inverse shape having negative values of n passes high frequencies and attenuates low ones. **Figure 6.31** shows the effect of shaping the frequency cutoff on the quality of the high- and low-pass-filtered images from **Figure 6.28**.

To illustrate the effects of these filters on ringing at edges, **Figure 6.32** shows a simple test shape and its two-dimensional FFT power-spectrum image. The orientation of principal terms perpendicular to the major edges in the spatial-domain image is evident. Performing a reconstruction using a simple aperture with a radius equal to 25 pixels (called an ideal filter) produces the result shown in **Figure 6.33a**. The oscillations in brightness near the edges are quite visible.

Ringing can be reduced by shaping the edge of the filter, as discussed above. The magnitudes of frequency terms near the cutoff value are multiplied by factors less than 1, whose values are based on a simple function. If a cosine function is used, which varies from 1 to 0 over a total width of 6 pixels, the result is improved (**Figure 6.33b**). In this example, the original

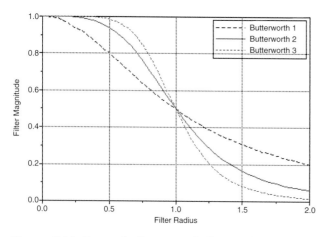

Figure 6.30 *Shapes for Butterworth filter profiles of order 1, 2, and 3.*

25-pixel radius used for the ideal filter (the sharp cutoff) is the point at which the magnitude of the weighting factor drops to 50%. The weights drop smoothly from 1.0 at a radius of 22 pixels to 0.0 at a radius of 28 pixels.

Increasing the distance over which the transition takes place further reduces the ringing, as shown in **Figure 6.33c**. Here, the 50% point is still at 25 pixels, but the range is from 15 to 35 pixels. Note that the improvement is not achieved simply by increasing the high-frequency limit, which would improve the sharpness of the feature edges but would not by itself reduce the ringing. **Figure 6.33d** shows the

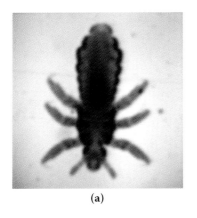

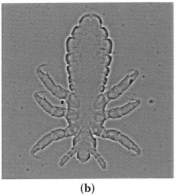

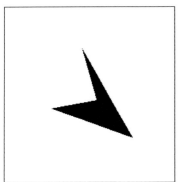

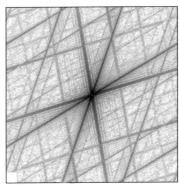

(a) (b)

Figure 6.31 Shaping the frequency cutoff with a Butterworth filter: (a) low-pass filter (compare with Figure 6.28c); (b) high-pass filter (compare with Figure 6.28d).

Figure 6.32 Test shape with its frequency-transform power spectrum, used in Figure 6.33.

same reconstruction using a second-degree Butterworth filter shape whose 50% point is set at 25 pixels.

Figure 6.34 shows an image with both fine detail and some noise along with its frequency transform. Applying Butterworth low-pass filters with radii of 10 and 25 pixels in the frequency-domain image smoothes the noise with some blurring of the high-frequency detail (**Figure 6.35**), while the application of Butterworth high-pass filters with the same radii emphasizes the edges and reduces the contrast in the large (low frequency) regions (**Figure 6.36**). All of these filters were applied to the amplitude values as multiplicative masks. Adjusting the radius of the filter cutoff controls the range of frequencies in the inverse-transformed image, just as changing the size of the convolution kernel alters the degree of smoothing or sharpening when the equivalent procedure is carried out in the spatial or pixel domain.

Of course, the magnitude need not vary from 1 to 0. Sometimes the lower limit is set to a fraction, so that the high (or low) frequencies are not completely attenuated. It is also possible to use values greater than 1. A high-frequency emphasis filter with the low-frequency value set to a reduced value, such as 0.5, and a high-frequency value greater than 1, such as 2, can be applied to an image whose brightness values have previously been converted to their logarithms. The use of the log-of-brightness data is important because it converts the multiplicative effect of illumination and reflectance into additive terms. The high-pass filter applied to these values suppresses the (large) variation in illumination and emphasizes the (smaller) variation in reflectance, sharpening the appearance of detail. **Figure 3.12** in **Chapter 3** illustrates the result. While the physical reasoning behind this homomorphic filter is the separation of illumination and reflectance components in the image, the real justification (as with most of these

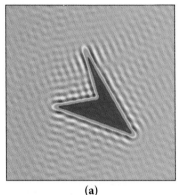

(a)

Figure 6.33 *Reconstruction of shape from its frequency transform in* Figure 6.32, *using a 25-pixel aperture (mask or filter) diameter:*
(a) ideal filter in which the cutoff is exact and abrupt;
(b) cosine-weighted edge shape with a half-width of 3 pixels;
(c) cosine-weighted edge shape with a half-width of 10 pixels;
(d) Butterworth second-degree shape. False color has been added to increase the visibility of small variations.

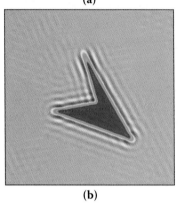

(b)

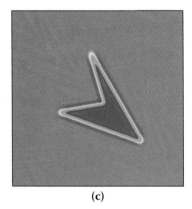

(c)

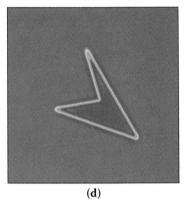

(d)

filters) is that it improves the appearance of many images of practical interest. When a similar procedure is carried out in the pixel domain, rather than by using a Fourier transform, this approach is called a "retinex" filter.

It is also possible to select a region of the Fourier-transform image that is not centered on the origin. **Figure 6.37** shows a selection of intermediate frequency values lying in a particular direction on the transform in **Figure 6.20**, along with the resulting reconstruction. This kind of filtering can be useful in selecting directional information from images. Removing selected frequencies and orientations is performed in the same way, as discussed below. This figure also demonstrates the basic characteristic of Fourier-transform images: locations in the Fourier-transform image identify periodicity and orientation information in any or all parts of the spatial-domain image. Note that the correct shape for off-centered regions is a combination of annuli and wedges that have cutoffs corresponding to frequencies and angles, rather than the more easily constructed circles or rectangles, and that the edges require the same type of shaping or smoothing shown previously.

Selective masks and filters

Once the location of periodic noise in an original image is isolated into a few points in the Fourier-transform image, it becomes possible to remove the noise by removing those sinusoidal terms. A filter removes selected frequencies and orientations by reducing the magnitude values for those terms, either partially or to zero, while leaving the phase information alone (which is important in determining where that information appears in the image).

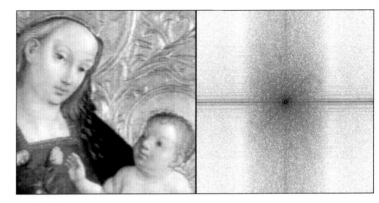

Figure 6.34 Image and its transform used for filtering in Figure 6.35 and Figure 6.36.

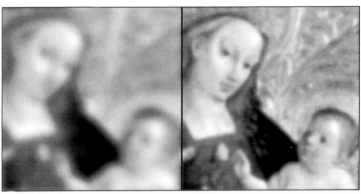

Figure 6.35 Filtering of Figure 6.34 with low-pass Butterworth filters having 50% cutoff diameters of 10 (left) and 25 pixels (right).

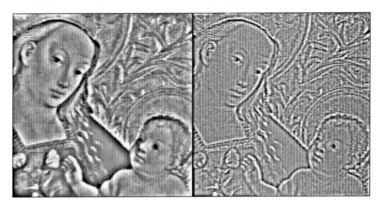

Figure 6.36 Filtering of Figure 6.34 with high-pass Butterworth filters having 50% cutoff diameters of 10 (left) and 25 pixels (right).

There are many different ways to specify and apply this reduction. Sometimes it is practical to specify a range of frequencies and orientations numerically, but most often it will be convenient to do so using the magnitude or the power-spectrum display of the Fourier-transform image. Manually or automatically selecting regions on this display allows specific peaks in the power spectrum, corresponding to the periodic information, to be selected for elimination. The terms "filter" and "mask" as used here are essentially synonymous. In a few cases a filter can be constructed mathematically and applied directly to the stored transform, but usually it is created as an array of pixels as large as the transform, containing values that are multiplied by the magnitude of the FFT data. The values often consist of just "on" or "off" to remove or leave the original terms unchanged, but in many cases they can have intermediate values, and they are typically represented by the same 0 to 255 range of values as used in an image. This

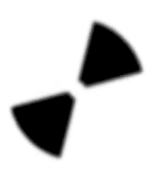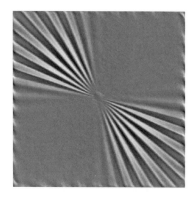

Figure 6.37 Inverse transform of the Fourier transform of Figure 6.20b through a filter selecting a range of frequencies and angles.

means that the mask or filter can itself be treated like an image, and thus all of the tools for processing images, such as Gaussian filters to smooth edges, can be applied to it.

Instead of using combinations of arcs and radial lines for isolated noise peaks (often referred to as noise "spikes"), it is convenient and usually acceptable to use small circles to define the regions when they consist of small points. However, it is important to use a smoothing function to modify the edges of the regions. When the transition takes place over a distance of only a few pixels, the differences between the previously described transition curves are of little importance, and a simple Gaussian smooth is most commonly applied.

Figure 6.38 illustrates the removal of periodic noise from an image by removing the corresponding frequencies from the Fourier transform. A square region with power-of-two dimensions within the original image is selected and the FFT computed. The two dark "spikes" correspond in orientation and radius to the dominant noise in the image. Removing the spikes eliminates the noise, which is still visible in the region around the processed area. Notice that all of the fine lines and details are preserved because they are composed of different frequencies.

Usually there are multiple spikes, and it is only by first examining the transform-image power spectrum that the presence and exact location of these points can be determined. **Figure 6.39** shows an image of a halftone print from a magazine. The pattern results from the halftone screen used in the printing process. In the frequency transform of the image, this regular pattern shows up as well-defined narrow peaks or spikes. Filtering removes the peaks by setting the magnitude at those locations to zero (but not altering any of the phase information). This allows the image to be retransformed without the noise.

It is interesting to note that image compression does not necessarily remove these noise spikes in the Fourier transform. Compression is generally based on discarding the small-magnitude terms in the transform (Fourier, cosine, etc.). These compression methods interpret halftone patterns or other periodic noise as an important feature of the image. The need to preserve the periodic noise spikes actually reduces the amount of other useful detail that can be retained.

The effects of compression are best examined in the frequency transform. **Figure 6.40** shows the FFT power spectrum for the "flowers" image (**Figure 3.30, Chapter 3**) before and after compression by the JPEG (Joint Photographers Expert Group) algorithm. Visually, the outer regions (higher frequencies) in the power spectrum appear lighter (lower magnitude). A plot of the values as a function of radius confirms that, while there are few differences in the average magnitude at low frequencies, there is an abrupt drop-off at high frequencies as the information corresponding to fine details is removed.

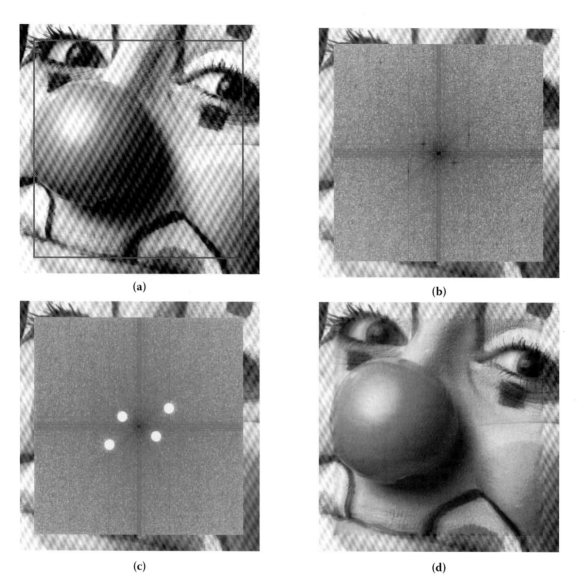

Figure 6.38 *Removal of periodic noise: **(a)** original image with outline of processed region; **(b)** frequency-transform power spectrum; **(c)** removal of noise spikes; **(d)** retransformed result. (Courtesy of Media Cybernetics, Silver Springs, MD.)*

The example in **Figure 6.39** relied on human observation of the peaks in the Fourier-transform image, recognition that the peaks were responsible for the periodic noise, and selection of the peaks to produce the filter. In some cases, it is possible to construct an appropriate image filter automatically from the Fourier-transform power spectrum. The guiding principle is that peaks in the power spectrum that are narrow and rise significantly above the local background should be removed. If the magnitude of the Fourier-transform image is treated like an ordinary spatial-domain gray-scale image, this peak removal can often be accomplished automatically using a rank-based filter like the top hat.

Figure 6.41 shows the power spectrum from the image in **Figure 6.38** and the result of applying a top-hat filter with an inner radius of 3 pixels, an outer radius of 5 pixels, and a height of

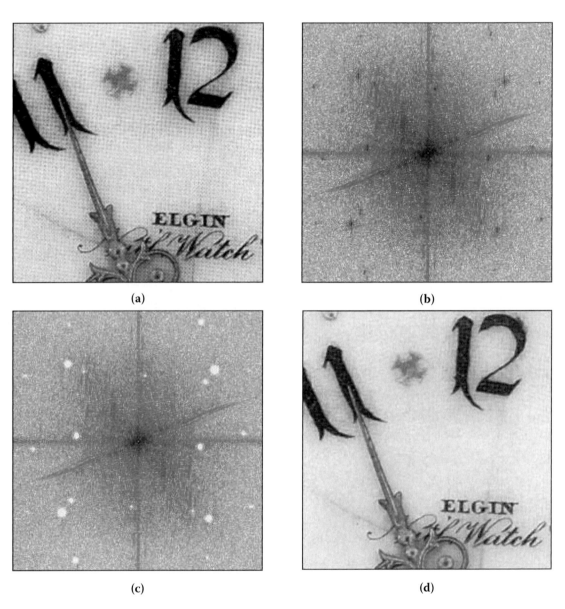

(a)   (b)

(c)   (d)

Figure 6.39 *Removal of complex periodic noise:* **(a)** *original halftoned printed image;* **(b)** *the frequency transform;* **(c)** *removal of the spikes from the FFT;* **(d)** *retransformed result.*

eight gray-scale values. The brim of the hat rests on the background, which drops off gradually and smoothly as frequency (radius) increases. The located features correspond to the noise spikes. A mask that removes these spikes can be created by enlarging the spots by a few pixels, applying a smoothing to the edges, and then inverting this result. **Figure 6.41** shows the modified power spectrum and the retransformed result. As discussed previously, one of the major uses of the top-hat filter is for processing Fourier transforms.

Sometimes the process of determining where the noise peaks are located can be simplified by selecting a region of the image that exhibits the noise pattern in an otherwise uniform area. This sequence is demonstrated in **Figure 6.42** for the same image as in **Figure 6.38** and **Figure 6.41**. A region of halftone periodic noise is selected, and the rest of the image cleared. The

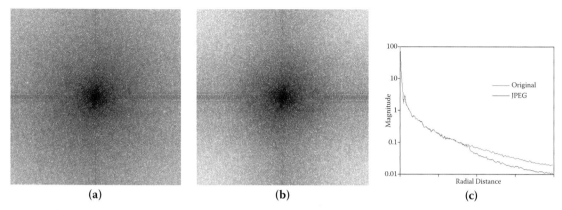

Figure 6.40 *Comparison of power spectra from the "flowers" image from* **Chapter 3** *(***Figure 3.30***): (a) original; (b) after JPEG compression; (c) plot of circularly averaged magnitude vs. radius.*

transform of this image is then processed by smoothing and leveling, and then thresholded to locate the peaks. The inverse of this mask is then smoothed and multiplied by the frequency transform of the original image to produce the filtered result.

Removal of noise spikes is not always enough to restore an image completely. The example in **Figure 6.43** shows an example of an image scanned from a newspaper; the halftone dots are very evident. The dark spots (spikes) in the power spectrum (**Figure 6.43c**) correspond to the periodic structure in the image. They align with the repetitive pattern of dots, and their darkness indicates the presence of the various frequencies. Removing them is equivalent to removing the periodic component. In this case, a top-hat filter was used to locate the spikes and create a mask (**Figure 6.43d**). The application of this mask as a filter to remove the spikes shows that the periodic noise has been removed without affecting any of the information present (**Figure 6.43e**). There is still some pixel-to-pixel noise because the image has been scanned at a higher resolution than the printed resolution, and the halftone cells in the original image are separated.

An additional filter can be employed to fill in the space between cells. A Butterworth second-order filter keeps low frequencies (gradual variations in gray scale) while progressively cutting off higher ones. In this case, the midpoint of the cutoff was set to the spacing of the halftone dots in the original image. The final version of the power spectrum (**Figure 6.43g**) shows the periodic spots removed and the high frequencies attenuated. An inverse transform produces the final image (**Figure 6.43h**). Note that even the cat's whiskers, which are barely discernible in the original image, are clearly visible.

A common recommendation (found in Internet newsgroups, for instance) for dealing with scanned halftone images or ones with moiré patterns from the scanner is to use smoothing to eliminate the pattern (sometimes by scanning the image at an angle and rotating it in software, using the interpolation as a low-pass filter; sometimes by scanning at a larger size and again depending on the filtering effects of interpolation as the image size is reduced; and sometimes by the overt application of a smoothing algorithm). This is a flawed strategy. The use of a smoothing or blur function in this image would have erased these fine lines long before the halftone dots were smoothed out.

When the original image has been scanned from a color print, the situation is slightly more complicated. As mentioned in **Chapter 3** and shown in **Figure 6.44**, colored halftone prints are typically made using cyan, magenta, yellow, and black (CMYK) inks, with each color having

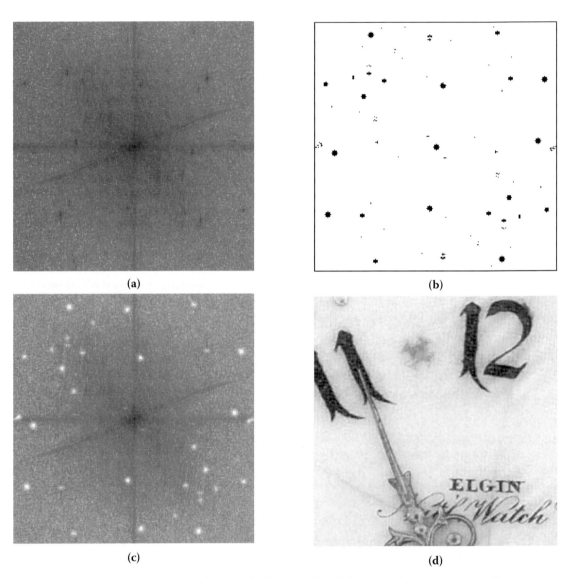

(a)

(b)

(c)

(d)

Figure 6.41 Automatic location and removal of noise spikes: (a) original power spectrum from Figure 6.39; (b) top-hat filter applied to image a; (c) modified power spectrum after removal of spikes found in image b; (d) retransformed image.

a halftone screen oriented at a different angle. The required procedure is to separate the color channels, processing each one and then recombining them for the final result. In **Figure 6.44**, the power spectra for each of the channels is shown superimposed, in the corresponding color, to illustrate the different screen orientations. A top-hat filter was applied to the Fourier-transform power spectrum from each channel to select the noise peaks, which were then removed. Recombining the resultant color-channel images produces the result shown.

Selection of periodic information

In some types of images, it is the periodic information that is useful and the nonperiodic noise that must be suppressed. The methods for locating the periodic peaks, constructing filters, smooth-

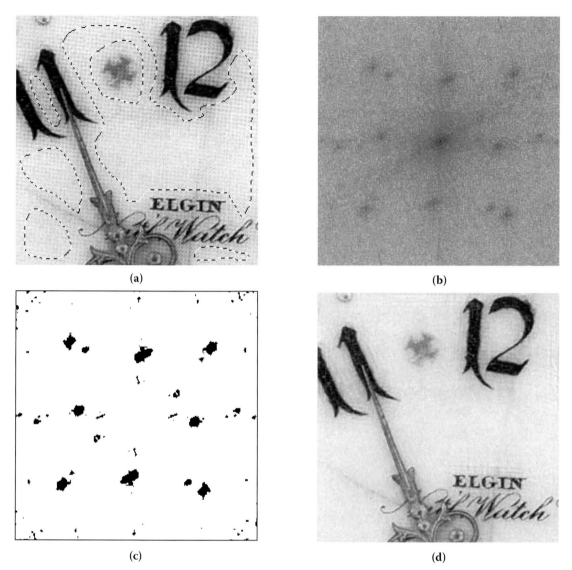

Figure 6.42 *(a) Identification of noise spikes by selecting image regions that exhibit the noise pattern; (b) Fourier-transform power spectrum from the selected areas; (c) mask created by processing image **b**; (d) result of applying the filter from image **c** to the Fourier transform of the entire original image.*

ing the filter edges, and so forth, are unchanged. The only difference is that the filter sense is changed, and in the case of a multiplicative mask, the values are inverted.

Figure 6.45 shows a one-dimensional example. The image is a light micrograph of stained skeletal muscle, in which there is a just-visible band spacing that is difficult to measure because of the spotty staining contrast (even with contrast expansion). The Fourier-transform image shows the spots that identify the band structure. The spacing can be easily and accurately determined by measuring the radius of the first major peak. Reconstruction with only the first harmonic shows the basic band structure, and adding the second and third harmonics defines the band shape fairly well.

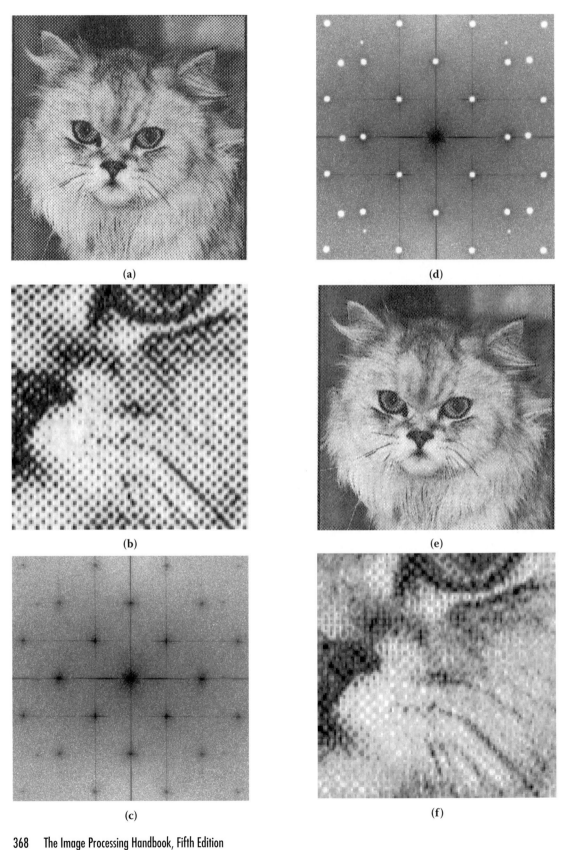

(a)

(b)

(c)

(d)

(e)

(f)

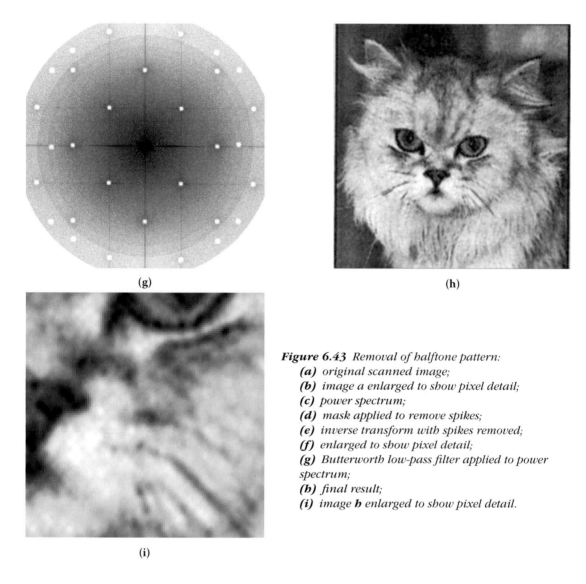

(g)

(h)

Figure 6.43 *Removal of halftone pattern:*
  (a) *original scanned image;*
  (b) *image a enlarged to show pixel detail;*
  (c) *power spectrum;*
  (d) *mask applied to remove spikes;*
  (e) *inverse transform with spikes removed;*
  (f) *enlarged to show pixel detail;*
  (g) *Butterworth low-pass filter applied to power spectrum;*
  (h) *final result;*
  (i) *image b enlarged to show pixel detail.*

(i)

Figure 6.46 shows a high-resolution TEM lattice image from a crystalline ceramic (mullite). The two-dimensional periodicity of the lattice can be seen, but it is superimposed on a variable and noisy background that alters the local contrast, making it more difficult to observe the details in the rather complex unit cell of this material. The Fourier-transform image has peaks that correspond to the periodic structure. As noted before, this image is essentially the same as would be recorded photographically using the TEM to project the diffraction pattern of the specimen to the camera plane. Of course, retransforming the spatial-domain image from the photographed diffraction pattern is not possible because the phase information has been lost. In addition, more control over the Fourier-transform display is possible because a log scale or other rule for converting magnitude to screen brightness can be selected.

A filter or mask is constructed to select a small circular region around each of the periodic spots. This was done, as before, by using a top-hat filter with size just large enough to cover the peaks. In this case, the filter is used to keep the amplitude of terms in the peaks while reducing all of the other terms to zero, which removes the random or nonperiodic noise,

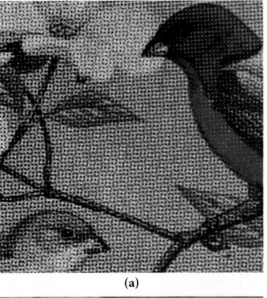

(a)

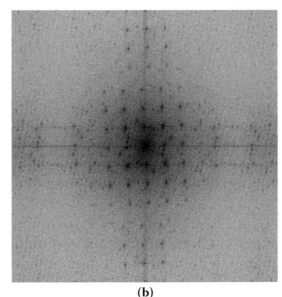

(b)

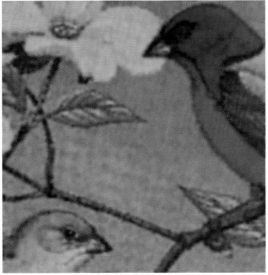

(c)

Figure 6.44 *Halftone removal in a color image:*
  (a) *original image (a magnified portion of a postage stamp, printed in CMYK);*
  (b) *Fourier-transform power spectra for each color channel, superimposed in color;*
  (c) *removal of noise from each channel and recombination of the color channels. Of course, since this book is printed using CMYK inks and halftoning, another set of frequencies and spacings is introduced in the printing process, which limits the performance of the result displayed here.*

both the short-range (high frequency) graininess and the gradual (low frequency) variation in overall brightness. Retransforming this image produces a spatial-domain image that shows the lattice structure clearly. It is equivalent to averaging together the several hundred repetitions of the basic unit cell structure that is present in the original image, to improve the signal-to-noise ratio.

Figure 6.47 shows an even more dramatic example. In the original image (a cross section of muscle myofibrils), it is practically impossible to discern the periodic structure due to the presence of noise. There are isolated locations where a few of the fibrils can be seen to have a regular spacing and arrangement, but human observers do not easily see through the noise and variability to find this regularity. However, the Fourier-transform image shows the peaks from the underlying regularity. Selecting only these peak points in the magnitude image (with their original phase information) and reducing all other magnitude values to zero produces the

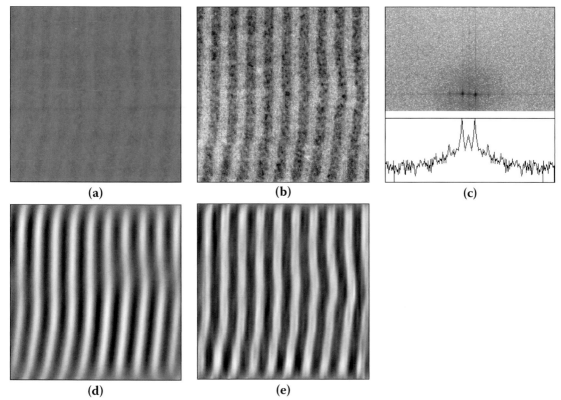

Figure 6.45 *Light micrograph of stained (toluidine blue) 1-μm section of skeletal muscle: **(a)** original image; **(b)** expanded contrast (the band spacing is still difficult to measure due to spotty stain contrast); **(c)** Fourier-transform power spectrum shows spots that identify the band spacing; **(d)** reconstruction with just the first harmonic shows the basic band spacing; **(e)** adding the second and third harmonics defines the band shape well.*

result shown in **Figure 6.48.** The retransformed image clearly shows the six-fold symmetry expected for the myofibril structure. The inset shows an enlargement of this structure in even finer detail, with both the thick and thin filaments shown. The thin filaments, especially, cannot be seen clearly in the original image.

A caution is needed in using this type of filtering to extract periodic structures. It is possible to construct a mask that will eliminate real information from the image while keeping artifacts and noise. Selecting points in the power spectrum with six-fold symmetry ensured that the filtered and retransformed spatial image would show that type of structure. This means that the critical step is the recognition and selection of the peaks in the Fourier-transform image. Fortunately, there are many suitable tools for finding and isolating such points, since they are narrow peaks that rise above a gradually varying local background. The top-hat filter illustrated above is an example of this approach.

It is also possible to construct a filter to select a narrow range of spacings, such as the inter-atomic spacing in a high-resolution image. This annular filter makes it possible to enhance a selected periodic structure. **Figure 6.49** shows a high-resolution TEM image of an atomic lattice. Applying an annular filter that blocks both the low and high frequencies produces the result shown, in which the atom positions are more clearly defined. However, if the filter also

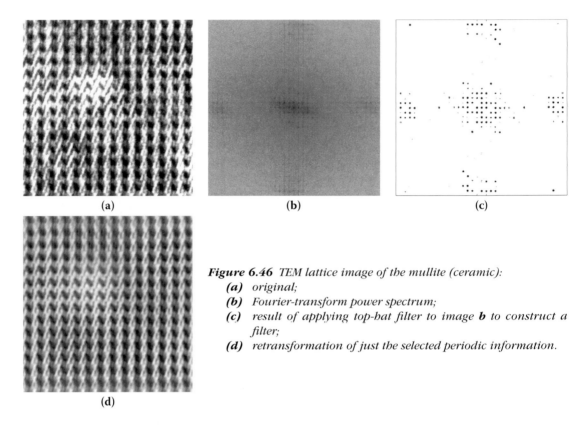

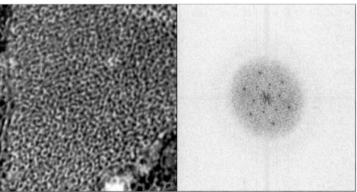

Figure 6.46 *TEM lattice image of the mullite (ceramic):*
(a) original;
(b) Fourier-transform power spectrum;
(c) result of applying top-hat filter to image **b** to construct a filter;
(d) retransformation of just the selected periodic information.

Figure 6.47 *TEM image of cross section of muscle myofibrils (left) and the frequency transform (right). (Courtesy of Arlo Reeves, Dartmouth College, Hanover, NH.)*

Figure 6.48 *Retransformation of* **Figure 6.47** *(left), with only the principal periodic peaks in the frequency transform (right). The points in the filter mask have been enlarged for visibility.*

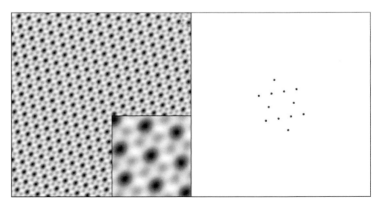

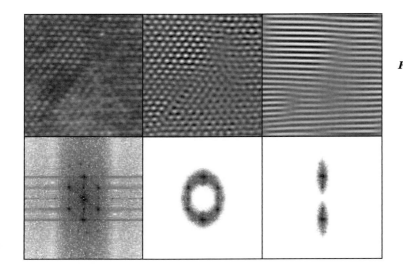

Figure 6.49 Noisy high-resolution TEM image (left), with the results of applying an annular filter to select atomic spacings (center), and a slit filter to select vertical spacings only (right). Top images show the spatial domain, and bottom row shows FFT power spectrum.

selects a particular orientation (a slit or wedge filter), then the dislocation that is difficult to discern in the original image becomes clearly evident.

As for the case of removing periodic noise, a filter that selects periodic information and reveals periodic structure can often be designed by examining the Fourier-transform power-spectrum image itself to locate peaks. The mask or filter can be constructed either manually or automatically. In some cases, there is *a priori* information available (such as lattice spacings of crystalline specimens).

In **Figure 6.50**, the structure (of graphitized carbon in particles used for tire manufacture) shows many atomic lattices in different orientations. In this case, the diffraction pattern shows the predominant atom plane spacing of slightly less than 3.5 Å, in the form of a ring of spots. Applying an annular filter to select just that spacing, retransforming, and then adding the atom positions to the original image enhances the visibility of the lattice structure. This is an example of a "band-pass" filter that keeps a selected range of frequencies. (In the spatial domain, the difference of Gaussians is an equivalent band-pass filter.)

The use of filtering in Fourier-transform space is also useful for isolating structural information when the original image is not perfectly regular. **Figure 6.51** shows the same skeletal muscle tissue shown in **Figure 6.45**, but cross-sectioned and stained with uranyl acetate/lead citrate. The black dots are immunogold labeling for fast myosin, involved in muscle contraction. The spots are more or less regularly spaced because of the uniform diameters of the muscle fibers, but have no regular order to their arrangement. Sharpening the image using a top-hat filter, as discussed above and in **Chapter 5**, improves the visibility of the spots compared with the original image. So does the use of an annular Fourier filter that selects just the ring of spots corresponding to the fiber diameter.

Convolution

One of the classes of operations on images performed in the spatial domain (and described in the preceding chapters) is convolution, in which a kernel of numbers is multiplied by each pixel and its neighbors in a small region, the results summed, and the result placed in the original pixel location. This is applied to all of the pixels in the image. In all cases, the original

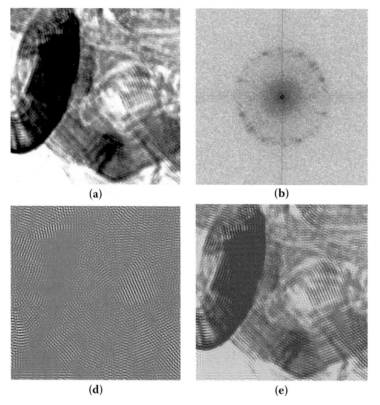

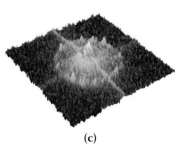

(a)

(b)

(c)

(d)

(e)

Figure 6.50
(a) *TEM image of graphitized carbon;*
(b) *the FT power spectrum from image **a**, showing the broken ring of spots corresponding to the 3.5-Å plane spacing in the graphite;*
(c) *the power spectrum plotted as a perspective drawing to emphasize the ring of peaks;*
(d) *inverse transform of just the ring of spots;*
(e) *image **d** added to the original image **a** to enhance the visibility of the lattice.*

pixel values are used in the multiplication and addition, and the newly derived values are used to produce a new image, although as a practical matter of implementation the operation can be performed by duplicating a few lines at a time, so that the new image ultimately replaces the old one.

This type of convolution is particularly common for the smoothing and derivative operations illustrated in **Chapter 4** and **Chapter 5**. A brief review of the information may be useful here. For instance, a simple smoothing kernel might contain the following values:

$$
\begin{array}{ccc}
1 & 2 & 1 \\
2 & 4 & 2 \\
1 & 2 & 1
\end{array}
$$

There are many spatial-domain kernels, including ones that apply Gaussian smoothing (to reduce noise), that take first derivatives (for instance, to locate edges), or that take second derivatives (for instance, the Laplacian, which is a nondirectional operator that acts as a high-pass filter to sharpen points and lines). They are usually presented as a set of integers, although greater accuracy is attainable with floating-point numbers, with it understood that there is

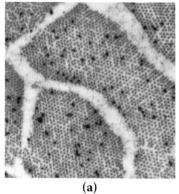

(a)

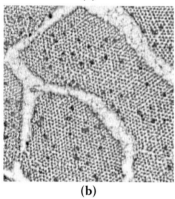

(b)

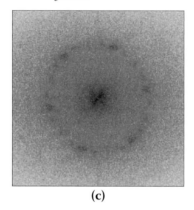

(c)

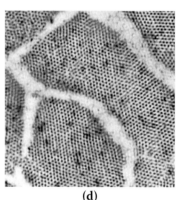

(d)

Figure 6.51 *Light micrograph of cross section of the same skeletal muscle as in **Figure 6.45**, cross sectioned and uranyl acetate/lead citrate stained. Black dots are immunogold labeling for fast myosin:*
(a) original;
*(b) top-hat filter applied to the image in the spatial domain, as shown in **Chapter 5**;*
(c) the power spectrum from the Fourier transform, showing a broken ring of spots corresponding to the average diameter of the fibers;
(d) retransforming the ring of spots with an annular filter that selects just the spacings of the gold particles and adding this back to the original image increases the contrast of the fibers.

a divisor (usually equal to the sum or largest of all the positive values) that normalizes the result. Kernels of numbers that include negative numbers can produce results that are negative, so an offset value such as 128 (medium gray for images that use a 0 to 255 range for pixel values) can be added to the result. Some of these operators can be significantly larger than the 3 × 3 example shown above, involving the adding together of the weighted sum of neighbors in a much larger region that is usually, but not necessarily, square.

Applying a large kernel takes time. **Figure 6.52** illustrates the process graphically for a single placement of the kernel. Even with very fast computers and with careful coding of the process to carry out additions and multiplications in the most efficient order, performing the operation with a 25 × 25 kernel on a 1024 × 1024 image would require a significant amount of time (and even larger kernels and images are often encountered). Though it can be sped up somewhat by the use of special hardware, such as a pipelined array processor, a special-purpose investment is required. A similar hardware investment can be used to speed

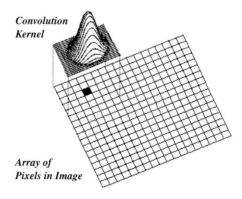

Convolution Kernel

Array of Pixels in Image

Figure 6.52 *Illustration of applying a convolution kernel to an image in the spatial domain. (Courtesy of Arlo Reeves, Dartmouth College, Hanover, NH.)*

up the Fourier transform. Our interest here is in the algorithms, rather than in their implementation.

For any computer-based system, increasing the kernel size eventually reaches a point at which it is more efficient to perform the operation in the Fourier domain. The time needed to perform the FFT transformation from the spatial domain to the frequency domain and back is more than balanced by the speed with which the convolution can be carried out. If there are any other reasons to perform the transformation to the frequency-domain representation of the image, then even small kernels can be most efficiently applied there.

This is because the operation after the Fourier transform that is equivalent to spatial-domain convolution is a single multiplication of each magnitude value by the corresponding value in a transform of the kernel. The transform of the kernel can be obtained and stored beforehand just as the kernel is stored. If the kernel is smaller than the image, it is padded with zeroes to the full image size. Convolution in the spatial domain is exactly equivalent to multiplication in the frequency domain. Using the notation presented before, in which the image is a function $f(x,y)$ and the kernel is $g(x,y)$, we describe the convolution operation, in which the kernel is positioned everywhere on the image and multiplied by it, as

$$g(x,y) * f(x,y) = \iint (f(\alpha,\beta) \cdot g(x-\alpha, y-\beta) d\alpha \, d\beta$$

(6.9)

where α and β are dummy variables for the integration, the range of which is across the entire image, and the symbol * indicates convolution. If the Fourier transforms of $f(x,y)$ and $g(x,y)$ are $F(u,v)$ and $G(u,v)$, respectively, then the convolution operation in the Fourier domain is simple point-by-point multiplication, or

$$g(x,y) * f(x,y) \Leftrightarrow G(u,v)F(u,v)$$

(6.10)

There are a few practical differences between the two operations. The usual application of a kernel in the spatial domain applies special rules to the edge pixels (those nearer to the edge than the half-width of the kernel), since their neighbors do not exist. But in transforming the image to the frequency domain, the assumption is made that the image wraps around at edges, so that the left edge is contiguous with the right and the top edge is contiguous with the bottom. Applying a convolution by multiplying in the frequency domain is equivalent to addressing pixels in this same wraparound manner when applying the kernel to the spatial image. It will usually produce some artifacts at the edges. The most common solution for this problem is to embed the image of interest in a larger one in which the borders are either filled with the mean brightness value of the image or smoothly interpolated from the edge values. As noted previously, this is called "padding."

Figure 6.53 shows the equivalence of convolution in the spatial domain and multiplication in the frequency domain for the case of a smoothing kernel. The kernel, a Gaussian filter with standard deviation of 2.0 pixels, is shown as an array of gray-scale values, along with its transform. Applying the kernel to the image in the spatial domain produces the result shown in the example. Multiplying the kernel transform by the image transform produces the frequency-domain image, whose power spectrum is shown. Retransforming this image produces the identical result to the spatial-domain operation.

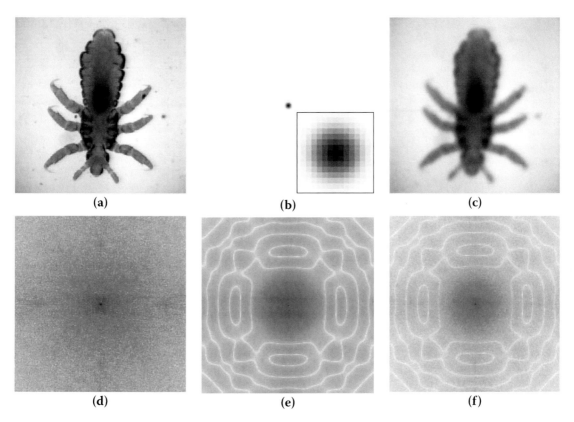

Figure 6.53 *Smoothing by applying a large kernel in the spatial domain and convolution in the frequency domain: (a) original image; (b) smoothing kernel (Gaussian, standard deviation = 2.0 pixels), with enlargement to show pixel detail; (c) smoothed image produced by spatial convolution with kernel or inverse Fourier transform of image e; (d) Fourier transform of image a; (e) Fourier transform of image b; (f) product of images d and e.*

Notice that the equivalence of frequency-domain multiplication to spatial-domain convolution is restricted to multiplicative filters, which are also known as "linear" filters. Other neighborhood operations, such as rank-based filtering (saving the brightest, darkest, or median brightness value in a neighborhood) and histogram modification (e.g., local adaptive equalization), are nonlinear and have no frequency-domain equivalent.

Deconvolution

Convolution can also be used as a tool to understand how imaging systems alter or degrade images. For example, the blurring introduced by imperfect lenses can be described by a function $H(u,v)$, which is multiplied by the frequency transform of the image, as shown schematically in **Figure 6.54**. The operation of physical optics is readily modeled in the frequency domain. Sometimes it is possible to determine the separate characteristics of each component of the system; often it is not. In some cases, determining the point-spread function of the system (the degree to which a perfect point in the object plane is blurred in the image plane) can make it possible to sharpen the image by removing some of the blur. This is called deconvolution and is done by dividing by $H(u,v)$, the transform of the point-spread image.

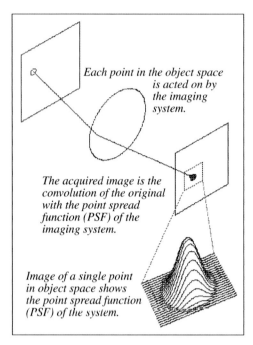

Each point in the object space is acted on by the imaging system.

The acquired image is the convolution of the original with the point spread function (PSF) of the imaging system.

Image of a single point in object space shows the point spread function (PSF) of the system.

Figure 6.54 *System characteristics introduce a point-spread function into the acquired image. (Courtesy of Arlo Reeves, Dartmouth College, Hanover, NH.)*

(A side note for any optical engineers: the point-spread function, or PSF, is the spread of an ideal point as measured in the spatial domain of the image. The modulation transfer function, or MTF, of an optical system, which is often used to describe its resolution and performance, is simply the absolute magnitude of the Fourier transform of the point-spread function. One of the many reasons that a Gaussian shape is often used as a convenient model for the PSF is that its Fourier transform is also a Gaussian shape; another reason comes from the central limit theorem of statistics, which says that whenever you have a large number of independent variables, their combined effect tends toward a Gaussian shape, and so in a real system comprising illumination, specimen or subject, optics, camera, and electronics, a Gaussian shape is often a pretty good approximation.)

Figure 6.55 shows the relationship between convolution and deconvolution. In **Figure 6.55a**, a Gaussian point-spread function is convolved with an image to produce a blurred result. The "*" indicates the convolution operation, which is akin to multiplication but performed with complex arithmetic. **Figure 6.55b** illustrates the deconvolution of the blurred image (the "/" indicates deconvolution, akin to division) with the same point-spread function. This recovers a less blurred image. Note, however, that the noise in the deconvolved image is increased, that not all of the original resolution can be recovered (some data are lost in the blurring process), and that there are artifacts around the edges of the image. These are all features of deconvolution that will be dealt with below.

To illustrate this sharpening, we can use the one of the best-known examples of correction of an out-of-focus condition due to an imperfect imaging system. As originally deployed, the Hubble telescope had an incorrectly figured main mirror that produced poorly focused images. Eventually a compensating optical device (an altered secondary mirror) was installed in the imaging system to correct most of the defect, but even with the original telescope it was possible to obtain high-resolution results by using deconvolution with the known point-spread function (or PSF). The corrected optical package, however, restored much of the telescope's light-gathering power, which was severely reduced due to the incorrect mirror curvature.

In this particular instance, it was possible to calculate the PSF from available measurement data on the mirror. But in many astronomical situations the problem is simplified because the point-spread function can be measured by examining the image of a single star, which is effectively a point as seen from Earth. This requires a considerable gray-scale depth to the image, but in astronomy, cooled cameras often deliver at least 14 bits of information, which is also important for obtaining enough precision to perform the deconvolution.

Figure 6.56 shows the result of this method. The original, blurred image is sharpened by dividing its Fourier transform by that of the measured PSF, and the resulting inverse transform

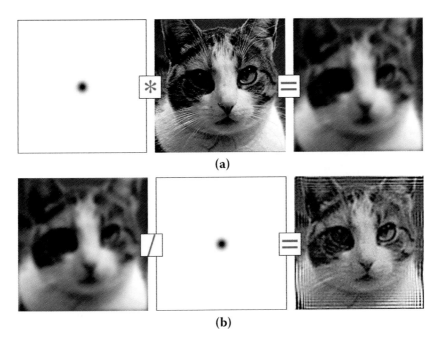

(a)

(b)

Figure 6.55 *The processes of convolution **(a)** and deconvolution **(b)**.*

shows a considerably sharpened image. Notice that unlike operations such as the unsharp mask (a high-pass filter) that increase the contrast at edges and make the image appear to be sharper visually, deconvolution actually recovers additional resolution and reveals faint details not visible in the original.

For deconvolution, we divide the complex frequency-domain image from the out-of-focus test pattern by that for the point-spread function (as indicated in **Figure 6.55**). This is complex division, performed by dividing the magnitude values and subtracting the phase values. One of the problems with division is that division by very small values can cause numeric overflow problems, and the Fourier transform of a symmetrical and well-behaved point-spread function often contains zero values. The usual solutions to this problem are either apodization to restrict

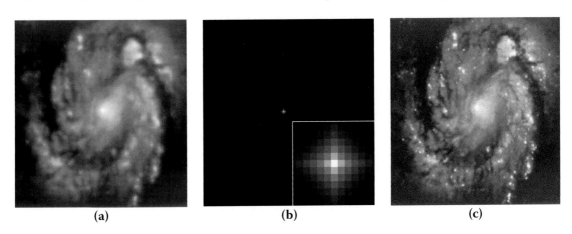

(a)   **(b)**   **(c)**

Figure 6.56 *Hubble telescope image sharpening: **(a)** original; **(b)** measured point-spread function, with enlargement to show pixel detail; **(c)** deconvolution result.*

the division operation to those pixels in the complex transform images that will not cause overflow, or adding a small constant to the denominator. Both will be shown below.

Deconvolution of image blur — which can arise from out-of-focus optics, motion, the size and arrangement of transistors in the camera chip, insufficient bandwidth in the electronics, or other causes — is an imperfect science. There is no mathematically optimum procedure, nor even a proof that one exists in all cases. The practical techniques that are used have been developed under a variety of assumptions and apply to many real situations, producing impressive improvements in image quality. But the results, while good, represent trade-offs between different limitations, one of which is the time required for the computations. Successful application of the method also requires images with as little random noise as possible and sufficient numerical precision in the arithmetic, as discussed below.

Deconvolution is discussed here in terms of gray-scale images. In most cases, color images need to be separated into discrete color channels that correspond to the physics of the acquisition device, usually red, green, and blue, and each one deconvolved separately. It is not uncommon to find that the point-spread function is different for each channel, especially if a single-chip camera with a Bayer pattern color filter has been used for acquisition.

It is important to always start with the best image possible. This means obtaining the best focus, least motion blur, etc., that you can achieve. Deconvolution is never as good a solution as correcting the source of the problem beforehand. Next, capture the image with the best possible range of contrast, from nearly full white to nearly full black without clipping. The tonal or gray-scale range should have good precision and a wide dynamic range. Eight-bit images from uncooled digital cameras are marginal, and poorer images from video cameras are usually unacceptable unless special procedures such as averaging multiple frames are used. It is particularly important to have high precision and bit depth for the point-spread function, whether it is obtained by measurement or by calculation.

Finally, random pixel noise (speckle) must be minimized. Noise in either the acquired image or (especially) in the point-spread function is significantly amplified in the deconvolution process and will dominate the result if it is too great. Long exposures and image averaging can be useful in some cases. The usual description of the magnitude of image noise is a signal-to-noise ratio expressed in decibels. This is defined in terms of the standard deviation of values in the blurred image and in the noise (which of course may not be known).

$$SNR[\mathrm{dB}] = 10 \cdot \log_{10}\left(\frac{\sigma_{image}}{\sigma_{noise}}\right)$$

(6.11)

When the signal-to-noise ratio is greater than 50 dB, the noise is, practically speaking, invisible in the image and has a minimal effect on deconvolution. On the other hand, a low signal-to-noise ratio of 10 to 20 dB makes the noise so prominent that deconvolution becomes quite impractical.

The ideal and simplest form of deconvolution is to measure (or in a few cases calculate from known optical parameters) the point-spread function of the system. Computing the Fourier transform of the blurred image and that of the PSF, dividing the second into the first, and performing an inverse transform, produces the deconvolved result, as shown above. The key requirement is that the blur due to the imaging system is assumed to be the same everywhere in the image, which is a good assumption for telescope images. When some portion of the blur is due to the passage of light through the sample itself, as occurs in thick sections examined in the light microscope, the blur can vary from point to point, and this method becomes less useful.

An indirect measurement of the PSF can be accomplished by capturing an image of a precisely known object using the same optical setup as that used for the real image. Dividing the Fourier transform of the image of the object by that of the ideal shape, and inverse-transforming the result, produces the system PSF, which can then be used to deconvolve images obtained with the optical system.

In some microscope situations, the insertion of fluorescing microbeads, or even an image of a small dust particle on the slide, can be useful as an estimate of the PSF. In the atomic force microscope, a direct measurement of the PSF can be accomplished by scanning an image of a known shape, usually a circular test pattern produced expressly for this purpose by the same methods used to etch integrated circuits. As shown in **Figure 6.57**, if the resulting image is deconvolved by dividing its Fourier transform by that for the ideal shape, the result is an image of the point-spread function, which in this case corresponds to the shape of the scanning tip. This shape can then be used to deconvolve other images, at least until the tip is further damaged or replaced.

If an image contains many edges oriented in different directions, and if the actual edge shape is known (ideally a perfectly sharp knife-edge transition in gray level), then the PSF can be determined at least in principle by measuring the actual transition across each edge and combining the various profiles to form a PSF image. In practice, this usually requires assuming that the function is symmetrical and of known shape (often a Gaussian as a convenient approximation to the central portion of the Airy disk produced by real optics), so that measurements on a few edges can be generalized to an entire two-dimensional PSF image.

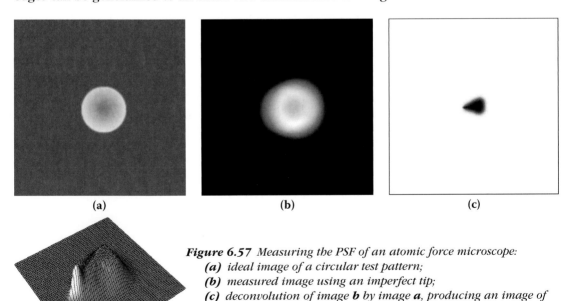

(a)   (b)   (c)

Figure 6.57 *Measuring the PSF of an atomic force microscope:*
  (a) *ideal image of a circular test pattern;*
  (b) *measured image using an imperfect tip;*
  (c) *deconvolution of image **b** by image **a**, producing an image of the tip;*
  (d) *perspective view of the shape in image **c**.*

(d)

If it is not possible to obtain a PSF by measurement, it may be possible to calculate a useful approximation based on assumptions such as a Gaussian blur function or straight-line motion. Real optical defocusing does not produce an ideal Gaussian blur, but it is not necessary in many cases to have the exact PSF, just a sufficiently useful approximation to remove most of the blur by deconvolution. A comparison of several shapes for the PSF is shown below.

Sometimes important insight into the nature of the PSF can be obtained by examining the Fourier transform of the blurred image. The presence of zeroes (or near-zero values) in lines, arcs, etc., is a powerful clue to the nature of the blur. Straight lines indicate motion blur, in a direction orthogonal to the lines. Arcs indicate non-Gaussian blurring (e.g., by a uniform disk). These can be used to estimate a PSF that can be used to perform a deconvolution, perhaps iterating the estimated PSF either automatically using one of the convergence methods discussed below, or by interactive selection, to reach a satisfactory result.

The blur produced by purely optical effects is frequently uniform in all directions, although astigmatism can modify this. However, the tip shape in scanned-probe microscopes can produce arbitrarily shaped point-spread functions. In many cameras the shape and spacing of the transistors produces different blur magnitudes in the horizontal and vertical directions, and the effects of the color filter pattern used can also alter the shape of the PSF. In any scanned image acquisition, the electronic parameters of the amplifiers used can produce different amounts of blur in the fast scan direction (generally horizontal) as compared with the slow scan direction (vertical). Time constants in phosphors, amplifiers, or other components can also produce asymmetrical blurs (comet tails) in the output signal.

Noise and Wiener deconvolution

If there is significant noise content in the image to be sharpened, or worse yet in the measured PSF, it can exacerbate the numerical precision and overflow problems and greatly degrade the resulting inverse transform. Removal of more than a portion of the blurring in a real image is almost never possible, but of course there are some situations in which even a small improvement can be of considerable practical importance.

Division by the frequency transform of the blur is referred to as an inverse filter. Using the notation introduced previously, this "ideal" deconvolution procedure can be written as

$$F(u,v) \approx \left[\frac{1}{H(u,v)} \right] G(u,v)$$

(6.12)

If the presence of noise in the blurred image prevents satisfactory deconvolution by simply dividing the Fourier transforms, then it may be practical to perform a Wiener deconvolution. Instead of calculating the deblurred image by dividing the Fourier transform of the original image by that of the blur function, a scalar value is used to increase the denominator. Theoretically, the additive factor K is dependent on the statistical properties of the images and their relative noise contents (technically, it is the ratio of the power of the image noise component to the image signal component), but in practice these are not usually known, and so the additive constant is typically treated as an adjustable parameter that controls the trade-off between sharpening and noise.

$$F(u,v) \approx \left[\frac{1}{H(u,v)} \right] \cdot \left[\frac{|H(u,v)|^2}{|H(u,v)|^2 + K} \right] \cdot G(u,v)$$

(6.13)

Figure 6.58 shows an example of the effect of random noise on an image with out-of-focus blur. An ideal inverse filter amplifies the noise so that it dominates the result and obscures any useful detail, although the edges are sharp. Apodization (skipping those frequency terms for which the division would produce numeric overflow) achieves a better result, but there is evidence of ringing, and some blur remains. Wiener filtering (**Figure 6.59**) reduces this problem and allows adjustment that trades off the sharpness of the restoration (higher K values leave more blurring) against the amount of noise (higher K values reduce the noise). Because of the low signal-to-noise ratio and large amount of blurring in the original, it is not possible in this case to recover all the internal details of the original image.

The Wiener deconvolution has a long history as a practical method for achieving useful, if not perfect, blur removal. The Wiener method is an optimal restoration technique when the signal (the image) is blurred and corrupted by random additive noise, in the statistical sense that it minimizes the errors between the actual (true) image and the reconstructed result. Another approach of long standing is the Van Cittert iterative technique. This method has apparently been discovered many times and is also known as a Bially or Landweber iteration. Instead of trying to remove the entire blur in one step, a series of iterative removal steps is performed. In the limit, this iteration would reach the same result as an ideal deconvolution, but instead it is terminated before convergence, resulting in a (partially) deblurred image that does not exhibit an unacceptable noise level. The quality of the results is generally similar to that of the Wiener method.

There are many other methods, most of them much more complicated mathematically (and requiring much more computation and time). Many of them are iterative, trying to find the best form of the blur function and the deblurred image. Typically, this involves trying to solve a very large number of simultaneous equations, which may be over- or underdetermined. The techniques for such solutions occupy a significant mathematical literature, and arise again in the context of three-dimensional imaging (**Chapter 12**). One of the issues is how to efficiently guide the iteration and how to determine when to terminate it. Another related question is the

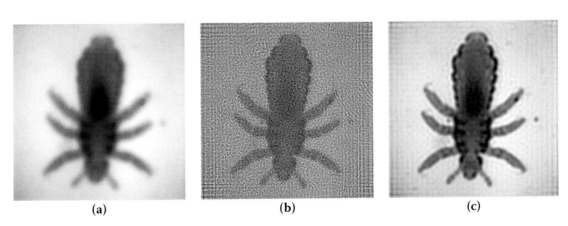

(a) (b) (c)

Figure 6.58 *Effect of noise on deconvolution: **(a)** severely blurred image of the bug in **Figure 6.53** with added random noise; **(b)** ideal inverse deconvolution with noise present; **(c)** deconvolution with apodization.*

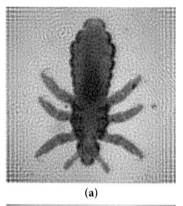

(a)

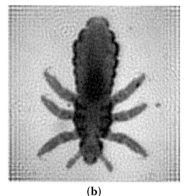

(b)

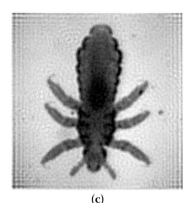

(c)

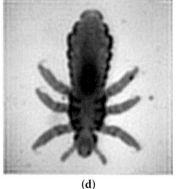

(d)

Figure 6.59 Wiener filtering of the image in *Figure 6.58a*: images *a* through *d* show that increasing the empirical K value reduces noise at the expense of sharpness.

best measure of image quality, which in different implementations may be based on Bayesian statistics, maximization of entropy, etc. The calculations can be performed in either the frequency or the spatial domain. Even a small PSF in the spatial domain becomes as large as the entire image in the frequency domain, and the number of simultaneous equations is the number of pixels in the image.

Most of these methods are highly specific to particular types of applications and depend on the *a priori* information that can be supplied, usually in the form of constraints on the solution of the equations. For example, a commonly used constraint is that negative values for pixels have no physical meaning, and so values are not permitted to become negative. If more information on the image can be incorporated, such as the presence of a constant background over much of the image area (as in astronomical or fluorescence images) or known specific pixel values that should be permitted, it improves the quality of the result and the efficiency of reaching it. The details of these methods are far beyond the scope of this text, but a very clear and comprehensive review and comparison can be found in Lagendijk and Biemond (1991).

Another area of current interest is the deconvolution of multiple images that are related to each other. This includes multiple channel images (e.g., different wavelengths or colors) of the same scene or a series of images from parallel, closely spaced planes in semitransparent specimens (e.g., a series of focal planes in the light microscope). Using information from one channel or plane can be used to guide the deconvolution of another.

If the blur is not known *a priori*, it can often be estimated from the power spectrum or by trial and error to find an optimum (or at least useful) result. A recent development in deconvolution that has great efficiency because it is not an iterative method has been published by Carasso (2001). Interactive adjustment of the Wiener *K* constant and the shape of the PSF function is practical using Wiener deconvolution. **Figure 6.60** shows an example in which a basic Gaussian shape with adjustable width and astigmatism is manipulated while viewing the deconvolved result. The Gaussian shape is convenient, but other mathematical functions are also used. For example, a simple disk (intended to model the aperture of a camera) is used in the deconvolution (called the "smart sharpening" method) in Adobe Photoshop 9. Functions that have a peak "sharper" than a Gaussian with a broad "skirt" often produce good results with real images. **Figure 6.61** shows one example and compares the results with a Gaussian.

Analysis of the shape of the radial profile of the values in the Fourier transform of the blurred image (avoiding the regions dominated by noise) allows constructing an approximate PSF that can be used for deconvolution. This method cannot be used for all types of blur functions (particularly motion blur), but produces very good results for those situations where it is applicable.

One application for these image restoration techniques is deblurring the images formed by optical sectioning. This is the technique in which a series of images are recorded from different depths of focus in a semitransparent specimen using a light microscope. The passage of light through the overlying layers of the specimen cause a blurring that adversely affects the sharpness and contrast of the images, preventing their being assembled into a three-dimensional stack for visualization and measurement of the three-dimensional structures present.

The confocal light microscope overcomes some of these problems by rejecting light from points away from the point of focus, which improves the contrast of the images. (It also reduces the depth of field of the optics, producing higher resolution in the depth axis, which is important particularly at the highest magnifications.) But the scattering and diffraction of light by the upper layers of the specimen still degrades the image resolution.

In principle, the images of the upper layers contain information that can be used to deconvolute those from below. This would allow sharpening of those images. The entire process is iterative and highly computer-intensive, the more so because the blurring of each point on each image may be different from other points. In practice, it is usual to make some assumptions about the blurring and noise content of the images that are used as global averages for a given specimen or for a given optical setup.

Even with these assumptions, the computations are still intensive and iterative. There is a considerable theoretical and limited practical literature in this field (Carrington 1990; Dey

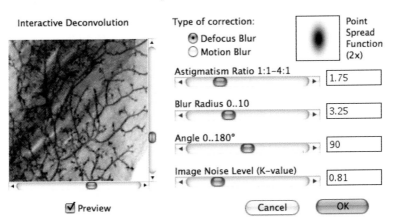

Figure 6.60 *An interactive dialog for Wiener deconvolution with adjustments for the shape of the Gaussian PSF. (Courtesy of Reindeer Graphics, Asheville, NC.)*

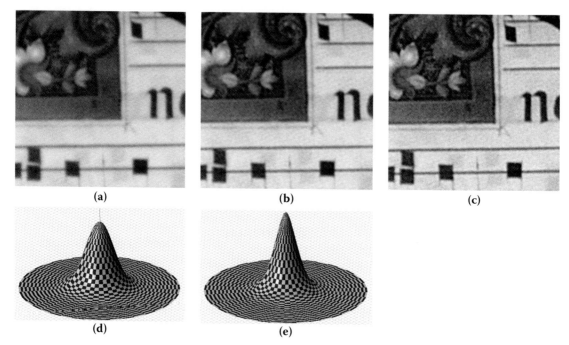

Figure 6.61 *Comparison of deconvolution results using different PSF functions: (a) original (macro photo of an illuminated manuscript with significant pixel noise); (b) best result using the Gaussian PSF shown in image d; (c) best result using the function shown in image e; (d) Gaussian PSF shape $z = exp(-r^2)$; (e) mathematical function with sharper peak $z = exp(-r^{1.7})$.*

et al. 2006; Holmes et al. 1995; Holmes et al. 2000; Joshi and Miller 1993; Monck et al. 1992; Richardson 1972; Snyder et al. 1992; von Tiedemann et al. 2006; Willis et al. 1993). A review of several of the leading methods can be found in Van Kempen et al. (1997). The examples shown deal only with idealized structures and averaging assumptions about the noise characteristics of the images and the point-spread function of the microscope, which suggests that restoration of real images may not be as good as those examples. Similar concerns and methods can in principle be applied to other *in situ* three-dimensional imaging techniques such as tomography and seismic imagery.

On a simpler level, many digital cameras store images with more pixels than correspond to the actual resolution of the chips, for instance because of the interpolation of color information from a filtered single chip (as described in **Chapter 1**). Even when the images are well focused optically, significant improvement in the image sharpness and resolution can often be produced by deconvolution, as shown in **Figure 6.62**. As noted previously, the improvement in resolution is quite distinct from the effect of a high-pass filter such as the unsharp mask. **Figure 6.63** compares the results of the two procedures. The unsharp mask increases contrast for existing edges (and creates halos adjacent to edges) but does not resolve additional detail, as deconvolution does.

Additional defects besides out-of-focus optics can be corrected by deconvolution as well. These operations are not always performed in the frequency domain, but the basic understanding of the process of removing the blur convolution imposed by the system is most clearly illustrated there. One of the most common defects is blur caused by motion. This is rarely a problem in microscopy applications (except perhaps for stage drift at very high magnifications), but it can

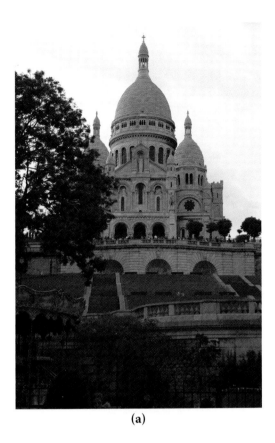

(a)

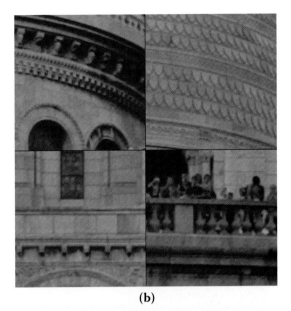

(b)

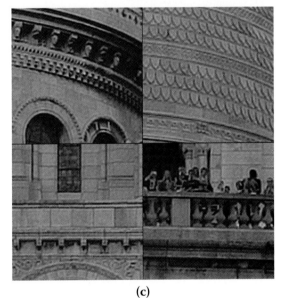

(c)

Figure 6.62 Deconvolution sharpening of an image from a digital still camera:

(a) original image, captured without compression with a high-end single-lens-reflex Nikon digital still camera (the original image file is 38.7 MB);

(b) enlarged details from image **a**;

(c) same areas as image **b** after Wiener deconvolution with a Gaussian PSF with standard deviation of 0.95 pixels.

be very important in remote sensing, in which light levels are low and the exposure time must be long enough for significant camera motion to occur with respect to the scene.

Fortunately, in most of these circumstances the amount and direction of motion is known. That makes it possible to draw a line in the spatial domain that defines the blur. The frequency transform of this line is then divided into the transform of the blurred image. Retransforming the resulting image restores the sharp result. **Figure 6.64** illustrates the possibilities. Notice in this example that a slight rotational motion of the camera during the exposure has caused imperfect restoration at the top and bottom edges of the image. The deconvolution process assumes that the same PSF applies to the entire image area.

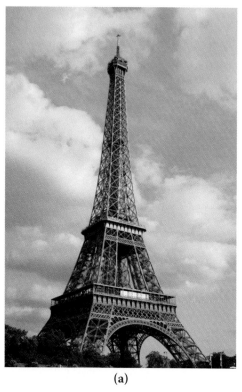

(a)

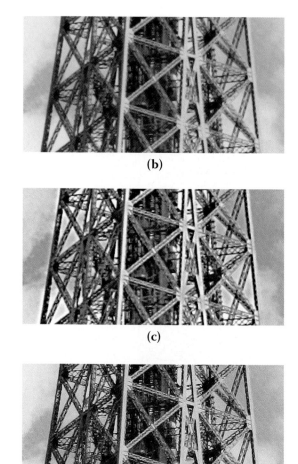

(b)

(c)

(d)

Figure 6.63 *Comparison of deconvolution with a high-pass filter:*
(a) *original image;*
(b) *enlarged detail from image **a**;*
(c) *same area as image **b** after the application of an unsharp mask;*
(d) *same area as image **b** after Wiener deconvolution.*

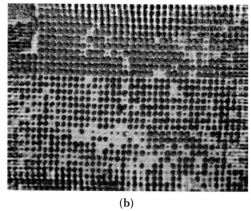

(a)

(b)

Figure 6.64 *Removal of motion blur: **(a)** original image (aerial photo of an orchard) with superimposed motion vector (enlarged); **(b)** deconvolved result.*

It is important to note the similarity and the difference between this example and the removal of out-of-focus blur. Both involve dividing the transform of the blurred image by that of the defect. This follows directly from the equation presented for convolution, in which the transform of the convolved image is the product of those from the original image and the defect. The major difference is that in the motion blur case we can sometimes calculate the exact blurring vector to be removed, or at least estimate the blur vector from the image. As in the example shown above for out-of-focus blur, the use of a Wiener deconvolution can partially alleviate the effects of noise.

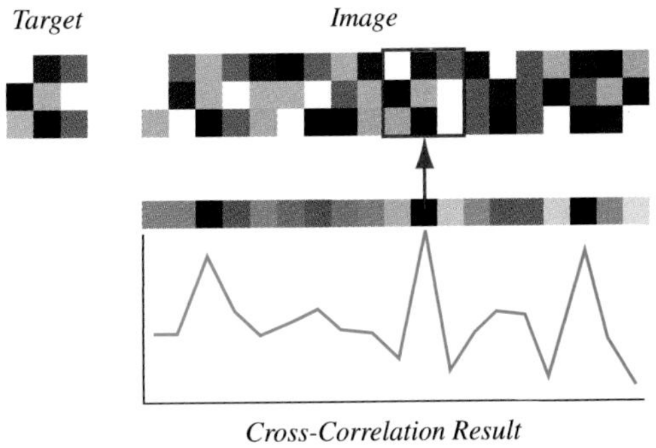

Figure 6.65 *Cross-correlation matches a pattern of gray-scale values to many points in the target image to find the location with the best match. In the tiny example shown here, the 3 × 3 target is applied to every possible position in the image to produce the line of values shown. The marked location is most similar (but not identical) to the target.*

Template matching and correlation

Closely related to the spatial-domain convolution application of a kernel for smoothing, derivatives, etc., is the idea of template matching or cross-correlation. In this case, a target pattern is shifted to every location in the image, the values are multiplied by the pixels that are overlaid, and the total is stored at that position to form an image showing where regions identical or similar to the target are located. **Figure 6.65** illustrates this process. The multiplication and summation process is identical to convolution, except that the target is rotated 180° first so that the upper left corner value in the target pattern is multiplied by the lower right value in the neighborhood on the image, and so forth. When the process is performed in frequency space, this is equivalent to convolution but with a 180° phase shift of the Fourier-transform values.

This method is used in many contexts to locate features within images. One is searching reconnaissance images for particular objects such as vehicles. Tracking the motion of hurricanes in a series of weather satellite images or cells moving on a microscope slide can also use this approach. Modified to deal optimally with binary images, it can be used to find letters in text. When the target is a pattern of pixel brightness values from one image in a stereo pair and the searched image is the second image from the pair, the method can be used to perform fusion (locating matching points in the two images) to measure parallax and calculate elevation, as shown in **Chapter 13**, **Figure 13.8**.

For continuous two-dimensional functions, the cross-correlation image is calculated as

$$c(i,j) = \iint f(x,y)g(x-i, y-j)dx\,dy \tag{6.14}$$

Replacing the integrals by finite sums over the dimensions of the image gives **Equation 6.15**. To normalize the result of this template matching or correlation without the absolute brightness value of the region of the image biasing the results, the operation in the spatial domain is usually calculated as the sum of the products of the pixel brightnesses divided by their geometric mean.

$$\frac{\displaystyle\sum_{i,j} f_{x+i,y+j} \cdot g_{i,j}}{\sqrt{\displaystyle\sum_{i,j} f_{x+i,y+j}^2 \cdot \sum_{i,j} g_{i,j}^2}} \tag{6.15}$$

When the dimensions of the summation are large, this is a slow and inefficient process compared with the equivalent operation in frequency space. The frequency-space operation is simply

$$C(u,v) = F(u,v)G*(u,v) \tag{6.16}$$

where * indicates the complex conjugate of the function values. The complex conjugate affects only the phase of the complex values, so the operation is very similar to convolution, and indeed it is often performed using many of the same program subroutines. Operations that involve two images (division for deconvolution, multiplication for convolution, and multiplication by the conjugate for correlation) are sometimes called dyadic operations, to distinguish them from filtering and masking operations (monadic operations) in which a single frequency-transform image is operated on. (The filter or mask image is not a frequency-domain image and does not contain complex values.)

Usually, when correlation is performed, the wraparound assumption joining the left and right edges and the top and bottom of the image is not acceptable. In these cases, each image should be padded by surrounding it with zeros or the mean value of the image to bring it to the next larger size for transformation (the next exact power of 2, required by many FFT routines). Since the correlation operation also requires that the actual magnitude values of the transforms be used, slightly better mathematical precision can be achieved by padding with the average values of the original image brightnesses rather than with zeros. It can also be useful to subtract the average brightness value from each pixel, which removes the zeroth (DC) term from the transformation. Since this value is usually the largest in the transform (it is the value at the central pixel), its elimination allows the transform data greater dynamic range.

Correlation is primarily used for locating features in one image that also appear in another. **Figure 6.66** shows an example. The image contains text with some random noise, while the target contains the letter A by itself. The result of the cross-correlation (after retransforming the image to the spatial domain) shows peaks where the target letter is found, which may be more apparent when the same image is presented as an isometric display. The brightest points in the correlation image correspond to the occurrences of the letter A in the same size and font as the target. There are lower but still significant peaks corresponding to two of the other letter As, in different fonts, but in general cross-correlation is quite size- and shape-specific.

When combined with other image processing tools to analyze the cross-correlation image, this is an extremely fast and efficient tool for locating known features in images. In the example of **Figure 6.67**, a very large number of SEM images of Nuclepore filters with latex spheres presented a problem for automatic counting because of the variation in contrast and noise, the presence of dirt, and the texture presented by the filters themselves. Also, the contrast of an isolated sphere is consistently different than that of one surrounded by other spheres.

A target image (**Figure 6.67a**) was created by averaging together ten representative latex spheres. This was then cross-correlated with each image, a top-hat filter (inner radius = 3 pixels, outer radius = 5 pixels, height = 8 gray-scale values) applied to isolate each peak in the image, and the resulting spots counted automatically. The figure shows a few example images from the set, with marks showing the particles that were found and counted. After the top-hat

EABCDEABCDI
ABCDEABCDE
BCDE ABCDE A
CDEABCDEAB
DE *ABCDE* ABC
EABCDEABCD
ABCDEABCDE

(a)

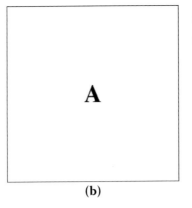

(b)

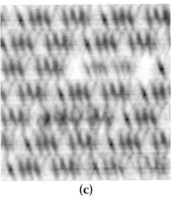

(c)

Figure 6.66 *Cross-correlation example:*

(a) image containing many letters with superimposed random noise;

(b) target letter;

(c) cross-correlation result (gray-scale representation of goodness of match);

(d) isometric view of image showing peaks on the A's in the original;

(e) thresholded peaks in image c superimposed on image a. Note that only the letters in the same size and font have been located.

(d)

EABCDEABCDI
ABCDEABCDE
BCDE ABCDE A
CDEABCDEAB
DE *ABCDE* ABC
EABCDEABCD
ABCDEABCDE

(e)

filter has been applied to select the peaks in the cross-correlation image, the resulting spots can be convolved with the stored target image to produce the result shown in **Figure 6.68**, which shows just the latex spheres without the other features (dirt, background texture, etc.) present in the original image.

Cross-correlation is also used as a tool for aligning serial-section images. Even if the images are not identical (as in general they are not), there are usually enough common features that a sharp cross-correlation peak occurs when two successive images are in best x,y alignment. The location of the peak can be determined to subpixel accuracy and used to shift the images into optimum alignment. **Figure 6.69** shows an example. The two sequential slices of Swiss cheese have subtle differences in the position and size of holes, and in fact several small holes present in each slice are not present in the other, which is an important requirement for a stereological measurement tool (the Disector) discussed in **Chapter 9**. However, comparisons are difficult to make until the two slices have been properly aligned, as shown.

Alignment is important for all of the serial-section reconstruction methods described in **Chapter 12** and **Chapter 13**. It is also necessary for the merging of multiple focal planes into an extended-focus image, as described in **Chapter 5**. **Figure 6.70** shows an example of a focal series from a light microscope in which the successive planes are offset because of mechanical and optical effects in the microscope. Superposition of the edge-filtered images (using

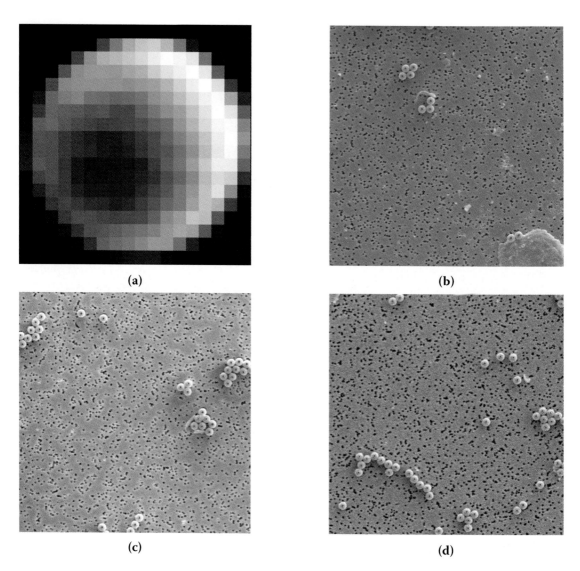

(a)

(b)

(c)

(d)

Figure 6.67 *Cross-correlation to detect and count latex spheres on Nuclepore filters: **(a)** average of ten representative latex spheres, used as a target; **(b–d)** representative example images, with red spots marking the result of the procedure described in the text.*

a Sobel edge-delineation filter as described in **Chapter 5**) in the red and green channels of **Figure 6.70c** shows the offset. Automatically correcting this offset for each plane to subpixel accuracy by cross-correlation allows an extended-focus image to be formed from the entire set of images.

Standard video consists of alternate fields containing the even- and odd-numbered scan lines. If the camera is rapidly panned or the image subject is moving, this can produce an offset between the fields, which shows up in the digitized image as shown in **Figure 6.71**. By treating the two fields (i.e., the even- and odd-numbered scan lines) as separate images, cross-correlation can be used to correct the offset, as shown in **Figure 6.71b**. Notice that there are still some residual local differences between the even and odd lines because the motion of the subject is not perfectly uniform.

In extreme cases, such as a video of a running person, many different subregions of the image (body, arms, legs, etc.) will move in different ways. In some cases it is possible to break the image into regions and align each one separately. Also, the cross-correlation method does not deal with rotation, but it is possible to iteratively rotate the images and use the peak cross-correlation value as a measure of quality to determine the best value, or for small rotations to perform alignment on subregions of the image and from the offsets calculate an overall rotation amount. Alignment of serial sections that include arbitrary shifts, rotations, and distortions can also be performed based on a small number of matched points between images, as described in **Chapter 13**.

Autocorrelation

In the special case when the image functions f and g (and their transforms F and G) are the same, the correlation operation is called autocorrelation. This is used to combine all parts of the image to find

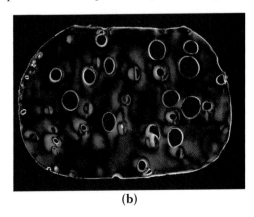

Figure 6.68 Convolution of the target image from *Figure 6.67a*, with the binary image of peaks found by the top-hat filter applied to the cross-correlation image (the red marks superimposed on *Figure 6.67d*), showing just the latex spheres.

repetitive structures. Interpretation of the autocorrelation image can be understood by imagining the image to be printed on transparency and placed on top of itself. By sliding the top image laterally in any direction, the degree of match with the underlying original is measured by the autocorrelation function. When features still reside on themselves, the match is high. Likewise, when a large shift brings a feature onto another similar one, the match is again high.

For images in which there is a more-or-less regular arrangement of features, the autocorrelation image finds this pattern and also facilitates its measurement, as shown in **Figure 6.72**. In the image, the darkness and shape of each spot shows the probability of finding another

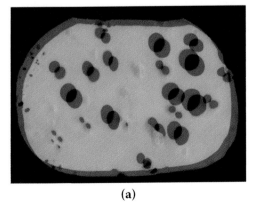

(a)

(b)

Figure 6.69 Automatic alignment using cross-correlation: *(a)* two superimposed images of sequential slices of Swiss cheese; *(b)* absolute-difference combination of the two images after alignment, showing slight differences in hole position and size that are useful for measurement.

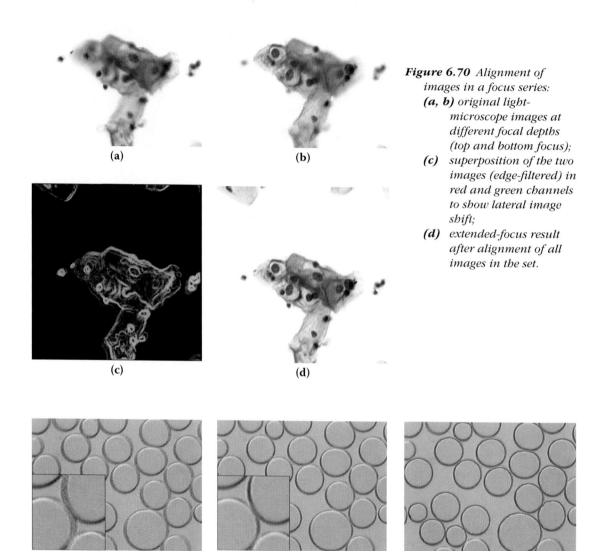

Figure 6.70 Alignment of images in a focus series: **(a, b)** original light-microscope images at different focal depths (top and bottom focus); **(c)** superposition of the two images (edge-filtered) in red and green channels to show lateral image shift; **(d)** extended-focus result after alignment of all images in the set.

Figure 6.71 De-interlacing a video image: **(a)** original image of bubbles moving in a flowing channel, producing offset of even and odd scan lines (with inset showing enlarged detail); **(b)** result after automatic alignment of the fields by correlation; **(c)** thresholding and processing of the binary image (using procedures from **Chapter** 7 and **Chapter** 8) produces bubble outlines for measurement.

particle at a given distance and direction. The circularly averaged radial plot shows the gradual increase in the disorder of the arrangement with distance.

For images in which individual particles partially obscure each other, so that individual measurements of size is impractical, autocorrelation sometimes provides a simple and powerful way to measure the size, shape, and even size distribution. **Figure 6.73** shows the surfaces of two different cheeses, produced with different pH. Visually, there is a difference in the size of the structuring element present in the two specimens, but because this is a rough surface and

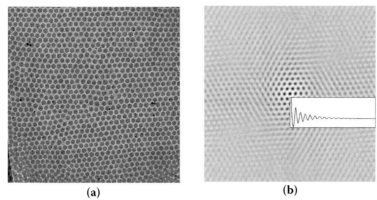

(a)   **(b)**

Figure 6.72 *Finding a regular arrangement pattern with autocorrelation: **(a)** TEM image of latex spheres, which are arranged in an approximately hexagonal pattern; **(b)** autocorrelation image showing the pattern of neighbor distance and direction, with an inset showing the measurement of a circularly averaged radial profile.*

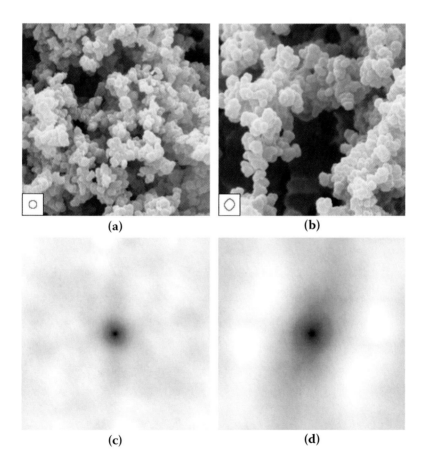

(a)   **(b)**

(c)   **(d)**

Figure 6.73 *Measurement of overlapped features: **(a, b)** SEM images of two cheeses, produced with different pH, and consisting of different size structures (insets show outlines of mean feature size obtained by thresholding the peaks in images **c** and **d**, as described in the text); **(c, d)** autocorrelation results for images **a** and **b**.*

the particles are piled up rather than dispersed, traditional feature measurements are not possible. The autocorrelation images are also shown.

As noted above, the central peak represents the distance that the image can be shifted laterally before features no longer lie on top of themselves. The dimension of the central peak thus provides a handy measure for the size of the structuring elements in the cheese. In the figure, this is shown for the two structures by drawing a contour line on the autocorrelation image at the 50% magnitude level, to represent an average size. The intensity profile of the peak also provides information on the size distribution of the particles.

In **Chapter 14**, autocorrelation is used to measure the texture of surface roughness in terms of the characteristic distance over which the amplitude of the peak drops. **Figure 6.74** shows another use of the autocorrelation function, to measure preferred orientation. The image is a felted textile material. Due to the fabrication process, the fibers do not have a randomized or uniform orientation; neither are they regularly arranged. The intensity profiles of the autocorrelation central spot along its major and minor axes measure the preferred orientation quantitatively.

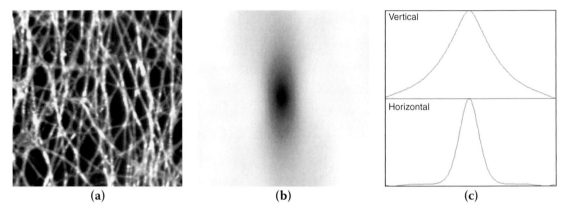

(a)   (b)   (c)

Figure 6.74 *Measurement of preferred orientation: **(a)** image of felted textile fibers; **(b)** the autocorrelation peak (enlarged); **(c)** horizontal and vertical intensity profiles of the peak.*

Segmentation and Thresholding

Thresholding

Selecting features within a scene or image is an important prerequisite for most kinds of measurement or analysis of the scene. Traditionally, one simple way this selection has been accomplished is to define a range of brightness values in the original image, select the pixels within this range as belonging to the foreground, and reject all of the other pixels to the background. Such an image is then usually displayed as a binary or two-level image, using black and white (or sometimes other colors) to distinguish the regions. There is no standard convention on whether the features of interest are white or black; the choice depends on the particular display hardware in use and the designer's preference; in the examples shown here, the features are black and the background is white, which matches most modern computer displays and printing that show black text on a white background.

The selection process is usually called thresholding. Thresholds can be set interactively by a user watching the image and using a colored overlay to show the result of turning a knob or otherwise adjusting the settings. As a consequence of the ubiquitous use of a mouse as the human interface to a graphical computer display, the user can adjust virtual sliders or mark a region on a histogram to select the range of brightness values. The brightness histogram of the image (or a region of it) is often used for making adjustments. As discussed in earlier chapters, the histogram is a plot of the number of pixels in the image having each brightness level. For a typical 8-bit monochrome image, this equals 2^8 or 256 gray-scale values. The plot can be presented in a variety of formats, either vertical or horizontal, and some displays use color or gray-scale coding to assist the viewer in distinguishing the white and black sides of the plot. **Figure 7.1** illustrates the basics of the technique; many programs add provisions to adjust the color of the preview, to enlarge and scroll the image, and sometimes to implement automatic threshold settings, as discussed later in this chapter.

Systems that handle images with a greater tonal range than 256 levels (8 bits per color channel) — as are obtained from scanners, some digital cameras, and other instruments — can have as many as 16 bits (65,536 distinct pixel values). As a matter of convenience and consistency, both for thresholding purposes and to preserve the meaning of the various numeric constants introduced in preceding chapters, such images can still be described as having a brightness range of 0 to 255 to cover the range from black to white. But instead of being limited to integer

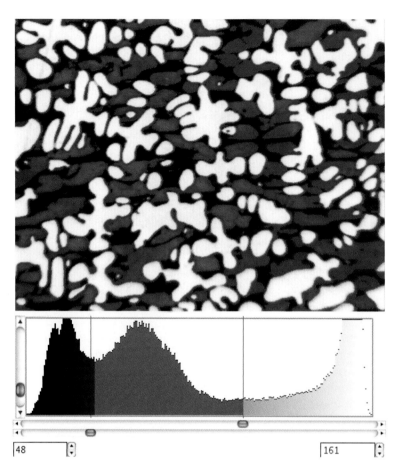

Figure 7.1 *Example of thresholding an image by setting brightness limits on the histogram. A mouse is used to drag the sliders, the selected pixels are shaded in color, and the numeric values of the limits are shown.*

brightness values, the greater precision of the data allows brightnesses to be reported as real numbers (e.g., a pixel value of 31,605 out of 65,536 would be divided by 256 and reported as 123.457). This makes it possible to compare values independent of the original image depth or dynamic range, but it does not solve the problem of displaying such a range of values in a histogram. A full histogram of more than 65,000 values would be too wide for any computer screen, and for a typical image size would have so few counts in each channel as to be uninterpretable. Generally, the counts are binned into a smaller number of channels for viewing, but still more than the 256 bins used for 8-bit images. **Figure 7.2** shows the additional detail and the visibility of additional peaks that appear as more channels are used for the histogram.

Examples of histograms have been shown in earlier chapters. Note that the histogram counts pixels in the entire image (or in a defined region of interest), losing all information about the original location of the pixels or the brightness values of their neighbors. Peaks in the histogram can identify the various homogeneous regions (often referred to as phases, although they correspond to a phase in the chemical sense only in a few applications), and thresholds can then be set between the peaks. There are also automatic methods to adjust threshold settings (Kittler et al. 1985; Lee et al. 1990; Melgani 2006; Otsu 1979; Prewitt and Mendelsohn 1966; Rigaut 1988; Russ 1995c; Russ and Russ 1988a; Sahoo et al. 1988; Weszka 1978), using

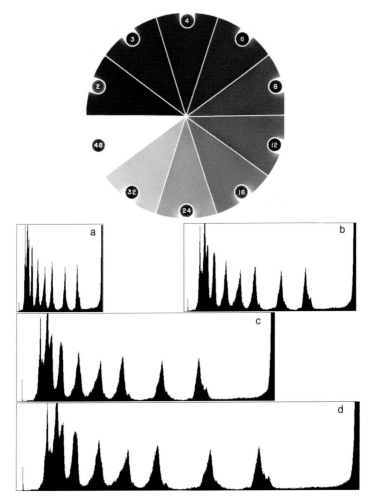

Figure 7.2 *A 16-bit image of a density calibration standard, and the histogram of brightness values: (a) conventional 256-channel histogram; (b) 512 channels; (c) 768 channels; (d) 1024 channels. Larger arrays generally do not fit well on a computer monitor.*

either the histogram or the image itself as a guide, as we will see below. Specialized methods are available to compare *a priori* knowledge with the measurement parameters obtained from features in the image at many threshold levels (Wolf 1991).

The presumption that a peak in the histogram corresponds to a structure in the image may be true in some settings, but it often does not hold for real-world images such as **Figure 7.3**. Under the more controlled lighting conditions of a microscope, and with sample preparation that includes selective staining or other procedures, this situation is more likely to be met. In some of the difficult cases, direct thresholding of the image is still possible, but the settings are not obvious from examination of the histogram peaks (if indeed the histogram has distinct peaks). In many circumstances, the brightness levels of individual pixels are not uniquely related to structure. In some of these instances, prior image processing, as described in **Chapter 5**, can be used to transform the original brightness values in the image to a new image, in which pixel brightness represents some derived parameter such as the local texture, brightness gradient, or direction.

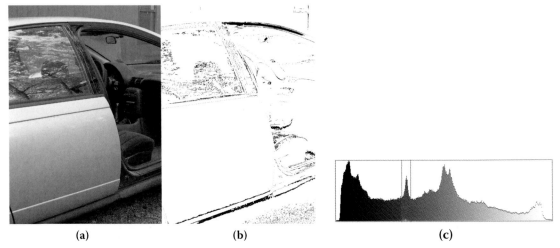

(a)   (b)   (c)

Figure 7.3 *Thresholding a real-world image based on a histogram peak: **(a)** the original image and the pixels selected by setting the levels shown in image **b**; **(c)** histogram showing a peak with threshold limits. The locations of pixels with the selected brightness values do not correspond to any obvious structural unit in the original scene.*

It is not always necessary to threshold the image to make measurements such as determining the area fraction of each structure. Histogram analysis can be done by fitting Gaussian (or other shape) functions to the histogram. Given the number of Gaussian peaks to combine for a best overall fit, the position, width, and height of each can be determined by multiple regression. This permits estimating the area of each phase, but of course cannot determine the spatial position of the pixels in each phase if the peaks overlap. The result is generally poor because few real imaging situations produce ideally Gaussian peaks (or any other consistent shape). One exception is MRI (magnetic resonance imaging) images, where this method has been applied to produce images in which pixels in the overlap areas are not converted to black or white, but shaded according to the relative contributions of the two overlapping Gaussian peaks at that brightness value (Frank et al. 1995). This does not, of course, produce a segmented image in the conventional sense, but it can produce viewable images that delineate the overlapped structures (e.g., dark matter and white matter in brain scans).

Automatic settings

Manual adjustment of thresholds to produce a result that is considered to be correct based on visual inspection by a human operator is common, but in most cases this should be avoided if possible. In addition to taking time and being incompatible with automatic processing, different results are likely to be obtained at different times or by different people. Manual thresholding errors are probably responsible for more problems in subsequent image analysis than any other cause.

A number of algorithms have been developed for automating the thresholding procedure, as discussed below. Some of them, primarily used in machine-vision setups for industrial quality control, are more concerned with reproducibility than with absolute accuracy. Most of the automatic methods utilize the histogram in their calculations, but some also involve the image itself to make use of the location information for the pixels (and their neighbors). All automatic

methods make some assumptions about the nature of the image, and if one is to choose the proper algorithm it is important to know as much as possible about the nature of the image, how it was acquired, and what kinds of scenes or subjects are dealt with.

In machine-vision systems, it is rarely practical to set constant threshold levels to select the features of interest. Changes over time in the illumination, the camera, or the positioning or cleanliness of the parts being examined make it necessary to have a method that adapts to the actual images. However, it is sometimes possible, by controlling the placement and color of the lighting, to produce images that have simple histograms. If the histogram has a fixed number of well-defined peaks, automatic tracking of peak locations can adjust the threshold values for changes such as those listed above.

Probably the simplest method of all is to locate the peaks in the histogram and set the thresholds midway between them. This approach is robust, because the peaks usually have well-defined shapes and easily found positions. While it is a very reproducible method, it is not very accurate at defining the actual structures present. There is no particular reason to expect the midpoint to correspond to the boundary between regions, and as pointed out in **Chapter 1**, some cameras have a linear and others a logarithmic response. But if the goal is consistency, a simple method like this has obvious appeal.

Another method that is sometimes used is selecting a fixed percentage of the brightest or darkest pixels to produce a binary image. The procedure is to start at one end of the histogram and sum the histogram bins until the intended fraction of the image area is reached. The threshold setting is then the brightness level of the last bin counted. This approach works well in applications such as locating holes in a backlit workpiece, where the position of the holes may vary but their total area will remain constant.

Many of the algorithms developed for automatic setting of thresholds were intended for the discrimination of printed text on paper, as a first step in optical character recognition (OCR) programs that scan pages and convert them to text files for editing or communication. **Figure 7.4** shows an example of a page of scanned text with the results of several of these algorithms. Note that there is no "valley between two peaks" present in this histogram, so methods that look for a bimodal histogram cannot be used. All of the statistical methods assume that there are two populations of pixels, and each method applies a statistical test to select a threshold that "best" distinguishes these populations.

Each method makes different assumptions about the nature of the histogram and the appropriate statistical or other tests that can be used to divide it into two parts, each representing one of the two structures present (paper and ink). An excellent summary of the more widely used methods can be found in Parker (Parker 1997) and in other works (Otsu 1979; Trussell 1979; Yager 1979), and a recent comprehensive survey of all techniques is available in Sezgin and Sankur (2004). Only a brief summary of a few methods is given here.

The Trussell algorithm (Trussell 1979) is probably the most widely used automatic method because it usually produces a fairly good result (**Figure 7.4d**) and is easy to implement. It finds the threshold setting that produces two populations of pixels (brighter and darker) with the largest value of the Student's t-statistic, which is calculated from the means of the two groups (μ), their standard deviations (σ), and the number of pixels in each (n), as shown in **Equation 7.1**. This is a standard statistical test that measures the probability that the two populations are indeed different, so finding the threshold setting that produces the maximum value for t should correspond to the desired separation of the two groups of pixels. But it makes the hidden assumption that the populations are properly represented by the mean and standard

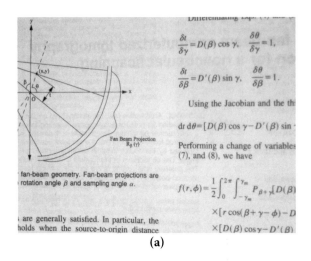

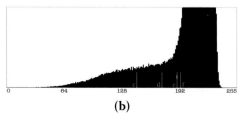

(b)

fan-beam geometry. Fan-beam projections are rotation angle β and sampling angle α.

$$\frac{\delta t}{\delta\gamma} = D(\beta)\cos\gamma, \quad \frac{\delta\theta}{\delta\gamma} = 1,$$

$$\frac{\delta t}{\delta\beta} = D'(\beta)\sin\gamma, \quad \frac{\delta\theta}{\delta\beta} = 1.$$

Using the Jacobian and the th

$$dt\, d\theta = [D(\beta)\cos\gamma - D'(\beta)\sin$$

Performing a change of variables (7), and (8), we have

$$f(r,\phi) = \frac{1}{2}\int_0^{2\pi}\int_{-\gamma_m}^{\gamma_m} P_{\beta+}[D(\beta)$$
$$\times [r\cos(\beta+\gamma-\phi)-D$$
$$\times [D(\beta)\cos\gamma - D'(\beta)$$

are generally satisfied. In particular, the holds when the source-to-origin distance

(a)

Figure 7.4 Automatic thresholding of printed text on paper using algorithms from Parker (1997): **(a)** original gray-scale scan; **(b)** histogram, showing the settings used in the following examples; **(c)** Yager algorithm, threshold = 134; **(d)** Trussell algorithm, threshold = 172; **(e)** Shannon entropy algorithm, threshold = 184; **(f)** Kittler algorithm, threshold = 196.

Using the Jacobian and the th

$$dt\, d\theta = [D(\beta)\cos\gamma - D'(\beta)\sin$$

Performing a change of variables (7), and (8), we have

(c)

Using the Jacobian and the thi

$$dt\, d\theta = [D(\beta)\cos\gamma - D'(\beta)\sin$$

Performing a change of variables (7), and (8), we have

(d)

Using the Jacobian and the thi

$$dt\, d\theta = [D(\beta)\cos\gamma - D'(\beta)\sin$$

Performing a change of variables (7), and (8), we have

(e)

Using the Jacobian and the thi

$$dt\, d\theta = [D(\beta)\cos\gamma - D'(\beta)\sin$$

Performing a change of variables (7), and (8), we have

(f)

deviation — in other words, that they are normally distributed — and many histograms do not consist of Gaussian peaks.

$$t = \frac{|\mu_F - \mu_B|}{\sqrt{\dfrac{\sigma_F^2}{n_F} - \dfrac{\sigma_B^2}{n_B}}} \tag{7.1}$$

Another approach that often produces good (but slightly different) results and is nonparametric (i.e., does not assume a shape for the histogram) uses the entropy of the two sets of pixels (above and below the threshold setting), and is illustrated in **Figure 7.4e**. There are several different models for calculating the relevant entropy, which produce somewhat different results (Abutaleb 1989; Brink and Pendcock 1989; Kapur et al. 1985). **Equation 7.2** shows the calculation for the simplest form, in which the total entropy H for the foreground and background is maximized by selecting a threshold value t. The p_i values are calculated from the actual histogram counts $h(i)$ by dividing by the total number of pixels in that portion of the histogram.

$$H = H_B + H_F$$

$$H_B = -\sum_{i=0}^{t} p_i \log(p_i)$$

$$H_F = -\sum_{i=t+1}^{255} p_i \log(p_i) \tag{7.2}$$

$$p_i = \frac{h(i)}{\sum_k h(k)}$$

Many of the algorithms summarized in Parker produce similar results on this image, but some of the results do not separate the characters entirely, and others cause them to break up. There is no one method that works for all types of printing, paper, and image-acquisition settings. And even if there were, the problem being addressed is much more specialized than the general range of images containing just two types of structures, and many images contain more than two. Some of these methods can be generalized to more than two populations of pixels. For example, the Student's t-test method, when applied to more than two groups, becomes the well-known analysis of variance. But in general it is necessary to have *a priori* knowledge of the number of groups present.

The accuracy and precision of automatic thresholding depends on choosing the appropriate method, which amounts to using independent knowledge about the specimen or scene and the imaging hardware. For example, von Bradke et al. (2004) reported that manual settings produced more consistent (in the sense of reproducible, not necessarily accurate) results than automatically setting the threshold to the minimum point in the histogram. Of course, the selection of the minimum is an inherently flawed method anyway, because the minimum point is noisy and unstable, and will move relative to the peaks when the area fractions vary (exactly what you do not want to happen). In addition, changing the overall image brightness (contrast, gain, and gamma), as was done for this series of SEM (scanning electron microscope) images, would also change the minimum point.

However, in this case the most noteworthy problem was that the histogram for a typical image had a large bright peak (corresponding to the polished surface) and a long, nearly flat tail for darker values, including the porosity. In many cases there was no evident minimum, so the technique simply chose a value based on the statistical fluctuations in the counts, with the predictable result that the threshold bounced around wildly. When the values were set by hand, while looking at the image, a different algorithm (probably something based on the smoothness of the periphery of the pores) was used by the operator. Note that achieving reproducibility in this case does not imply accuracy; the low image magnification (many pores were only one or a few pixels across), and questions about rounding of edges in sample preparation as well as considerations of electron beam penetration in the sample, would also produce bias in the results. Other critical tests of automatic methods (e.g., Francus and Pinard 2004; Jalba et al. 2004; Ozkaya et al. 2005) have also examined the performance of specific algorithms on real-world images.

Methods that take into account more than just the shape of the histogram — such as the brightness differences between each pixel and its neighbors, or the brightness values of pixels along the boundaries between foreground and background regions, or the shape of those boundaries — are discussed later in this chapter. They can be more successful in automatically selecting accurate values for thresholding, but also require somewhat more knowledge about the nature of the image to choose the proper algorithm.

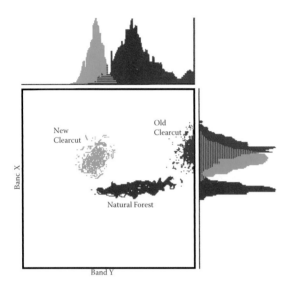

Figure 7.5 Example of terrain classification from satellite imagery using multiple spectral bands. Overlaps between classes in each band require that both be used to distinguish the types of terrain.

Multiband images

In some cases, segmentation can be performed using multiple original images of the same scene. The most familiar example is that of color imaging, which uses different wavelengths of light. For satellite imaging in particular, this may include several infrared bands containing important information for selecting regions according to vegetation, types of minerals, and so forth (Haralick and Dinstein 1975). **Figure 7.5** shows an example in which the measured values in each band contain overlaps between different types of terrain, but they are fully separated by using the combination of two channels.

A series of images obtained by performing different processing operations on the same original image can, in some cases, also be used in this way. Examples include combining one image containing brightness data, a second containing local texture information, etc., as shown below.

In general, the greater the number of available independent color bands or other images, the better the job of segmentation that can be performed. Points that are indistinguishable in one image may be fully distinct in another. However, with multispectral or multilayer images, it can be difficult to specify the selection criteria. The logical extension of thresholding is simply to place brightness thresholds on each image, for instance to specify the range of red, green, and blue (RGB) intensities. These multiple criteria are then usually combined with a Boolean AND operation (i.e., the pixel is defined as part of the foreground if its three RGB components all lie within the selected ranges). This is logically equivalent to segmenting each image channel individually, creating separate binary images, and then combining them with a Boolean AND operation afterward. Such operations to combine multiple binary images are discussed in **Chapter 8**.

The reason for wanting to combine the various selection criteria in a single process is to assist the user in defining the ranges for each. The optimum settings and their interactions are not particularly obvious when the individual color bands or other multiple image brightness values are set individually. Indeed, simply designing a user interface that makes it possible to select a specific range of colors for thresholding a typical visible-light image (usually specified by the RGB components) is not easy. A variety of partial solutions to aid in setting threshold criteria for colored images are in use.

This problem has several aspects. First, while red, green, and blue intensities represent the way the detector works and the way the data are stored internally, they do not correspond to the way that people recognize or react to color. As discussed in **Chapter 1**, a system based on hue, saturation, and intensity or lightness (HSI) is more familiar. It is sometimes possible to perform satisfactory thresholding using only one of the hue, saturation, or intensity channels, as shown in **Figure 7.6**, or a principal-components channel, as described in **Chapter 5**, but in the general case it may be necessary to use all of the information. A series of histograms for each of the RGB color channels may show peaks, but the user is not often able to judge which of the peaks corresponds to individual features of interest.

Even if the RGB pixel values are converted to the equivalent HSI values and histograms are constructed in that space, the use of three separate histograms and sets of threshold levels does little to help the user see which combinations of values are present or which pixels have those combinations.

For a three-dimensional color space, either RGB or HSI, interactive thresholding is more difficult than for the two-dimensional situation shown in **Figure 7.5**. There is no easy or obvious way with present display or control facilities to interactively enclose an arbitrary region in three-dimensional space and see which pixels are selected, or to adjust that region and see the effect on the image. It is also helpful to mark a pixel or region in the image and see the color values (RGB or HSI) labeled directly in the color space. For more than three colors (e.g., the multiple bands sensed by satellite imagery), the situation is even worse.

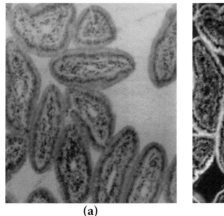
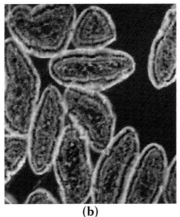
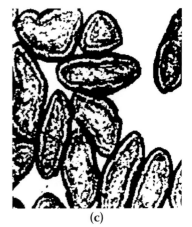

(a)   (b)   (c)

Figure 7.6 *Thresholding a color image using a single channel: **(a)** original stained biological thin section; **(b)** hue values calculated from stored RGB values; **(c)** thresholding on the hue image delineates the stained structures.*

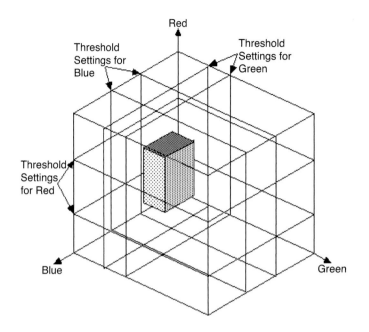

Red

Threshold Settings for Blue

Threshold Settings for Green

Threshold Settings for Red

Blue

Green

Figure 7.7 Illustration of the combination of separate thresholds on individual color channels. The shaded area is the Boolean AND of the three threshold settings for RGB. The only shape that can be formed in the three-dimensional space is a rectangular prism.

Using three one-dimensional histograms and sets of threshold levels, for instance in the RGB case, and combining the three criteria with a logical Boolean AND selects pixels that lie within a portion of the color space that is a simple prism, as shown in **Figure 7.7**. If the actual distribution of color values has some other shape in the color space, for instance if it is elongated in a direction not parallel to one axis, then this simple rectangular prism is inadequate to select the desired range of colors.

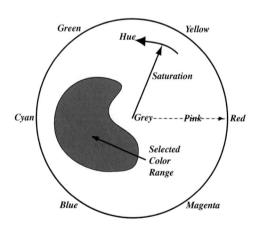

Green   Yellow

Hue

Saturation

Cyan   Grey- - - - - - Pink - - - ► Red

Selected Color Range

Blue   Magenta

Figure 7.8 Schematic illustration of selecting an arbitrary region in a two-dimensional parameter space (here the hue/saturation circle) to define a combination of colors to be selected for thresholding.

Two-dimensional thresholds

A somewhat better bound can be set by using a two-dimensional threshold (Russ 1991). This can be done in any color coordinates (RGB, HSI, etc.), but in RGB space it is difficult to interpret the meaning of the settings. This is one of the (many) arguments against the use of RGB for color images. However, the method is well suited for color images encoded by hue and saturation. The HS plane can be represented as a circle in which direction (angle) is proportional to hue and radius is proportional to saturation (**Figure 7.8**). The intensity or lightness of the image is perpendicular to this plane and requires another dimension to show or to control.

Instead of a one-dimensional histogram of brightness in a monochrome image, the figure represents a two-dimensional display in the HS plane. The number of pixels with each pair of values of hue and saturation can be plotted as a gray-scale value on this plane, representing a histogram with dark

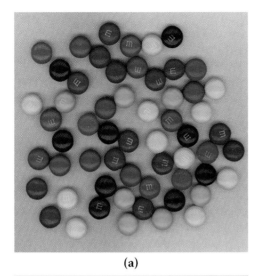

(a)

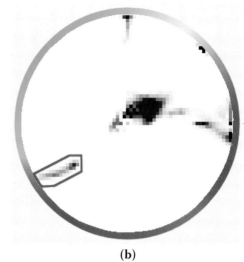

(b)

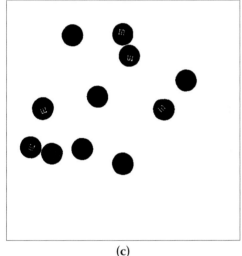

(c)

Figure 7.9 *Example of hue-saturation selection:*

(a) *original image;*

(b) *selection of the HS values for a single candy color (blue) from the histogram (which is shown on the hue-saturation circle as gray-scale values representing the number of image pixels; note the clusters for each color including the low-saturation gray background close to the center of the circle);*

(c) *resulting binary image.*

peaks. Thresholds can be selected as a region that is not necessarily simple, convex, or even connected, and so can be adapted to the distribution of the actual data. **Figure 7.9** illustrates this method; note that a narrow range of hue values is selected (but with a greater range of saturations) to deal with the variations introduced by the rounded shape of each candy piece. It is also possible to find locations in this color space, as a guide to the user in the process of defining the boundary, by pointing to pixels in the image so that the program can highlight the location of the color values on the HS circle.

Similar histogram displays and threshold settings can be accomplished using other channels and coordinates. For color images, the HS plane is sometimes shown as a hexagon (with red, yellow, green, cyan, blue, and magenta corners) rather than a circle. The CIE (Commission Internationale de L'Éclairage) color diagram shown in **Chapter 1** is also a candidate for this purpose. For some satellite images, the near- and far-infrared intensities form a plane in which combinations of thermal and reflected infrared can be displayed and selected.

As a practical matter, the HS plane can be plotted as a square face on a cube that represents the HSI space. This is simpler for the computer graphics display and is used in several of the examples that follow. However, the HSI cube with square faces is topologically different from the cone or bi-cone used to represent HSI space in **Chapter 1**, and the square HS plane is topologically different from the circle in **Figure 7.8**. In the square, the minimum and maximum hue values (orange-red and magenta-red) are far apart, whereas in the circle, hue is a continuous function that wraps around. This makes using the square for thresholding somewhat less intuitive, but it is still superior in most cases to the use of RGB color space.

For the two-dimensional square plot, the axes may have unfamiliar meanings, but the ability to display a histogram of points based on the combination of values and to select threshold boundaries based on the histogram is a significant advantage over multiple one-dimensional histograms and thresholds, even if it does not generalize easily to the *n*-dimensional case.

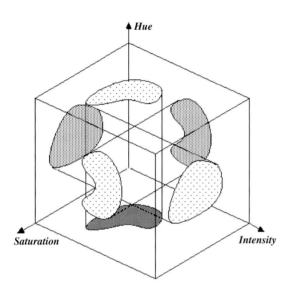

Figure 7.10 *Illustration of the combination of two-parameter threshold settings. Outlining of regions in each plane defines a shape in the three-dimensional space that is more adjustable than the Boolean combination of simple one-dimensional thresholds in Figure 7.7 but that still cannot conform to arbitrary three-dimensional cluster shapes.*

The dimensions of the histogram array are usually somewhat reduced from the actual resolution (typically at least one part in 256) of the various RGB or HSI values for the stored image. This is not only because the array size would become very large (256^2 = 65,536 for the square, 256^3 = 16,777,216 for the cube). Another reason is that for a typical real image, there are simply not that many distinct pairs or triples of values present, and a useful display showing the locations of peaks and clusters can be presented using fewer bins. The examples shown here use 32 × 32 or 64 × 64 bins for each of the square faces of the RGB or HSI cubes, each of which thus requires 32^2 = 1024 or 64^2 = 4096 storage locations.

It is possible to imagine a system in which each of the two-dimensional planes defined by pairs of signals is used to draw a contour threshold, then project all of these contours back through the multidimensional space to define the thresholding, as shown in **Figure 7.10**. However, as the dimensionality increases, so does the complexity for the user, and the Boolean AND region defined by the multiple projections still cannot fit irregular or skewed regions very satisfactorily.

Multiband thresholding

Figure 7.6 showed a color image from a light microscope. The microtomed thin specimen of intestine has been stained with two different colors, so that there are variations in shade, tint, and tone. The next series of figures illustrates how this image can be segmented by thresholding to isolate a particular structure using this information. **Figure 7.11** shows the original red, green, and blue color channels in the image and their individual brightness histograms. **Figure 7.12** shows the histograms of pixel values, projected onto the red/green, green/blue, and

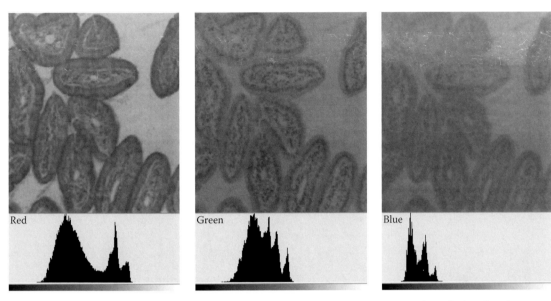

Figure 7.11 *Red, green, and blue color channels from the image in* *Figure 7.6*, *with their brightness histograms.*

blue/red faces of the RGB color cube. Notice that there is a trend on all faces for the majority of pixels in the image to cluster along the central diagonal in the cube. In other words, for most pixels, the trend toward more of any one color is part of a general increase in brightness by increasing the values of all colors. This means that RGB space poorly disperses the various color values and does not facilitate setting thresholds to discriminate the different regions present.

Figure 7.13 shows the conversion of the color information from **Figure 7.11** into hue, saturation, and intensity images as well as the individual brightness histograms for these channels. **Figure 7.14** shows the values projected onto individual two-dimensional hue/saturation, saturation/intensity, and intensity/hue square plots. Notice how the much greater dispersion of peaks in the various histograms uses more of the color space and separates several different clusters of values. In general, for stains used in biological samples, the hue image identifies where a particular stain is located, while the saturation image corresponds to the amount of the stain, and the intensity image indicates the overall density of the stained specimen.

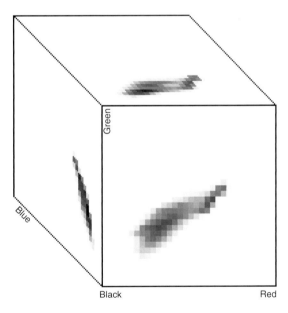

Figure 7.12 *Pairs of values for the pixels in the images of* *Figure 7.11*, *plotted on RG, BG, and RB planes and projected onto the faces of a cube.*

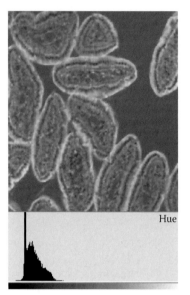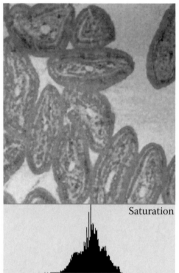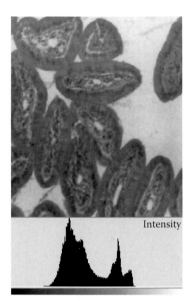

Figure 7.13 *Hue, saturation, and intensity channels from the image in* Figure 7.6, *with their brightness histograms.*

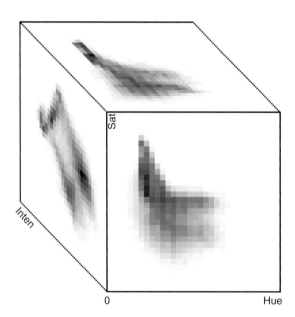

Figure 7.14 *Pairs of values for the pixels in the images of* Figure 7.13, *plotted on HS, SI, and HI planes and projected onto the faces of a cube.*

Principal components analysis (PCA) processing of images, as shown in **Chapter 5**, also produces images in which the various derived channels have more-dispersed values, which are often more suitable for thresholding than the original red, green, and blue channels. **Figure 7.15** shows the principal components channels and their histograms, and **Figure 7.16** shows the two-dimensional plots. **Figure 5.66b** in **Chapter 5** showed this same image displayed with the three principal components channels assigned arbitrarily to red, green, and blue.

Multiband images are not always different colors. A very common example is the use of multiple elemental X-ray maps from the SEM, which can be combined to select phases of interest based on composition. In many cases, this combination can be accomplished simply by separately thresholding each individual image and then applying Boolean logic to combine the images. Of course, the rather noisy original X-ray maps may first require image processing (such as smoothing) to reduce the statistical variations from pixel to pixel (as discussed in **Chapter 4**), and binary image processing (as illustrated in **Chapter 8**).

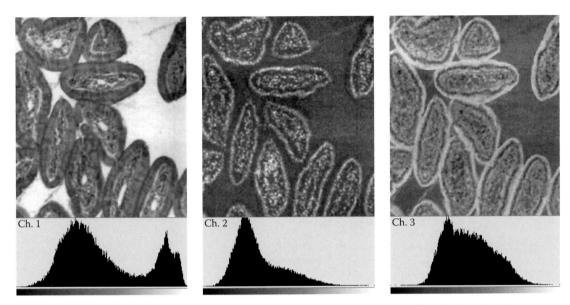

Figure 7.15 Principal components channels from the image in *Figure 7.6*, with their brightness histograms.

Using X-rays or other element-specific signals, such as secondary ions or Auger electrons, essentially the entire periodic table can be detected. It becomes possible to specify very complicated combinations of elements that must be present or absent, or the approximate intensity levels needed (since intensities are generally roughly proportional to elemental concentration) to specify the region of interest. Thresholding these combinations of elemental images produces results that are sometimes described as chemical maps. Of course, the fact that several elements may be present in the same area of a specimen, such as a metal, mineral, or block of biological tissue, does not directly imply that they are chemically combined.

In principle, it is possible to store an entire analytical spectrum (e.g., from an X-ray spectrometer, a mass spectrometer, or a spectrophotometer) for each pixel in an image and then use appropriate computation to derive actual compositional information at each point, which is eventually used in a thresh-

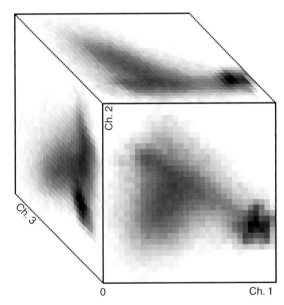

Figure 7.16 Pairs of values for the pixels in the images of *Figure 7.15*, projected onto the faces of a cube.

olding operation to select regions of interest. At present, this approach is limited in application by the large amount of storage and lengthy calculations required. However, as faster and larger computers and storage devices become common, such methods are becoming more widely used.

Visualization programs used to analyze complex data may also employ Boolean logic to combine multiple parameters. A simple example would be a geographical information system in which such diverse data as population density, mean income level, and other census data were recorded for each city block (which would be treated as a single pixel). Combining these different values to select regions for test marketing commercial products is a standard technique. Another example is the rendering of calculated tensor properties in metal beams subject to loading, as modeled in a computer program. Supercomputer simulations of complex dynamic systems, such as evolving thunderstorms, produce rich data sets that can benefit from such analysis.

There are other uses of image processing that derive additional information from a single original gray-scale image to aid in performing selective thresholding of a region of interest. The processing produces additional images that can be treated as multiband images useful for segmentation.

Thresholding from texture

Few real images of practical interest can be satisfactorily thresholded using simply the original brightness values in a monochrome image. The texture information present in images is one of the most powerful additional tools available. Several kinds of texture may be encountered, including different ranges of brightness, different spatial frequencies, and different orientations (Haralick et al. 1973). The next few figures show images that illustrate these variables and the tools available to utilize them.

Figure 7.17 shows a test image containing five irregular regions that can be visually distinguished by texture. The average brightness of each of the regions is identical, as shown by the brightness histograms. Region e contains pixels with uniformly random brightness values covering the entire 0 to 255 range. Regions a through d have Gaussian brightness variations, which for regions a and d are also randomly assigned to pixel locations. For region b, the values have been spatially averaged with a Gaussian smooth, which also reduces the amount of variation. For region c, the pixels have been averaged together in one direction to create a directional texture.

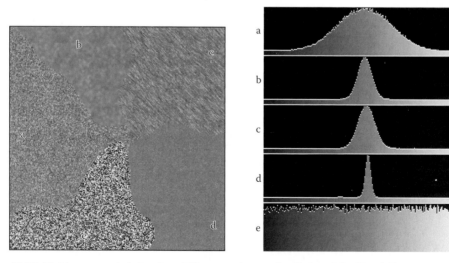

Figure 7.17 *Test image containing five different regions to be distinguished by differences in the textures. The brightness histograms are shown; the average brightness of each region is the same.*

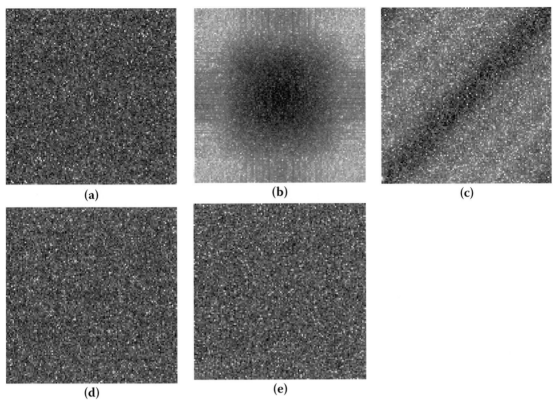

Figure 7.18 *Two-dimensional FFT power spectra of the pattern in each area of* **Figure 7.17**. *While some minor differences are seen (e.g., the loss of high frequencies in region **b** and the directionality in region **c**), these cannot be used for satisfactory segmentation.*

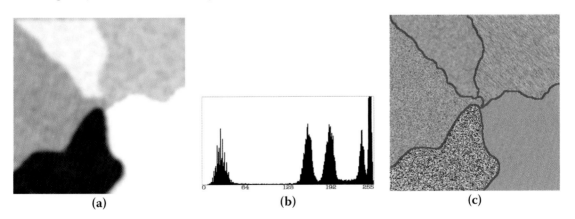

Figure 7.19 *(a) Result of applying a variance operator to the image in* **Figure 7.17**, *(b) with the histogram in which the five regions are distinct in brightness. (c) Thresholding can now separate the regions.*

One tool that is often suggested (and occasionally useful) for textural characterization is the two-dimensional frequency transform introduced in **Chapter 6**. **Figure 7.18** shows these power spectra for each of the patterns in **Figure 7.17**. The smoothing in region b acts as a low-pass filter, so the high frequencies are attenuated. In region c, the directionality is visible in the frequency-transform image. For the other regions, the random pixel assignments do not create any distinctive patterns in the frequency transforms. They cannot be used to select the different regions in this case.

The variance in a moving 4-pixel-radius neighborhood is calculated for this image as a spatial-domain texture-sensitive operator in **Figure 7.19**. This operation, introduced in **Chapter 5**, produces a derived image that has unique gray-scale values for each region, as shown in the brightness histogram The five peaks are separated and allow direct thresholding. The figure shows an image with outlines of the regions selected by thresholding the variance image superimposed on the original. Notice that because the spatial scale of the texture is several pixels wide, the location of the boundaries of regions is necessarily uncertain by several pixels. It is also difficult to estimate the proper location visually, for the same reason.

Figure 5.50 in **Chapter 5** shows an image typical of many obtained in microscopy in which regions that have no distinct brightness difference are visually distinguished by a textural difference. Converting that texture to a brightness with a suitable texture operator converts the original image to one that can be thresholded. **Chapter 5** illustrated several texture operators that can be used for this purpose.

Multiple thresholding criteria

Figure 7.20 shows a somewhat more complex test image in which some of the regions are distinguished by a different spatial texture and some by a different mean brightness. No

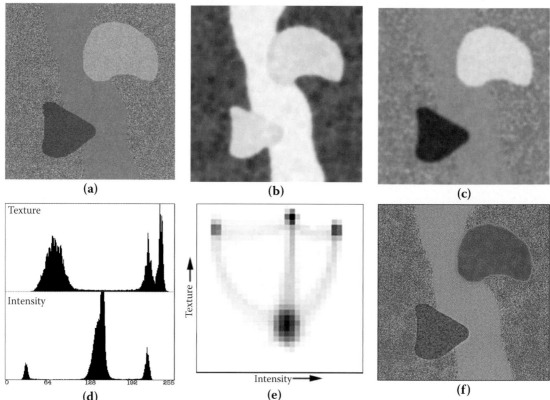

*Figure 7.20 Segmenting with multiple criteria: (a) original image; (b) texture image produced by variance operator; (c) intensity image produced by smoothing; (d) histograms of images **b** and **c**; (e) two-dimensional histogram; (f) color composite as described in text.*

single parameter can be used to discriminate all four regions. The texture can be extracted by applying a variance operator to produce a useful gray-scale distinction. Smoothing to eliminate the texture creates an image in which the brightness differences stand out. It is necessary to use both images to select individual regions. This could be done by thresholding each region separately and then using Boolean logic (discussed in **Chapter 8**) to combine the two binary images in various ways. Another approach is to use the same kind of two-dimensional histogram as described above for color images (Panda and Rosenfeld 1978). The figure shows the individual image histograms and the two-dimensional histogram. In each of the individual histograms, only three peaks are present because the regions are not all distinct in either brightness or variance. In the two-dimensional histogram, individual peaks are visible for each of the four regions.

The situation is analogous to the use of different color channels shown in **Figure 7.5**. In practice, the different derived images used to successfully segment an image such as this one are sometimes displayed using different color channels. This is purely a visual effect, of course, since the data represented have nothing to do with color. However, it does take advantage of the fact that human vision distinguishes colors well (for most people, at least) and uses color information for segmentation. It also reveals the similarity between this example of thresholding based on multiple textural and brightness criteria and the more commonplace example of thresholding color images based on the individual color channels. **Figure 7.20f** shows the information with the original image in the luminance (L*) channel, the smoothed brightness values in the a* (red-green) channel, and the texture information from the variance operator in the b* (blue-yellow) channel of an L*a*b* color image.

Figure 7.21 shows an application of thresholding using two criteria, one of them being texture, to a real image. The image shows ice crystals in a food product. The fractal texture operator partially delineates the ice crystals, as does the use of the hue channel. Thresholding

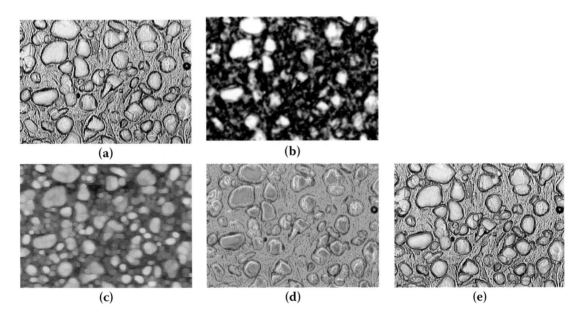

(a) (b)

(c) (d) (e)

Figure 7.21 *Segmentation of ice crystals in a food product:* **(a)** *original image;* **(b)** *fractal texture operator applied to the intensity channel;* **(c)** *hue channel;* **(d)** *color composite with original brightness in the luminance (L*) channel, texture in the a* channel, and hue in the b* channel of an L*a*b* image;* **(e)** *final thresholded result shown as outlines on the original image.*

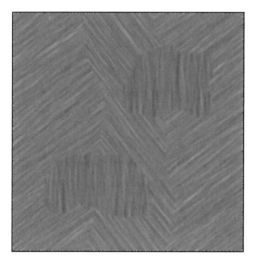

Figure 7.22 An image containing regions with different textural orientations but the same average brightness, standard deviation, and spatial scale.

each, and then combining them with Boolean logic and applying a closing (discussed in **Chapter 8**) produces a useful segmentation of the crystals, as shown by the outlines on the figure.

Textural orientation

Figure 7.22 shows another test image containing regions having identical mean brightness, brightness distribution, and spatial scale of the local variation, but with different textural orientations. This is evident in a two-dimensional frequency transform, as shown in **Figure 7.23a**. The three ranges of spatial-domain orientation are revealed in the three spokes in the transform.

Using a selective wedge-shaped mask with smoothed edges (as described in **Chapter 6**) to select each of the spokes and retransform the image produces the three spatial-domain images shown in **Figure 7.23**. Each texture orientation in the original image is isolated, having a uniform gray background in other locations. These images cannot be directly thresholded because the brightness values in the textured regions cover a range that includes the surroundings. Applying a range operator to a 5 × 5-pixel octagonal neighborhood, as shown in **Figure 7.24**, suppresses the uniform background regions and highlights the individual texture regions.

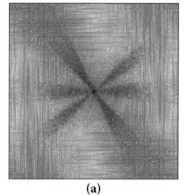

(a)

Figure 7.23 Isolating the directional texture in frequency space: (a) two-dimensional frequency transform of the image in Figure 7.22, showing the radial spokes corresponding to each textural alignment; (b, c, d) retransformation using masks to select each of the orientations.

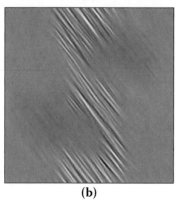

(b)

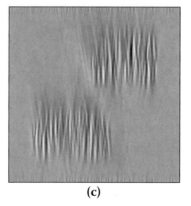

(c)

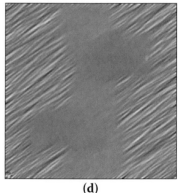

(d)

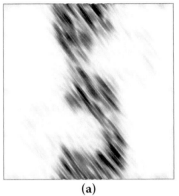
(a)

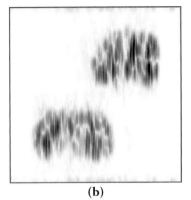
(b)

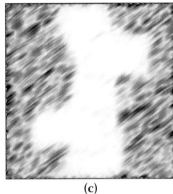
(c)

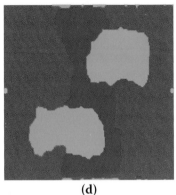
(d)

Figure 7.24 *Application of a range operator to the images in Figure 7.23 b, c, and d (a, b, c) and the color combination (d) of the regions selected by thresholding these images.*

Thresholding these images and applying a closing operation (discussed in **Chapter 8**) to fill in internal gaps and smooth boundaries produces images of each region. **Figure 7.24d** shows the composite result. Notice that the edges of the image are poorly handled, a consequence of the inability of the frequency transform to preserve edge details, as discussed in **Chapter 6**. Also, the boundaries of the regions are rather irregular and only approximately rendered in this result.

In most cases, spatial-domain processing is preferred for texture orientation. **Figure 7.25** shows the result from applying a Sobel operator to the image, as discussed in **Chapter 5**. Two directional first derivatives in the x and y directions are obtained using a 3×3-neighborhood operator. These are then combined using the arctangent function to obtain an angle that is the direction of maximum brightness gradient. The resulting angle is scaled to fit the 0 to 255 brightness range of the image, so that each step in brightness corresponds to about $1.4°$.

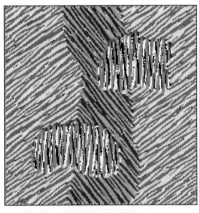

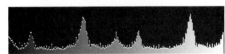

Figure 7.25 *Application of the Sobel direction operator to the image in Figure 7.22, calculating the orientation of the gradient at each pixel by assigning a gray level to the arctangent of $(\partial B/\partial y)/(\partial B/\partial x)$. The brightness histogram shows six peaks, in pairs for each principal textural orientation, since the directions are complementary.*

The brightness histogram shown in **Figure 7.25b** shows six peaks. These occur in pairs 180° apart, since in each texture region the direction of maximum gradient can lie in either of two opposite directions. This image can be reduced to three directions in several ways. One is to

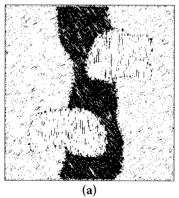

(a)

Figure 7.26 Thresholded binary images from **Figure 7.25***, selecting the gray values corresponding to each pair of complementary directions (a, b, c), and the outlines (d) showing the regions defined by applying a closing operation to each of the binary images.*

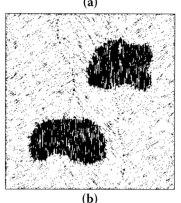

(b)

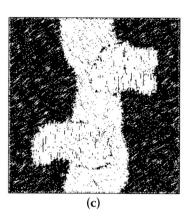

(c)

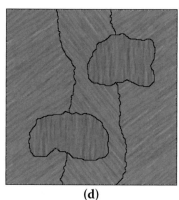

(d)

use a gray-scale lookup table (LUT), as discussed in **Chapter 5** and illustrated below, that assigns the same gray-scale values to the highest and lowest halves of the original brightness (or angle) range; this converts the 0 to 360° range to 0 to 180° and permits thresholding a single peak for each direction. A second method is to set two different threshold ranges on the paired peaks and then combine the two resulting binary images using a Boolean OR operation (see **Chapter 8**). A third approach is to set a multiple-threshold range on the two complementary peaks. All of these are functionally equivalent.

Figure 7.26 shows the results of three thresholding operations to select each of the three textural orientations. There is some noise in these images, consisting of white pixels within the dark regions and vice versa, but these are much fewer and smaller than in the case of thresholding the results from the frequency-transform method shown above. After applying a closing operation (a dilation followed by an erosion, as discussed in **Chapter 8**), the regions are well delineated, as shown by the superposition of the outlines on the original image (**Figure 7.26d**). This result is superior to the frequency transform and has smoother boundaries, better agreement with the visual judgment of location, and no problems at the image or region edges.

Figure 7.27 illustrates the use of this procedure with a real image. The herringbone cloth has two predominant orientation regions, which are otherwise identical in color and brightness. The Sobel orientation operator assigns gray-scale values representing orientations from 0 to 360°. To reduce this to a more meaningful 0 to 180°, a special LUT is used, as shown in the figure. The resulting image can be thresholded and processed to delineate the regions in the original image.

Note that applying any neighborhood processing operation such as smoothing or median filtering to an image in which gray scale represents direction requires special rules to account for

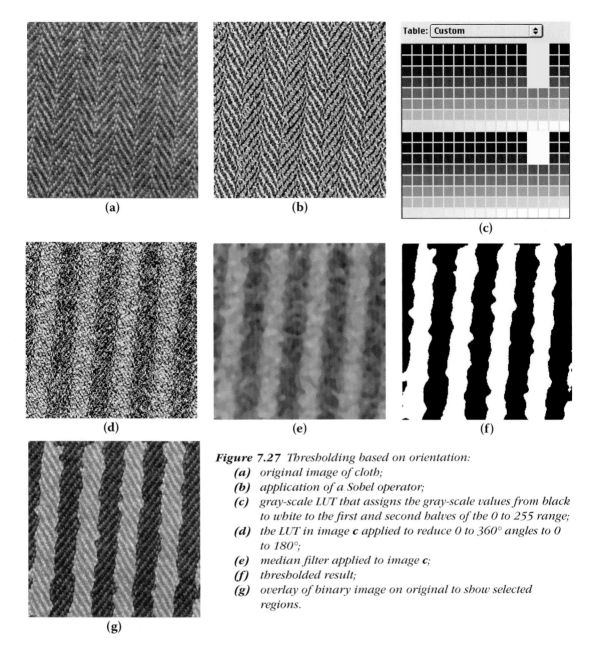

Figure 7.27 *Thresholding based on orientation:*
- **(a)** *original image of cloth;*
- **(b)** *application of a Sobel operator;*
- **(c)** *gray-scale LUT that assigns the gray-scale values from black to white to the first and second halves of the 0 to 255 range;*
- **(d)** *the LUT in image **c** applied to reduce 0 to 360° angles to 0 to 180°;*
- **(e)** *median filter applied to image **c**;*
- **(f)** *thresholded result;*
- **(g)** *overlay of binary image on original to show selected regions.*

the modulo change in values at 0. For example, the average value in a neighborhood containing pixel values of 15 and 251 is 5, not 133. A simple but effective way to accomplish this is to process each neighborhood twice, once with the stored values and once with the values shifted to become (P + 128) mod 255, and then keep whichever result is smaller.

Figure 7.28 shows another compound example, a metallographic sample with a lamellar structure. This requires several steps to segment into the various regions. Brightness thresholding can delineate the texture-free region directly. Applying the Sobel orientation operator produces an image that can be thresholded to delineate the other two regions, but as before, each region has pairs of gray-scale values that are 180° or 128 gray values apart. Thresholding the various regions produces a complete map of the sample, as shown.

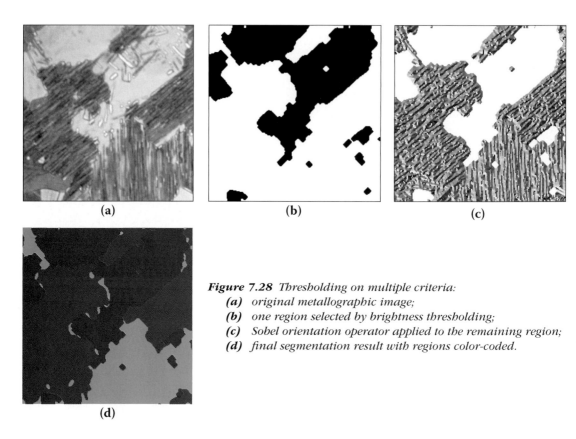

(a)

(b)

(c)

(d)

Figure 7.28 Thresholding on multiple criteria:
  (a) original metallographic image;
  (b) one region selected by brightness thresholding;
  (c) Sobel orientation operator applied to the remaining region;
  (d) final segmentation result with regions color-coded.

Region boundaries

Since pixel-based images represent at best an approximation to the continuous real scene being represented, and since thresholding classifies each pixel as either part of the foreground or the background, only a finite level of accuracy can be achieved. An alternative representation of features based on boundary lines can be more accurate. These can be polygons with many sides and corner points defined as *x,y* coordinates of arbitrary accuracy, or spline curves, etc., as compared with the comparatively coarse pixel spacing.

Such boundary-line representation is superior for accurate measurement because the line itself has no width. However, determining the line is far from easy. The location of individual points can be determined by interpolation between pixels, perhaps fitting mathematical functions to pixels on either side of the boundary to improve the results. This type of approach is commonly used in geographic applications in which elevation values measured at discrete points are used to construct topographic maps. It is also used in metrology applications, such as measuring dimensions of microelectronic circuit elements on silicon wafers, and is possible because the shapes of those features (usually consisting of straight lines) is known *a priori*. This type of application goes beyond the typical image processing operations dealt with in this chapter.

One approach to interpolating a smoothed boundary line through the pixels is used by the superresolution perimeter measurement routine used in **Chapter 10** for feature measurement. This uses neighborhood processing (the Laplacian of a Gaussian [LoG] operator mentioned in **Chapter 5**) to fit an adaptive boundary line through each pixel, thereby achieving improved precision and fractional-pixel accuracy. There is a further discussion of boundary contours below.

Thresholding produces a pixel-based representation of the image that assigns each pixel to either the feature(s) or the surroundings. The finite size of the pixels allows the representation only a finite accuracy, but we would prefer to have no bias in the result. This means that performing the same operation on many repeated images of the same scene should produce an average result that approaches the true value for size or other feature measurements. The question is always what to do with the pixels along the boundaries between regions, whose brightness values typically lie between the peaks in the brightness histogram. In most instances, these are pixels that straddle the boundary and have averaged together the two principal brightness levels in proportion to the area subtended within the pixel, as indicated in **Figure 7.29**.

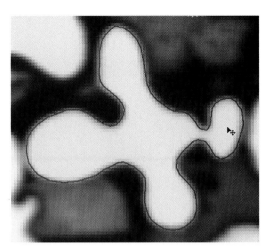

Figure 7.29 Example of finite pixels straddling a boundary line, with brightness values that average those of the two sampled regions.

As noted previously, the histogram shows only the frequency of occurrence of different values and does not preserve any information about position, the brightness of neighboring pixels, and other factors. Yet it is this spatial information that is important for determining boundary location. It is possible, in principle, to build a co-occurrence matrix for the image in which all possible combinations of pixel brightness are counted in terms of the distance between them. This information is used to select the pixels that are part of the feature instead of simply the pixel brightness values; this is equivalent to a processing operation that uses the same co-occurrence matrix to construct a texture image for which simple thresholding can be used.

Using the shape of the histogram to select a threshold generally places that value between peaks. The difficulty is that because this region of the histogram is (hopefully) very low, with few pixels having these values, the counting statistics are poor and the shape of the curve in the histogram is poorly defined. Consequently, the threshold value is hard to locate and may move about considerably with only tiny changes in overall illumination, with a change in the field of view to include objects with a different shape, or with more or fewer pixels along the boundary. Smoothing the histogram with a polynomial fit may provide a somewhat more robust location for a minimum point.

Figure 7.30 shows an image having two visibly distinguishable regions. Each contains a Gaussian noise pattern with the same standard deviation but a different mean, though the brightness values in the two regions overlap. This means that setting a threshold value at the minimum between the two peaks causes some pixels in each region to be misclassified, as shown. This image is used again in several examples below to compare thresholding and processing methods.

This type of image often results from situations in which the total number of photons or other signals is low and counting statistics cause a variation in the brightness of pixels in uniform areas, resulting in broad peaks in the histogram. Counting statistics produce a Poisson distribution, but when moderately large numbers are involved, this is very close to the more convenient Gaussian function used in these images. For extremely noisy images, such as X-ray dot maps from the SEM, some additional processing in the spatial domain may be required before attempting thresholding (O'Callaghan 1974).

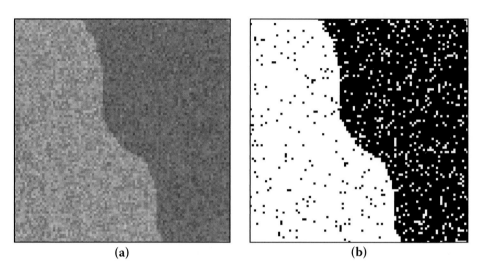

(a)   (b)

*Figure 7.30 A test image containing two regions whose mean brightness levels are different, but which have variations in individual pixels that overlap: **(a)** original image (enlarged to show pixels); **(b)** result of setting a simple threshold at the minimum point.*

Figure 7.31 shows a typical sparse-dot map. Most of the pixels contain 0 counts, and a few contain 1 count. The boundaries in the image are visually evident, but their exact location is at best approximate, requiring the human visual computer to group the dots together. Image processing can do this by counting the number of dots in a circular neighborhood around each pixel. Convolution with a kernel consisting of 1s in a 15-pixel-diameter circle accomplishes this, producing the result shown. This gray-scale image can be thresholded to locate the boundaries shown, but there is inadequate data to decide whether the small regions, voids, and irregularities in the boundaries are real or simply due to the limited counting statistics. Typically, the threshold level will be set by determining the mean brightness level in the background region, and then setting the threshold several standard deviations above this to select just the significant regions.

The figure compares this approach with one based on the binary editing operations discussed in **Chapter 8**. Both require making some assumptions about the image. In the smoothing and thresholding case (**Figure 7.31b** and **Figure 7.31c**), some knowledge about the statistical meaning of the data is required. For X-rays, the standard deviation in the count rate is known to vary in proportion to the square root of the number of counts, which is the brightness in the smoothed image. Erosion and dilation (discussed in **Chapter 8**) are based on assumptions about the distances between dots in the image. Closing (dilation followed by erosion) fills in the gaps between dots to create solid areas corresponding to the features, as shown in **Figure 7.31d**. In the background regions, this does not produce a continuous dark region, and so an opening (erosion followed by dilation) can remove it (**Figure 7.31e**). Adding and then removing pixels produces the final result shown. The boundaries are slightly different from those produced by smoothing and thresholding, but the original image does not contain enough data to distinguish between them.

Several possible approaches can be used to improve the segmentation of noisy regions, using **Figure 7.30** as a test case. **Chapter 8** discusses binary image-editing operations, including morphological processing. The sequence of a dilation followed by an erosion, known as a closing, fills holes, erases isolated pixels, and smoothes the boundary line to produce the result shown in **Figure 7.32a**. In contrast, a much more complicated operation reassigns pixels from

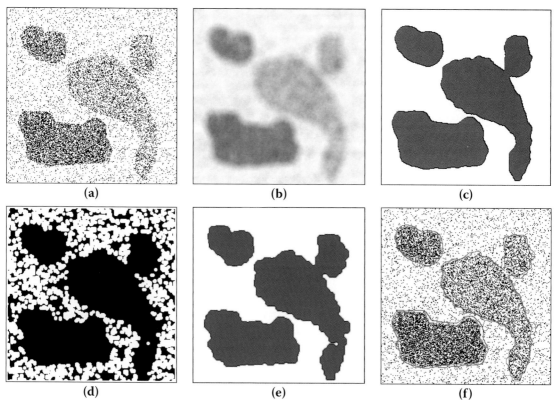

Figure 7.31 *Thresholding a sparse-dot image: (a) X-ray dot map; (b) gray-scale image formed by counting the dots within a 15-pixel-diameter circle centered on each pixel; (c) boundary determined by thresholding image b at 4 standard deviations above the mean background level; (d) application of a closing operation (dilation followed by erosion) to fill the gaps between closely spaced pixels in image a; (e) application of an opening operation (erosion followed by dilation) to remove small dark regions in the background in image d; (f) comparison of the feature outlines determined by the smoothing and thresholding (red) vs. closing and opening (blue) methods.*

one region to the other based on the entropy in both regions. Such methods are generally very computer-intensive.

In this case, the collection of pixels into two regions can be described as an entropy problem (Kapur et al. 1985): The total entropy in each region is calculated as $-\Sigma p_i \log_e p_i$, where p_i is the fraction of pixels having brightness i. Solving for the boundary that classifies each pixel into one of two groups to minimize this function for the two regions, subject to the constraint that the pixels in each region must touch each other, produces the boundary line shown in **Figure 7.32b**. Additional constraints, such as minimizing the number of touching pixels in different classes, would smooth the boundary. The problem is that such constraints assume that something is known about the specimen (for instance, that the boundary is smooth), they make the solution of the problem very difficult, and they can usually be applied more efficiently in other ways (for instance by smoothing the binary image).

Setting a threshold value at the minimum in the histogram is sometimes described as "selecting for minimum area sensitivity" in the value (Wall et al. 1974; Weszka 1978). This means that changing the threshold value causes the least change in the feature (or background) area, although as noted above, this says nothing about the spatial arrangement of the pixels that are

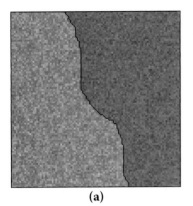

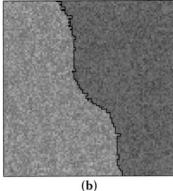

(a) (b)

Figure 7.32 *The boundary in the image of **Figure 7.30** determined by various methods:*
(a) *thresholding at the minimum point in the histogram followed by closing (dilation and erosion);*
(b) *iteratively setting the minimum entropy point.*

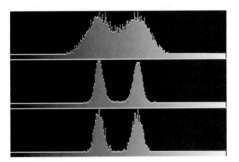

Figure 7.33 *Histogram of the image in* **Figure 7.30**:
(a) *original, with overlapped peaks;*
(b) *after smoothing;*
(c) *after median filtering.*

thereby added to or removed from the features. Indeed, the definition of the histogram makes any minimum in the plot a point of minimum area sensitivity.

For the image shown in **Figure 7.30,** processing can change the histogram to produce a minimum that is deeper, broader, and has a more stable minimum value. **Figure 7.33** shows the results of smoothing the image (using a Gaussian kernel with a standard deviation of 1 pixel) or applying a median filter. (Both of these methods involve the neighborhood around each pixel and are discussed in **Chapters 4** and **5**.) The peaks are narrower and the valley is broader and deeper. The consequences for the image, and the boundaries that are selected by setting the threshold level between the resulting peaks, are shown in **Figure 7.34**.

These methods seem not to be the criteria used by skilled human operators when they watch an image and interactively adjust a threshold value. Instead of the total area of features changing least with adjustment, which is difficult for humans to judge, another approach is to use the total change in perimeter length around the features (Russ and Russ 1988a), which corresponds to the "smoothest" boundary. The variation in total perimeter length with respect to threshold value provides an objective criterion that can be efficiently calculated. The minimum in this response curve provides a way to set the thresholds that is reproducible, adapts to varying illumination, etc., and mimics to some extent the way humans set the values when they assume that the boundaries should be smooth. For the case in which both upper and lower threshold levels are to be adjusted, this produces a response surface in two dimensions (the upper and lower values), which can be solved to find the minimum point, as indicated in **Figure 7.35**.

Figure 7.36 shows an image whose brightness threshold has been automatically positioned to minimize the variation in total boundary length. The specimen (oil droplets in mayonnaise) is one in which boundaries are expected to be smooth because of surface tension at the oil-water interface. Similar smooth boundaries occur in many situations, including membranes in biological tissue and phase changes in materials (solidification or melting), but such an assumption would not be appropriate for, e.g., abraded or fractured surfaces that are rough.

The brightness histogram shown in the figure has a valley between two peaks, neither of which has a symmetric or Gaussian shape. The selected threshold point is not at the lowest

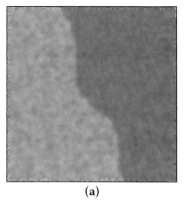

(a)

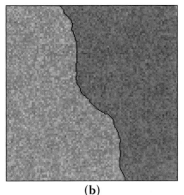

(b)

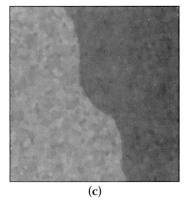

(c)

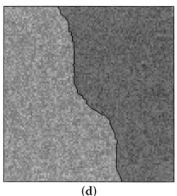

(d)

Figure 7.34 Processing the image in *Figure 7.30* to modify the histogram:
- *(a)* smoothing with a Gaussian kernel, standard deviation = 1 pixel;
- *(b)* the boundary produced by thresholding image *a*, superimposed on the original;
- *(c)* median processing (iteratively applied until no further changes occurred);
- *(d)* the boundary produced by thresholding image *c*, superimposed on the original.

point in the histogram. Repeated measurements using this algorithm on many images show that the reproducibility in the presence of moderate image noise and changing illumination is rather good. Length variations for irregular objects varied less than 0.5%, or 1 pixel in 200, across the major diameter of the object.

Selective histograms

Most of the difficulties with selecting the optimum threshold brightness value between two peaks in a typical histogram arise from the intermediate brightness values of the histogram. Many of these pixels lie along the boundaries of the two regions, so methods that eliminate them from the histogram will ideally leave only peaks from the uniform regions and facilitate selecting the proper threshold value (Milgram and Herman 1979; Weszka and Rosenfeld 1979).

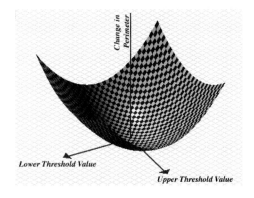

Figure 7.35 A two-way plot of the absolute change in perimeter length vs. the settings of upper- and lower-level brightness thresholds. The minimum indicates the optimal settings.

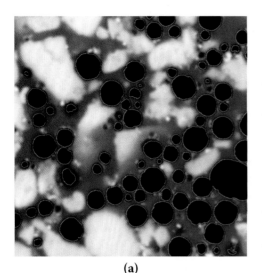

(a)

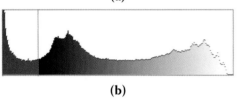

(b)

Figure 7.36 *Test image for automatic threshold adjustment:*

(a) *original image (oil droplets in mayonnaise), with outlines corresponding to the threshold setting shown in image **b**;*

(b) *brightness histogram showing the optimum threshold point based on minimizing the change in perimeter length.*

One way to perform this selection is to use another derived image, such as the Sobel gradient or any of the other edge-finding operators discussed in **Chapter 5**. Pixels having a high gradient value can be eliminated from the histogram of the original image to reduce the background level in the range between the two phase peaks. **Figure 7.37** shows an example. The original image contains three phases with visually distinct gray levels. Several methods can be used to eliminate edge pixels. It is most straightforward to threshold a gradient image, selecting pixels with a high value. This produces a binary image that can be used as a mask that restricts the pixels in the original image from being used in the histogram to be analyzed.

In the example, the 20% of the pixels with the largest magnitude in the Sobel gradient image were selected to produce a mask used to remove those pixels from the original image and the histogram. The result is the reduction of those portions of the histogram between pcaks, with the peaks themselves little affected. This makes it easier to characterize the shapes of the peaks from the phases and select a consistent point between them.

Of course, this method requires setting a threshold on the gradient image to select the pixels to be bypassed. The most often used technique is simply to choose some fixed percentage of the pixels with the highest gradient value and eliminate them from the histogram of the original image. In the example shown, however, the gradient operator responds more strongly to the larger difference between the white and gray regions than to the smaller difference between the gray and dark regions. Hence the edge-straddling pixels (and their background in the histogram) are reduced much more between the white and gray peaks than between the gray and black peaks.

Figure 7.38 shows another method that alleviates the problem in this image. Beginning with a range image (the difference between the darkest and brightest pixels in a 5-pixel-wide octagonal neighborhood), nonmaximum suppression (also known as gray-scale thinning, skeletonization, or ridge-finding) is used to narrow the boundaries and eliminate pixels that are not actually on the boundary. This line is uniformly dilated to 3 pixels wide and used as a mask to remove edge-straddling pixels from the original. The plot of the resulting histogram, also in **Figure 7.37d**, shows a much greater suppression of the valley between the gray and black peaks. All of these methods are somewhat *ad hoc*; the particular combination of different region brightnesses present in an image will dictate what edge-finding operation will work best and what fraction of the pixels should be removed.

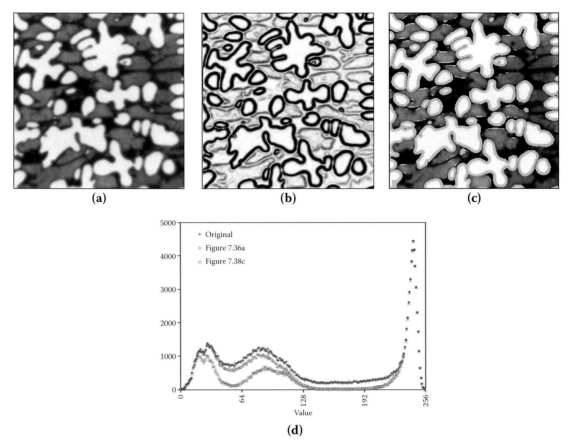

(a)   (b)   (c)

(d)

Figure 7.37 *Thresholding by ignoring boundary pixels:* ***(a)*** *original image containing three visually distinct phase regions with different mean gray levels;* ***(b)*** *application of a gradient operator (Sobel) to image* ***a****;* ***(c)*** *the image without the 20% of the pixels having the largest gradient value, which eliminates the edge-straddling pixels in the original;* ***(d)*** *comparison of histograms from the original image in* ***Figure 7.46a*** *and the masked image in image* ***c*** *as well as the image in* ***Figure 7.38c****, showing the reduction of number of pixels with brightness in the ranges between the main peaks.*

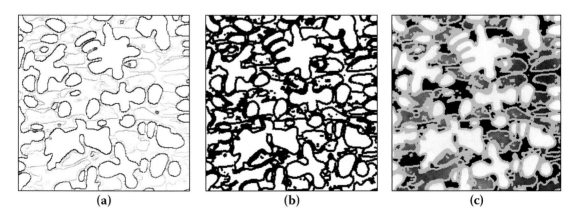

(a)   (b)   (c)

Figure 7.38 *Removal of edge pixels:* ***(a)*** *nonmaximum suppression (gray-scale thinning) applied to* ***Figure 7.37b****;* ***(b)*** *dilation of lines to 3 pixels wide;* ***(c)*** *removal of edges leaving uniform interior regions in the original. The histogram of the resulting masked image is shown in* ***Figure 7.37d****.*

Boundary lines

One of the shortcomings of selecting pixels by brightness or color, and only secondarily by location, is that there is no requirement for regions to be continuous. Instead of defining a region as a collection of pixels whose brightness values are similar in one or more images, an alternative definition can be based on a boundary.

Manually outlining regions for measurement is one way to use this approach. Various interactive pointing devices — such as graphics tablets (also called drawing pads), touch screens, mice, or light pens — can be used, and the drawing can take place while the viewer looks at the computer screen, at a photographic print on a tablet, or through an optical device such as a microscope, with the pointer device optically superimposed. None of these methods is without problems. Display monitors have rather limited resolution. Drawing on a screen representation of a live image does not provide a record of where you have been unless the software draws in a line. Mice are clumsy pointing devices, light pens lose precision in dark areas of the display, touch screens have poor resolution (and your finger gets in the way), and so on. Drawing tablets that incorporate displays are costly, but these are used to some extent in creating graphic arts.

It is beyond the purpose here to describe the operation or compare the utility of these different approaches. Regardless of what physical device is used for manual outlining, the method relies on the human visual image processor to locate boundaries and produces a result that consists of a polygonal approximation to the region outline. Many people tend to draw just outside the actual boundary of whatever features they perceive to be important, making dimensions larger than they should be, and the amount of error is a function of the contrast at the edge. (There are exceptions to this, of course. Some people draw inside the boundary. But bias is commonly present in all manually drawn outlines.)

Attempts to emulate the human outlining operation with a computer algorithm require a starting point, usually provided by the human. Then the program examines each adjoining pixel to find which has the characteristics of a boundary, usually defined as a step in brightness. Whichever pixel has the highest value of local gradient is selected and added to the growing polygon, and then the procedure is repeated. Sometimes a constraint is added to minimize sharp turns, such as weighting the pixel values according to direction.

Automatic edge following suffers from several problems. First, the edge definition is essentially local. People have a rather adaptable capability to look ahead various distances to find pieces of edge to be connected together. Gestalt psychologists describe this as grouping, and it is discussed in **Chapter 2**. Such a response is difficult for an algorithm that looks only within a small neighborhood. Even in rather simple images, there may be places along boundaries where the local gradient or other measure of edgeness drops.

In addition, edges may touch where regions abut. The algorithm is equally likely to follow either edge, which of course gives a nonsensical result. There may also be a problem of when to end the process. If the edge is a single, simple line, then it ends when it reaches the starting point. If the line reaches another feature that already has a defined boundary (from a previous application of the routine), or if it reaches the edge of the field of view, then there is no way to complete the outline.

The major problems with edge following are: (a) it cannot by itself complete the segmentation of the image because it has to be given each new starting point and cannot determine whether there are more outlines to be followed and (b) the same edge-defining criteria used for following edges can be applied more easily by processing the entire image and then thresholding. This produces a line of pixels that may be broken and incomplete (if the edge following would have been unable to continue) or may branch (if several boundaries touch). However, there are methods discussed in **Chapter 8** that apply erosion/dilation or watershed logic to deal with some of these deficiencies. The global application of the processing operation finds all of the boundaries.

Figure 7.39 illustrates a few of these effects. The image consists of several hand-drawn dark lines, to which a small amount of random noise is added and a ridge-following algorithm applied (Van Helden 1994). Each of the user-selected starting points is shown with the path followed by the automatic routine. The settings used for this example instruct the algorithm to consider points out to a distance of 5 pixels in deciding which direction to move at each point. Increasing this number produces artificially smooth boundaries and also takes more time, as more neighbors must be searched. Conversely, reducing it makes it more likely to follow false turnings. Many of the paths are successful, but a significant number are not. By comparison, thresholding the image to select dark pixels, and then skeletonizing the resulting broad outline as discussed in **Chapter 8**, produces good boundary lines for all of the regions at once.

The same comparison can be made with a real image. **Figure 7.40** shows a fluorescence image from a light microscope. In this case, the inability of the fully automatic ridge-following method to track the boundaries has been supplemented by a manually assisted technique. The user draws a line near the boundary, and the algorithm moves the points onto the nearest (within some preset maximum distance) darkest point. This method — sometimes called "active contours," "balloons," or "snakes" — allows the user to overcome many of the difficulties in which the automatic method might wander away from the correct line, never to return. But it is still faster to use thresholding and skeletonizing to get the boundary lines, and while the details of the lines differ, it is not evident that either method is consistently superior for delineation.

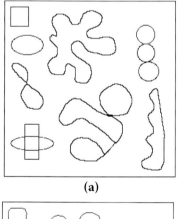
(a)

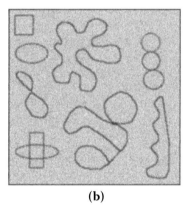
(b)

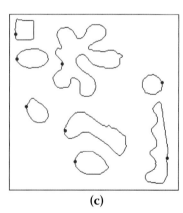
(c)

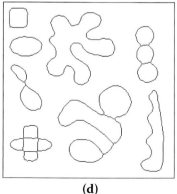
(d)

Figure 7.39 *Test image for automatic line following:*
  (a) *hand-drawn lines;*
  (b) *addition of random noise to image **a**;*
  (c) *lines found by automatic tracing, showing the starting points for each (notice that some portions of crossing or branching line patterns are not followed);*
  (d) *lines found by thresholding and skeletonization.*

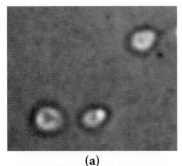

(a)

Figure 7.40 *Light-microscope fluorescence image with three features:*
(a) *original;*
(b) *edge-following algorithm (red shows fully automatic results, purple shows a feature that required manual assistance to outline), with outlines from superimposed on the original;*
(c) *brightness thresholding the original image;*
(d) *skeletonized outlines from image c superimposed on the original.*

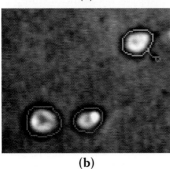

(b)

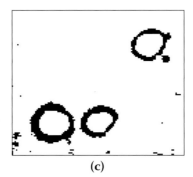

(c)

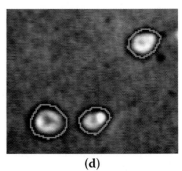

(d)

Contours

One type of line that can provide boundary information and is guaranteed to be continuous is a contour line. This is analogous to the isoelevation contour lines drawn on topographic maps. The line marks a constant elevation or, in the case of images, a constant brightness in the image. These lines cannot end, although they can branch or loop back upon themselves. In a continuous image or an actual topographic surface, there is always a point through which the line can pass. For a discrete image, the brightness value of the line may not happen to correspond to any specific pixel value. Nevertheless, if there is a pair of pixels with one value brighter than and one value darker than the contour level, then the line must pass somewhere between them.

The contour line can, in principle, be fit as a polygon through the points interpolated between pixel centers for all such pairs of pixels that bracket the contour value. This permits measuring the locations of these lines, and the boundaries that they may represent, to less than the dimensions of one pixel, called subpixel sampling or measurement. This is used in **Chapter 10** for feature measurement, but it is rarely used to represent an entire image because of the need to represent each boundary by such a series of points, which must be assembled into a polygon.

The most common use of contour lines is to mark the pixels that lie closest to, or closest to and above, the line. These pixels approximate the contour line to the resolution of the pixels in the original image, form a continuous band of touching pixels (touching in an eight-neighbor sense, as discussed below), and can be used to delineate features in many instances. Creating the line from the image is simply a matter of scanning the pixels once, comparing each pixel and its neighbors above and to the left to the contour value, and marking the pixel if the values bracket the test value.

Figure 7.41 shows an image with contour lines drawn at a selected brightness value to mark the boundaries of the pores. **Chapter 9** introduces the relationship between the length of these

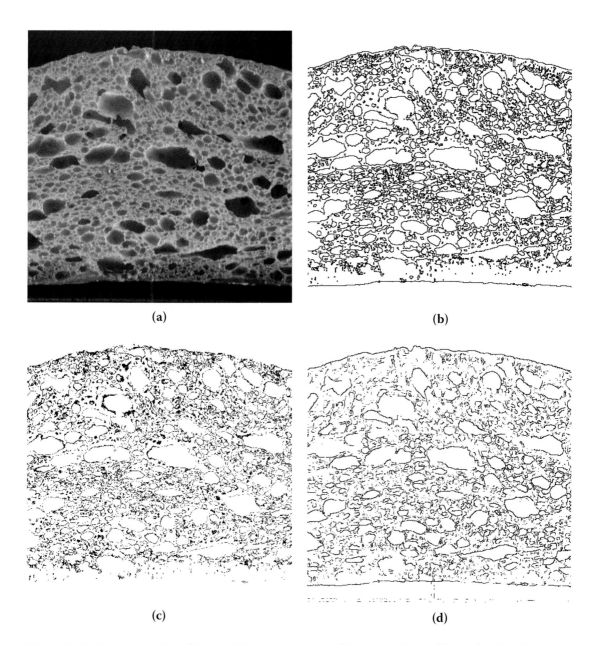

Figure 7.41 *Pores in a slice of bread:* **(a)** *original image;* **(b)** *contour lines;* **(c)** *pixels selected by thresholding;* **(d)** *edges from a Canny edge detector.*

lines and the total surface area of the pores. Notice that setting a threshold range around this same brightness level, even with a fairly large range, does not produce continuous lines, because the brightness gradient in some regions is quite steep and no pixels fall within the range. The brightness gradient is very gradual in other regions, so an edge-finding operator such as the Canny does not show all of the same boundaries, and does introduce more noise.

Drawing a series of contour lines on an image can be an effective way to show minor variations in brightness, as shown in **Figure 7.42**. Even for complex three-dimensional scenes

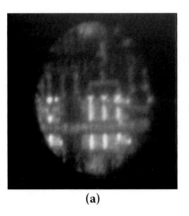

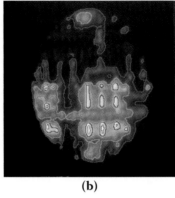

(a)   (b)

Figure 7.42 *Ion microprobe image of boron implanted in a silicon wafer:*
(a) *original image, in which brightness is proportional to concentration;*
(b) *isobrightness or isoconcentration contour lines superimposed, which make it easier to compare values in different parts of the image.*

such as **Figure 7.43**, a series of contour lines is often able to delineate regions of similarity or convey structural meaning. For one important class of images, range images in which pixel brightness measures elevation, such a set of lines is the topographic map. Such images can result from radar imaging, the CSLM (confocal scanning laser microscope), interferometry, the STM (scanning tunneling microscope) or AFM (atomic force microscope), and other devices. **Figure 7.44** shows a scanned stylus image of a coin, with contour lines drawn to delineate the raised surfaces, and a similar image of a ball bearing. The contour lines on the ball show the roughness and out-of-roundness of the surface, and these can be measured quantitatively for such a purpose. **Chapter 14** illustrates the measurement of such range images.

Image representation

Different representations of the binary image are possible; some are more useful than others for specific purposes. Most measurements, such as feature area and position, can be directly calculated from a pixel-based representation by simple counting procedures. This can be stored in less space than the original array of pixels by using run-length encoding (also called chord encoding). This treats the image as a series of scan lines. For each sequential line across each region or feature, it stores the line number, start position, and length of the line. **Figure 7.45** illustrates this schematically.

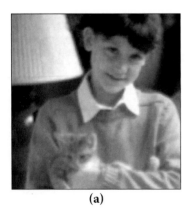

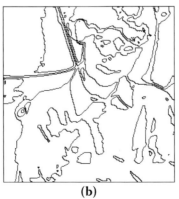

(a)   (b)

Figure 7.43
(a) *Real-world image and*
(b) *four contour lines drawn at selected brightness values. However irregular they become, the lines are always continuous and distinct.*

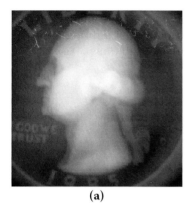

(a)

Figure 7.44 *Range images and contour lines:*
(a) *range image of a coin;*
(b) *contour lines delineating raised areas on the surface;*
(c) *range image of a ball bearing;*
(d) *contour lines showing roughness and out-of-roundness (color-coded according to elevation).*

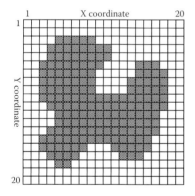

(b)

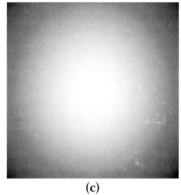

(c)

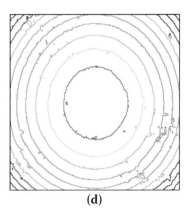

(d)

1   X coordinate   20

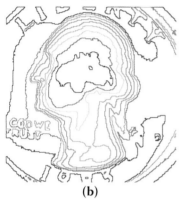

Y coordinate

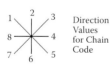

Direction Values for Chain Code

Chain Code

4444546776664444223244566676
676788118877781123321 12222323

Run-Length Encoded			Boundary Coord.	
Y	X	Length	X	Y
3	5	5	5	3
4	4	8	9	3
5	4	8	11	4
6	3	8	11	5
6	15	3	9	7
7	3	7	9	10
7	15	4	14	10
8	3	7	14	8
8	14	5	15	7
9	3	7	15	6
9	14	5	17	6
10	3	16	18	7
11	4	15	18	11
12	5	14	17	14
13	5	14	16	16
14	4	15	15	17
15	3	15	13	17
16	3	6	11	15
16	12	5	9	15
17	4	4	6	18
17	13	3	5	18
18	5	2	3	16
			3	15
			5	13
			5	12
			3	10
			3	6
			4	5
			4	4
			5	3

Figure 7.45 *Encoding the same region in a binary image by run-length encoding, boundary polygonal representation, or chain code.*

For typical images, the pixels are not randomly scattered, but collected together into regions or features so that the run-length-encoded table is much smaller than the original image. This is the method used, for instance, to transmit fax messages over telephone lines. **Figure 7.46** shows how a black and white image is encoded for this purpose. In this example, the original image is $256 \times 256 = 65,536$ pixels, while the run-length table is only 1460 bytes long. The run-length table can be used directly for area and position measurements, with even less arithmetic than the pixel array. Since the chords are in the order in which the raster crosses the features, some logic is required to identify the chords with the features, but this is often done as the table is built.

The chord table is poorly suited for measuring feature perimeters or shape. Boundary representation, consisting of the coordinates of the polygon comprising the boundary, is superior for this task. However, it is awkward for dealing with regions containing internal holes, since

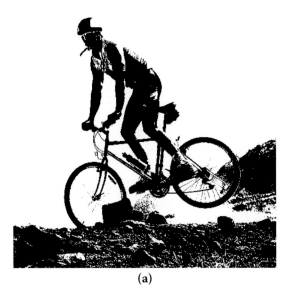

(a)

Figure 7.46 Representing a black-and-white image for fax transmission:
(a) original;
(b) run-length encoded (each horizontal line is marked with a red point at its start, just the position of the red point and the length of the line are sent);
(c) representing the same image with formed characters, a graphic trick that was in common use several decades ago.

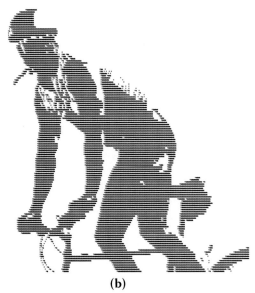

(b)   (c)

there is nothing to relate the interior boundary to the exterior. Again, logic must be used to identify the internal boundaries, keep track of which ones are exterior and which are interior, and construct a hierarchy of features within features, if needed.

A simple polygonal approximation to the boundary can be produced when it is needed from the run-length table by using the endpoints of the series of chords shown in **Figure 7.45**. A special form of this polygon can be formed from all of the boundary points, consisting of a series of short vectors from one boundary point to the next. On a square-pixel array, each of these lines is either 1 or √2 pixels long and can only have one of eight directions. Assigning a digit from 1 to 8 (or 0 to 7, or −3 to +4, depending on the particular implementation) to each direction and writing all of the numbers for the closed boundary in order produces chain code, also shown in **Figure 7.45**.

This form is particularly well suited for calculating perimeter or describing shape (Cederberg 1979; Freeman 1961, 1974). The perimeter is determined by counting the number of even and odd digits, multiplying the number of odd ones by the square root of 2 to correct for diagonal directions, and adding. The chain code also contains shape information, which can be used to locate corners, simplify the shape of the outline, match features independent of orientation, or calculate various shape descriptors.

Most current-generation imaging systems use an array of square pixels, because it is well suited both to raster-scan acquisition devices and to processing images and performing measurements. If rectangular pixels are acquired by using a different pixel spacing along scan lines than between the lines, processing in either the spatial domain with neighborhood operations or in the frequency domain becomes much more difficult, because the different pixel distances as a function of orientation must be taken into account. The use of rectangular pixels also complicates measurements.

With a square-pixel array, there is a problem that we have already seen in the previous chapters on image processing: the four pixels diagonally adjacent to a central pixel are actually farther away than the four sharing an edge. An alternative arrangement that has been used in a few systems is to place the pixels in a hexagonal array. This has the advantage of equal spacing between all neighboring pixels, and makes all of the neighboring pixels equivalent in sharing an edge, which simplifies processing and calculations. Its great disadvantage, however, is that standard cameras and other acquisition and display devices do not operate that way.

For a traditional square-pixel array, it is necessary to decide whether pixels adjacent at a corner are actually touching. This will be important for the binary processing operations in **Chapter 8**. It is necessary in order to link pixels into features or follow the points around a boundary, as discussed previously. While it is not obvious that one choice is superior to the other, whichever one is made for the pixels that compose a feature, the background (the pixels that surround the features) must have the opposite relationship.

Figure 7.47a shows this dual situation. If pixels within a feature are assumed to touch any of their eight adjacent neighbors (called eight-connectedness), then the line of pixels in the figure separates the background on either side, and the background pixels that are diagonally adjacent do not touch. They are therefore four-connected (touch only their four edge-sharing neighbors). Conversely, if the background pixels touch diagonally, the pixels are isolated and would only touch along their edges. For the fragment shown in **Figure 7.47b**, choosing an eight-connected rule for features (dark pixels) produces a single feature with an internal hole. If a four-connected rule is used, there are four features, and the background, now eight-connected, is continuous. Most systems use an eight-connected rule for features and a four-connected rule for background.

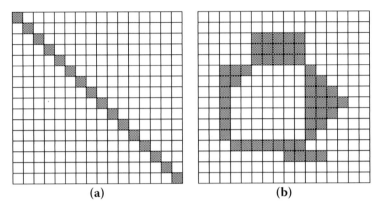

(a)   (b)

Figure 7.47 Ambiguous images: (a) If the pixels are assumed to touch at their corners, then this shows a line that separates the background pixels on either side; but those pixels also touch at their corners; if eight-connectedness or four-connectedness is selected for feature pixels, then the opposite convention applies to background pixels; (b) example showing either four separate features or one containing an internal hole, depending on the touching convention.

This duality means that simply inverting an image (interchanging white and black) does not reverse the meaning of the features and background. **Figure 7.48** shows a situation in which the holes within a feature (separated from the background) become part of a single region in the reversed image. This can cause confusion in measurements and binary image processing. When feature dimensions as small as one pixel are important, there is some basic uncertainty. This is unavoidable and argues for using large arrays of small pixels to define small dimensions and feature topology accurately.

Other segmentation methods

There are other methods used for image segmentation besides the ones based on thresholding discussed so far. These are generally associated with fairly powerful computer systems and with attempts to understand images in the sense of machine vision and robotics (Ballard and Brown 1982; Wilson and Spann 1988). Two of the most widely described are split-and-merge and region-growing methods, which seem to lie at opposite extremes.

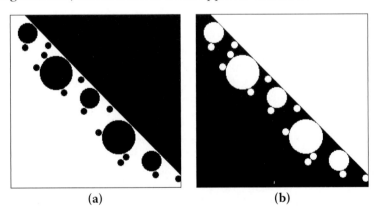

(a)   (b)

Figure 7.48 Reversing an image (interchanging features and background) without changing the connectedness rules alters meaning. In image (a) the black pixels all touch at corners (eight-connectedness), and so this is one feature with an irregular boundary; (b) the white pixels do not touch (four-connectedness), and so these are separate holes within the feature.

Split-and-merge is a top-down method that begins with the entire image. Some image property is selected as a criterion to decide whether everything is uniform. This criterion is often based on the statistics from the brightness histogram, although color information or local statistical properties can also be used. If the histogram is multimodal, or has a high standard deviation, etc., then the region is assumed to be nonuniform and is divided into four quadrants. Each quadrant is examined in the same way and subdivided again if necessary. The procedure continues until the individual pixel level is reached. The relationship between the parent region and the four quadrants, or children, is typically encoded in a quadtree structure, another name sometimes applied to this approach.

This is not the only way to subdivide the parent image and encode the resulting data structure. Thresholding can be used to divide each region into arbitrary subregions, which can be subdivided iteratively. This can produce final results having less blocky boundaries, but the data structure is much more complex, since all of the regions must be defined, and the time required for the process is much greater.

Subdividing regions alone does not create a useful image segmentation. After each iteration of subdividing, each region is compared with adjacent ones that lie in different squares at a higher level in the hierarchy. If they are similar, they are merged together. The definition of "similar" can use the same tests applied to the splitting operation, or comparisons can be made only for pixels along or near the common edge. The latter has the advantage of tolerating gradual changes across the image.

Figure 7.49 shows an example in which only four iterations have been performed. A few large areas have already merged, and their edges will be refined as the iterations proceed. Other parts of the image contain individual squares that require additional subdivision before regions become visible.

An advantage of this approach is that a complete segmentation is achieved after a finite number of iterations (for instance, a 512-pixel-square image takes nine iterations to reach individual pixels, since $2^9 = 512$). Also, the quadtree list of regions and subregions can be used for some measurements, and the segmentation identifies all of the different types of regions at one time. By comparison, thresholding methods typically isolate one type of region or feature at a time. They must be applied several times to deal with images containing more than one class of objects.

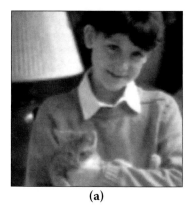 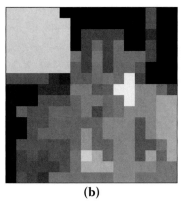 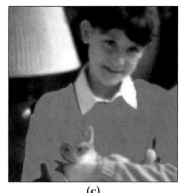

(a)   (b)   (c)

Figure 7.49 *Other segmentation methods: (**a**) original gray-scale image; (**b**) split and merge after four iterations; (**c**) region growing from a point in the girl's sweater.*

On the other hand, the split-and-merge approach depends on the quality of the test used to detect inhomogeneity in each region. Small subregions within large uniform areas can easily be missed with this method. Standard statistical tests that assume, for example, a normal distribution of pixel brightness within regions are rarely appropriate for real images, so more complicated procedures must be used (Yakimovsky 1976). Tests used for subdividing and merging regions can also be expressed as image processing operations. A processed image can reveal the same edges and texture used for the split-and-merge tests in a way that allows direct thresholding. This is potentially less efficient, since time-consuming calculations can be applied to parts of the image that are uniform, but the results are the same. Thresholding also has the advantage of identifying similar objects in different parts of the field of view as the same, which may not occur with split-and-merge.

Conversely, region growing starts from the bottom, or individual pixel level, and works upward. Starting at some seed location (usually provided by the operator but in some cases located by image processing tools such as the top-hat filter), neighboring pixels are examined one at a time and added to the growing region if they are sufficiently similar. Again, the comparison can be made to the entire region or just to the local pixels, with the latter method allowing gradual variations in brightness. It is also possible, but more time consuming, to make the test "adaptive" in the sense that the tolerance for adding another pixel depends on the standard deviation of pixels in the growing region. The procedure continues until no more pixels can be added. **Figure 7.49c** shows an example in which one region has been identified; notice that it includes part of the cat as well as the girl's sweater, and does not include an arm of the sweater. Then a new region is begun at another location.

The seed-fill algorithm is logically equivalent (although usually implemented quite differently) to a point-sampled dilation, constrained to regions within a set threshold range. Dilation is a morphological procedure described in detail in **Chapter 8**.

If the same comparison tests are implemented to decide whether a pixel belongs to a region, the result of this procedure is the same region as top-down split-and-merge produces. The difficulty with this approach is that the starting point for each region must be provided. Depending on the comparison tests employed, different starting points may not grow into identical regions. **Figure 7.50** shows several different starting points (shown by the blue marks) within what is visually the same structure (the unbrowned cheese on a pizza), and the resulting different regions (red outlines) are obtained with the same tolerance value. Also, there is no ideal structure to encode the data from this procedure, beyond keeping the entire pixel array until classification is complete; and the complete classification is slow, since each pixel must be examined individually.

Region growing also suffers from the conflicting needs to keep the test local, to see if an individual pixel should be added to the growing region, and to make it larger in scale, if not truly global, to ensure that the region has some unifying and distinct identity. If too small a test region is used, a common result is that regions leak out into adjoining areas or merge with different regions. This leaking or merging can occur if even a single pixel on the boundary can form a bridge.

Finally, there is no easy way to decide when the procedure is complete and all of the meaningful regions in the image have been found. Region growing (also known as a seed-fill technique) can be a useful method for selecting a few regions in an image, as compared with manual tracing or edge following, for example, but it is rarely the method of choice for complex images containing many regions (H-S. Wu et al. 2005; Zucker 1976).

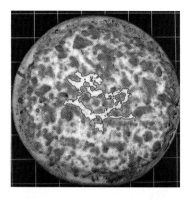 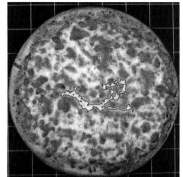 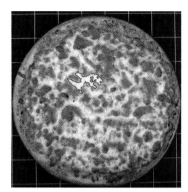

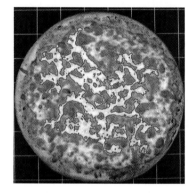

Figure 7.50 *Region growing from various seeds. The blue marks indicate the original seed, and the red lines show the boundaries of the contiguous selected regions, all using the same tolerance values.*

Edge following was mentioned previously in terms of an algorithm that tries to mimic a human drawing operation by tracing along a boundary and, at each point, selecting the next pixel to step toward based on local-neighborhood values. Human vision does not restrict itself to such local decisions but can use remote information to bridge over troublesome points. A machine-vision approach, which does the same, constructs outlines of objects as deformable polygons. The sides of the polygon can be splines rather than straight lines, to achieve a smoother shape. These deformable boundaries are referred to as "snakes" (Kass et al. 1987). Other arbitrary fitting constants — the minimum length of any side, the maximum angular change at any vertex, etc. — must reflect some independent knowledge about the region that is to be fitted. They must generally be adjusted for each application until the results are acceptable compared with visual judgment.

Since fitting is accomplished for all of the points on the boundary at once using a minimization technique, the snakes can accommodate some missing or confusing points. They are particularly useful for tracking moving boundaries in a sequence of images, since the deformation of the snake from one moment to the next must be small. This makes them useful for tracking moving objects in robotics vision. When applied to three-dimensional arrays of voxels, as in medical imaging, they become deformable polyhedra and are called "balloons."

The general classification problem

The various methods described so far have relied on human judgment to recognize the presence of regions and to define them by delineating the boundary or selecting a range

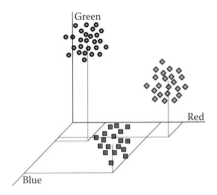

Green

Red

Blue

Figure 7.51 *Schematic illustration of pixel classification in color space. Each pixel is plotted according to its color values, and clusters identify the various regions present.*

of brightness values. Methods have been discussed that can start with an incomplete definition and refine the segmentation to achieve greater accuracy or consistency. There are also fully automatic techniques that determine how many classes of objects are present and then fully subdivide the image to isolate them. However, they are little used in small computer-based systems and are often much less efficient than using some human input. The task of general image segmentation can be treated as an example of a classification problem. Like most techniques involving elements or artificial intelligence, this may not use the same inputs or decision methods that a human employs, but it seeks to duplicate the results (and often succeeds).

One successful approach to general classification has been used with satellite imagery, in which many wavelength bands of data are available (Reeves 1975). If each pixel in the image is plotted in a high-dimensionality space, where each axis is the measured brightness in one of the wavelength bands, it is expected that points corresponding to different classes of land use, crop type, soil or rock type, and so forth, will cluster together and that the clusters will be well separated from each other, as indicated in **Figure 7.51**. The problem then reduces to finding the clusters and fitting boundaries between them that can be used for classification. Finding clusters and boundaries between regions is discussed in a more general context in **Chapter 11**.

Reduced to a single dimension (a simple gray-scale image), this classification begins with the brightness histogram. The cluster analysis looks for peaks and tries to draw thresholds between them. This is successful in a few specialized tasks, such as counting cells of one type on a microscope slide. As the number of dimensions increases, for instance using the RGB or HSI data from color imagery or adding values from a derived texture or gradient image, the separation of the clusters usually becomes more distinct while the location of a "peak" and the definition of its boundaries become more difficult. Satellite imagery with several discrete visible and infrared wavelength bands is especially well suited to this approach.

Clusters are easier to recognize when they contain many similar points, but minor regions or uncommon objects may be overlooked. Also, the number of background points surrounding the clusters (or more often lying along lines between them) confuse the automatic algorithms. These points arise from the finite size of pixels that straddle the boundaries between regions. Finding a few major clusters may be straightforward. Being sure that all have been found is not.

Even after the clusters have been identified (and here some *a priori* knowledge or input from a human can be of great assistance, particularly the number of clusters expected), there are different strategies for using this information to classify new points. One is to surround each cluster with a boundary, typically either a polyhedron formed by planes lying perpendicular to the lines between the cluster centers, or *n*-dimensional ellipsoids. Points falling inside any of these regions are immediately classified.

Particularly for the ellipsoid case, it is also possible to have a series of concentric boundaries that enclose different percentages of the points in the cluster, which can be used to give a probability of classification to new points. This is sometimes described as a "fuzzy" classification method. If the new pixels added to a cluster change the mean value and the limits, this becomes an iterative method.

A third approach is to find the nearest classified point to each new point and assign that identity to the new one. This method has several drawbacks, particularly when there are some densely populated clusters and others with very few members, or when the clusters are close or overlapping. It requires considerable time to search through a large universe of existing points to locate the closest one, as well. An extension of this technique is also used, in which a small number of nearest neighbors are identified that "vote" for the identity of the new point. It is even possible to weight the existing values inversely by their distance from the pixel being tested (Chen et al. 2005).

Segmentation of gray-scale images into regions for measurement or recognition is probably the most important single problem area for image analysis. Many novel techniques have been used that are rather *ad hoc* and narrow in their range of applicability. Review articles by Fu and Mui (1981) and Haralick and Shapiro (1988) present good guides to the literature. Most standard image-analysis textbooks, such as Rosenfeld and Kak (1982), Castleman (1979), Gonzalez and Wintz (1987), Russ (1990b), and Pratt (1991), also contain sections on segmentation.

All of these various methods and modifications are used extensively in other artificial-intelligence situations (see, for example, Fukunaga 1990). They can be implemented in hardware, software, or some combination of the two. Only limited application of any of these techniques has been made to the segmentation problem. However, it is likely that the use of such methods will increase in the future as more color or multiband imaging is done and as computer power continues to increase.

Processing Binary Images

Binary images, as discussed in the preceding chapter, consist of pixels and groups of pixels selected on the basis of some property. The selection can be performed by thresholding brightness values, perhaps using several gray-scale images containing different color channels, or processed to extract texture or other information. The goal of binarization is to separate features from background so that counting, measurement, or matching operations can be performed.

However, as shown by the examples in **Chapter 7**, the result of the segmentation operation is rarely perfect. For images of realistic complexity, even the most elaborate segmentation routines misclassify some pixels as foreground or background. These can be pixels along the boundaries of regions, or patches of noise within regions, or pixels that happen to share the specific property or properties used for thresholding with the intended target. The major tools for working with binary images to correct these thresholding errors fit broadly into two groups: Boolean operations for combining images, and morphological operations that modify individual pixels within an image.

Boolean operations

In the section on thresholding color images, in **Chapter 7**, a Boolean AND operation was introduced to combine the data from individual color-channel images. Setting thresholds on brightness values in each of the RGB (red, green, blue) channels allows pixels to be selected that fall into those ranges. This technique produces three binary images (one for each channel), which can then be combined with a logical AND operation. The procedure examines the three images pixel by pixel, keeping pixels for the selected regions if, and only if, they are selected in all three images.

The color-thresholding example illustrates a situation in which pixel brightness values at the same location in several different images (the color channels) must be compared and combined. In some situations it is useful to compare the location and brightness value of pixels in two or more images. **Figure 8.1** shows an example. Two X-ray maps of the same area on a mineral sample show the intensity distributions, and hence represent the concentration distributions for aluminum and silicon. A colocalization (or co-occurrence) plot uses the pixel brightness values for each location in both images as coordinates to produce a histogram

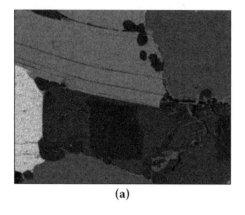
(a)

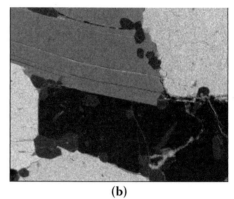
(b)

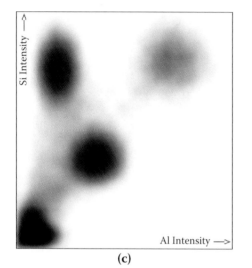
(c)

Figure 8.1 Colocalization:
(a, b) X-ray maps showing the intensity distribution for Al and Si in a mineral;
(c) colocalization plot.

display in which the darkness of each point represents the number of pixels having that combination of values. Regions in the resulting plot that have many pixels represent combinations of elemental concentrations in the original sample. In the example plot, there are four regions present based on Si/Al combinations, and these can be observed in the original images.

Colocalization is also used for biological samples prepared with multiple stains or imaged with multiple wavelengths of light, and it was used in **Chapter 5** as part of the discussion of principal-components analysis. When a colocalization plot shows specific combinations of intensity values that share the same location, each image can be thresholded and the two binary images combined with an AND operation to produce an image of the selected regions.

An aside: The terminology used here will be that of foreground, selected, or ON pixels and unselected, background, or OFF pixels. There is no accepted standard for whether the selected pixels are displayed as white, black, or some other color. In many cases, systems that portray the selected regions as white on a black background on the display screen may reverse this and print hard copy of the same image with black features on a white background. This reversal apparently arises from the fact that, in each case, the selection of foreground pixels is associated with some positive action in the display (turning on the electron beam) or printout (depositing ink on the paper). This inconsistency seems to cause most users little difficulty, provided that something is known about the image. Since many of the images used here are not common objects and some are illustrative examples, it is important to consistently define the foreground pixels (those of interest) in each case. The convention used here is that ON or selected pixels (which will constitute features for subsequent measurement) are shown as black, while OFF pixels (background) are white.

Returning to our desire to combine the information from several images or channels, the AND operation requires that a pixel at location i,j be ON in each individual channel to show up in the result. Pixels having the correct amount of blue but not of red will be omitted, and vice versa. As was noted before, this marks out a rectangle in two-dimensional color space, or a rectangular prism in higher dimensions, encompassing the pixel values to be included. More complicated combinations of color values can be described by delineating an irregular region in n dimensions for pixel selection, as was shown in the preceding chapter. The advantage of simply ANDing discrete ranges is that it can be performed very efficiently and quickly using binary images.

Other Boolean logical rules can be employed to combine binary images. The four possibilities are AND, OR, Ex-OR (exclusive OR), and NOT. **Figure 8.2** illustrates each of these basic operations. **Figure 8.3** shows a few of the possible combinations. All are performed pixel by pixel. The illustrations are based on combining two images at a time, since any logical rule involving

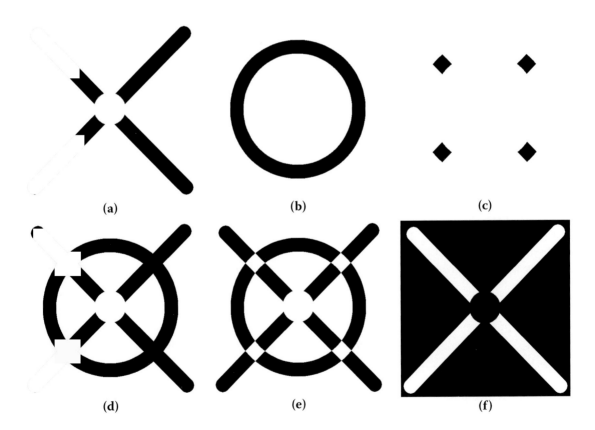

(a)   (b)   (c)

(d)   (e)   (f)

Figure 8.2 Simple Boolean operations: **(a, b)** two binary images; **(c)** A OR B; **(d)** A AND B; **(e)** A Ex-OR B; **(f)** NOT A.

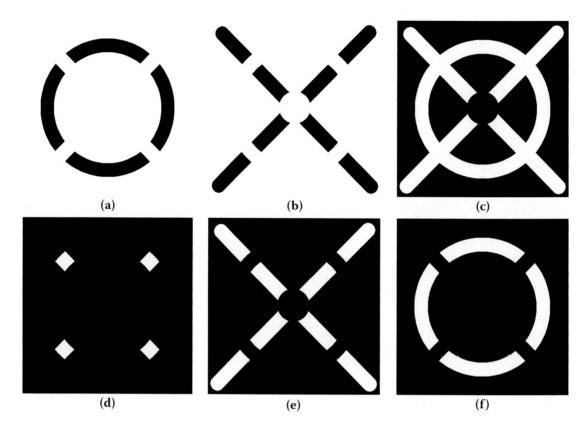

(a) (b) (c)

(d) (e) (f)

Figure 8.3 Combined Boolean operations: **(a)** (NOT A) AND B; **(b)** A AND (NOT B); **(c)** (NOT A) AND (NOT B); **(d)** NOT (A AND B); **(e)** (NOT A) OR B; **(f)** A OR (NOT B).

more than two images can be broken down to a series of steps using just two at a time. The illustrations in the figures are identical to the Venn diagrams used in logic.

As described above, AND requires that pixels be ON in both of the original images to be ON in the result. Pixels that are ON in only one or the other original image are OFF in the result. The OR operator turns a pixel ON in the result if it is ON in either of the original images. In the example shown in **Figure 7.25** of **Chapter 7**, complementary directions and hence different gray-scale values result from the Sobel direction operator as it encounters opposite sides of each striation. Thresholding each direction separately would require an OR to combine them to show the correct regions.

Ex-OR turns a pixel ON in the result if it is ON in either of the original images, but not if it is ON in both. That means that combining (with an OR) the results of ANDing together two images with those from Ex-ORing them produces the same result as an OR in the first place. There are, in fact, many ways to arrange different combinations of the four Boolean operators to produce identical results.

AND, OR, and Ex-OR require two original images and produce a single image as a result. They are also commutative, meaning that the order of the two images is unimportant. A AND B produces the same result as B AND A. The NOT operator requires only a single image. It simply reverses each pixel, turning pixels that were ON to OFF and vice versa. Some systems implement NOT by swapping black and white values for each pixel. As long as we are dealing with pixel-level detail, this works correctly. Later, when feature-level combinations are described, the difference between an eight-connected feature and its four-connected background (discussed in **Chapter 7**) will have to be taken into account.

Given two binary images A and B, the combination (NOT A) AND B will produce an image containing pixels that lie within B but outside A. This is quite different from NOT (A AND B), which selects pixels that are not ON in both A and B. It is also different from A AND (NOT B), as shown in **Figure 8.3**. The order in which the operators is applied is important, and the liberal use of parentheses to clarify the order and scope of operations is crucial. Actually, the four operations discussed above are redundant. Three would be enough to produce all of the same results. Consequently, some systems may omit one of them (usually Ex-OR). For clarity, however, all four will be used in the examples that follow.

Combining Boolean operations

When multiple criteria are available for selecting the pixels to be kept as foreground, they can be combined using any of these Boolean combinations. The most common situations are multi-band or multichannel images, such as produced by a satellite. **Figure 8.4** shows an example.

Another multichannel situation arises in the SEM (scanning electron microscope), where an X-ray detector is often used to create several images (usually called X-ray dot maps, and similar to the examples shown in **Figure 8.1**), each showing the spatial distribution of a selected element. These images can be quite noisy (**Chapter 4**) and difficult to threshold (**Chapter 7**). However, by suitable long-term acquisition or image processing, they can produce useful binary images that indicate locations where the concentration of the element is above some user-selected level.

This selection is usually performed by comparing the measured X-ray intensity to an arbitrary threshold, since there is a finite level of background signal resulting from the process of slowing down the electrons in the sample. The physical background of this phenomenon is not important here. The very poor statistical characteristics of the dot map (hence the name) make it difficult to directly specify a concentration level as a threshold. The X-ray intensity in one part of the image may vary from another region for several reasons: (a) a change in that element's concentration, (b) a change in another element that selectively absorbs or fluoresces the first element's radiation, or (c) a change in specimen density or surface orientation. Comparison of one specimen with another is further hampered by the difficulty in exactly reproducing

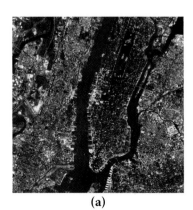

(a)

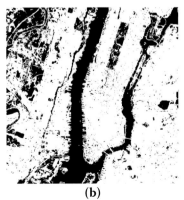

(b)

Figure 8.4 Satellite image:
(a) New York City;
(b) the combination of water (thresholded from a visible light channel) OR vegetation (thresholded from an infrared channel).

instrument conditions. These effects all complicate the relationship between elemental concentration and recorded intensity.

Furthermore, the very poor statistics of the images (due to the extremely low efficiency for producing X-rays with an electron beam and the low-beam intensity required for good spatial resolution in SEM images) mean that these images often require processing, either as gray-scale images (e.g., smoothing) or after binarization (using the morphological tools discussed below). For our present purpose, we will assume that binary images, each showing the spatial distribution of some meaningful concentration level of one of several elements, can be obtained.

As shown in **Figure 8.5**, the SEM also produces more conventional images using secondary or backscattered electrons. These have superior spatial resolution and better feature-shape definition, but with less elemental specificity. The binary images from these sources can be combined with the X-ray or elemental information, as shown in **Figure 8.6**. The X-ray maps for iron (Fe) and silicon (Si) were obtained by smoothing the dot map and thresholding the gray-scale image. Notice that in the gray-scale images, there is a just-discernible difference in the intensity level of the Fe X-rays in two different areas. This is too small a difference for reliable thresholding. Even the larger differences in Si intensity are difficult to separate. However, Boolean logic easily combines the images to produce an image of the region containing Fe but not Si.

Figure 8.7 shows another example from the same data. The regions containing silver (Ag) are generally bright in the backscattered electron image, but some other areas are also bright. On the other hand, the Ag X-ray map does not have precise region boundaries because of the poor statistics. Combining the two binary images with an AND operation produces the desired regions. More complicated sequences of Boolean logical operations can easily be imagined (**Figure 8.7d** shows an example).

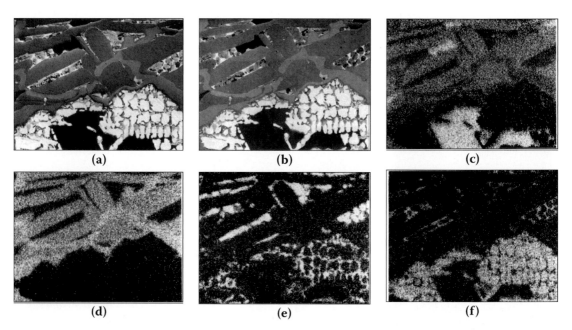

Figure 8.5 *SEM results from a mineral:* **(a)** *backscattered electrons;* **(b)** *secondary electrons;* **(c)** *silicon (Si) X-ray map;* **(d)** *iron (Fe) X-ray map;* **(e)** *copper (Cu) X-ray map;* **(f)** *silver (Ag) X-ray map.*

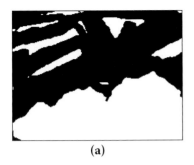

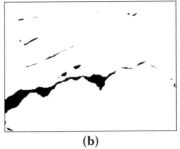

Figure 8.6 *Combining binary images:*
(a) iron;
(b) iron AND NOT silicon.

(a) (b)

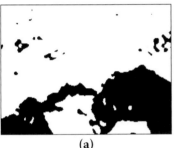

Figure 8.7 *Combining binary images:*
(a) silver;
(b) bright levels from backscattered electron image;
(c) image a AND image b;
(d) a further combination: (Cu OR Ag) AND NOT (Fe).

(a)

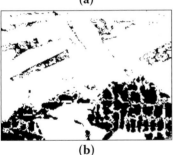

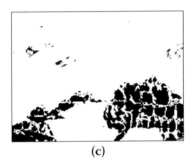

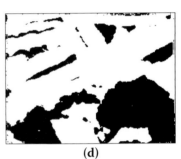

(b) (c) (d)

It is straightforward to imagine a complex specimen containing many elements. Paint pigment particles with a diverse range of compositions provide one example. To count or measure a particular class of particles (pigments, as opposed to brighteners or extenders), it might be necessary to specify those containing iron or chromium or aluminum, but not titanium or sulfur. This would be written as

(Fe OR Cr OR Al) AND (NOT (Ti OR S))

The resulting image might then be combined with a higher-resolution binary produced by thresholding a secondary or backscattered electron image to delineate particle boundaries. Performing these operations can be cumbersome to keep the order of operations straight, but is not difficult.

Most of the examples shown in earlier chapters that used multiple image channels (e.g., different colors or elements) or different processing operations (e.g., combining brightness and texture) use a Boolean AND to combine the separately thresholded binary images. As described above, the AND requires that the pixels to be kept meet all of the criteria. There are some cases in which the Boolean OR is more appropriate. One is illustrated in **Chapter 5**, **Figure 5.68**. This is an image of sand grains in a sandstone, viewed through polarizers. Each rotation of the analyzer causes different grains to become bright or colored. In the earlier chapter, it was shown that keeping the brightest pixel value at each location as the analyzer is rotated gives an image that shows all of the grains.

Figure 8.8 shows an alternative approach to the same problem. Each individual image is thresholded to select those grains that are bright for that particular analyzer rotation angle. Then all of the binary images are combined using a Boolean OR. The resulting combination delineates most of the grains, although the result is not as good as the gray-level operation for the same number of analyzer rotations. In general, image processing, including combining multiple images, is best performed before thresholding whenever possible, because there is more information available from the original pixel values than remains after thresholding.

Masks

The above description of using Boolean logic to combine images makes the assumption that both images are binary (that is, black and white). It is also possible to use a binary image as a mask to modify a gray-scale image. This is most often done to blank out (i.e., set to background) some portion of the gray-scale image, either to create a display in which only the

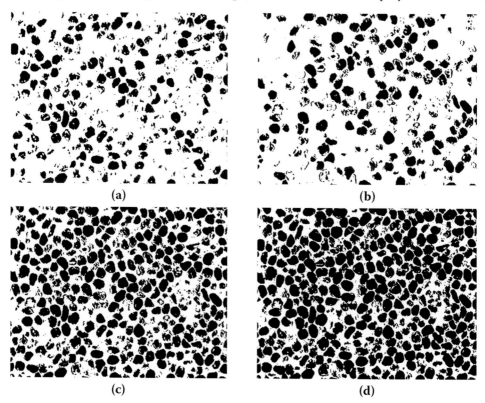

(a)

(b)

(c)

(d)

Figure 8.8 *Combining multiple binary images: (a, b) binary images obtained by thresholding two of the polarized light images of a petrographic thin section of a sandstone (Figure 5.68 in Chapter 5); (c) the result of ORing together six such images from different rotations of the analyzer; (d) comparison binary image produced by thresholding the gray-scale image obtained by combining the same six color images to keep the brightest pixel at each location.*

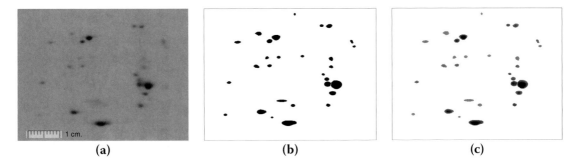

Figure 8.9 *Preserving feature intensity values:* **(a)** *original two-dimensional gel;* **(b)** *thresholded spots;* **(c)** *masked image in which pixels within the spots retain their original brightness values but the background is erased.*

regions of interest are visible or to select regions whose brightness, density, and so forth, are to be measured. **Figure 8.9** shows an example (a protein-separation gel) in which the dark spots are isolated by thresholding, and then the thresholded binary image is applied as a mask to produce separated features for measurement that retain the original density values.

There are several physical ways that this operation can be performed. The binary mask can be used in an overlay, or alpha channel, to select pixels to be displayed, or the mask can be used to modify the stored image. This can done by multiplying the gray-scale image by the binary image, with the convention that the binary image values are 0 (OFF) or 1 (ON) at each pixel. In some systems this result is implemented by combining the gray-scale and binary images to keep whichever value is darker or brighter. For instance, if the mask is white for background and black for foreground pixels, then the brighter pixel values at each location will erase all background pixels and keep the gray value for the foreground pixels.

This capability is often used to display the results of various processing and thresholding operations. It is easier to judge the performance of thresholding by viewing selected pixels with the original gray-scale information rather than just looking at the binary image. It is also useful to apply a mask obtained by thresholding one version of an image to view another version. **Figure 8.10** shows an example in which values representing the orientation angle (from the Sobel derivative) of grain boundaries in the aluminum alloy are masked by thresholding the magnitude of the gradient to isolate only the boundaries.

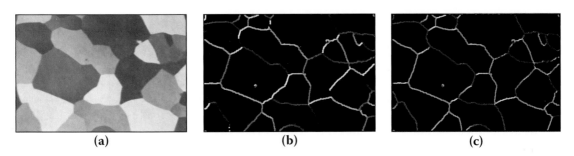

Figure 8.10 *Masking one image with another. The direction of a Sobel gradient applied to the light-microscope image of an aluminum alloy is shown only in the regions where the magnitude of the gradient is large:* **(a)** *original image;* **(b)** *orientation values (gray scale) shown only along grain boundaries;* **(c)** *color lookup table applied to assign colors to the orientation values.*

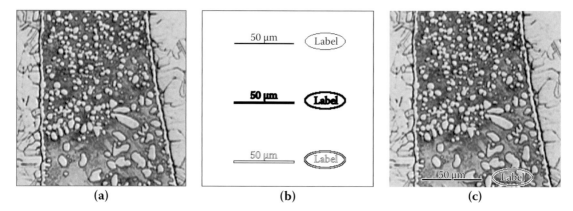

Figure 8.11 *Using a mask to apply a label to an image. The original image **(a)** contains both white and black areas, so that simple superimposition of text will not be visible. A mask is created by dilating the label and Ex-ORing that with the original **(b)**. The composite is then superimposed on the gray-scale image **(c)**.*

Another use of masking and Boolean image combination is shown in **Figure 8.11**. An essentially cosmetic application, it is still useful and widely employed. A label superimposed on an image using either black or white can be difficult to read if the image contains a full range of brightness values. In this example, using dilation (discussed later in this chapter), the label is used to create a mask that is one pixel larger in all directions. This mask is then used to erase the pixels in the gray-scale image to white before writing in the label in black (or vice versa). The result maintains legibility for the label while obscuring a minimum amount of the image.

From pixels to features

The Boolean operations described above deal with individual pixels in the image. For some purposes it is necessary to identify the pixels forming part of a connected whole. As discussed in **Chapter 7**, it is possible to adopt a convention for touching that is either eight-connected or four-connected for the pixels in a single feature (sometimes referred to as a "blob" to indicate that no interpretation of the connected group of pixels has been inferred as representing anything specific in the image). Whichever convention is adopted, grouping pixels into features is an important step (Levialdi 1972; Ritter and Wilson 2001).

It is possible to imagine starting with one pixel (any ON pixel, selected at random) and checking its four- or eight-neighbor positions, labeling each pixel that is ON as part of the same feature, and then iteratively repeating the operation until no neighbors remain. Then a new unlabeled pixel would be chosen and the operation repeated, continuing until every ON pixel in the image was labeled as part of some feature. The usual way of proceeding with this deeply recursive "seed-fill" operation is to create a stack in which to place pixel locations as they are found to be neighbors of already labeled pixels. Pixels are removed from the stack as their neighbors are examined. The process ends when the stack is empty and all connected pixels have been located and identified.

It is more efficient to deal with pixels in groups. If the image has already been run-length or chord encoded, as discussed in **Chapter 7**, then all of the pixels within the chord are known to touch, that touching any of them is equivalent to touching all, and that the only candidates for touching are those on adjacent lines above or below. This fact makes possible a straightforward labeling algorithm that passes one time through the image. Each chord's endpoints are compared with those of chords in the preceding line; if they touch or overlap (based on a simple comparison of values), the label from the preceding line is attached to this chord. If not, then a new label is used.

If a chord touches two chords in the previous line that had different labels, then the two labels are identified with each other (this handles the bottom of a letter *U* for example). All of the occurrences of one label can be changed to the other, either immediately or later. When the pass through the image or the list of chords is complete, all of the chords, and therefore all of the pixels, are identified, and the total number of labels (and therefore features) is known. **Figure 8.12** shows this logic in the form of a flow chart.

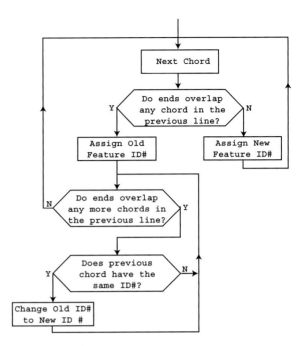

Figure 8.12 *Flow chart for grouping touching pixels in a run-length- or chord-encoded array into features and assigning identification numbers.*

For boundary representation (including the special case of chain code), the analysis is partially complete, since the boundary already represents a closed path around a feature. If features contained no holes and no feature could ever be surrounded by another, this would provide complete information. Unfortunately, this is not always the case. It is usually necessary to reconstruct the pixel array to identify pixels with feature labels (Kim et al. 1988).

In any case, once the individual features have been labeled, several additional Boolean operations are possible. One is to find and fill holes within features. Any pixel that is part of a hole is OFF (i.e., part of the background) but is surrounded by ON pixels. For boundary representation, that means the pixel is within a boundary. For pixel representation, it means it is not connected to other pixels that eventually form a path to the edge of the field of view.

Recalling that the convention for touching (eight- or four-connectedness) must be different for the background than for the foreground, we can identify holes most easily by inverting the image (replacing white with black and vice versa) and labeling the resulting pixels as though they were features, as shown step by step in **Figure 8.13**. Features in this inverted image that do not touch any side of the field of view are the original holes. If the pixels are added back to the original image (using a Boolean OR), the result is to fill any internal holes in the original features.

One very simple example of the application of this technique is shown in **Figure 8.14**. In this image of spherical particles, the center of each feature has a brightness very close to that of the substrate due to the lighting. Thresholding the brightness values gives a good delineation of the outer boundary of the particles, but the centers have holes. Filling them as described produces a corrected representation of the particles, which can be measured. This type of processing is commonly required for SEM images, whose brightness varies as a function of local

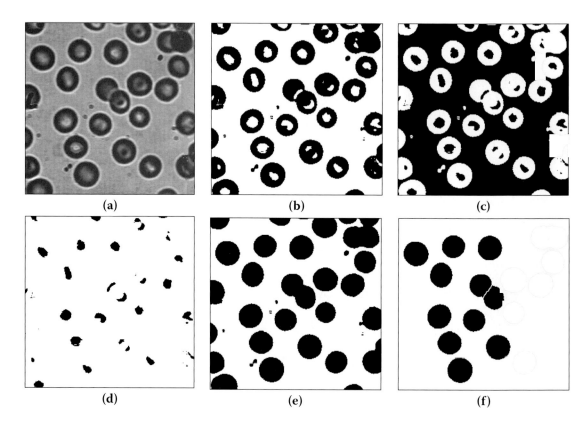

(a)   (b)   (c)

(d)   (e)   (f)

Figure 8.13 *Light-microscope image of red blood cells:* **(a)** *original;* **(b)** *thresholded, which shows the thicker outer edges of the blood cells but not the thinner central regions;* **(c)** *image* **b** *inverted;* **(d)** *removing the edge-touching background from image* **c**; **(e)** *combining the features in image* **d** *with those in image* **b** *using a Boolean OR;* **(f)** *removing small features (dirt), edge-touching features (which cannot be measured), and separating touching features in image* **e**.

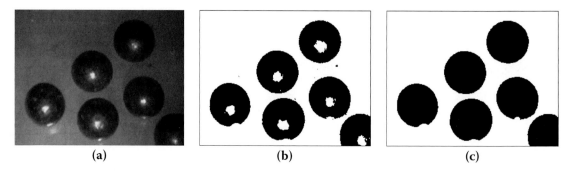

(a)   (b)   (c)

Figure 8.14 *Image of metal spheres with near-vertical incident illumination:* **(a)** *original gray-scale image;* **(b)** *brightness thresholded after leveling illumination;* **(c)** *internal holes filled and small regions (noise) in background removed by erosion.*

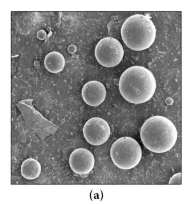 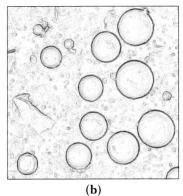 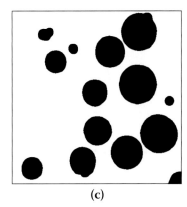

Figure 8.15 *SEM image of spherical particles:* **(a)** *original image;* **(b)** *edges obtained with a Sobel operator;* **(c)** *particles delineated by thresholding the edges and filling the centers.*

surface slope so that particles frequently appear with bright edges and dark centers. **Figure 8.15** shows an example.

This problem is not restricted to convex surfaces or to the SEM. **Figure 8.16** shows a light-microscope image of spherical pores in an enamel coating. The light spots in the center of many of the pores vary in brightness, depending on the depth of the pore. They must be corrected by filling the features in a thresholded binary image.

Figure 8.17 shows a more complicated situation requiring several operations. The SEM image shows the boundaries of the spores clearly to a human viewer, but they cannot be directly revealed by thresholding because the shades of gray are also present in the substrate. Applying an edge-finding algorithm (in this example, a Frei and Chen operator) delineates the boundaries, and it is then possible to threshold them to obtain feature outlines, as shown. These must be filled using the method described above. Further

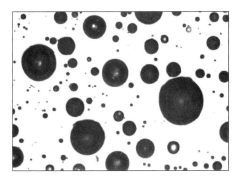

Figure 8.16 *Light-microscope image of a polished section through an enamel coating on steel shows bright spots of reflected light within many pores (depending on their depth). (Courtesy of V. Benes, Research Institute for Metals, Panenské Brezany, Czechoslovakia.)*

operations are then needed before measurement: an erosion operation to remove the other thresholded pixels in the image, and watershed segmentation to separate the touching objects. Both are described later in this chapter.

The use of edge-enhancement routines, discussed in **Chapter 5**, is often followed by thresholding the outlines of features and then filling in the interior holes. In some situations, several different methods must be used and the information combined. **Figure 8.18** shows a difficult example, bubbles in epoxy resin. Some of the concave pores are dark, some light, and some bounded by a bright edge. Processing and thresholding each type of pore and then combining the results with a Boolean OR is required to obtain an image delineating all of the pores.

The Boolean AND operation is extremely useful for applying measurement templates to images. For instance, consider the measurement of coating thickness on a wire or plate viewed

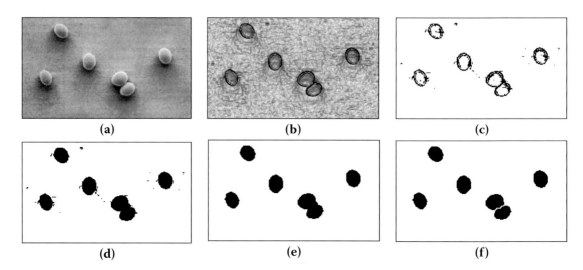

(a)   (b)   (c)

(d)   (e)   (f)

Figure 8.17 Segmentation of an image using multiple steps: (a) original SEM image of spores on a glass slide; (b) application of a Frei and Chen edge operator to image a; (c) thresholding of image b; (d) filling of holes in the binary image of the edges; (e) erosion to remove the extraneous pixels in image d; (f) watershed segmentation to separate touching features in image e.

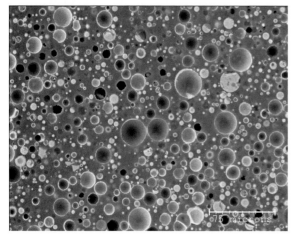

Figure 8.18 Section through an epoxy resin containing bubbles. To delineate the bubbles for measurement, the bright, dark, and outlined pores must be processed in different ways and the results combined with a Boolean OR.

in cross section. In the examples of **Figure 8.19** and **Figure 8.20**, the layer can be readily thresholded, but it is not uniform in thickness. To obtain a series of discrete thickness values for statistical interpretation, it is convenient to AND the binary image of the coating with a template or grid consisting of lines normal to the coating. These lines can be easily measured. In **Figure 8.19**, for the case of a coating on a flat surface, the lines are vertical. For a cylindrical structure such as a similar coating on a wire, or the wall thickness of a tube, a set of radial lines can be used.

In the example of **Figure 8.20**, the vein is approximately circular in cross section and the lines do not perpendicularly intersect the wall, introducing a cosine error in the measurement that may or may not be acceptable. A nonround cross section could indicate that the section plane is not perpendicular to the vein axis, which would introduce another error in the measurement. The measurement of three-dimensional structures from two-dimensional section images is dealt with by stereological techniques, discussed in more detail in **Chapter 9**.

Figure 8.21 illustrates a situation in which the length of the lines gives the layer thickness indirectly, requiring stereological interpretation. The image shows a section plane through coated particles embedded in a metallographic mount and polished. Since the section plane

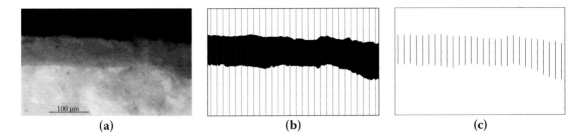

(a)   **(b)**   **(c)**

Figure 8.19 *Measurement of layer thickness: **(a)** paint layer viewed in cross section; **(b)** thresholded layer, with superimposed grid of vertical lines; **(c)** AND of lines, with layer producing line segments for measurement.*

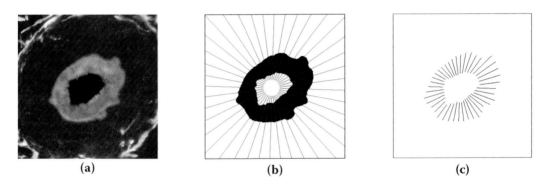

(a)   **(b)**   **(c)**

Figure 8.20 *Measurement of layer thickness: **(a)** cross section of vein in tissue; **(b)** thresholded wall with superimposed grid of radial lines; **(c)** AND of lines with layer producing line segments for measurement (note the cosine errors introduced by nonperpendicular alignment of grid lines to wall, which is not exactly circular).*

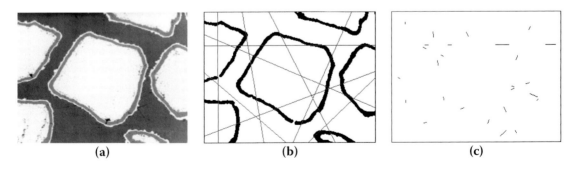

(a)   **(b)**   **(c)**

Figure 8.21 *Measuring coating thickness on particles: **(a)** original gray-scale image of a random section through embedded, coated particles; **(b)** thresholded binary image of the coating of interest with superimposed grid of random lines; **(c)** AND of the lines, with the coating producing line segments for measurement.*

does pass perpendicularly through the coating, the coating can appear thicker than the actual perpendicular or three-dimensional thickness. This is handled by using a grid of random lines. The distribution of line-intercept lengths is related to that of the coating thickness in the normal direction. The average of the inverse intercept lengths is two-thirds the inverse of the true coating thickness, so this value can be obtained even if the image does not include a perpendicular cross section through the coating.

Selection of an appropriate grid is crucial to the success of measurements. **Chapter 9** discusses the principal stereological measurements made on structures to determine the volumes, surface areas, lengths, and topological properties of the components present. Many of these procedures are performed by counting the intersections made by various grids within the structures of interest. The grids typically consist of arrays of points or lines, and the lines used include regular and random grids of straight lines, circular arcs, and cycloids, depending on the type of measurement desired, the procedure used to select and prepare the specimens being imaged, and particularly the orientation of the sections used to generate the surfaces for examination. In all cases, if the image can be thresholded successfully to delineate the structure, then a Boolean AND with the appropriate grid produces a result that can be measured. In some situations this requires measuring the lengths of lines, but in most cases this can be accomplished by simply counting the number of intersections produced by the grid.

Even for complex or subtle images for which automatic processing and thresholding cannot delineate the structures of interest, the superimposition of grids as a mask may be important. Many stereological procedures require only counting of intersections of various types of grids with features of interest, and these can be extremely efficient, providing unbiased estimates of valuable structural parameters. Combining image capture and processing to enhance the visibility of structures with overlays of the appropriate grids — arrays of points or lines, the latter including straight lines, circles, and cycloids — allows the human user to recognize the important features and intersections (Russ 1995a). The counting can be performed manually, or the computer can assist by tallying mouse-clicks or counting marks that the user places on the image. The combination of human recognition with computer assistance to acquire, process, and display the image and generate the appropriate grid provides efficient solutions to many image-analysis problems.

Boolean logic with features

Having identified or labeled the pixel groupings as features, it is possible to carry out Boolean logic at the feature level rather than at the pixel level. **Figure 8.22** shows the principle of a feature-based AND. Instead of simply keeping the pixels that are common to the two images, entire features are kept if any part of them touches. This preserves the entire feature, so that it can be correctly counted or measured if it is selected by the second image.

This method is also called a "marker-based" approach, which uses features in one image as a set of markers to select features in a second one (Russ 1993b). Efficient implementation applies a feature-labeling operation to at least one of the images to be combined. Touching pixels in one image are identified as features, as described previously. Then each pixel that is "ON" in one of those features is checked against the second image. If any of the pixels in the feature match an "ON" pixel in the second image, the entire feature in the first image is copied to the result.

This is not the only possible implementation. It would be equally possible to check each pixel in the second image against the first, but that is less efficient. The method outlined limits the

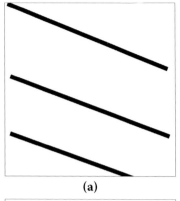
(a)

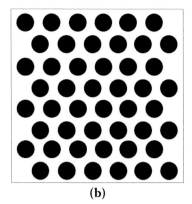
(b)

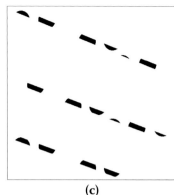
(c)

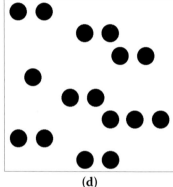
(d)

Figure 8.22 *Schematic diagram of feature-based AND:*
  (a) marker image;
  (b) test image;
  *(c) conventional pixel-based Boolean AND of images **a** and **b**;*
  *(d) feature-based AND in which features in image **a** select ones in image **b**.*

comparison to those pixels that are ON and halts the test for each feature whenever any pixel within it is matched. Still another way to accomplish the same result is to perform dilation (as described later in this chapter) of the markers while only allowing the dilation to propagate within a mask defined by the features in the second image. This method is also slow (because it is iterative), and for features that are very intricate or have tortuous shapes, it may take many iterations to reach an unchanging endpoint.

Notice that unlike the more common pixel-based AND, this statement does not commute; this means that (A Feature-AND B) does not produce the same result as (B Feature-AND A), as illustrated in **Figure 8.23**. The use of NOT with Feature-AND is straightforwardly implemented, for instance by carrying out the same procedure and erasing each feature in the first image that is matched by any pixel in the second. There is no need for a Feature-OR statement, since this would produce the identical result as the conventional pixel-based OR.

A major use for the Feature-AND capability is to use markers within features to select them. For example, these might be cells containing a stained organelle or fibers in a composite containing a characteristic core. In any case, two binary images are produced by thresholding. In one image, the entire features are delineated, and in the second the markers are defined. Applying the Feature-AND logic then selects all of the features that contain one or more markers.

This use of markers to select features is a particularly valuable capability in an image-analysis system. **Figure 8.24** illustrates one way that it can be used. The original image has several red features, only some of which contain darker regions within. If one copy of the image is thresholded for dark spots and a second copy is thresholded for red features, then the first can be used as a set of markers to select the features of interest. A Feature-AND can be used to perform that operation.

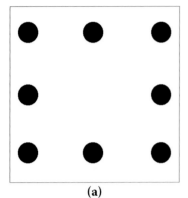

(a)

Figure 8.23
  (a, b) *Feature-based Boolean logic used to combine two test images;*
  (c) *using image **b** as a marker to select features in image **a**;*
  (d) *using image **a** as a marker to select features in image **b**.*

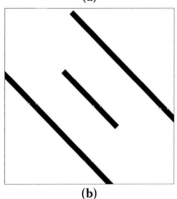

(b)

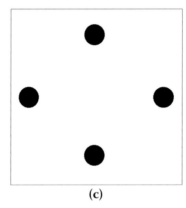

(c)

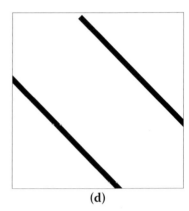

(d)

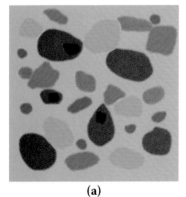

(a)

Figure 8.24 *Example of feature selection using markers:*
  (a) *red features and dark spots in the original image are thresholded to produce*
  (b, c) *separate binary images;*
  (d) *dark spots are used as markers to select only those red features that contain dark markers.*

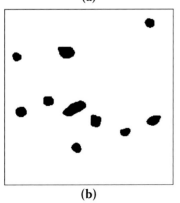

(b)

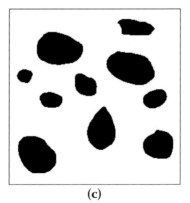

(c)

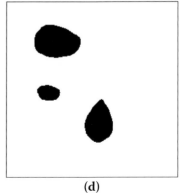

(d)

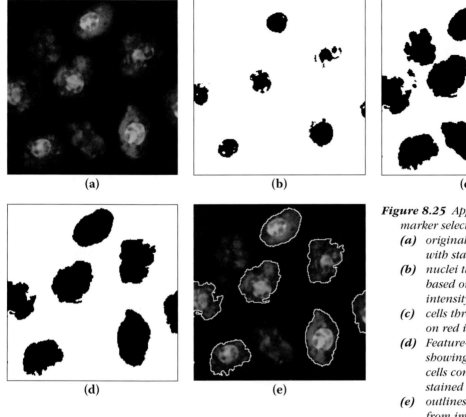

(a)   (b)   (c)

(d)   (e)

Figure 8.25 Application of marker selection:
- *(a) original image of cells with stained nuclei;*
- *(b) nuclei thresholded based on green intensity;*
- *(c) cells thresholded based on red intensity;*
- *(d) Feature-AND result showing only those cells containing green-stained nuclei;*
- *(e) outlines of features from image **d** superimposed on original.*

In real applications, the marker image that selects the features of interest can be obtained by processing or by using another channel in a multichannel image. **Figure 8.25** shows an example. Only those cells containing green-stained nuclei are selected, but they are selected in their entirety so that they can be measured. A related procedure that uses the Feature-AND capability is the use of the nucleator (Gundersen et al. 1988), a stereological tool that selects and counts cells in thin sections of tissue according to the presence of a unique marker within the cell, such as the nucleus.

At a very different scale, the method might be used with aerial photographs to select and measure all building lots that contain any buildings or fields that contain animals. The technique can also be used with X-ray images to select particles in SEM images, for instance if the X-ray signal comes only from the portion of the particle that is visible to the X-ray detector. The entire particle image can be preserved if any part of it generates an identifying X-ray signal.

Marker selection is also useful for isolating features that are within or partially within some region, or adjacent to it. For example, in **Figure 8.26** the colonies contain bacterial cells that are to be counted and measured, although some of them extend beyond the boundaries of the colony. The logic of Feature-AND allows them to be assigned to the appropriate colony and counted, and not to be counted more than once if they exit and reenter the region. And in **Figure 8.27** the outline of a region has been generated (using dilation as discussed below) and used as a marker to select features that are adjacent to the substrate so that they can be measured.

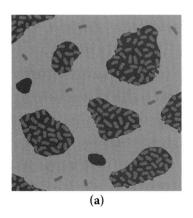 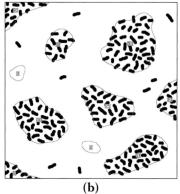

Figure 8.26 Colony counting:
(a) *image representing colonies of bacterial cells, some of which extend beyond the stained area;*
(b) *counted results showing the number of cells in each colony.*

(a) (b)

Selecting features by location

In a generalization of the method for identification of boundary-touching features shown in **Figure 8.27**, marker selection is also useful when applied in conjunction with images that map regions according to distance. We will see below that dilating a line, such as a grain boundary or cell wall, can produce a broad line of selected thickness. Using this line to select

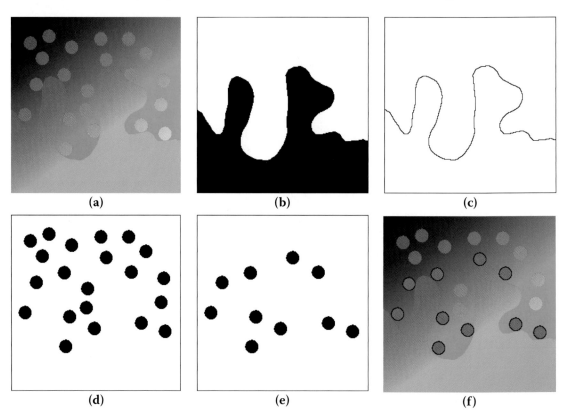

(a) (b) (c)

(d) (e) (f)

Figure 8.27 *Identifying adjacent features: (a) diagram showing cross section of a blue substrate with some orange features touching it; (b) thresholded substrate; (c) pixels immediately adjacent to the substrate, produced by dilating and Ex-ORing; (d) thresholded orange features; (e) selection of features from image d using the line in image c as the marker; (f) features identified in image e superimposed on the original for confirmation.*

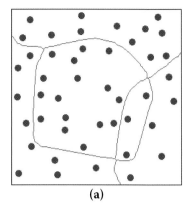

(a)

Figure 8.28 Comparison of pixel- and feature-AND:
- *(a)* diagram of an image containing features and a boundary;
- *(b)* the boundary line, made thicker by dilation;
- *(c)* pixel-based AND of image *b* with blue features in image *a* (incomplete features and one divided into two parts);
- *(d)* feature-AND selection of blue features in image a using image *b* as a marker (all features within a specified distance of the boundary.

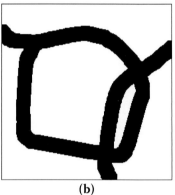

(b)

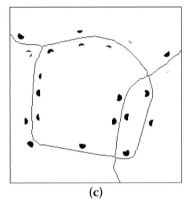

(c)

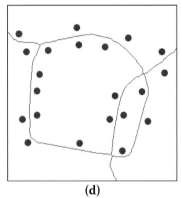

(d)

features that touch it selects those features that, regardless of size or shape, come within that distance of the original boundary. Counting these for different thickness lines provides a way to classify or count features as a function of distance from irregular boundaries. **Figure 8.28** shows an example, and **Figure 8.29** shows an actual image of grain-boundary depletion. The method works at any scale and, for instance, could locate all shopping centers within a specified distance from major highways.

Figure 8.30 shows a situation in which the pixel-based AND is appropriate. The image shows a metallurgical cross section of a plasma-sprayed coating applied to a turbine blade. There is always a certain amount of oxide present in such coatings, which in general causes no difficulties. But if the oxide, which is an identifiable shade of gray, is preferentially situated at the coating-substrate interface, it can produce a region of weakness that may fracture and cause spalling failure of the coating. Thresholding the image to select the oxide and then ANDing this with the line representing the interface (itself obtained by thresholding the metal substrate phase, dilating, and Ex-ORing to

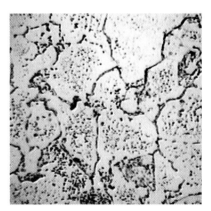

Figure 8.29 Light-microscope image of polished section through steel used at high temperature in boiler tubes. Notice the depletion of carbides (black dots) in the region near grain boundaries. This effect can be measured using procedures described in the text.

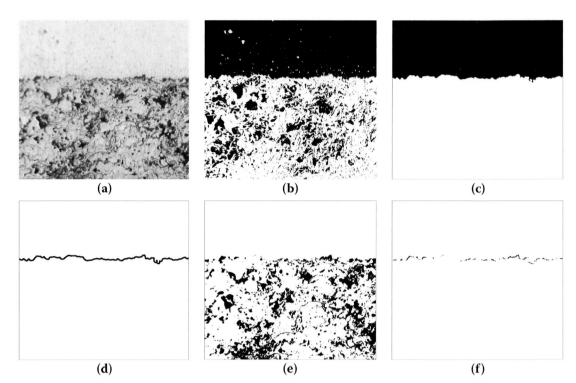

Figure 8.30 *Isolating the oxide in a coating/substrate boundary:* **(a)** *original gray-scale microscope image of a cross section of the plasma-sprayed coating on steel;* **(b)** *thresholding of the metal in the coating and the substrate;* **(c)** *applying erosion and dilation (discussed later in this chapter) to image **b** to fill holes and remove small features, producing a representation of the metal substrate;* **(d)** *boundary line produced by dilating image **c** and Ex-ORing with the original;* **(e)** *thresholding the oxide in the coating, including that lying in the interface;* **(f)** *a pixel-based AND of image **d** with image **b**, showing just the fraction of the interface that is occupied by oxide.*

get the "custer," discussed more extensively later in this chapter) gives a direct measurement of the contaminated fraction of the interface.

An aperture or mask image can be used to restrict the analysis of a second image to only those areas within the aperture. Consider counting spots on a leaf: either spots due to an aerial spraying operation to assess uniformity of coverage, or perhaps spots of fungus or mold to assess the extent of disease. The acquired image is normally rectangular, but the leaf is not. There may well be regions outside the leaf that are similar in brightness to the spots. Creating a binary image of the leaf and then Feature-ANDing it with the total image selects those spots lying on the leaf itself. If the spots are small enough, this could be done as a pixel-based AND. However, if the spots can touch the edge of the leaf, the feature-based operation is safer, since systems may not count or measure edge-touching features (as discussed in **Chapter 10**). Counting can then provide the desired information, normally expressed as number-per-unit-area where the area of the leaf forms the denominator. This procedure is similar to the colony-counting problem in **Figure 8.26**.

Figure 8.31 shows another situation in which two different thresholding operations and a logical combination are used to select features of interest. The micrograph shows tissue containing immunogold particles. Some of these are located on the dark organelles, while others are in the lighter cytoplasm. To select only those that are on the organelles, two images are

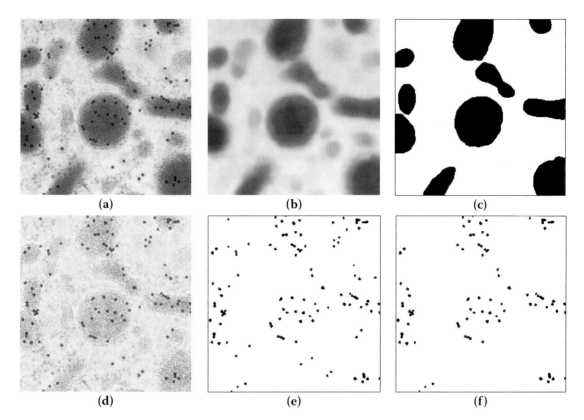

Figure 8.31 *Selecting immunogold particles: (a) original image; (b) gray-scale opening applied to remove small dark particles, leaving the organelles; (c) thresholded binary from image b; (d) dividing image b into image a produces uniform image contrast for the particles; (e) thresholded binary from image d; (f) combining image c AND image e leaves just the particles on the organelles.*

needed, both derived from the same original. Applying a gray-scale opening to the image (as discussed in **Chapter 5**) produces an image of just the organelles by eliminating the smaller gold particles. This can be divided into the original image to produce a second image of just the gold particles. Thresholding each and combining the two isolates the gold particles that were originally on the organelles. A pixel-based AND would retain only portions of the particles at the edges of the organelles, so a Feature-AND is used with the organelles as markers to select particles.

Similar procedures allow identifying grains in ores that are contained within other minerals, for instance to determine the fraction that is "locked" within a harder matrix that cannot easily be recovered by mechanical or chemical treatment, as opposed to grains that are not so enclosed and are easily liberated from the matrix.

A rather different use of feature-based Boolean logic implements the Disector, a stereological tool discussed in **Chapter 9** that gives an unbiased and direct measure of the number of features per unit volume (Sterio 1984). It requires matching features in two images that represent parallel planes separated by a distance *T*. The features represent the intersection of three-dimensional objects with those planes. Those objects that intersect both planes are ignored, but those that intersect only one plane or the other are counted. The total number of objects per unit volume is then

$$N_V = \frac{Count}{2 \cdot Area \cdot T}$$

(8.1)

where Area is the area of each of the images. This method has the advantage of being insensitive to the shape and size of the objects, but it requires that the planes be close enough together that no information is lost between the planes. In effect, this means that the distance T must be small compared with any important dimension of the objects.

When T is small, most objects intersect both planes. The features in those planes will not correspond exactly, but are expected to overlap at least partially. In the case of a branching three-dimensional object, both of the intersections in one plane are expected to overlap with the intersection in the second plane. Of course, since most of the objects do pass through both planes when T is small, and only the few that do not are counted, it is necessary to examine a large image area to obtain a statistically useful number of counts. That requirement makes the use of an automated method based on the Feature-AND logic attractive.

Since the features that overlap in the two images are those that are not counted, a candidate procedure for determining the value of N to be used in the calculation of number of objects per unit volume might be to first count the number of features in each of the two plane images (N_1 and N_2). Then the Feature-AND can be used to determine the features that are present in both images, and a count of those features (N_{common}) obtained, giving

$$N = N_1 + N_2 - 2 \cdot N_{common}$$

(8.2)

However, this is correct only for the case in which each object intersects each plane exactly once. For branching objects, it will result in an error.

A preferred procedure is to directly count the features in the two planes that are not selected by the Feature-AND. Since the logical operation does not commute, it is necessary to perform both operations: (#1 NOT Feature-AND #2) and (#2 NOT Feature-AND #1), and count the features remaining. This is illustrated schematically in **Figure 8.32**.

Figure 8.33 shows a typical application. The two images are separated optical slices from confocal light-microscope imaging of oil droplets in a food product. Each image is thresholded to generate a binary image of particle intersections, and touching features are separated with a watershed (described below). Each of the Feature-AND operations is performed, and the final image is the OR combination showing those features that appear in one (and only one) of the two slices. It would be appropriate to describe this image as a feature-based version of the exclusive-OR operation between the two images.

Double thresholding

Another application for marker selection logic arises in the thresholding of difficult images such as grain boundaries in materials or cell boundaries in tissue. It is not unusual to have nonuniform etching or staining of the cell or grain boundaries in specimen preparation. In the example of **Figure 8.34**, this is due to thermal etching of the interiors of the grains. The result is that direct thresholding of the image cannot produce a complete representation of the etched boundaries that does not also include "noise" within the grains.

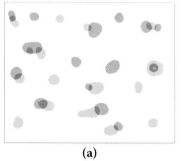

(a)

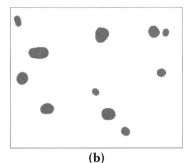

(b)

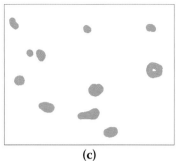

(c)

(d)

Figure 8.32 Implementation of the Disector:
(a) *two section images, overlaid in different colors to show matching features;*
(b) *1 Feature-AND 2 showing features in plane 2 matched with plane 1;*
(c) *2 Feature-AND 1 showing the features matched in the other plane;*
(d) *ORing together the 1 NOT Feature-AND 2 with 2 NOT Feature-AND 1 leaves just the unmatched features in both planes that area to be counted.*

A technique for dealing with such situations has been described as "double thresholding" by Olsson (1993), but it can also be implemented by using a Feature-AND operation. As illustrated in **Figure 8.34**, the procedure is first to threshold the image to select only the darkest pixels that are definitely within the etched boundaries, even if they do not form a complete representation of the boundaries. Then a second binary image is produced to obtain a complete delineation of all the boundaries, accepting some noise within the grains. In the example, a variance operator was applied to a copy of the original image to increase the contrast at edges. This process allows thresholding more of the boundaries, but also some of the intra-grain structures. Then a morphological closing (discussed later in this chapter) was applied to fill in noise within the boundaries. The increase in apparent width of the boundaries is not important, since skeletonization (also discussed below) is used to reduce the boundary lines to minimum width (the actual grain boundaries are only a few atoms thick).

The two binary images are combined with a Feature-AND to keep any feature in the second image that is selected by the markers in the first. This uses the few dark pixels that definitely lie within the boundaries to select the broader boundaries, while rejecting the noise within the grains. Finally, as shown in the figure, the resulting image is skeletonized and pruned to produce an image useful for stereological measurements of grain boundary area, grain size, and so forth.

In the preceding example, the grain boundary network is a continuous tessellation of the image. Hence, it could be selected by using other criteria than the double-threshold method (for instance, touching multiple edges of the field). **Figure 8.35** shows an example that requires the double-threshold method. The acoustic microscope image shows a cross section through a fiber-reinforced material. These images are inherently noisy, but double-thresholding (in this example selecting the bright pixels) allows the boundaries around the fibers to be selected. Since the fibers touch each other, it is also necessary to separate them for measurement using a watershed segmentation, as discussed below.

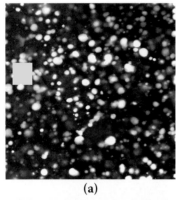

(a)

Figure 8.33 *Applying Disector logic:*
(a, b) two parallel section images from a confocal light
  microscope;
*(c, d) thresholded and separated particles in images **a** and **b**;*
(e, f) using marker selection to keep just the features in images
  ***c** and **d** that do NOT touch features in the other image;*
*(g) OR of images **e** and **f**, showing the more than 200 features*
  that are counted.

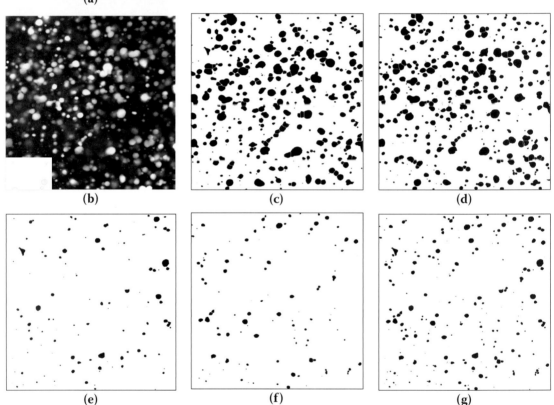

(b)   (c)   (d)

(e)   (f)   (g)

Erosion and dilation

The most widely used processing procedures for binary images are often collectively described as morphological operations (Coster and Chermant 1985; Dougherty and Astola 1994, 1999; Serra 1982; Soille 1999). These include erosion and dilation as well as modifications and combinations of these operations. The classic versions of these are fundamentally neighbor operations, as discussed in **Chapter 4** and **Chapter 5**, where similar procedures that rank pixel values in a neighborhood are used to process gray-scale and color images in the spatial domain. Because the values of pixels in the binary images are restricted to black and white, the operations are simpler and usually involve counting rather than sorting. However, the basic ideas are the same.

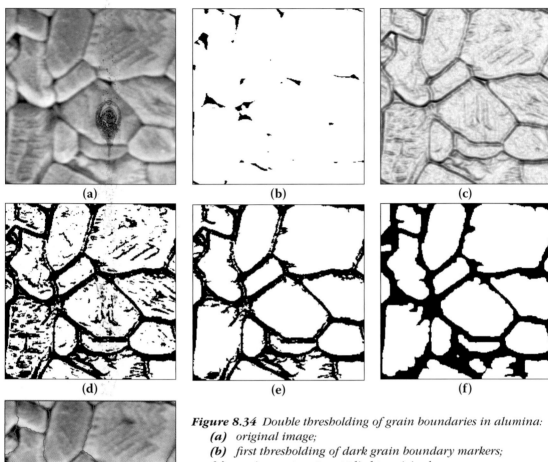

Figure 8.34 *Double thresholding of grain boundaries in alumina:*
  (a) *original image;*
  (b) *first thresholding of dark grain boundary markers;*
  (c) *variance operator applied to original;*
  (d) *second thresholding of image **c** for all boundaries plus other marks;*
  (e) *marker selection of features in image **d** that touch features in image **b**;*
  (f) *closing applied to image **e**;*
  (g) *skeletonized and pruned boundary overlaid on original.*

There is a rich literature, much of it French, in the field of mathematical morphology. It has developed a specific language and notation for the operations and is generally discussed in terms of set theory. A much simpler and more empirical approach is taken here. Operations can be described simply in terms of adding or removing pixels from the binary image according to certain rules, which depend on the pattern of neighboring pixels. Each operation is performed on each pixel in the original image, using the original pattern of pixels. In practice, it may not be necessary to create an entirely new image; the existing image can be replaced in memory by copying a few lines at a time. None of the new pixel values are used in evaluating the neighbor pattern.

Erosion removes pixels from features in an image or, equivalently, turns pixels OFF that were originally ON. The purpose is to remove pixels that should not be there. The simplest example

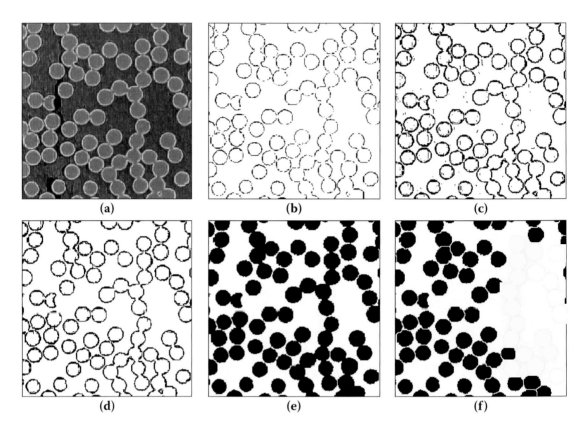

Figure 8.35 *Double thresholding of fiber boundaries:* **(a)** *original image;* **(b)** *first thresholding;* **(c)** *second thresholding,* **(d)** *marker selection result;* **(e)** *filled boundaries;* **(f)** *segmented fibers.*

is pixels that have been selected by thresholding because they fell into the brightness range of interest, but that do not lie within large regions with that brightness. Instead, they may have that brightness value either accidentally, because of finite noise in the image, or because they happen to straddle a boundary between a lighter and darker region and thus have an averaged brightness that happens to lie within the range selected by thresholding.

These pixels cannot be distinguished by simple thresholding because their brightness value is the same as that of the desired regions. It may be possible to remove them by using Boolean logic, for instance using the gray level as one criterion and the gradient as a second one, and requiring that the pixels to be kept have the desired gray level and a low gradient. However, for our purposes here we will assume that the binary image has already been formed and that extraneous pixels are present.

The simplest kind of erosion is to remove (set to OFF) any pixel touching another pixel that is part of the background (is already OFF). This removes a layer of pixels from around the periphery of all features and regions, which will cause some shrinking of dimensions and may create other problems if it causes a feature to break up into parts. We will deal with these difficulties below. Erosion can entirely remove extraneous pixels representing point noise or line defects (e.g., scratches) because these defects are frequently only 1 or 2 pixels wide.

Instead of removing pixels from features, a complementary operation known as dilation (or sometimes dilatation) can be used to add pixels. The classical dilation rule, analogous to that for erosion, is to add (set to ON) any background pixel that touches another pixel that is already part of a foreground region (is already ON). This will add a layer of pixels around the periphery of all features and regions, which will cause some increase in dimensions and may cause features to merge. It also fills in small holes within features.

Because erosion and dilation cause a reduction or increase in the size of regions, respectively, they are sometimes known as etching and plating or shrinking and growing. There are a variety of rules for deciding which pixels to add or remove and for forming combinations of erosion and dilation.

In the rather simple example described above and illustrated in **Figure 8.36**, erosion to remove the extraneous lines of pixels between light and dark phases causes a shrinking of the features. Following the erosion with a dilation will more or less restore the pixels around the feature periphery, so that the dimensions are (approximately) restored. However, isolated pixels and lines that have been completely removed do not cause any new pixels to be added. They have been permanently erased from the image.

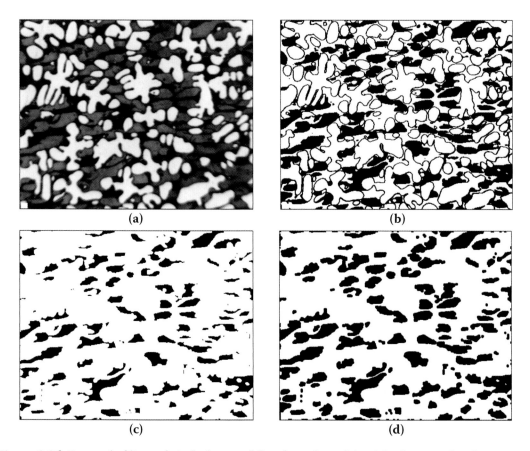

(a)

(b)

(c)

(d)

Figure 8.36 *Removal of lines of pixels that straddle a boundary: **(a)** original gray-scale microscope image of a three-phase metal; **(b)** binary image obtained by thresholding on the intermediate gray phase; **(c)** erosion of image **b** using two iterations; **(d)** dilation of image **c** using the same two iterations, restoring the feature size but without the lines.*

Opening and closing

The combination of an erosion followed by a dilation is called an opening, referring to the ability of this combination to open up gaps between just-touching features, as shown in **Figure 8.37**. It is one of the most commonly used sequences for removing pixel noise from binary images. Performing the same operations in the opposite order (dilation followed by erosion) produces a different result. This sequence is called a closing because it can close breaks in features. There are several parameters that can be used to adjust erosion and dilation operations, particularly the neighbor pattern or rules for adding or removing pixels and the number of iterations, as discussed below. In most opening or closing operations, these are kept the same for both the erosion and the dilation.

Openings can be used in some cases to separate touching features. In the example shown in **Figure 8.38**, the features are all similar in size. This fact makes it possible to continue the erosion until all features have separated but none have been completely erased. After the separation is complete, dilation grows the features back toward their original size. They would merge again unless logic is used to prevent it. A rule that prevents turning a pixel ON if its neighbors belong to different features maintains the separation shown in the figure. This requires performing feature identification for the pixels, so the logic discussed above is required at each step of the dilation. An additional rule prevents turning on any pixel that was not on in the original image, so that the features are restricted to their original sizes. If the features had different original sizes, the separation lines would not be positioned correctly at the junctions, and some features might disappear completely before others separated. The watershed segmentation technique discussed later in this chapter performs better in such cases.

As shown in **Figure 8.37**, the closing sequence is performed in the other order, a dilation followed by an erosion, and the result is not the same. Instead of removing isolated pixels that are ON, the result is to fill in places where isolated pixels are OFF, missing pixels within features, or narrow gaps between portions of a feature. **Figure 8.39** shows an example of a closing used to connect the parts of the cracked fibers shown in cross section. The cracks are all narrow, so dilation causes the pixels from either side to spread across the gap. The increase in fiber diameter is then corrected by erosion, but the cracks do not reappear.

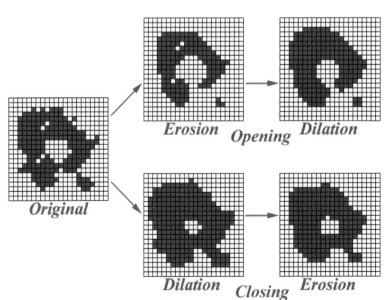

Erosion *Opening* *Dilation*

Original

Dilation *Closing* *Erosion*

Figure 8.37 Combining erosion and dilation to produce an opening or a closing. The result is different depending on the order of application of the two operations. Since the original image is ambiguous, it is necessary to use a priori knowledge to select the proper combination.

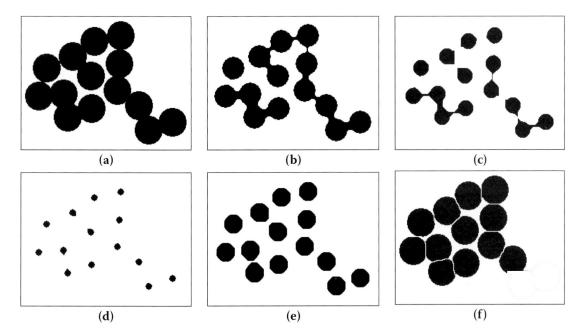

(a)   **(b)**   **(c)**

(d)   **(e)**   **(f)**

Figure 8.38 *Separation of touching features by erosion/dilation: **(a)** original test image; **(b)** after two cycles of erosion; **(c)** after four cycles; **(d)** after seven cycles (features are now all fully separated); **(e)** four cycles of dilation applied to image **d** (features will merge on next cycle); **(f)** additional cycles of nonmerging dilation restricted to the original pixel locations, which restores the feature boundaries.*

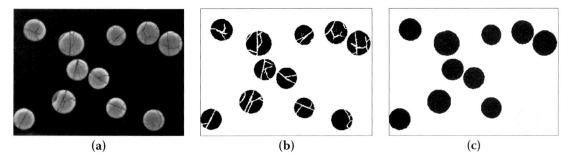

(a)   **(b)**   **(c)**

Figure 8.39 *Joining parts of features with a closing: **(a)** original image, cross section of cracked glass fibers; **(b)** brightness thresholding, showing divisions within the fibers; **(c)** after application of a closing.*

The classical erosion and dilation operations illustrated above turn a pixel ON or OFF if it touches any pixel in the opposite state. Usually, touching in this context includes any of the adjacent 8 pixels, although some systems deal only with the 4 edge-sharing neighbors. These operations would be much simpler and more isotropic on a hexagonal pixel array, because the pixel neighbor distances are all the same, but practical considerations lead to the general use of a grid of square pixels.

A wide variety of other rules are possible. One approach is to count the number of neighbor pixels with the opposite color, compare this number to some threshold value, and only change the state of the central pixel if that test coefficient is exceeded. In this method, classical erosion corresponds to a coefficient of zero. One effect of different coefficient values is to alter the rate at which features grow or shrink and, to some extent, to control the isotropy of the result. This will be illustrated below.

It is also possible to choose a large coefficient, from 5 to 7, to select only the isolated noise pixels and leave most features alone. For example, choosing a coefficient of 7 will cause only single isolated pixels to be reversed (removed or set to OFF in an erosion, and vice versa for a dilation). Erosion with a coefficient value of 5 or 6 may be able to remove lines of pixels (such as those straddling a boundary) without affecting anything else.

An example of this method is shown in **Figure 8.40**. Thresholding the original image of the pigment cell produces a binary image showing the features of interest and also leaves many smaller and irregular groups of pixels. Performing a conventional opening to remove them would also cause the shapes of the larger features to change and some of them to merge. Applying erosion with a neighbor coefficient of 5 removes the small and irregular pixel groups

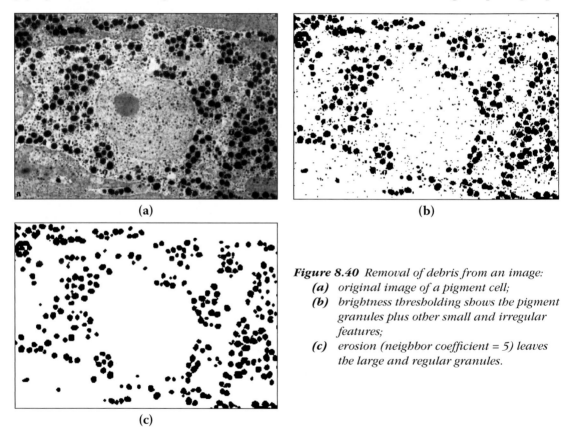

(a)

(b)

(c)

Figure 8.40 Removal of debris from an image:
 (a) original image of a pigment cell;
 (b) brightness thresholding shows the pigment granules plus other small and irregular features;
 (c) erosion (neighbor coefficient = 5) leaves the large and regular granules.

Figure 8.41 Illustration of the effect of different neighbor coefficients and the number of iterations: *(a)* original test image; *(b)* erosion (neighbor coefficient = 3, one iteration) removes isolated lines and points; *(c)* closing (neighbor coefficient = 2, two iterations) fills in gaps to connect features while removing isolated points; *(d)* closing using classical operations (neighbor coefficient = 0, one iteration) connects most features but leaves isolated points; *(e)* opening (neighbor coefficient = 7, one iteration) removes point noise without affecting anything else; *(f)* opening (neighbor coefficient = 1, four iterations) removes all small features, including the frame of the picture.

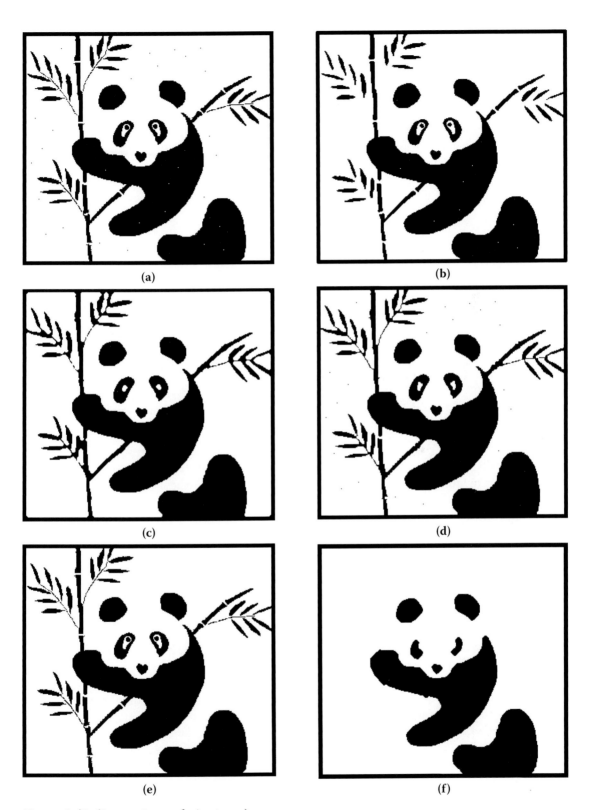

(a)

(b)

(c)

(d)

(e)

(f)

Figure 8.41 *(See caption on facing page.)*

without affecting the larger and more rounded features, as shown. The erosion is repeated until no further changes take place (the number of ON pixels in the binary image does not change). This procedure works because a corner pixel in a square has exactly five touching background neighbors and is not removed, while more irregular clusters have pixels with six or more background neighbors.

The test image in **Figure 8.41** shows a variety of fine lines and narrow gaps that can be removed or filled using different neighbor coefficients and a different number of iterations (number of erosions followed by dilations, or vice versa).

Isotropy

It is not possible for a small 3×3 neighborhood to define an isotropic neighbor pattern. Classic erosion applied to a circle will not shrink the circle uniformly, but will proceed at a faster rate in the $45°$ diagonal directions because the pixel spacing is greater in those directions. As a result, a circle will erode toward a diamond shape, as shown in **Figure 8.42**. Once the feature reaches this shape, it will continue to erode uniformly, preserving the shape. However, in most cases, features are not really diamond shaped, which represents a potentially serious distortion.

Likewise, classic dilation applied to a circle also proceeds faster in the $45°$ diagonal directions, so that the shape dilates toward a square (also shown in **Figure 8.42**). Again, square shapes are stable in dilation, but the distortion of real images toward a blocky appearance in dilation can present a problem for further interpretation.

A neighbor coefficient of 1 instead of 0 produces a markedly different result. For dilation, a background pixel that touches more than one foreground pixel (i.e., two or more out of the possible eight neighbor positions) will be turned ON and vice versa for erosion. Eroding a circle with this procedure tends toward a square and dilation tends toward a diamond, just the reverse of using a coefficient of 0. This is shown in **Figure 8.43**.

There is no intermediate test value between 0 and 1, since the pixels are counted as either ON or OFF. If the corner pixels were counted as 2 and the edge-touching pixels as 3, it would be possible to design a coefficient that better approximated an isotropic circle. This would produce a ratio of $3/2 = 1.5$, which is a reasonable approximation to $\sqrt{2}$, the distance ratio to the pixels. In practice, this is rarely done because of the convenience of dealing with pixels in binary images as black or white, with no need to take into account their neighborhood.

Another approach that can be used to achieve an intermediate result between the coefficients of 0 and 1 (with their directional bias) is to alternate the two tests. As shown in **Figure 8.44**, this alternating pattern produces a somewhat better octagonal approximation to a circular shape in both erosion and dilation. These examples illustrate the point that erosion or dilation need not be performed only once. The number of repetitions or iterations corresponds roughly to the distance that boundaries will grow or shrink radially. It can be expressed in pixels or as a scale dimension, but because of the effect of different neighbor coefficients on the process, the number of iterations does not directly correspond to an actual distance on the image.

Using a larger neighborhood can also moderate the anisotropy. In **Figure 8.45** a 5-pixel-wide circular neighborhood is used with ten iterations of erosion and dilation. As for the alternating

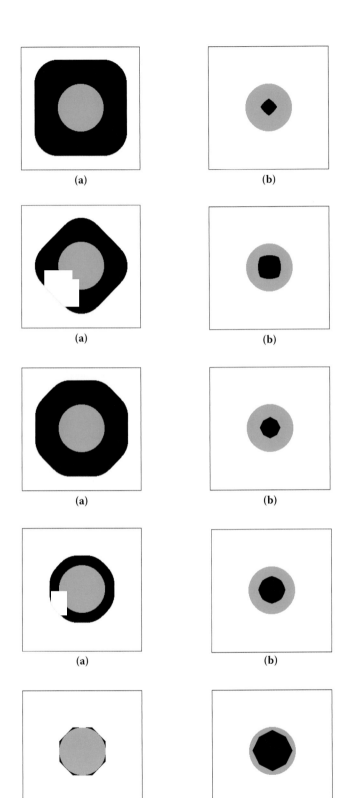

Figure 8.42 Anisotropy of classical dilation and erosion (neighbor coefficient = 0) applied to a circle:
(a) after 50 iterations of dilation;
(b) after 25 iterations of erosion.

Figure 8.43 Anisotropy of dilation and erosion (neighbor coefficient = 1) applied to a circle:
(a) after 50 iterations of dilation;
(b) after 25 iterations of erosion.

Figure 8.44 Improved isotropy by alternating neighbor coefficients of 0 and 1 applied to a circle:
(a) after 50 iterations of dilation;
(b) after 25 iterations of erosion.

Figure 8.45 Using a larger neighborhood size (a 5-pixel wide approximation to a circle):
(a) after 10 iterations of dilation;
(b) after 10 iterations of erosion.

Figure 8.46 Octagonal shape and slow rate of addition or removal using a coefficient of 3:
(a) circle after 50 iterations of dilation (no further changes occur);
(b) circle after 25 iterations of erosion.

(a)   (b)
(a)   (b)
(a)   (b)
(a)   (b)
(a)   (b)

0 and 1 coefficients, the shapes evolve toward octagons. However, the larger neighborhood provides less control over the distance affected by erosion and dilation.

Each neighbor pattern or coefficient has its own characteristic anisotropy. **Figure 8.46** shows the rather interesting results using a neighborhood coefficient of 3. Like an alternating 0,1 pattern, this operation produces an eight-sided polygon. However, the rate of erosion is much lower, and in dilation the figure grows to the bounding octagon and then becomes stable, with no further pixels being added. This coefficient is sometimes used to construct bounding polygons around features.

Measurements using erosion and dilation

Erosion performed n times, using either a coefficient of 0 or 1, or alternating them, will cause features to shrink radially by about n pixels (with local variations depending on the shape of the original feature). This will cause features whose smallest dimension is less than $2n$ pixels to disappear altogether. Counting the features that have disappeared (or subtracting the number that remain from the original) gives an estimate of the number of features smaller than that size. This means that erosion and counting can be used to get an estimate of size distributions without actually performing feature measurements (Ehrlich et al. 1984). The same methodology can be applied using gray-scale morphology (a ranking operation that, as described in **Chapter 5**, replaces each feature with its brighter or darker neighbor) and counting features as they disappear. This is illustrated below.

For irregularly shaped and concave features, the erosion process may cause a feature to subdivide into parts. Simply counting the number of features as a function of the number of iterations of erosion is therefore not a good way to determine the size distribution. One approach to this problem is to follow erosion by a dilation with the same coefficient(s) and number of steps. This will merge together many (but not necessarily all) of the separated parts and give a better estimate of their number. However, there is still considerable sensitivity to the shape of the original features. A dumbbell-shaped object will separate into two parts when the handle between the two main parts erodes; they will not merge. This separation may be desirable if, indeed, the purpose is to count the two main parts.

A second method is to use Feature-AND or marker selection, discussed previously. After each iteration of erosion, the remaining features are used to select only those original features that touch them. The count of original features then gives the correct number. This is functionally equivalent to keeping feature labels on each pixel in the image and counting the number of different labels present in the image after each cycle of erosion. This method of estimating size distributions without actually measuring features, using either of these correction techniques, has been particularly applied to measurements in geology, such as mineral particle sizes or sediments.

The opposite operation, performing dilations and counting the number of separate features as a function of the number of steps, is less common. It provides an estimate of the distribution of the nearest distances between features in the image. When this is done by conventional feature measurement, the x,y location of each feature is determined; then sorting in the resulting data file is used to determine the nearest neighbor and its distance. In this case, the distance is from center to center. When the features are significantly large compared with their spacing or when their shapes are important, it can be more interesting to characterize the distances between their boundaries (the edge-to-edge distance). This dilation method can provide that information.

The methods described in the preceding paragraphs were used despite problems with anisotropy when computer power was limited and more accurate methods were impractical. However, these methods have largely been replaced by methods using the Euclidean distance map, which are discussed later in this chapter.

Instead of counting the number of features that disappear at each iteration of erosion, it is much easier simply to count the number of ON pixels remaining, which provides some information about the shape of the boundaries. Smooth Euclidean boundaries erode at a constant rate. Irregular and especially fractal boundaries do not, since many more pixels are exposed and touch opposite neighbors. This effect has been used to estimate fractal dimensions, although more accurate methods are available, as discussed below.

Fractal dimensions and the description of a boundary as fractal based on a self-similar roughness is a fairly new idea that is finding many applications in science and art (Feder 1988; Mandelbrot 1982; Russ 1994). No description of the rather interesting background and uses of the concept is included here. The basic idea behind measuring a fractal dimension by erosion and dilation comes from the Minkowski definition of a fractal boundary dimension. By dilating a region and Ex-ORing the result with another image formed by eroding the region, the pixels along the boundary are obtained. For a minimal distance of a single pixel for erosion and dilation, this will be called the "custer" and is discussed below.

To measure the fractal dimension, the operation is repeated with an increasing number of iterations of erosion and dilation (Flook 1978), and the effective width (total number of pixels divided by length and number of cycles) of the boundary is plotted vs. the number of iterations on a log-log scale. For a Euclidean boundary, this plot shows no trend; the number of pixels along the boundary selected by the Ex-OR increases linearly with the number of erosion/dilation cycles. However, for a rough boundary with self-similar fine detail, the graph shows a linear variation on log-log axes whose slope gives the fractal dimension of the boundary directly. **Figure 8.47** shows an example.

There are a variety of other methods for determining the boundary fractal dimension, including (a) box-counting or mosaic amalgamation (Kaye 1986; Russ 1990a), in which the number of pixels through which the boundary passes (for boundary representation) are counted as the pixel size is increased by coarsening the image resolution and (b) a structured walk method (Schwarz and Exner 1980), which requires the boundary to be represented as a polygon instead of as pixels. For a fractal boundary, these also produce straight-line plots on a log-log scale, from whose slope the dimension is determined. Newer and more accurate techniques for performing the measurement are shown in **Chapter 10**.

Counting the number of pixels as a function of dilations provides a rather indirect measure of feature clustering, since as nearby features merge, the amount of boundary is reduced and the region's rate of growth slows. Counting only the pixels and not the features makes it difficult to separate the effects of boundary shape and feature spacing. If all of the features are initially very small or if they are single points, this method can provide a fractal dimension (technically a Sierpinski fractal) for the clustering.

Extension to gray-scale images

In **Chapter 5**, one of the image processing operations described was the use of a ranking operator, which finds the brightest or darkest pixel in a neighborhood and replaces the central pixel with that value. This operation is sometimes described as a gray-scale erosion or dilation, depending on whether the use of the brightest or darkest pixel value results in a

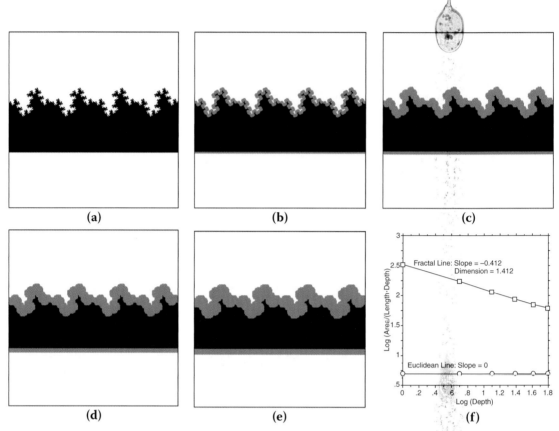

Figure 8.47 *Measurement of Minkowski fractal dimension by erosion/dilation: (a) test figure with upper boundary a classical Koch fractal and lower boundary a Euclidean straight line; (b) gray pixels show difference between erosion and dilation by one iteration; (c, d, e) differences between erosion and dilation after two, three, and four iterations; (f) plot of log of effective width (area of gray pixels divided by length and number of iterations) vs. log of number of iterations (approximate width of gray band).*

growth or shrinkage of the visible features. Morphological operations on gray-scale and colored images are analogous to those performed in binary images, and if the routines for gray-scale morphology are applied to binary images, they correspond to the classical erosion/dilation operations.

Just as an estimate of the distribution of feature sizes can be obtained by eroding features in a binary image, the same technique is also possible using gray-scale erosion on a gray-scale image. **Figure 8.48** shows an example. The lipid spheres in this SEM image are partially piled up and touch one another, which is a problem for conventional image-measurement techniques. Applying gray-scale erosion reduces the feature sizes, and counting the bright central points that disappear at each step of repeated erosion provides a size distribution (which is shown below in **Figure 8.68**).

The assumption in this approach is that the features ultimately separate before disappearing. This works for relatively simple images with convex features, none of which are more than about half hidden by others. No purely two-dimensional image processing method can count the number of cannon balls in a pile if the inner ones are hidden. It is possible to estimate the volume of the pile and guess at the maximum number of balls contained, but impossible to know whether they are actually there or whether something else is underneath the topmost layer.

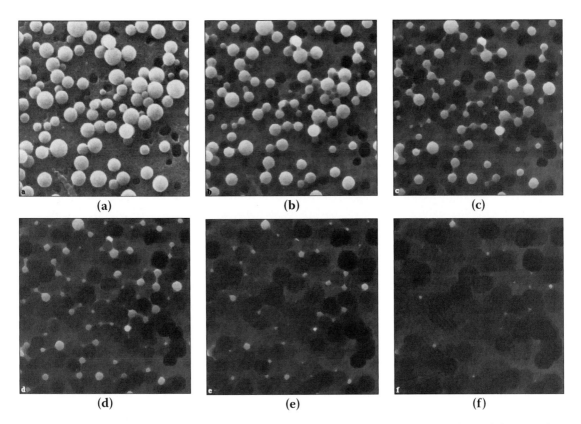

(a) (b) (c)

(d) (e) (f)

Figure 8.48 Use of gray-scale erosion to estimate size distribution of overlapped spheres: (a) original SEM image of lipid droplets; (b, c, d, e, f) result of applying repetitions of gray-scale erosion by keeping the darkest pixel value in a 5-pixel-wide octagonal neighborhood.

Morphology neighborhood parameters

The important parameters for erosion and dilation are the neighborhood size and shape, the comparison test that is used, and the number of times the operation is repeated. The use of a simple test coefficient based on the number of neighbors, irrespective of their location in the neighborhood, provides considerable flexibility in the functioning of the operation as shown above, although each coefficient produces results having a characteristic shape that distorts the original features. Also, the greater the number of iterations in the operation, the greater is this effect.

Specific neighbor patterns can also be used for erosion and dilation operations. The most common are those that compare the central pixel with its four edge-touching neighbors (usually called a "+" pattern because of the neighborhood shape) or to the four corner-touching neighbors (likewise called an "x" pattern), changing the central pixel if any of those four neighbors is of the opposite color. They are rarely used alone, but can be employed in an alternating pattern to obtain greater directional uniformity than classical erosion, similar to the effects produced by alternating coefficient tests of 0 and 1.

Any specific neighbor pattern can be used if it is appropriate to the specific application. It is not even required to restrict the comparison to immediately touching neighbors. As for gray-scale operations, larger neighborhoods make it possible to respond to more subtle textures and achieve greater control over directionality. **Figure 8.49** shows a simple example. The general case for this type of operation is called the hit-or-miss operator, which specifies a pattern of neighboring pixels divided into three classes: those that must be ON, those that must be OFF, and those that do not matter (are ignored). If the pattern is found, then the pixel is set to the specified state (Serra 1982; Coster and Chermant 1985).

This operation is more generally called template matching. The same type of operation carried out on gray-scale images (usually implemented with Fourier transforms) is called correlation and is a way to search for specific patterns in the image. This is also true for binary images; in fact, template matching with thresholded binary images was one of the earliest methods for optical character reading and is still used for situations in which the character shape, size, and location are tightly controlled (such as the characters at the bottom of bank checks). Much more flexible methods are needed to read more general text, however. In practice, most erosion and dilation are performed using only the eight nearest-neighbor pixels for comparison.

A method for implementing neighborhood comparison that makes it easy to use any arbitrary pattern of pixels is the fate table. The eight neighbors are considered to each have a value of 1 or 0, depending on whether the pixel is ON or OFF. Assembling these eight values into a number produces a single byte, which can have any of 256 possible values. This value is used as an address into a table, which provides the result (i.e., turning the central pixel ON or OFF). Efficient ways to construct the address by bitwise shifting of values, which takes advantage of the machine-language idiosyncrasies of specific computer processors, makes this method very fast. The ability to create several tables of possible fates to deal with different erosion and dilation rules, perhaps saved on disk and loaded as needed, makes the method very flexible. However, it does not generalize well to larger neighborhoods or to three-dimensional voxel-array images because the tables become too large.

Applications for specific erosion/dilation operations that are not symmetrical or isotropic always require some independent knowledge of the image, the desired information, and the selection of operations that will selectively extract it. However, this is not as important a criticism or limitation as it may seem, since all image processing is to some extent knowledge-directed. The human observer tries to find operations to extract information he or she has some reason to know or expect to be present.

Figure 8.50 shows an example. The horizontal textile fibers vary in width as they weave above and below the vertical ones. Measuring this variation is important in modeling the mechanical

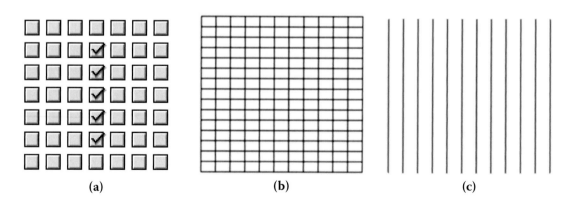

(a)   (b)   (c)

Figure 8.49 Example of specifying the neighborhood pixels for morphological operations: (a) a vertical neighborhood for erosion; (b) original pattern; (c) eroded result.

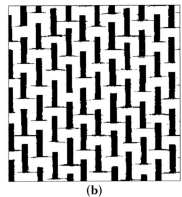
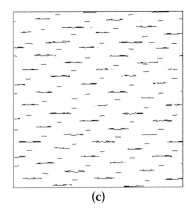

(a)   (b)   (c)

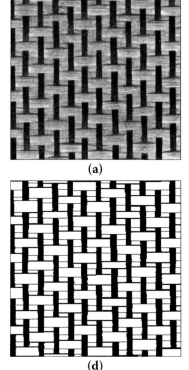

Figure 8.50 *Using directional erosion and dilation to segment an image:*
- *(a)* *original gray-scale image of a woven textile;*
- *(b)* *brightness thresholding of image **a**;*
- *(c)* *end pixels isolated by performing a vertical erosion and Ex-ORing with the original;*
- *(d)* *completed operation by repeated horizontal dilation of image **c** and then ORing with the original.*

(d)

properties of the weave, which will be embedded into a composite. The dark vertical fibers can be thresholded based on brightness, but delineating the horizontal fibers is very difficult. The procedure shown in the figure uses the known directionality of the structure.

After thresholding the dark fibers, an erosion is performed to remove only those pixels whose neighbor immediately below or above is part of the background. These pixels, shown in **Figure 8.50c**, can then be isolated by performing an Ex-OR with the original binary. They include the few points distinguishable between horizontal fibers and the ends of the vertical fibers where they are covered by horizontal ones.

Next, a directional dilation is performed in the horizontal direction. Any background pixel whose left or right touching neighbor is ON is itself set to ON, and this operation is repeated enough times to extend the lines across the distance between vertical fibers. Finally, the resulting horizontal lines are ORed with the original binary image to outline all of the individual fibers (**Figure 8.50d**). Inverting this image produces measurable features.

The use of a nonisotropic neighborhood for erosion/dilation operations is particularly useful for removing known patterns from an image. The most common example is the removal of scratches from scanned photographic negatives. The scratches are usually narrow and oriented parallel to the film strip. A neighborhood that is longer than the width of the scratch and oriented perpendicular to it will replace the dark pixels in the scratch with values from the adjacent image. This method is also useful for removing other linear structures, as shown in **Figure 8.51**. In this case, the procedure uses the methods described in **Chapter 4** for ranking in color images to perform erosion and dilation.

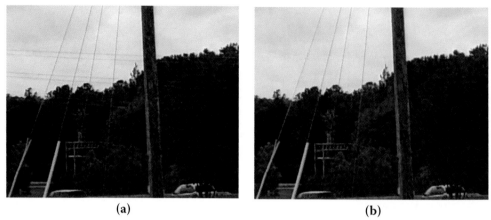

(a)   (b)

Figure 8.51 *Removing power lines: **(a)** original image; **(b)** result of applying an opening and closing using a vertical neighborhood. Only the horizontal lines are removed; a different neighbor pattern would be needed to remove the other wires.*

Examples of use

Some additional examples of erosion and dilation operations illustrate typical applications and methods. One area of use is for X-ray maps from the SEM. These are usually so sparse that even though they are recorded as gray-scale images, they are virtually binary images even before thresholding because most pixels have zero photon counts and a few pixels have one. Regions containing the element of interest are distinguished from those that do not by a difference in the spatial density of dots, which humans are able to interpret by a gestalt grouping operation. This very noisy and scattered image is difficult to use for locating feature boundaries. Dilation may be able to join points together to produce a more useful representation.

Figure 8.52 shows a representative X-ray map from an SEM. Notice that the dark bands in the aluminum dot map represent the shadows where the gold grid blocks the incident

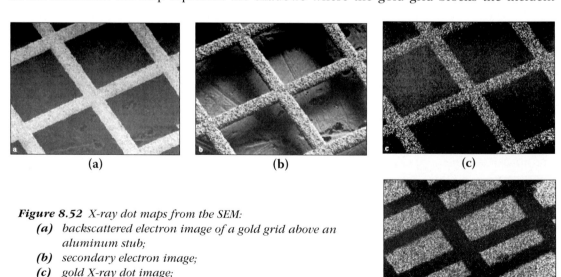

(a)   (b)   (c)

Figure 8.52 *X-ray dot maps from the SEM:*
  - ***(a)*** *backscattered electron image of a gold grid above an aluminum stub;*
  - ***(b)*** *secondary electron image;*
  - ***(c)*** *gold X-ray dot image;*
  - ***(d)*** *aluminum X-ray image (note shadows of grid).*

(d)

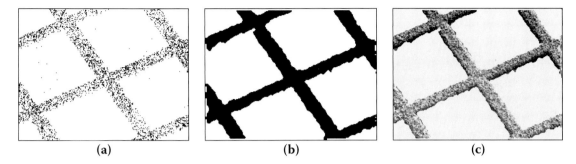

Figure 8.53 *Delineating the gold grid: **(a)** thresholded X-ray map; **(b)** image a after two repetitions of closing; **(c)** the backscattered electron image masked to show the boundaries from image **b** (notice the approximate location of edges).*

electron beam or the emitted X-rays en route to the detector. **Figure 8.53** shows the result of thresholding the gold map and applying a closing to merge the individual dots. **Figure 8.54** illustrates the results for the aluminum map. Because it has more dots, it produces a somewhat better definition of the region edges. Notice, however, that superior results are obtained in this case by smoothing the gray-scale image and then thresholding, as described in **Chapter 7**. In general, processing the gray-scale image before thresholding can produce results superior to processing the binary image after thresholding, because more information is available in the gray-scale image.

Other images from the light and electron microscope sometimes have the same essentially binary image as well. Examples include ultrathin biological tissue sections stained with heavy metals and viewed in the TEM (transmission electron microscope) and chemically etched metallographic specimens. The dark regions are frequently small, corresponding to barely resolved individual particles whose distribution and clustering reveal the desired microstructure (membranes in tissue, eutectic lamellae in metals, etc.) to the eye. As for the case of X-ray dot maps, it is sometimes possible to utilize dilation operations to join such dots to form a well-defined image.

Combinations of closings and openings are often useful for defining regions for measurement. In **Figure 8.55**, iron carbide particles in a steel specimen are etched to appear dark. However, it is not the individual dark features that are important for measurement. The size of the

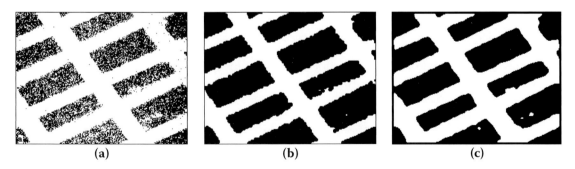

Figure 8.54 *Delineating the aluminum map: **(a)** thresholding (notice the isolated continuum or background X-rays recorded between the grids); **(b)** after erosion with a neighborhood coefficient of 7 to remove the isolated pixels and dilation (two cycles) to fill the regions; **(c)** result of smoothing the gray-scale image **(Figure 8.52d)** and thresholding.*

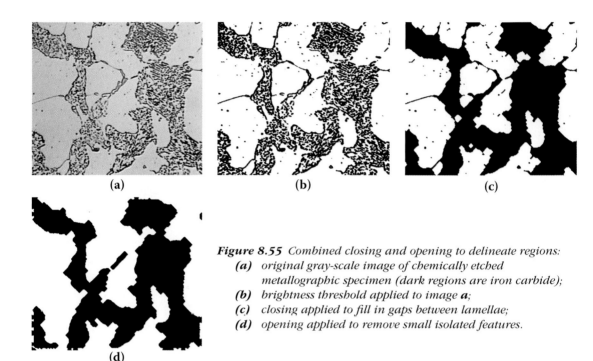

(a) (b) (c)

(d)

Figure 8.55 *Combined closing and opening to delineate regions:*
(a) *original gray-scale image of chemically etched metallographic specimen (dark regions are iron carbide);*
(b) *brightness threshold applied to image **a**;*
(c) *closing applied to fill in gaps between lamellae;*
(d) *opening applied to remove small isolated features.*

islands of lamellar structure and those without such structure control the properties of the alloy, but these are not well defined by the individual dark carbide particles. Dilation followed by erosion (closing) merges the individual lamellae, but there are also dark regions within the essentially white grains because of the presence of a few dark points in the original image. Following the closing with an opening (for a total sequence of dilation, erosion, erosion, dilation) produces a useful result, as shown.

In the example, the closing and opening used a neighborhood coefficient of 1 and six iterations. The number of iterations is based on the size of the gap to be filled or feature to be removed. The presence of primarily 45° orientations of the edges of features in the processed binary images reveals the anisotropic effects of the erosion/dilation operations. Using different coefficients in the various operations sometimes lessens the obvious geometric bias. The choice of appropriate parameters is largely a matter of experience with a particular type of image and human judgment of the correctness of the final result. A more isotropic result for this same image using a different approach to erosion and dilation is shown below (**Figure 8.61**).

There is a basic similarity between using these morphological operations on a thresholded binary image and some of the texture operators used in **Chapter 5** on gray-scale images. In most cases, similar (but not identical) results can be obtained with either approach (provided the software offers both sets of tools). For instance, **Figure 8.56** shows the same image of curds used earlier to compare several gray-scale texture-processing operations. Background leveling and thresholding the smooth, white areas (the curds) produces the result shown. Clearly, there are many regions in the textured portion of the image that are just as bright as the curds. In gray-scale texture processing, these were eliminated based on consideration of the local variation in pixel brightness. In this image, that variation produces narrow and irregular thresholded regions. An opening, consisting of an erosion to remove edge-touching pixels and a dilation to restore pixels smoothly to boundaries of features that are still present, effectively removes the background clutter, as shown in the figure. The erosion/dilation

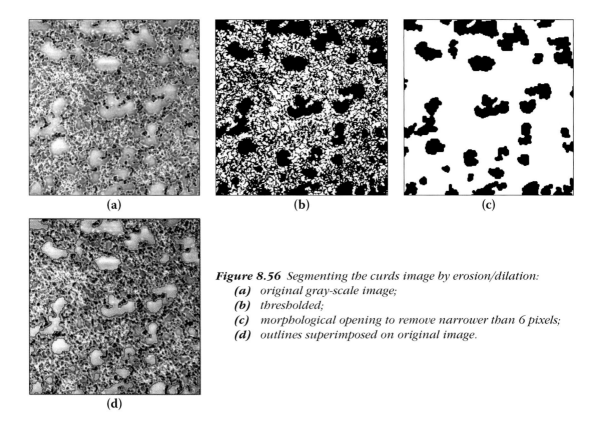

Figure 8.56 *Segmenting the curds image by erosion/dilation:*
(a) original gray-scale image;
(b) thresholded;
(c) morphological opening to remove narrower than 6 pixels;
(d) outlines superimposed on original image.

approach to defining the structure in this image amounts to making some assumptions about the characteristic dimensions of the features, their boundary irregularities, and their spacings, but a similar decision about the spatial scale of the texture was required for successful gray-scale processing in **Chapter 5**.

Erosion/dilation procedures are often used along with Boolean combinations. In the examples of **Figure 8.27**, **Figure 8.28**, **Figure 8.29**, and **Figure 8.30**, the lines used to test for adjacency were obtained by dilating the binary image and then Ex-ORing the result with the original. The superimposed outlines shown in **Figure 8.56d** and many others to compare the results of processing with the original image can be produced by performing an erosion followed by an Ex-OR with the original binary image. This leaves the outlines of pixels that were originally adjacent to the background. It is also possible to obtain this image directly, by a specialized erosion operation that erases any pixel that does *not* have an adjacent background pixel. However it is produced, the outline is called the "custer" of a feature, perhaps in reference to George Armstrong Custer, who was also surrounded back in 1876.

The custer can be used to determine neighbor relationships between features or regions. As an example, **Figure 8.57** shows a three-phase metal alloy imaged in the light microscope. Each of the individual phases can be readily delineated by thresholding (and in the case of the medium-gray image, applying an opening to remove lines of pixels straddling the white-black boundary). Then the custer of each phase can be formed as described above.

Combining the custer of each phase with the other phases using an AND keeps only the portion of the custer that is common to the two phases. The result is to mark the boundaries as white-gray, gray-black, or black-white, so that the extent of each type can be determined. In

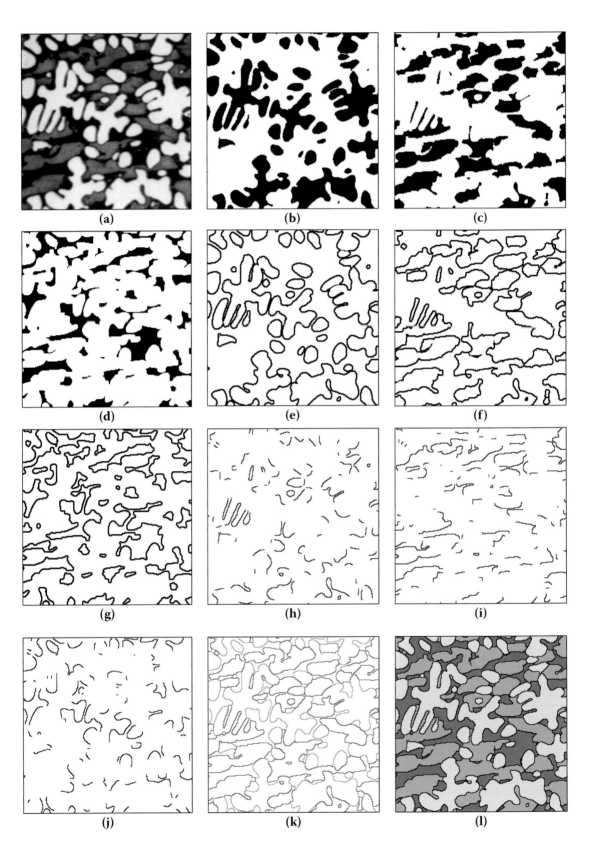

other cases, the marker-selection or Feature-AND logic can be used to select the entire features that are adjacent to one region (and hence touch its custer), as illustrated previously.

Euclidean distance map

The directional bias present in morphological operations because of their restriction to pixels on a square grid can be overcome by performing equivalent operations (erosion, dilation, opening, closing, etc.) using a different technique. It makes use of a gray-scale image, produced from the original binary, in which every pixel within a feature is assigned a value that is its distance from the nearest background pixel. This is called the Euclidean distance map (EDM).

Most of the image processing functions discussed in this and preceding chapters operate either on gray-scale images (to produce other gray-scale images) or on binary images (to produce other binary images). The EDM is a tool that works on a binary image to produce a gray-scale image. The definition is simple enough: each point in the foreground is assigned a brightness value equal to its straight-line (hence "Euclidean") distance from the nearest point in the background. In a continuous image, as opposed to a digitized one containing finite pixels, this is unambiguous. In most pixel images, the distance is taken from each pixel in the feature to the nearest pixel in the background.

Searching through all of the background pixels to find the nearest one to each pixel in a feature and calculating the distance in a Pythagorean sense would be an extremely inefficient and time-consuming process for constructing the EDM. Some researchers have implemented a different type of distance map in which distance is measured in only a few directions. For a lattice of square pixels, this can either be restricted to the 90° directions or extended to include the 45° directions (Rosenfeld and Kak 1982). This measuring convention is equivalent to deciding to use a four-neighbor or eight-neighbor convention for considering whether pixels are touching. In either case, the distance from each pixel to one of its four or eight neighbors is taken as 1, regardless of the direction. Consequently, as shown in **Figure 8.58**, the distance map from a point gives rise to either square or diamond-shaped artifacts and is quite distorted compared with the correct Pythagorean distance. These measuring conventions are sometimes described as city-block models (connections in four directions) or chessboard models (eight directions), because of the limited moves available in those situations. These versions of a distance map do not offer any advantage over classical erosion and dilation in terms of being more isotropic.

A conceptually straightforward iterative technique for constructing such a distance map can be programmed as follows.

1. Assign a brightness value of 0 to each pixel in the background.
2. Set a variable N equal to 0.
3. For each pixel that touches (in either the four- or eight-neighbor sense, as described above) a pixel whose brightness value is N, assign a brightness value of $N + 1$.
4. Increment N and repeat step 3 until all pixels in the image have been assigned.

Figure 8.57 (See facing page.) Use of Boolean logic to measure neighbor-adjacency relationships: (a) an original light-microscope image of a three-phase metal; (b, c, d) thresholded white, gray, and black phases; (e, f, g) surrounding outlines of each phase produced by dilation and Ex-OR with original; (h, i, j) AND of outlines of pairs of phases; (k) OR of all ANDed outlines using different colors to identify each phase/phase interface; (l) outlines filled to show idealized phase regions.

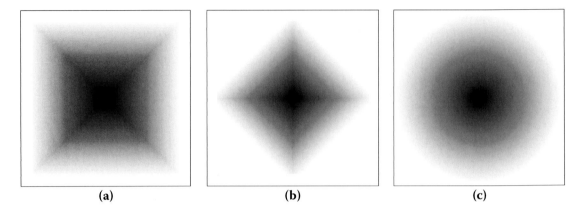

Figure 8.58 Gray-scale images showing the distance from the center pixel measured in different ways: *(a)* city block or four-neighbor paths; *(b)* chessboard or eight-neighbor paths; *(c)* Pythagorean distance.

The time required for this iteration depends on the size of the features (the maximum distance from the background). A more efficient method is available that gives the same result with two passes through the image (Danielsson 1980). This technique uses the same comparisons, but propagates the values through the image more rapidly.

1. Assign the brightness value of 0 to each pixel in the background and a large positive value (greater than the maximum feature width) to each pixel in a feature.
2. Proceeding from left to right and top to bottom, assign each pixel within a feature a brightness value one greater than the smallest value of any of its neighbors.
3. Repeat step 2, proceeding from right to left and bottom to top.

A further modification provides a better approximation to the Pythagorean distances between pixels (Russ and Russ 1988b). The diagonally adjacent pixels are neither a distance 1 (eight-neighbor rules) nor $\sqrt{2}$ = 1.414 (four-neighbor rules) away. The latter value is an irrational number, but closer approximations than 1.00 or 2.00 are available. For instance, modifying the above rules so that a pixel brightness value must be larger than its 90° neighbors by 2 and greater than its 45° neighbors by 3 is equivalent to using an approximation of 1.5 for the square root of 2.

The disadvantage of this method is that all of the pixel distances are now multiplied by 2, increasing the maximum brightness of the EDM image by this factor. For images capable of storing a maximum gray level of 255, this represents a limitation on the largest features that can be processed in this way. However, if the EDM image is 16 bits deep (and can hold values up to 65,535), this is not a practical limitation. It also opens the way to selecting larger ratios of numbers to approximate $\sqrt{2}$, getting a correspondingly improved set of values for the distance map, for instance 7/5 = 1.400 and 58/41 = 1.415.

It takes no longer to compare or add these values than it does any others, and the ratio 58/41 allows dimensions larger than 1024 pixels. Since this dimension is the half-width, features or background up to 2048 pixels wide can be processed (1024 × 41 = 41,984, which is less than $2^{16} - 1$ = 65,535). Of course, the final image can be divided down by the scaling factor (41 in this example) to obtain a result in which pixel brightness values are the actual distance to the boundary (rounded or truncated to integers) and the total brightness range is within the range of 0 to 255 that most displays are capable of showing.

The accuracy of an EDM constructed with these rules can be judged by counting the pixels whose brightness values place them within a specified distance. This is just the same as constructing a cumulative histogram of pixel brightness in the image. **Figure 8.59** plots the error in the number of pixels vs. integer brightness for a distance map of a circle 99 pixels in diameter; the overall errors are not large. Even better accuracy for the EDM can be obtained by performing additional comparisons with pixels beyond the first eight nearest neighbors. Adding a comparison to the eight neighbors in the 5 × 5 neighborhood whose Pythagorean distance is √5 produces values having even less directional

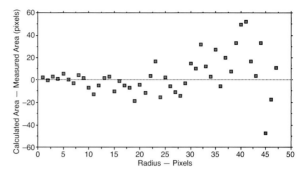

Figure 8.59 *Difference between theoretical area value (πr^2) and the actual area covered by the EDM as a function of brightness (distance from boundary) shows increasing but still small errors for very large distances.*

sensitivity and more accuracy for large distances. If the integer values 58 and 41 mentioned above are used to approximate √2, then the path to these pixels consisting of a "knight's move" of one 90° and one 45° pixel step would produce a value of 58 + 41 = 99. Substituting a value of 92 gives a close approximation to the Pythagorean distance (92/41 = 2.243; √5 = 2.236) and produces even more accurate and isotropic results.

There is another algorithm that produces a Euclidean distance map with real number values. During the passes through the image, the x and y distances from the nearest background point are accumulated separately for each pixel within the features, and then the actual Pythagorean distance is calculated as the square root of the sum of squares. Of course, it is still necessary to convert to an integer representation for display purposes. In general, the better the quality of the EDM values, the better the results obtained using the EDM for erosion, dilation, and watershed segmentation, as described below. Many of the cases in which watershed segmentation produces poor results are in fact cases in which the EDM is of poor quality because of limited accuracy and the use of integer arithmetic, which is a hangover from the days when computer power was less than currently available.

Comparison of the pixel-by-pixel classic erosion and dilation with the circular-pattern-provided thresholding by the EDM of either the foreground (erosion) or background (dilation) to select pixels that are farther from the edge than any desired extent of erosion shows that the EDM method is much more isotropic (**Figure 8.60**). Furthermore, the distance map is constructed quickly and the thresholding requires no iteration, so the execution time of the method does not increase with feature size (as do iterative classical erosion methods) and is preferred for large features or distances.

When more irregular shapes are subjected to erosion and dilation, the difference between the iterative methods and thresholding by the EDM is also apparent, with EDM methods avoiding the 90° or 45° boundaries present with the traditional morphological tools. **Figure 8.61** shows the same example of closing and opening applied to the image in **Figure 8.55**. The distance used for both closing and opening was 5.5 pixels (note that with the EDM it is possible to specify that distances are real numbers rather than being restricted to integers), and the final outlines trace the edges of the structures with much greater fidelity.

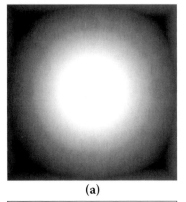

(a)

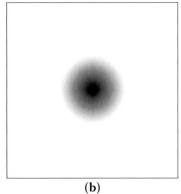

(b)

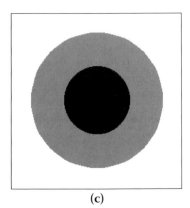

(c)

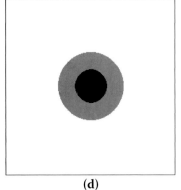

(d)

Figure 8.60 Isotropic erosion and dilation achieved by using the EDM for dilation and erosion (compare with *Figures 8.42–8.46*):

(a) the EDM of the background around the circle;

(b) the EDM of the circle,

(c) dilation achieved by thresholding the background EDM at a value of 50;

(d) erosion achieved by thresholding the circle EDM at a value of 25.

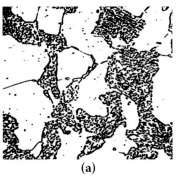

(a)

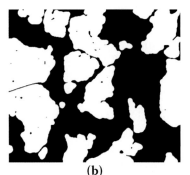

(b)

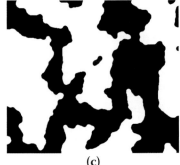

(c)

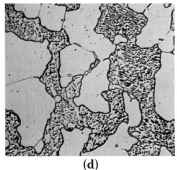

(d)

Figure 8.61 Closing and opening using the EDM:

(a) thresholded original image (same as *Figure 8.55*);

(b) closing, distance of 5.5 pixels;

(c) opening; distance of 5.5 pixels;

(d) outlines superimposed on original image.

Watershed segmentation

A common difficulty in measuring images occurs when features touch and therefore cannot be separately identified, counted, or measured. This situation can arise when examining an image of a thick section in transmission, where feature overlap may occur, or when particles resting on a surface tend to agglomerate and touch each other. The method that is usually preferred for separating touching, but mostly convex, features in an image is known as watershed segmentation (Beucher and Lantejoul 1979; Lantejoul and Beucher 1981).

The classical method for accomplishing this separation (Jernot 1982) is an iterative one. The image is repetitively eroded, and at each step those separate features that disappeared from the previous step are designated ultimate eroded points (UEPs) and saved as an image, along with the iteration number. Saving these is necessary because the features will in general be of different sizes and would not all disappear in the same number of iterations. The process continues until the image is erased.

Then, beginning with the final image of UEPs, the image is dilated using classical dilation, but with the added logical constraint that no new pixel can be turned ON if it causes a connection to form between previously separate features or if it was not ON in the original image. At each stage of the dilation, the image of UEPs that corresponds to the equivalent level of erosion is added to the image using a logical OR. This process causes the features to grow back to their original boundaries, except that lines of separation appear between the touching features.

The method just described has two practical drawbacks: the iterative process is slow, requiring each pixel in the image to be processed many times, and the amount of storage required for all of the intermediate images is quite large. The same result can be obtained more efficiently using an EDM. Indeed, the name "watershed" comes directly from the EDM implementation. Imagine that the brightness values of each pixel within features in an EDM correspond to a physical elevation. The features then appear as a mountain peak. **Figure 8.62** illustrates this for a circular feature.

If two features touch or overlap slightly, the EDM shows two peaks, as shown in **Figure 8.63**. The slope of the mountainside is constant, so the larger the feature, the higher is the peak. The ultimate eroded points are the peaks of the mountains, and where features touch, the flanks of the mountains intersect. The saddles between these mountains are the lines selected as boundaries by the segmentation method. They are locations where water running down from

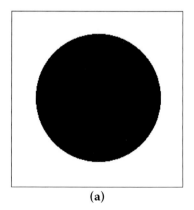 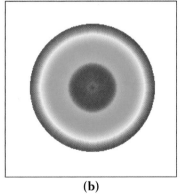 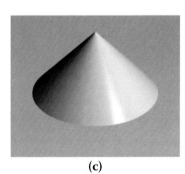

| (a) | (b) | (c) |

Figure 8.62 *Interpreting the EDM as the height of pixels: **(a)** binary image of a circular feature; **(b)** EDM with pixels color-coded to show distance from boundary; **(c)** rendered display showing pixel heights.*

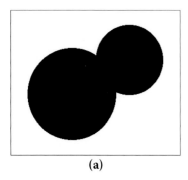 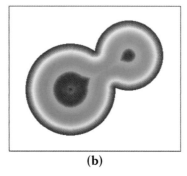 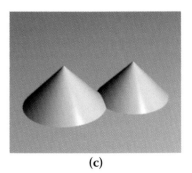

(a)   (b)   (c)

Figure 8.63 *EDM for touching features:* ***(a)*** *binary image of two touching circular features;* ***(b)*** *EDM with pixels color-coded to show distance from boundary;* ***(c)*** *rendered display showing pixel heights. Note the boundary between the two cones.*

the mountains arrives from two different peaks, and hence are called watershed lines. The placement of these lines according to the relative height of the mountains (size of the features) gives the best estimate of the separation lines between features, which are divided according the regions that belong to each mountaintop.

Implementing the segmentation process using an EDM approach (Russ and Russ 1988b) is very efficient, both in terms of speed and storage. The required distance map image is constructed without iteration. The ultimate eroded points are located as a special case of local maxima (there is a further discussion of UEPs below), and the brightness value of each directly corresponds to the iteration number at which it would disappear in the iterative method. Dilating these features is fast, because the distance map supplies a constraint. Starting at the maximum value and "walking down the mountain" covers all of the brightness levels. At each one, only those pixels at the current brightness level in the distance map need to be considered. Those that do not produce a join between features are added to the image. The process continues until all of the pixels in the features, except for those along the separation lines, have been restored.

Figure 8.64 shows an example of this method applied to an image consisting of touching circles. Since these are of different sizes, the method described previously in **Figure 8.38** does not work, but watershed segmentation separates the features. For an image of real particles, as shown in **Figure 8.65**, the method works subject to the assumption that the features are sufficiently convex that the EDM does not produce multiple peaks within each feature.

Watershed segmentation was used as part of several previous examples. Of course, this method is not perfect. Watershed segmentation cannot handle concave and irregular particles, nor does it separate particles whose overlap is so great that there is no minimum in the EDM between them. Depending on the quality of the original distance map, watershed segmentation may subdivide lines of constant width into many fragments because of the apparent minima produced by aliasing along the line edges. In most cases, the effort needed to correct such defects is much less than would have been required to perform manual separation of the original features.

The presence of holes within features confuses the watershed algorithm and breaks the features up into many fragments. It is therefore necessary to fill holes before applying the watershed. However, there may also be holes in the image between features as well as those within them. Normal hole filling would fill them in, since any region of background not connected to the edge of the image is considered a hole. This difficulty can be overcome if some difference in hole size or shape can be identified to permit filling only the holes within features and

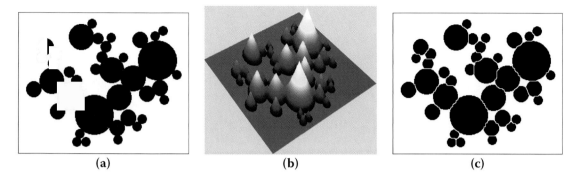

Figure 8.64 *Watershed segmentation on an image of touching circles of different sizes:* **(a)** *original;* **(b)** *"surface" representation of the EDM;* **(c)** *watershed result.*

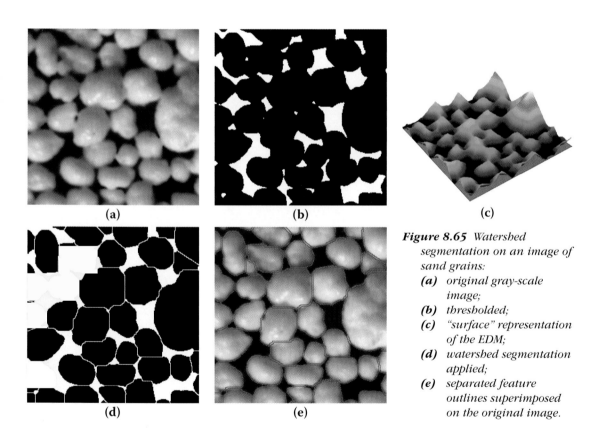

Figure 8.65 *Watershed segmentation on an image of sand grains:*
(a) *original gray-scale image;*
(b) *thresholded;*
(c) *"surface" representation of the EDM;*
(d) *watershed segmentation applied;*
(e) *separated feature outlines superimposed on the original image.*

not those between them (Russ 1995f). In the example shown in **Figure 8.66**, the holes within features (organelles within the cells) are much rounder than spaces between the touching cells. Isolating these holes by measurement, and ORing them with the original image, allows watershed segmentation to separate the cells.

Figure 8.67 shows another problem for the watershed method. The image shows cross sections of touching sheaths around nerve fibers. Filling the holes does not permit a watershed operation to separate them because of their irregular shapes. The watershed not only separates

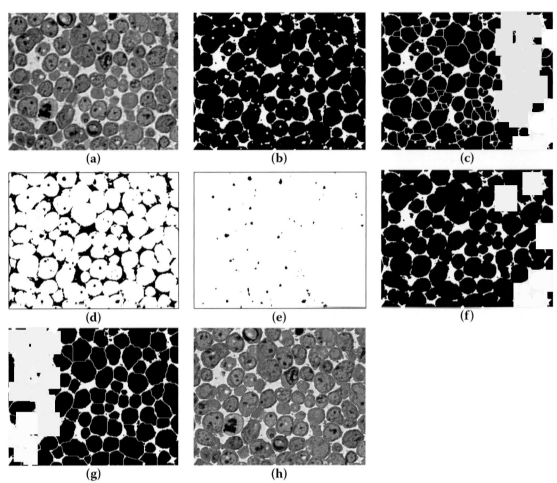

Figure 8.66 *Separation of touching cells: (a) original gray-scale image; (b) thresholded; (c) erroneous watershed segmentation produced by holes within cells; (d) inverting image b to show holes within and between cells; (e) holes within cells selected by their rounder shapes; (f) combining images b and e using a Boolean OR; (g) watershed segmentation of image f; (h) separated feature outlines superimposed on original image.*

the features, but also cuts them into pieces. Using the image of the interiors of the original sheaths as a set of markers to select the watershed lines that cut across the features (the Feature-AND introduced above) allows ORing those lines back into the image, so that the desired separation can be accomplished. Note that this procedure uses both pixel- and feature-based Boolean operations. Understanding the multiple steps in this sequence is a good test for general knowledge of these operations.

Ultimate eroded points

The ultimate eroded points (UEPs) described above in the watershed segmentation technique can be used as a measurement tool in their own right. The number of points gives the number of separable features in the image, while the brightness of each point gives a measure of the original feature size (the inscribed radius). In addition, the location of each point can be used

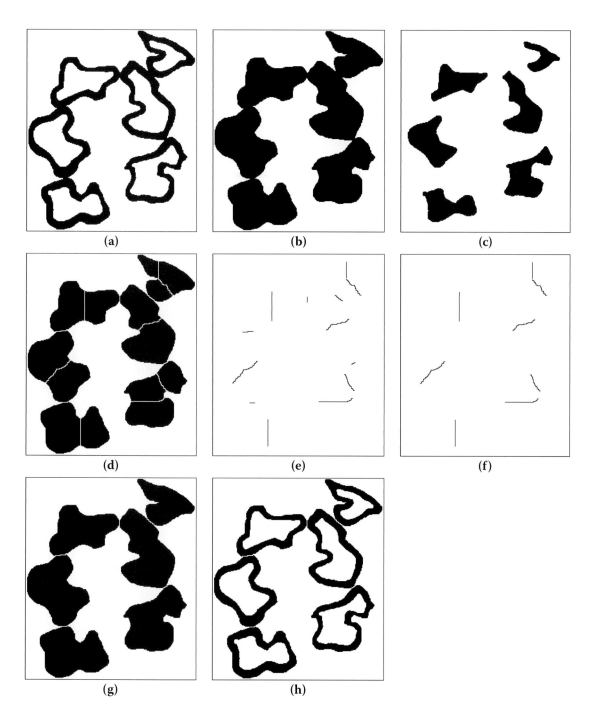

Figure 8.67 *Separation of touching nerve sheaths: (a) binary image of touching, irregular features; (b) holes filled; (c) interiors of features (image **a** Ex-ORed with image **b**); (d) watershed segmentation of image **b**; (e) watershed lines (image **b** Ex-ORed with image **d**); (f) lines in image **e** that cross the interiors of features (selected by markers in image **b**); (g) image **f** ORed with image **d**; (h) image **g** ANDed with image **a**, producing the intact and separated nerve sheaths.*

as a location for the feature if clustering or gradients are to be investigated. **Figure 8.68** shows an example and compares the measurement results with those produced by the successive erosion method described previously in **Figure 8.48**.

The formal definition of a UEP in a continuous, rather than pixel-based, image is simply a local maximum of brightness in the EDM image. Since the image is subdivided into finite pixels, the definition must take into account the possibility that more than one pixel may have equal brightness, forming a plateau. In other words, the set of pixels that are UEPs must be as bright or brighter than all neighbors; if the neighbors are equal in brightness, then they must also be part of the set.

The brightness of each pixel in the distance map is the distance to the nearest boundary. For a UEP, this must be a point that is equidistant from at least three boundary locations. Consequently, the brightness is the radius of the feature's inscribed circle. A histogram of the brightness values of the UEP pixels gives an immediate measure of the size distribution of the features. This is much faster than performing the watershed segmentation, since the dilation procedure is eliminated, and much faster than measurement, since no feature identification or pixel counting is required. For separate (nontouching) features, the maximum point of the EDM provides a measurement of the radius of an inscribed circle, a useful size parameter.

The EDM provides values that can be effectively used for many types of measurements. For example, the method described above for determining a fractal dimension from successive erosion and dilation operations has two shortcomings: it is slow and has orientational bias because of the anisotropy of the operations. The EDM offers a simple way to obtain the same information (Russ 1988), as will be discussed in detail in **Chapter 10**.

Because the distance map encodes each pixel with the straight-line distance to the nearest background point, it can also be used to measure the distance of many points or features from irregular boundaries. In the example shown in **Figure 8.69**, the image is thresholded to define the boundary lines (which might represent grain boundaries, cell membranes, roads on a map, etc.) and points (particles, organelles, structures, etc.). The image of the thresholded features is applied as a mask to the EDM of the interior so that all pixels in the features have the distance values. Measuring the brightness of the features gives the distance of each feature from the boundary. This is much faster and more accurate than the method shown previously in **Figure 8.28**.

EDM values can also be combined with the skeleton of features or of the background, as discussed below.

Skeletonization

Erosion can be performed with special rules that remove edge pixels, except when doing so would cause a separation of one region into two. The rule for this is to examine the touching neighbors; if they do not form a continuous group, then the central pixel cannot be removed (Davidson 1991; Lam et al. 1992; Nevatia and Babu 1980; Pavlidis 1980; Ritter and Wilson 2001). The definition of this condition is dependent on whether four- or eight-connectedness is used. In either case, the selected patterns can be used in a fate table to conduct the erosion (Russ 1984). The most common convention is that features, and hence skeletons, are eight-connected, while background is four-connected, and that is the convention used in the following examples.

Skeletonization by erosion is an iterative procedure, and the number of iterations required is proportional to the largest dimension of any feature in the image. An alternative method for

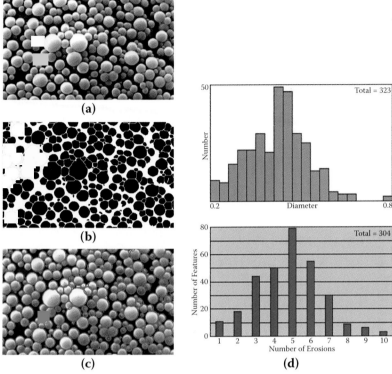

Figure 8.68 *Measurement of touching particles:*

(a) *original (SEM image of lipid particles);*

(b) *binary image produced by thresholding and watershed;*

(c) *estimated size and location (shown by red circles and green points) using the ultimate eroded points;*

(d) *comparison of size distributions measured by this procedure (top, in red) and the iterative gray-scale erosion method shown for the same image in* **Figure 8.48** *(bottom, blue).*

constructing the skeleton uses the EDM. The ridge of locally brightest values in the EDM contains those points that are equidistant from at least two points on the boundaries of the feature. This ridge constitutes the medial-axis transform (MAT). As for the UEPs, the MAT is precisely defined for a continuous image but only approximately defined for an image composed of finite pixels (Mott-Smith 1970).

In most cases, the MAT corresponds rather closely to the skeleton obtained by sequential erosion. However, since it is less directionally sensitive than any erosion pattern and because of the pixel limitations in representing a line, it may be shifted slightly in some cases. The uses of the MAT are the same as the skeleton, and in many cases, the MAT procedure is used because it is more isotropic and faster, but the result is still described as a skeleton.

Figure 8.70 shows several features with their (eight-connected) skeletons. The skeleton is a powerful shape factor for feature recognition, containing both topological and metric information. The topological values include the number of endpoints, the number of nodes where branches meet, and the number of internal holes in the feature (loops in the skeleton). The metric values are the mean length of branches (both those internal to the feature and those having a free end) and the angles of the branches. These parameters correspond closely to what human observers see as the significant characteristics of features. **Figure 8.71** shows the nomenclature used.

The numbers of each type of feature are related by Euler's equation

$$\# \text{ Loops} = \# \text{ Branches} - \# \text{ Ends} - \# \text{ Nodes} + 1 \tag{8.3}$$

There are a few specific cases that appear to violate this basic rule of topology, requiring careful interpretation of the digitized skeleton. **Figure 8.72** shows two of them. The ring skel-

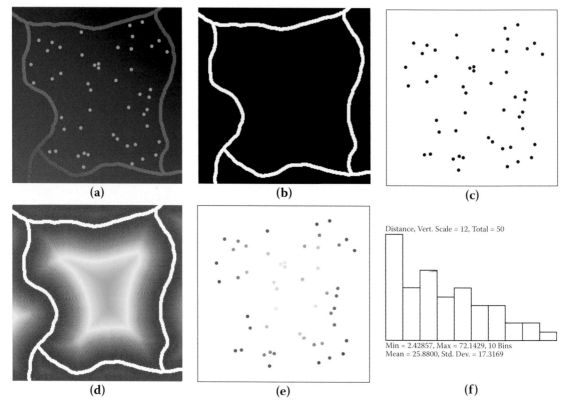

(a)   (b)   (c)

(d)   (e)   Distance, Vert. Scale = 12, Total = 50

Min = 2.42857, Max = 72.1429, 10 Bins
Mean = 25.8800, Std. Dev. = 17.3169

(f)

Figure 8.69 *Measurement of distance from a boundary:* **(a)** *example image;* **(b)** *thresholded interior region;* **(c)** *thresholded features;* **(d)** *EDM of the interior (color-coded);* **(e)** *distance value assigned to features;* **(f)** *histogram of distances for features.*

etonizes to a single circular branch that has one loop, a single branch, and no apparent node. However, the rules of topology require that there be a "virtual" node someplace on the ring where the two ends of the linear branch are joined. Likewise, the symmetrical circle figure

skeletonizes to a single point. which, having fewer than two neighbors, would be classified as an end. In reality, this point represents a short branch with two ends. Special rules can correctly deal with these special cases.

Locating the nodes and endpoints in a skeleton is simply a matter of counting neighbors. Points along the eight-connected skeleton branches have exactly two neighbors. Endpoints have a single neighbor, while nodes have more than two (either three or four). The topology of features is an instantly recognizable shape descriptor that can be determined quickly from the feature skeleton. For example, in **Figure 8.73** the number of points in each star is something that humans identify easily as a defining shape parameter. Count-

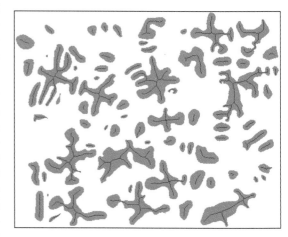

Figure 8.70 *A binary image containing multiple features, with their skeletons superimposed.*

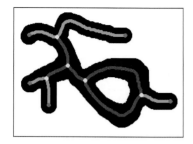

Figure 8.71 *The skeleton of a feature with five endpoints (magenta), five nodes (yellow), five external branches (green), five internal branches (red), and one loop. The skeleton has been dilated and features color-coded for visibility.*

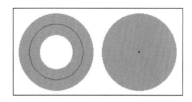

Figure 8.72 *Skeletons for a ring and a circle, as discussed in the text.*

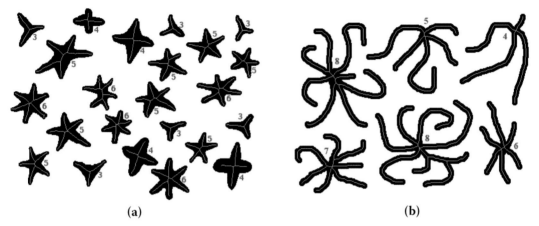

(a)   (b)

Figure 8.73 *Labeling star-shaped and branched features according to the number of endpoints in the skeleton: (a) a simple case; (b) complex shapes.*

ing the number of skeleton pixels that have just one neighbor allows labeling them with this topological property. This method also works (as shown in the figure) when the features are less easily recognized visually. Similarly, an easy distinction between the letters A, B, and C is the number of loops (1, 2, and 0, respectively). As topological properties, these do not depend on size, position, or distortion of the letters (for example by the use of different fonts).

Depending on how the skeleton is constructed (or the EDM from which the MAT can be derived), it may show some directional anisotropy. **Figure 8.74** shows the skeleton for an image of a gear. The number of endpoints (47) in the skeleton immediately provides a count for the number of teeth in the gear. The skeleton shown in **Figure 8.74a** was constructed from a high-precision EDM and has spokes that are correctly radial (within the limits of square pixels) from a circular core. The skeleton in **Figure 8.74b** was constructed with a widely used freeware program (NIH-Image) that uses successive erosions to form the skeleton, and results in lines that show strong directional bias. Examination of such a skeleton is often a good test of the underlying implementation used in image processing software.

Segment lengths are important measures of feature size, as will be discussed in **Chapter 10**. These can also be determined by counting, i.e., keeping track of the number of pixel pairs that are diagonally or orthogonally connected, or by fitting smoothed curves through the points to measure the length, which gives more accurate results. Notice that the skeleton does not extend to the end of each branch. The length of the external branch in a skeleton can be corrected to get the actual branch length of the feature by adding the value of the EDM for the pixel at the end of the skeleton. Counting the number of nodes, ends, loops, and branches

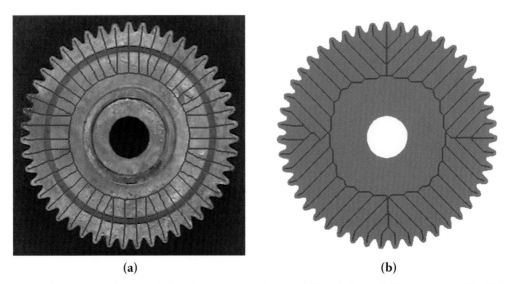

(a)   (b)

Figure 8.74 Skeleton of a gear: (a) skeleton and endpoints (dilated for visibility) generated by Reindeer Graphics Fovea Pro software superimposed on the original gear image; (b) skeleton (dilated for visibility) superimposed on the same binary image used in image a, as generated by NIH-Image software.

defines the topology of features. These topological events simplify the original image and assist in characterizing structure, as illustrated in **Figure 8.75**.

Skeletons are very useful for dealing with images of crossed fibers. **Figure 8.76** shows a diagrammatic example in which several fibers cross each other. Because these lines were drawn in different colors, counting them is not difficult, but in a typical real case with many indistinguishable fibers, counting can be difficult. In a few situations it is necessary to actually follow individual fibers in such a tangle. This can be done (generally using rather specialized software and some prior knowledge about the nature of the fibers) by skeletonizing the image. The regions around each of the nodes where the skeletons cross are then examined, and the branches that represent the continuation of a single fiber are identified (Beil et al. 2005; Talbot et al. 2000). The criteria are typically that the local direction change be small, and perhaps that the width, color, or density of the fiber be consistent. When fibers cross at a shallow angle, the skeleton often shows two nodes with a segment that belongs to both fibers. Images of straight fibers are much easier to disentangle than curved ones.

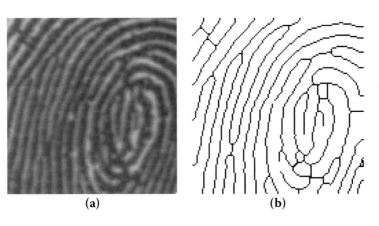

(a)   (b)

Figure 8.75 Simplification of a fingerprint image (a); by thresholding and (b) skeletonization.

A much simpler result is possible if the required information is just the total number and average length of the fibers. Regardless of the number of nodes or fiber crossings, the number of fibers is just half the number of endpoints, which can be counted directly (with a small error introduced by the probability that an end of one fiber will lie on a second fiber). Measuring the total length of the skeleton (with a correction for the endpoints, as mentioned above) and dividing by the number gives the average value. In **Figure 8.76** there are 12 ends, hence 6 fibers, and a total of 40.33 in. of skeleton length, for an average length of 6.72 in.

For images of fibers that extend beyond the image area, half the number of visible endpoints is still the correct value to give the number of fibers per unit area, because the other endpoint for each fiber would be counted in some other field of view, producing a result of one-half fiber in each field of view. **Figure 8.77** shows an example. Nonwoven or felted fabrics are characterized by the density of fibers. The figure shows cellulose fibers used in papermaking, with the skeleton superimposed. There are 193 ends (96.5 fibers) with a total length of 68.29 mm in an area of 6 mm².

In other situations, such as the example shown in **Figure 8.78**, it may be useful to separate the branches of the skeleton for individual measurements of parameters such as length or orientation angle. Removing the exact node pixels is not sufficient to accomplish this, because the remaining branches may still

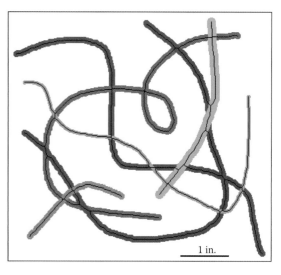

Figure 8.76 *Example of crossing fibers, as discussed in the text, with superimposed skeleton lines.*

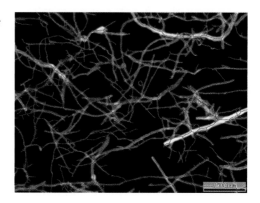

Figure 8.77 *Image of cellulose fibers with the superimposed skeleton.*

be connected. This arises from the nature of eight-connected logic. **Figure 8.79** shows an enlargement of a portion of a skeleton network from **Figure 8.78** in which the node points for topological counting and near-node points are color-coded for illustration. These adjacent points must also be removed to separate the branches This technique is particularly appropriate for branched structures such as the roots of plants, provided that they can be spread out to produce a two-dimensional image. There is also a stereological method for measuring the total length of three-dimensional structures from projections, as discussed in **Chapter 9**.

Just as the skeleton of features can be determined in an image, it is also possible to skeletonize the background. This is often called the "skiz" of the features. **Figure 8.80** shows an example. Consisting of points equidistant from feature boundaries, it effectively divides the image into regions of influence around each feature (Serra 1982). It may be desirable to eliminate from the skiz those lines that are equidistant from two portions of the boundary of

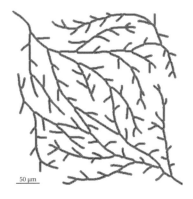

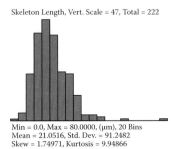

Skeleton Length, Vert. Scale = 47, Total = 222

Min = 0.0, Max = 80.0000, (μm), 20 Bins
Mean = 21.0516, Std. Dev. = 91.2482
Skew = 1.74971, Kurtosis = 9.94866

50 μm

Figure 8.78 Separating the branches of the skeleton of a network for measurement of their lengths.

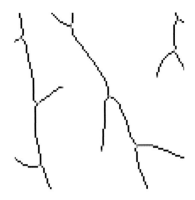

Figure 8.79 Detail of a skeleton showing nodes. Removing the red node points does not disconnect all of the branches; the green "near-node" points must also be deleted to ensure that no eight-connections remain between different branches.

the same feature. This elimination is easily accomplished, since branches have an end; other lines in the skiz are continuous and have no ends except at the image boundaries. Pruning branches from a skeleton (or skiz) simply requires starting at each endpoint (points with a single neighbor) and eliminating touching pixels until a node (a point with more than two neighbors) is reached. Pruning is also used to clean up tessellations, as shown below.

Boundary lines and thickening

A major use for skeletonization is to thin down boundaries that appear to be broad or of variable thickness in images. This phenomenon is particularly common in microscope images of metals whose grain boundaries are revealed by chemical etching, or cells whose bounding walls or membranes are stained. In order to produce continuous dark lines, the preparation and imaging also broadens them. A similar situation arises when digitizing and processing images of maps in which the printed boundaries may be thick. To measure the actual size of the cells, the adjacency

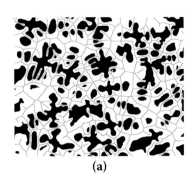

(a)

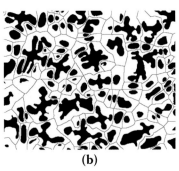

(b)

Figure 8.80 The "skiz" of the same image shown in Figure 8.70:
(a) complete skeleton of the background;
(b) pruned skeleton.

of different grain types, or the length of boundary lines, it is preferable to thin the lines by skeletonization.

Figure 8.81 shows an example. The original polished and etched metal sample has dark and wide grain boundaries as well as dark patches corresponding to carbides and pearlite. Thresholding the image produces broad lines, which can be skeletonized to reduce them to single-pixel width. Since this is properly a continuous tessellation, it can be cleaned up by pruning to remove all branches with endpoints.

The resulting lines delineate the grain boundaries, but because they are eight-connected, they do not separate the grains for individual measurement. Converting the lines to four-connected, called thickening, can be accomplished with a dilation that adds pixels only for a few neighbor patterns corresponding to eight-connected corners (or the skeleton could have been produced using four-connected rules to begin with). The resulting lines separate the grains, which can be identified and measured as shown.

Figure 8.82 shows how this approach can be used to simplify an image and isolate the basic structure for measurement. The original image is a light micrograph of cells in plant tissue. It might be used to measure the variation in cell size with the distance from the two stomata (openings). This process is greatly simplified by reducing the cell walls to single lines. Leveling the background brightness of the original image and then thresholding leaves boundary lines of variable width. Skeletonizing them produces a network of single-pixel-wide lines that delineate the basic cell arrangement.

Unfortunately, the grain boundary or cell tessellation produced by simple thresholding and skeletonization may be incomplete in some cases. Some of the boundaries may fail to stain or to show high density because of their angle with respect to the plane of section, or boundaries for metals may not etch because the crystallographic mismatch across the boundary is small or the concentration of defects or impurities is low. The result is a tessellation with some missing lines, which would bias subsequent analysis. **Figure 8.83** shows one approach to dealing with this situation. Skeletonizing the incomplete network is used to identify the endpoints (points with a single neighbor). It is reasoned that these points should occur in pairs, so each is dilated by some arbitrarily selected distance that, it is hoped, will span half of the gap in the network.

The resulting dilated circles are ORed with the original network, and the result is again skeletonized. Wherever the dilation has caused the circles to touch, the result is a line segment that joins the corresponding endpoints. This method is imperfect, however. Some of the points may be too far apart for the circles to touch, while in other places, the circles may obscure details by touching several existing lines, oversimplifying the resulting network. It is not easy to select an appropriate dilation radius, since the gaps are not all the same size (and not all of the cells are, either). In addition, unmatched ends, or points due to dirt or particulates within the cells, can cause difficulties.

Other methods are also available. A computationally intensive approach locates all of the endpoints and uses a relaxation method to pair them up, so that line direction is maintained, lines are not allowed to cross, and closer points are matched first. This method suffers some of the same problems as dilation if unmatched endpoints or noise are present, but it deals well with gaps of different sizes. A third approach, the use of watershed segmentation based on the EDM, is perhaps the most efficient and reasonably accurate method. As shown in **Figure 8.84**, it correctly draws in most of the missing lines, but erroneously segments grains or cells with concave shapes (which are fortunately rare in real cell or grain structures).

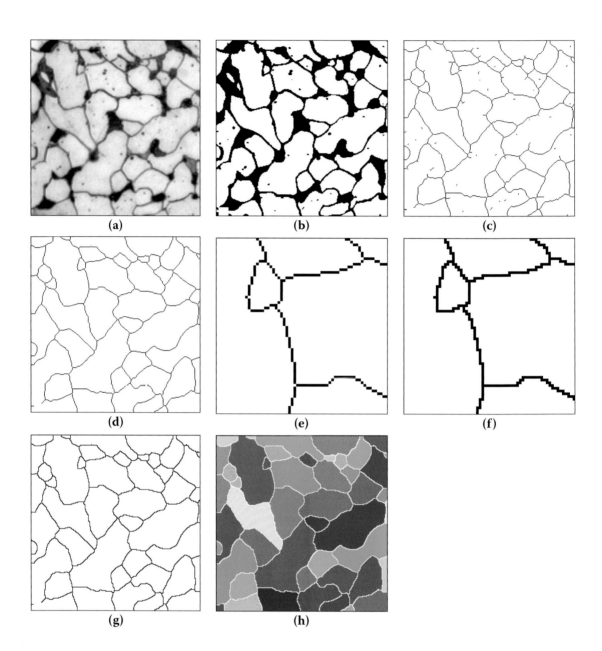

(a) (b) (c)

(d) (e) (f)

(g) (h)

Figure 8.81 *Skeletonization of grain boundaries:* **(a)** *metallographic image of etched 1040 steel;* **(b)** *thresholded image showing boundaries and dark patches containing iron carbide;* **(c)** *skeletonized result from image* **b**; **(d)** *pruned result from image* **c**; **(e)** *enlarged to show eight-connected line;* **(f)** *converted to four-connected line;* **(g)** *grains separated by thickened lines;* **(h)** *identification of individual grains.*

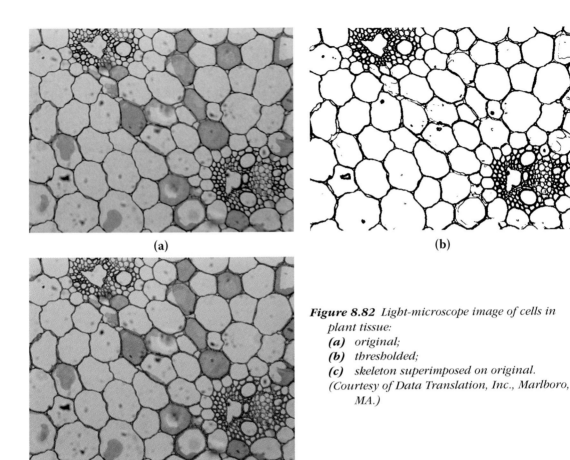

Figure 8.82 *Light-microscope image of cells in plant tissue:*
(a) *original;*
(b) *thresholded;*
(c) *skeleton superimposed on original.*
(Courtesy of Data Translation, Inc., Marlboro, MA.)

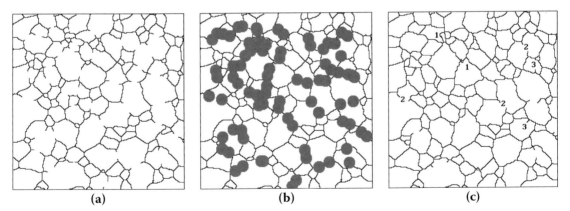

Figure 8.83 *Dilation method for completing grain boundary tessellation: (a) incomplete network;*
(b) dilation of endpoints by an arbitrary radius, shown as circles overlaid on the original;
(c) reskeletonization of network, showing typical errors such as removal of small grains (1), large gaps still not joined (2), and dangling single ends (3).

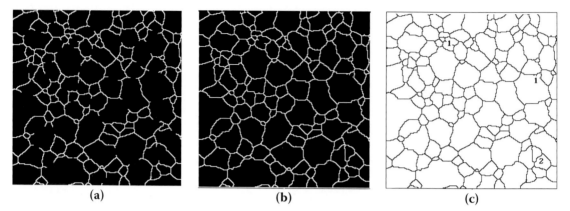

| (a) | (b) | (c) |

Figure 8.84 *Watershed segmentation applied to the same image as **Figure 8.83**: **(a)** the image is inverted to process the grains rather than the boundaries; **(b)** watershed lines are drawn in, connecting most of the broken boundaries; **(c)** in the reinverted result typical errors appear, such as large gaps not joined (1) and false segmentation of irregularly shaped grains (2).*

Combining skeleton and EDM

The skeleton and the EDM are both important tools for measuring images as well as processing them, and by combining the skeleton with the EDM in various ways it is possible to efficiently extract quite a variety of numeric values to quantify image data. A few examples will illustrate the variety of techniques available.

The EDM discussed above provides values that measure the distance of every pixel from the background. For features of irregular shape or width, the pixels along the center line correspond to the centers of inscribed circles, and their EDM values can be used to measure the width and its variation. The skeleton provides a way to sample these pixels, for example by using the skeleton as a mask and then examining the histogram, as shown in **Figure 8.85**. This facilitates the measurement of the width of irregular features, easily determining the mean, minimum, maximum, and standard deviation from the histogram.

The skeleton provides a basic tool for measuring the length of such irregular features, but in general it is too short. The EDM values for the pixels at the endpoints of the skeleton give the radii of the inscribed circles at the ends. As mentioned above, adding these values to the skel-

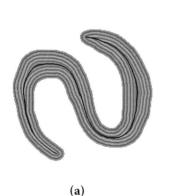

(a)

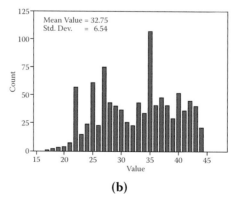

(b)

Figure 8.85 *An irregular feature with its skeleton superimposed on the EDM shown in* **(a)** *pseudocolor, and* **(b)** *the histogram of the EDM values selected by the skeleton.*

eton length corrects for the shortness of the skeleton and provides a more accurate measure of the length of the irregular feature.

The skeleton of the background (the skiz) can be combined with the EDM of the background to determine the minimum separation distance between features. Minimum EDM values along the pruned skiz correspond to the centers of circles that touch two features, and twice those values correspond to the separation distances.

The example in **Figure 8.86** shows a diagram representing a neuron with branching processes. Thresholding the central cell body, inverting the image, and creating the EDM produces a measurement of the distance of points from the cell body. The skeleton of the neurites can be separated into its component branches by removing the nodes, and the resulting segments that are terminal branches can be selected by using the original skeleton endpoints as markers. When these are applied as a mask to the EDM, the numeric values of the pixels in the branches correspond to the distance from the cell body. It may be desirable to use either the minimum or the mean value as an effective distance measurement. (The figure uses the minimum value as the closest distance to the cell body.) Plotting the skeleton length for each branch against the EDM values shows that the lengths are correlated with distance.

Measuring the distance of each feature in an image from the nearest point on the skiz (using the method shown in **Figure 8.69**) provides a measure of clustering in images. Many other combinations of the EDM and skeleton can be devised to solve measurement problems in images that combine distance and topological information.

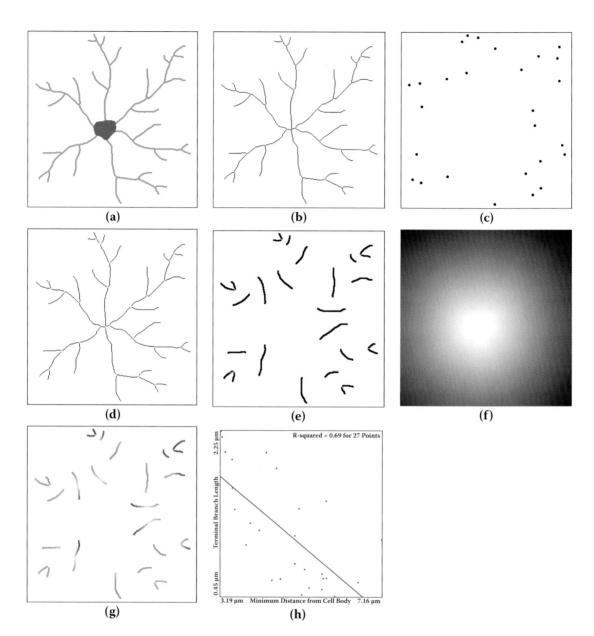

Figure 8.86 *Relating distance to length: (a) diagram of a neural cell; (b) skeleton; (c) terminal endpoints (dilated for visibility); (d) separated branches after removal of nodes in image b;(e) terminal branches, selected by markers in image c and dilated for visibility; (f) EDM of pixels outside the cell body; (g) skeleton segments of the terminal branches, color-coded according to distance from the cell body (values obtained from the EDM, as described in the text); (h) plot of distance vs. length.*

9

Global Image Measurements

The distinction between image processing, which has occupied most of the preceding chapters, and image analysis lies in the extraction of information from the image. As mentioned previously, image processing, like word processing (or food processing), is the science of rearrangement. Pixel values can be altered according to neighboring pixel brightnesses, or shifted to another place in the array by image warping, but the number of pixels is unchanged. So in word processing it is possible to cut and paste paragraphs, perform spellchecking, or alter type styles without reducing the volume of text. And food processing is also an effort at rearrangement of ingredients to produce a more palatable mixture, not to convert it to a list of those ingredients. Image analysis, by contrast, attempts to find those descriptive parameters, usually numeric, that succinctly represent the information of importance in the image.

The processing steps considered in earlier chapters are in many cases essential to carrying out this task. Defining the features to be measured frequently requires image processing to correct acquisition defects, enhance the visibility of particular structures, threshold them from the background, and perform further steps to separate touching objects or select those to be measured. And we have seen in several of the earlier chapters opportunities to use these processing methods themselves to obtain numeric information.

Global measurements and stereology

There are two major classes of image measurements: those performed on the entire image field (sometimes called the "scene"), and those performed on each of the separate features present. The latter feature-specific measurements are covered in the next chapter. The first group of measurements is typically involved in the characterization of three-dimensional (3-D) structures viewed as section planes in the microscope, although the methods are completely general. Indeed, some of the relationships have been discovered and are routinely applied by workers in Earth sciences and astronomy. The science of stereology relates the measurements that can be performed on two-dimensional images to the three-dimensional structures that are represented and sampled by those images. It is primarily a geometrical and statistical science, whose most widely used rules and calculations have a deceptive simplicity. Guides to modern stereological methods can be found in Russ and Dehoff (2001), Howard and Reed (1998), Mouton (2002),

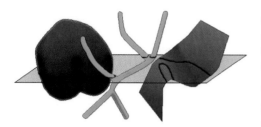

Figure 9.1 A section that passes through three-dimensional structures produces intersections. The volume (red), surface (blue), and linear structure (green) are intersected to produce an area, line, and point, respectively.

and Kurzydlowski and Ralph (1995), while classical methods are described in Dehoff and Rhines (1968), Underwood (1970), Weibel (1979), and Russ (1986).

The key to understanding stereological measurements is the relationship between a three-dimensional structure and a two-dimensional section through it, as used in most types of microscopy for examining materials and biological specimens. As shown in **Figure 9.1**, a section plane that intersects a volume presents an area, while an intersection with a surface presents a line and an intersection with a linear structure presents a point. Measuring and counting these "events" provides the raw data that are interpreted to provide estimates of the three-dimensional structures themselves.

The simplest and perhaps most frequently used stereological procedure is the measurement of the volume fraction that some structure occupies in a solid. This could be the volume of nuclei in cells, a particular phase in a metal, porosity in ceramic, mineral in an ore, etc. Stereologists often use the word "phase" to refer to the structure in which they are interested, even if it is not a phase in the chemical or thermodynamic sense. If a structure or phase can be identified in an image, and that image is representative of the whole, then the area fraction that the structure occupies in the image is a measure of the volume fraction that it occupies in the solid. This relationship is, in fact, one of the oldest known relationships in stereology, used in mineral analysis 150 years ago.

Of course, this requires some explanation and clarification of the assumptions. The image must be representative in the sense that every part of the solid has an equal chance of being examined, so the sections must be uniformly and randomly placed in the solid. Trying to measure the volume fraction of bone in the human body requires that head, torso, arms, and legs all have an equal chance of being viewed; that is the "uniform" part of the assumption. Random means, simply, that nothing is done to bias the measurements by including or excluding particular areas in the images. For example, choosing to measure only those images in which at least some bone was visible would obviously bias the measurements. More subtle, in many cases, is the tendency of microscopists to select areas for imaging that have some aesthetic quality (collecting pretty pictures). Almost certainly this will tend to bias the results. A proper random stereological sampling procedure does not allow the human to select or shift the view.

Many published papers in all fields of science, particularly ones that use microscopy, include images with the caption "representative microstructure" or "typical structure," and in no case is this likely to be true. Either the particular image selected has been chosen because it shows most clearly some feature of the structure that the author believes is important, or it displays the best qualities of specimen preparation and image contrast or some other characteristic that makes it (almost by definition) nontypical. In most real structures there is no such thing as one typical field of view in a true statistical sense. That is why it is important to collect many images from multiple fields of view, spread throughout the specimen in an unbiased way. Data are collected from many fields and combined to represent the entire structure.

Assuming that one image could be a uniform, random sample of the structure, then the "expected value" of the area fraction of the structure is equal to the volume fraction. Of course, in any given image, that may not be the result. In some images, the phase or structure of interest may not even be present, while in others it may occupy the entire field of view. In general it is necessary to select an appropriate magnification so that the structures are visible, to examine multiple fields of view, and to average the measurements. The average then approaches the true value as more measurements are included.

One way to measure the area fraction of a structure is, of course, to use the image histogram. If the phase has a unique gray scale or color value, then the area of peak in the histogram provides a direct measure of the number of pixels covered, and hence the total area, regardless of whether it occupies one large or many small regions in the image. However, as shown in previous chapters, it is common to require image processing before thresholding can selectively delineate a structure, and to require editing of the binary image after thresholding. These steps also affect the area measurement, so in most cases the determination of area fraction must be made from the final binary image. All that is required is to count the black and white pixels.

While this is a simple procedure, it is difficult to assess the accuracy of the measurement. Pixels along the boundaries of features or regions present a challenge because thresholding and subsequent morphological processing may include or exclude them from the total. An image consisting of a single large, compact region has many fewer edge pixels (and hence less potential measurement error) than an image in which the same total area is distributed as many small or irregular features (**Figure 9.2**).

There is a preferred way to determine area fraction (and hence volume fraction) that is very efficient and does allow an estimation of the measurement precision. Traditionally, this method has been performed manually, but it is also easy to accomplish using a computer. A grid of points is superimposed on the image, and the fraction of the points that fall on the structure of interest is counted. The expected value of this point fraction is also the volume fraction. Often, the number of points in the grid is very small so that manual counting can be done at a glance. The grid may be on an eyepiece reticule in the microscope, or overlaid on a video screen or photograph, or generated within the computer. The points should be far enough apart that they provide independent measures of the structure (in other words, at the image magnification being used, two points should rarely fall into the same feature). If the structure is random, then any grid of points can be used, and a regular square grid is convenient. If the structure is highly regular, then the grid itself should be randomized to prevent bias, as discussed previously.

Figure 9.2 *Two images with the same area fraction (26%) of black pixels:*
(a) *one large compact region;*
(b) *many small irregular features. The measurement precision depends on the total periphery of the black-white boundary. The number of edge pixels (black pixels adjacent to the white background) is 3.42% of the total black area in image a and 36.05% of the total black area in image **b**. It is also interesting to note that most human observers do not estimate area fractions very accurately, nor judge that these two images have the same area of black pixels.*

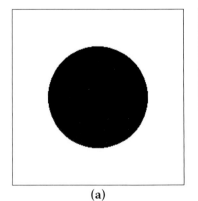
(a)

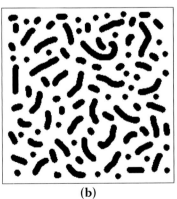
(b)

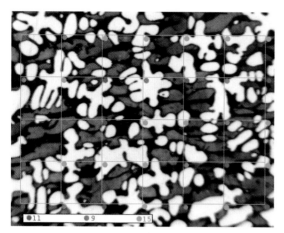

Figure 9.3 Computer counting of marks: a
human has placed color marks near the grid
points (intersection of the lines) that fall on
each phase of interest, and the computer
has counted them. For the white phase, the
estimated volume fraction is 15/35 = 42.8%.

When a grid is superimposed on the original gray-scale or color image (with whatever enhancement has been provided by processing), the human viewer can use independent knowledge and judgment to decide whether each point is within the region of interest. People are very good at this recognition. But they are not very good at counting, so it may still be useful to have the human mark the points and the computer perform the counting operation, as shown in **Figure 9.3**.

The points become a probe into the three-dimensional microstructure, and the number of points that "hit" the phase of interest allows an estimate of the measurement precision, since for independent events the standard deviation is just the square root of the count. This permits making a quick estimate of the number of images (multiple fields of view on multiple sections) that will be needed to achieve the desired final measurement precision. For example, if a grid of 35 points is used (a 7 × 5 array as shown in the figure), and about 11 points, on average, lie on the phase of interest, that corresponds to a volume fraction of about 30%. To determine the actual value with a relative precision of (for example) 5% (in other words 30 ± 1.5% volume fraction), it is only necessary to apply the grid to multiple fields of view until a total of 400 hits have been tallied (the square root of 400 is 20, or 5%). This would require about 36 fields of view (400/11). This is the proper way to design an experimental procedure.

A grid of points can also be efficiently applied to a thresholded and processed binary image using Boolean logic, as shown in **Chapter 8**. If the grid is combined with the binary image using a Boolean AND operation and the surviving points are counted, the result is just those points that fell onto the phase of interest, as shown in **Figure 9.4**. The usual notation for these relationships is

$$V_V = A_A = P_P$$

(9.1)

meaning that the volume of the phase of interest per unit volume of material, V_V, equals (or more precisely is measured by) the area fraction A_A or the point fraction P_P.

Volume fraction is a dimensionless ratio, so the magnification of the image need not be known exactly. However, it is also possible to measure the volume of a specific structure by cutting a series of sections through it and measuring the area in each section (Gundersen 1986). As shown in **Figure 9.5**, the volume of the sampled space is defined by the size and spacing of the sections, and the number of "hits" made by the grid points provides an absolute measure of the feature volume. Each grid point samples the structure and represents a volume in space equal to the area of a grid square times the section spacing. In this case, of course, the magnification must be calibrated.

In many cases, as shown in **Figure 9.6**, it is necessary to measure two volumes, that of the structure of interest and of an enclosing structure. In the example, a sectioned rat lung, the

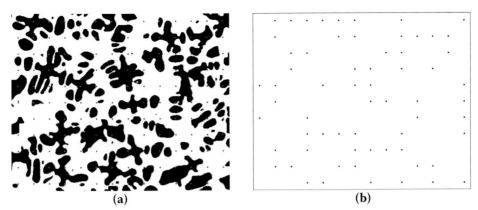

Figure 9.4 (a) *Binary image of the white phase in the metal structure from* Figure *9.3, with a superimposed point grid (points enlarged for visibility). A Boolean AND of the two images leaves just the points that lie on the phase* (b)*, which the computer then counts to determine $P_P = 64/154 = 41.5\%$. The density of points illustrated in this figure is somewhat too high for optimum precision estimation, as there are cases in which multiple points fall on the same feature. That affects the precision but not the accuracy of the measurement.*

area of lung tissue in each section is added including internal voids, and the net area is also summed. The void area within the lung is then calculated as

$$Volume = \frac{\sum Filled\ Area - \sum Net\ Area}{\sum Filled\ Area}$$

(9.2)

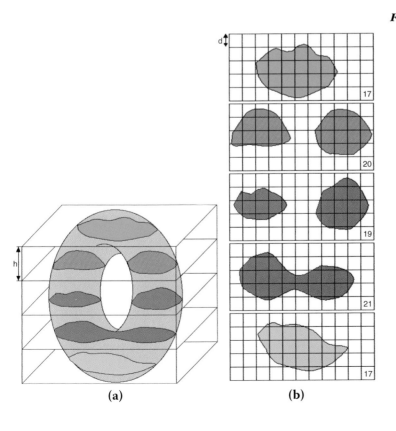

Figure 9.5 *Cavalieri's method for measuring the volume of an object. The grids on each section plane divide the object into cells. Counting the grid points that fall on the structure of interest provides a measure of the number of cells within the structure, and hence a measure of the volume. In the example, if the plane spacing* h *is 5 μm and the grid spacing* d *is 2 μm, then each cell has a volume of 5 × 2 × 2 = 20 μm³, and the total number of hits (17 + 20 + 19 + 21 + 17 = 94) estimates the total volume as 1880 μm³. Measuring the area of each intersection and integrating the volume with Simpson's rule gives an estimate of 1814 μm³.*

(a)　　　　　　(b)

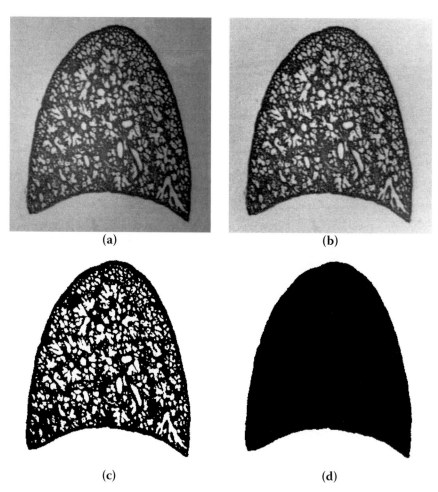

Figure 9.6 *One section of rat lung tissue:* ***(a)*** *original image;* ***(b)*** *leveled;* ***(c)*** *thresholded;* ***(d)*** *internal gaps filled. The areas of images* ***c*** *and* ***d*** *are used to determine the void volume within the lung.*

Surface area

Another global parameter that is measured stereologically is the surface area. Surfaces can be the boundary between two structures, such as the surface area of the nucleus, the total area of cell wall in plant tissue, the total grain boundary area in a metal, or the surface of porosity in a ceramic. Note that in some of these examples the surface separates two different phases or structures, while in others it separates different regions (cells or grains) that are the same in structure and composition. Surfaces are usually very important in structures because they are the interfaces where chemistry and diffusion take place, and they control many properties such as strength, fracture, light scattering, thermal and electrical conductivity, etc.

In a two-dimensional section image through a three-dimensional structure, boundaries and surfaces are seen as lines. The total length of these lines is proportional to the amount of surface area present in the three-dimensional solid. The surface will not in general intersect the section plane perpendicularly. If the surfaces are isotropic (have an equal probability of being oriented in any direction), or the section planes are randomly oriented with respect to the surfaces, then the relationship between total surface area per unit volume of sample and the total length of line per unit area of image is

$$S_V = \tfrac{4}{\pi} B_A \qquad (9.3)$$

where S_V is the accepted notation for the surface area per unit volume, and B_A denotes the total length of boundary per unit area of image. Notice that both terms have dimensions of 1/length, and that it is consequently important to know the image magnification. **Figure 9.7** shows an example. The boundary lines (colored) have a total length of 9886 μm, and the image area is 15,270 μm^2. This gives a calculated surface area per unit volume of 0.0824 μm^2/μm^3, or 82.4 mm^2/mm^3.

Once again, it is difficult to specify the precision of such a measurement. Measuring the length of a boundary line in a digitized image is one of the most error-prone tasks in image measurement because of

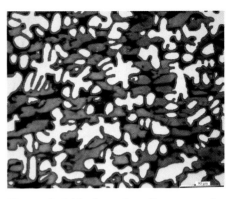

Figure 9.7 The boundary lines around the white phase in the same image as Figure 9.3 and Figure 9.4 can be isolated using the techniques from Chapter 8 and then measured to determine the surface area, as described in the text. (The lines are dilated here for visibility.)

(a) the pixelation of the image and (b) the observation that, as magnification is increased, more irregularities in the boundary may become visible so that the measured boundary length increases. The preferred method for determining surface area is consequently to place a grid of lines on the image and to count the number of intersection points that they make with the line representing the surface of interest. The relationship between the surface area per unit volume (S_V, square micrometers per cubic micrometer) and the number of intersections (P_L, number per micrometer) is just

$$S_V = 2 \cdot P_L \qquad (9.4)$$

where the factor 2 compensates for the various angles at which the grid lines can intersect the boundary. Again, because this is now a counting experiment, the measurement precision can be estimated from the square root of the number of intersection points, provided that the lines (which are the probes into the microstructure in this measurement) are far enough apart that the intersections are independent events.

Generating a grid of lines on the same image as in **Figure 9.7** and counting intersections (**Figure 9.8**) produces a measurement result similar to that of the boundary line technique. The total length of the grid lines is 4646 μm. Performing a Boolean AND and counting the intersections gives 197 hits (some are a single pixel and some more than one, depending on the angle between the boundary and the line, but the count is of intersection events, not pixels). Using **Equation 9.4**, this corresponds to a surface area per unit volume of 0.0848 μm^2/μm^3. Based on the number of counts, the estimated relative precision is ±7.2% (0.0848 ± 0.0061 μm^2/μm^3).

Placing grid lines on images and counting intersections can be performed in all of the same ways (manually, manual marking with computer counting, or automatically using Boolean logic), as discussed previously for point counting. The problem with this method as described is that it relies on the assumption that the surfaces being measured are isotropic or that the section planes and grid lines are randomly oriented with respect to the surfaces. In real structures this criterion is rarely met. Consequently, if the structure is not isotropic, then it is necessary

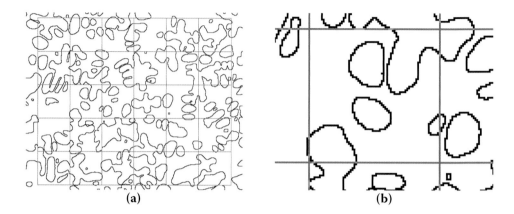

(a)   (b)

Figure 9.8 *ANDing a grid of lines with the boundary lines from* **Figure 9.7** *and counting the intersections also measures the surface area, as described in the text. Some of the intersections cover more than a single pixel, as shown in the enlarged detail* **(b)**, *but are counted as a single event.*

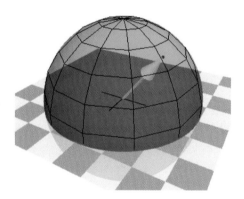

Figure 9.9 *A hemisphere showing a direction in three-dimensional space represented by a point on the sphere.*

to construct a grid of lines that does sample the structure isotropically (in addition to the requirements of uniform and random sampling noted above). Many of the developments in modern stereology are aimed at finding practical ways to meet this isotropic, uniform, random (IUR) requirement. To visualize the meaning of isotropic directions, consider a hemisphere as shown in **Figure 9.9**. Each direction in space is represented by a point on the sphere. Points should be distributed evenly across the spherical surface.

The most widely used approach to generating isotropic, uniform, and random lines to probe the surfaces in a three-dimensional structure is called "vertical sectioning" (Baddeley et al. 1986). It requires selecting some direction in the structure that can always be identified. This might be the axis of the backbone in an animal, or the normal to a surface in a rolled metal sheet, or the direction of gravity for sedimentary layers of rock. Then all sections are cut parallel to this direction, but rotated uniformly and randomly about it, as shown in **Figure 9.10**. Note that this is not the way most sections are cut when biological tissue is embedded and microtomed (those sections are all perpendicular to the same direction). It would also be possible to cut the vertical sections as a pie is normally cut, with radial slices, but these would oversample the center of the pie compared with the periphery.

The vertical axis direction is present on all sections, so these cut planes are directionally biased. If lines were drawn on these sections with uniform directions in the plane, as shown in **Figure 9.11**, they would cluster near the north pole on the hemisphere. Directions near the equator would be undersampled. That bias can be compensated by drawing lines that are sine-weighted, as shown in **Figure 9.12**. Instead of drawing lines in uniform angle steps, they are drawn with uniform steps in the sine of the angle. This produces more directions around the equator and spreads out the directions near the north pole so that the points are uniformly distributed on the sphere. However, while a set of radial lines shown in the figure produces

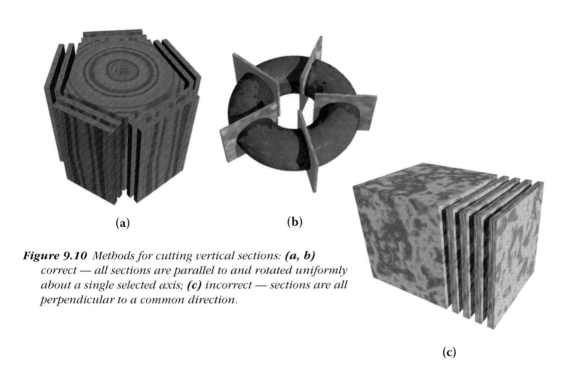

Figure 9.10 *Methods for cutting vertical sections: (a, b) correct — all sections are parallel to and rotated uniformly about a single selected axis; (c) incorrect — sections are all perpendicular to a common direction.*

(a)   **(b)**

(c)

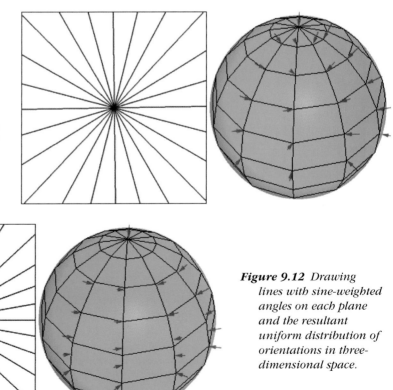

Figure 9.11 *Drawing lines with uniform angles on each plane and the resultant clustering of directions near the north pole of the hemisphere of orientations.*

Figure 9.12 *Drawing lines with sine-weighted angles on each plane and the resultant uniform distribution of orientations in three-dimensional space.*

isotropic directions, they do not produce uniform sampling (the center of each section is oversampled and the corners undersampled).

The most convenient way to draw sine-weighted lines that uniformly sample the area is to generate cycloids, as shown in **Figure 9.13**. The cycloid is the path followed by a point on the circumference of a rolling circle. It is sine-weighted and, when drawn on vertical sections, has exactly the correct set of orientations to provide isotropic sampling of directions in the three-dimensional solid from which the sections were cut. Counting the intersections made by the cycloid grid with the boundary lines in the image provides the P_L value needed to calculate the surface area per unit volume. The length of each quarter arc of the cycloid line is just twice its height.

If the specimen is actually isotropic, the method of cutting vertical sections and counting intersections using a grid of cycloids will produce the correct answer, at the expense of doing a bit more work (mostly in sample preparation) than would have been needed if the isotropy was known beforehand. But if the specimen has any anisotropy, the easy method of cutting parallel sections and drawing straight line grids would produce an incorrect answer with an unknown amount of bias, while the vertical section method gives the true answer.

There are many new and continually evolving techniques for using oriented sections and lines, including random lines as well as point-sampled lines, for stereological measurements (e.g., Cruz-Orive 2005; Howard and Reed 2005). These offer ways to measure volumes and surfaces of arbitrary (not necessarily convex) objects. The major difficulty with most of these methods lies in their practical implementation. When confocal microscopy is used to image samples with a transparent matrix, or when a series of parallel sections are imaged by computed tomography (CT) or magnetic resonance imaging (MRI), it is also possible to implement isotropic "virtual" probes such as cycloids or a spherical surface directly in the 3-D data set (Gokhale et al. 2004; Kubinova and Janacek 2001). A sphere, for example, is implemented as a set of circles of appropriately varying size in each of the parallel planes. Much of the emphasis in modern stereology is directed toward strategies for obtaining unbiased sampling of arbitrary structures.

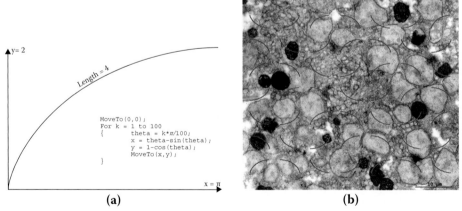

(a)   **(b)**

Figure 9.13 *Procedure for drawing an arc of the cycloid **(a)**, and a cycloid grid superimposed on a vertical section image **(b)**. The intersections (marked in color) of the cycloid lines with the membranes provide an unbiased measure of the total surface area per unit volume, $S_V = 2\,P_L = 2 \cdot 39/331.5\ \mu m = 0.235\ \mu m^2/\mu m^3$.*

ASTM Grain Size

More than 100 years ago, when naval gunnery was introducing larger and larger guns onto battleships, brass cartridge casings were used to hold the gunpowder and projectile, essentially an enlarged version of a modern rifle cartridge. It was observed that, after firing, it was sometimes difficult to extract the used brass cartridge from the gun chamber because the material fractured when it was pulled from the rear rim. The metal flowed and thinned when the charge was detonated, and clearly some difference in material structure was related to the tendency to tearing.

From that observation, a method for measuring a microstructural parameter known as the ASTM (American Society for Testing and Materials) "grain size" was developed and used for quality control of naval brass, and later applied to many other metals and nonmetals. In fact, there are several different standard techniques, which have been adjusted with appropriate constants so that they agree approximately with each other's numeric values. But in fact, the methods measure two entirely different characteristics of microstructure (neither of which is the "size" of the grains).

The first method proposed was to count the number of visible grains per square inch on a polished section at 100× magnification. The number of grains N is then related to the "grain size number" G by

$$N = 2^{(G-1)} \tag{9.5}$$

where the value G is never reported with a precision better than 0.5. An equivalent version adjusted to metric dimensions is also in use.

A second method for determining the value G is based on drawing a grid of lines on the image. Because many metals are anisotropic due to the forming processes, the grains are elongated in one direction. To avoid directional bias in the measurement, a circular grid is used. The number of intersections made by the line with the grain boundaries per unit length of the line (N_L, where length is in millimeters) can is used to calculate

$$G = 6.6457 \cdot \log_{10} N_L - 3.298 \tag{9.6}$$

The constants are needed to convert the metric units and to make the results approximately agree with the grain-count method. Again, the results are rounded to the nearest 0.5; **Figure 9.14** shows an example.

There are also other methods that are part of the ASTM standard (E112), such as counting the number of triple points (places where three grains meet at a point) per unit area, and most of these methods can be implemented either by hand count or by computer.

The intercept count method (**Equation 9.6**) in reality measures the total surface area of grain boundary. Note the use of N_L, which, like the P_L value in **Equation 9.4**, is proportional to the surface area per unit volume. The importance of grain boundary area makes sense from a mechanical property standpoint, since creep in materials occurs due to grain boundary sliding and grain rotation, and grain deformation occurs by motion of dislocations that start and end at these same boundaries. The grain count (**Equation 9.5**) and triple-point count methods actually measure the total length per unit volume of the edges of grains, which is a parameter related primarily to diffusion. Measurement of the length of structures is discussed below.

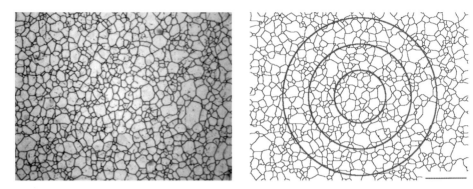

Figure 9.14 *Light-microscope image of a low-carbon steel **(a)**, which is prepared by leveling, thresholding, and skeletonizing to delineate the grain boundaries **(b)**. Counting the number of grains inside the largest circle (445, counting each one that intersects the circle as 1/2) gives a grain size number G = 8.8. Counting the intercepts with the concentric circle grids (147 with a grid length of 2300 µm) gives a grain size number G = 9.1. Both values would normally be reported as a grain size number of 9.*

The fact that one of these parameters can be even approximately tied to the other is due to the limited application of the method to metals that have been heat-treated so that they are fully recrystallized. In this condition, the distribution of actual three-dimensional grain sizes approaches a constant, more-or-less log-normal state in which the structure may coarsen with time (large grains grow and small ones vanish), but where the structure remains self-similar. Hence, there is an approximately consistent relationship between the length of edges of the grains and the area of their surfaces.

The same relationship does not apply to metals without this heat treatment, and so the notion of a single numerical value that can characterize the microstructure is flawed, even for quality control purposes, and the measurement method used does matter. But 100 years of use have sanctified the technique, and most practitioners are not aware of what their procedure actually measures in the microstructure, or that it is certainly not the grain size in a literal sense.

Actually measuring the "size" (usually the volume) of individual grains or cells in a three-dimensional solid is quite difficult. It has been done in a few cases by literally taking the material apart (e.g., by chemically dissolving a thin layer along the boundaries so the grains are separated) and measuring or weighing each grain. Other researchers have used an exhaustive serial-sectioning technique that produces a complete three-dimensional volumetric image of the structure, from which measurements of size can be made. Both of these approaches are far too laborious for routine practical use. Determining the mean volume of cells can be done using the Disector method described below. This actually measures the number per unit volume, but the inverse of that quantity is the mean volume per feature. This method relies heavily on computer-based image processing to deal with the large number of images.

It is also possible to measure the variance of the size distribution of the features using a point-sampled intercept method applied to IUR section planes, described below. But if the actual size distribution of the three-dimensional features is needed, then the more intensive methods must be undertaken.

The "grain size" of metals is by no means the only case in which an apparently obvious measure of feature size turns out to be a measure of something quite different. For example, drawing a grid of parallel lines on tissue sections of lung parenchyma and measuring the mean distance between intersections of the grid lines with air-tissue boundaries produces a mean chord length, which has been shown to correlate with the severity of emphysema (Rosenthal and Begum 2005). The chord length may seem to describe some characteristic size of the airways within the lung, but actually, since it is the inverse of the P_L value in **Equation 9.4**, it is a measure of the total alveolar surface area (which is involved in gas exchange efficiency).

Multiple types of surfaces

In most kinds of real samples, there are several different phases or structures present, and consequently many different types of boundary surfaces. In a three-phase material, containing regions which for convenience can be labeled as types α, β, and γ, there are six possible interfaces (α-α, α-β, α-γ, β-β, β-γ, and γ-γ), and the number goes up rapidly in more complex structures. Some of the possible interface types may be absent, meaning that those two phase regions never touch (e.g., nuclei in separate cells do not touch each other, it makes no sense to consider a contact surface between two pores, etc.). Measuring the amounts of each different type of interface can be very useful in characterizing the overall three-dimensional structure.

Figure 9.15 shows the phase boundaries in a three-phase metal structure. Notice that no white dendritic region touches another one, for example. **Chapter 9.8** showed how Boolean logic with the dilated region outlines can be used to delineate each type of interface. Once the image of the boundaries has been isolated, counting intersections with a grid provides the measurement of surface area per unit volume for each type of interface.

Figure 9.16 shows a simpler, idealized, two-phase microstructure. By thresholding each phase, using morphological operations such as a closing to eliminate boundaries between common regions, and Boolean logic to combine two derived images, each of the three distinct boundary types can be isolated (in the image, they have been combined as color channels for visualization purposes). Assuming that this is a vertical section, a cycloid grid such as the one shown can be used to estimate the surface area per unit volume as shown in the figure, using **Equation 9.4**.

It is instructive to illustrate and compare the various measurement procedures described above for volume and surface area measurement using the magnification calibration shown on the image in **Figure 9.16**. Counting pixels estimates the area fraction, and hence the volume fraction of the gray phase, at 17.3%. Placing a square grid of 90 points produces 14 hits, for a volume fraction estimate (using **Equation 9.1**) of 15.6 ± 4.2%. Measuring the length of the boundary lines for each type of interface and applying **Equation 9.3** produces the results listed in **Table 9.1**. Counting intersections of the grid lines with each type of boundary and applying **Equation 9.4** gives another estimate of surface area, also shown in **Table 9.1**. The image area is 5453.6 μm² and the grid used had a total length of 614 μm.

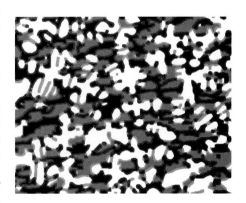

Figure 9.15 The three-phase aluminum-zinc alloy from *Figure 9.3*, with the region boundaries highlighted. The lines have been color-coded according to type and dilated for visibility.

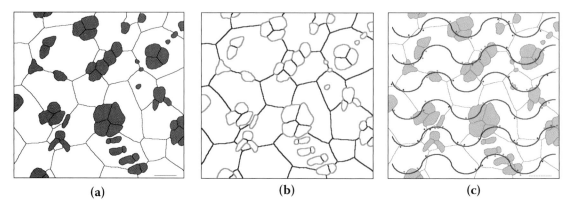

| (a) | (b) | (c) |

Figure 9.16 *Idealized drawing of a two-phase microstructure **(a)**, the three different types of interface boundaries present **(b)**, and the result of counting the intersections of these boundaries with a cycloid grid **(c)**. The measurements and calculated results are detailed in the text. (Courtesy of Robert Dehoff, University of Florida, Gainesville.)*

Table 9.1. Estimation of Surface Area

Boundary	Length (μm)	SV = (4/π) (Length/Area)	Grid counts	SV = 2 PL
White-white	441.96 μm	103.2 mm2/mm3	28	101.8 ± 19.2 mm2/mm3
Gray-white	551.24	128.7	37	134.5 ± 22.1
Gray-gray	123.30	28.8	8	29.1 ± 10.3

The agreement between these different methods is quite satisfying, but only the counting methods allow a simple estimate of the measuring precision to be made, from which it is straightforward to determine the number of sections that should be examined to obtain results with the desired final precision. Note that it is possible to squeeze a considerable amount of surface area into a small volume.

Length

Length measurement is usually applied to structures that are elongated in one direction and relatively small in lateral width, such as neurons or blood vessels in tissue, fibers in composites, or dislocations in metals. However, it is also possible to measure the total length of edges, such as the edges of polyhedral grains in a metal (as mentioned previously in connection with the ASTM grain size measurement) or any other line that represents the intersection of surfaces.

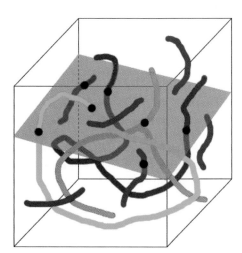

Figure 9.17 *Diagram of linear structures in a volume, intersected by a sampling plane to produce intersections that can be counted to measure the total length.*

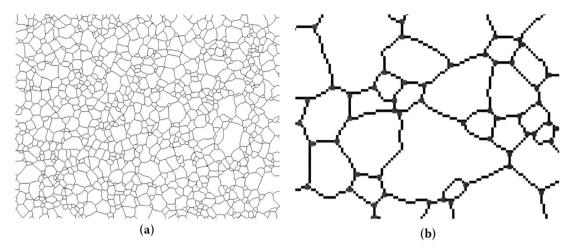

Figure 9.18 *The image from* **Figure 9.14**: *(a) thresholded and skeletonized with the 1732 branch points in the skeleton color-coded;* *(b) shows an enlarged portion with the points dilated for visibility.*

When a linear structure intersects the sampling plane, the result is a point, as shown in **Figure 9.17**. The number of such intersection points is proportional to the total length of the line. If the linear structures in the three-dimensional solid are isotropic, or if the section planes are randomly oriented with respect to the structures, then the relationship between the total length of line per unit volume L_V (with units of micrometers per cubic micrometer or length^{-2}) and the total number of points per unit area P_A (with units of number per square micrometer or length^{-2}) is:

$$L_V = 2 \cdot P_A$$

$$(9.7)$$

where the constant 2 arises, as it did in the case of surface area measurements, from considering all of the angles at which the plane and line can intersect. In some cases, a direct count of points can be made on a polished surface. For example, fibers in a composite are visible, and dislocations can be made so by chemical etching.

In the example of **Figure 9.14**, the triple points where three grains meet represent the triple lines in space that are the edges of the grains. These are paths along which diffusion is most rapid. To isolate them for counting, the skeleton of the grain boundaries can be obtained as shown in **Chapter 8**. The branch points in this tessellation can be counted as shown in **Figure 9.18** because they are points in the skeleton that have more than two neighbors. Counting them is another way (less commonly used) to calculate a "grain size" number.

One convenient way to measure the length of a structure, independent of its complexity or connectedness, is to image a thick section (considerably thicker than the breadth of the linear portions of the structure). In this projected image, the length of the features is not truly represented because they may incline upward or downward through the section. Any line drawn on the image represents a surface through the section (**Figure 9.19**), with area equal to the product of its length and the section thickness. Counting the number of intersections made by the linear structure with the grid line on the image, and then calculating the total length using the relationship in **Equation 9.7**, provides a direct measurement of the total length per unit volume.

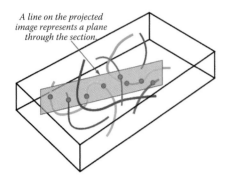

A line on the projected image represents a plane through the section.

Figure 9.19 Schematic diagram of a thick section containing linear structures. Drawing a line on the projected image and counting intersections of the line with the structures corresponds to counting the intersections of the structures with a plane through the section.

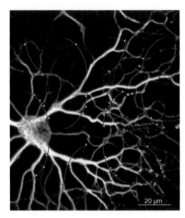

20 µm

Figure 9.20 Application of a cycloid grid to a TEM image of a section containing filamentous microtubules. Counting the number of intersections made with the grid allows calculation of the total length per unit volume, as discussed in the text.

If the sample is isotropic, any grid line can be used. If not, then if the sections have been taken with isotropic or random section planes, a circle grid can be used, since that samples all orientations in the plane. But the most practical way to perform the measurement without the tedium of isotropic section orientation or the danger of assuming that the sample is isotropic is to cut the sections parallel to a known direction (vertical sectioning) and then use cycloidal grid lines, as shown in **Figure 9.20**. In this case, since it is the normal to the surface represented by the lines that must be made isotropic in three-dimensional space, the generated cycloids must be rotated by 90° to the "vertical" direction.

In the example of **Figure 9.20**, the intersections of the grid lines with the projections of the microtubules allow the calculation of the total length per unit volume using **Equation 9.7**. There are 41 marked intersections; of course, these could also be counted by thresholding the image, skeletonizing the tubules, and ANDing them with the grid, as shown previously in this chapter and in **Chapter 8**. For an image area of 12,293 µm², an assumed section thickness of 3 µm, and a total length of grid lines of 331.2 µm, the length calculation from **Equation 9.7** gives:

$$L_V = 2 \cdot 41/(12293 * 3) \ \mu m/\mu m^3 = 2.22 \ mm/mm^3$$

It is rare to find a real three-dimensional structure that is isotropic. If the structure is (or is possibly) anisotropic, it may be necessary to generate section planes that are isotropic. Procedures for doing so have been published, but in general they are tedious, wasteful of sample material, and hard to make uniform (that is, they tend to oversample the center of the object as compared with the periphery).

Another way to generate isotropic samples of a solid, either for surface area or length measurement, is to subdivide the three-dimensional material into many small pieces, randomly orient each one, and then make convenient sections for examination. This is perhaps the most common approach that people really use. With such randomly isotropic section planes, it is not necessary to use a cycloid grid. Any convenient line grid will do. If there is preferred directionality in the plane, circular line grids can be used to avoid bias. If not, then a square grid of lines can be used. If the structure is highly regular, then it is necessary to use randomly generated lines (which can be conveniently performed by the computer). **Figure 9.21** shows examples of a few such grids. Much of the art of modern stereology lies in performing appropriate sample sectioning and choosing the appropriate grid to measure the desired structural parameter.

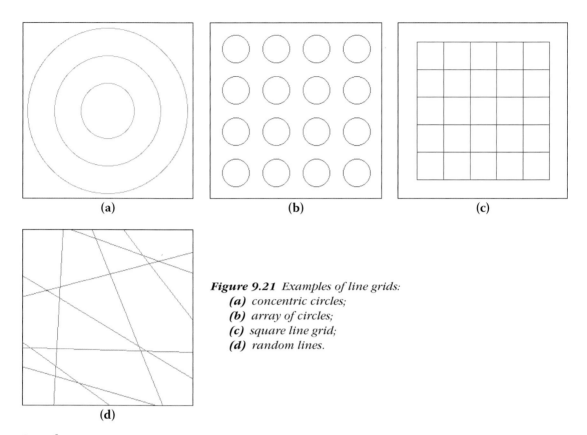

Figure 9.21 *Examples of line grids:*
(a) concentric circles;
(b) array of circles;
(c) square line grid;
(d) random lines.

Sampling strategies

Several of the examples shown thus far have represented the common method of microscopy in which views are taken through thin slices, generally using the light or electron microscope. The requirement is that the sections be much thinner than the dimensions of any structures of interest, except for the case above of thick sections used for length measurement. Confocal light microscopy does not require physical sectioning of thin slices, but produces equivalent images that are interpreted similarly.

For opaque materials, the same strategies are used for sectioning but the images are obtained by reflected light, or by scanning electron microscopy, or any other form of imaging that shows just the surface. Many imaging techniques actually represent the structure to some finite depth beneath the surface, and most preparation methods such as polishing produce some surface relief in which the softer structures are lower than the harder ones. Again, the criterion is that the depth of information (e.g., the depth from which electrons are emitted in the scanning electron microscope, or the depth of polishing relief) must be much less than the dimensions of any structures of interest. Corrections to the equations above for measuring volume, area, and length can be made for the case of finite section thickness or surface relief, but they are complicated and require exact determination of the depth or thickness (Overby and Johnson 2005; Weibel 1979).

While procedures for obtaining isotropic sampling have been outlined, little has been said thus far about how to achieve uniform, random sampling of structures. It is of course possible to cut the entire specimen up into many small pieces, select some of them by blind random sampling, cut each one in randomly oriented planes, and achieve the desired result. However, that is not the most efficient method (Gundersen and Jensen 1987; Gundersen 2002). A systematic or structured random sample can be designed that will produce the desired unbiased result with the fewest samples and the least work. The method works at every level through a hierarchical sampling strategy, from the selection of a few test animals from a population (or cells from a petri dish, etc.) to the selection of tissue blocks, the choice of rotation angles for vertical sectioning, the selection of microtomed slices for viewing, the location of areas for imaging, and the placement of grids for measurement.

Figure 9.22 illustrates the basic principle as it might be applied to selecting some apples from a population. Dividing the total population (30) by the number of desired samples (5) produces a value (6) that is used to control the sampling interval. A random number from 1 to 6 is generated to control the starting point for the sampling. Then every sixth apple after that is selected. This produces a uniform but randomized sampling of the population.

To illustrate the procedure as it applies to image measurement, consider the problem of determining the volume fraction of bone in the human body. Clearly, there is no single section location that can be considered representative of such a diverse structure: a section through the head would show proportionately much more bone than one at the waist. Let us suppose that in order to obtain sufficient precision, we have decided that eight sections are sufficient for each body. For volume fraction, it is not necessary to have isotropic sections, so we could use transverse sections. In practice, these could be obtained nondestructively using a CT or MRI scanner. If the section planes were placed at random, there would be some portions of the body that were not viewed, while some planes would lie close together and oversample other regions. The most efficient sampling would space the planes uniformly apart, but it is necessary to avoid the danger of bias in their placement, always striking certain structures and avoiding others.

Systematic random sampling would proceed by generating a random number to decide the placement of the first plane somewhere in the top one-eighth of the body. For a person 160 cm tall, that would be some position within the top 20 cm. Then position the remaining planes with uniform spacing of 20 cm, so that each has the same offset within its one-eighth of the body height. These planes constitute a systematic random sample. A different random number placement would be used on the next body, and the set of planes would be shifted as a unit. This procedure guarantees that every part of each body has an equal chance of being measured, which is the requirement for uniform random sampling.

When applied to the placement of a grid on each image, two random numbers are generated that specify the position of the first point (the upper left corner) of the grid. The other grid points then shift as a unit with uniform spacing. The same logic applies to selecting measurement positions on a slide in the microscope. For example, if it has been decided that adequate statistical sampling can be obtained by acquiring images from eight fields of view on a slide,

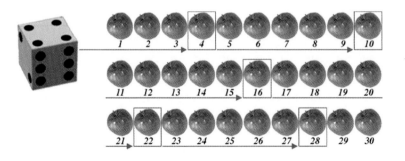

Figure 9.22 Example of systematic or structured random sampling, as described in the text.

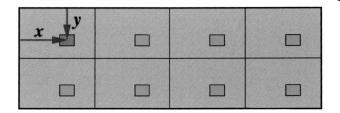

Figure 9.23 *Systematic random sampling applied to selecting fields of view on a slide. The area is divided into as many regions as the number of images to be acquired. Two random numbers are used to select the location for the first image in the first region (orange). Subsequent images (green) are then captured at the same relative position in each region.*

then the area is divided into eight equal areas as shown in **Figure 9.23**, two random numbers are generated to position the first field of view in the first rectangle, and the subsequent images are acquired at the same relative position in each of the other areas.

For rotations of vertical sections, if it is decided to use five orientations as shown in **Figure 9.10**, then a random number is used to select an angle between 0 and 72° for the first cut, and then the remaining orientations are placed systematically at 72° intervals. The method can obviously be generalized to any situation. It is uniform and random because every part of the sampled population has an equal probability of being selected. Of all of the possible slices and lines that could be used to probe the structure, each one has an equal probability of being used.

The goal of the stereologist in designing an experiment is to achieve IUR (isotropic, uniform, random) sampling of the structure. For some types of probes, the requirement of isotropy can be relaxed because the probe itself has no directionality, and hence is not sensitive to any anisotropy in the specimen. Using a grid of points, for example, to determine the volume fraction of a structure of interest does not require the vertical sectioning strategy described above because the point probe has no orientation. Any convenient set of planes that uniformly and randomly sample the structure can be probed with a uniformly and randomly placed grid to obtain an unbiased result.

The Disector, described below, is a volume probe and hence also has no directionality associated with it. Pairs of section planes can be distributed (uniformly and randomly) through the structure without regard to orientation. Being able to avoid the complexity of isotropic sectioning is a definite advantage in experimental design.

But, as noted previously, for measurement of length or surface area, the probes (surfaces and lines) do have orientation, so they must be placed isotropically as well as uniformly and randomly. It is in these cases that a strategy such as vertical sectioning and the use of cycloidal grids becomes desirable. Using a systematic random sampling approach reduces the number of such sections that need to be examined, as compared with a fully random sampling, but it does not alleviate the need to guarantee that all orientations have an equal probability of being selected. It bears repetition that unless it can be proven that the sample itself is isotropic (and uniform and random), then unless an appropriate IUR sampling strategy is employed, the results will be biased and the amount of the bias cannot be determined.

Determining number

Figure 9.24 shows several sections through a three-dimensional structure. Subject to the caveat that the sections must be IUR, it is straightforward to determine the total volume of the

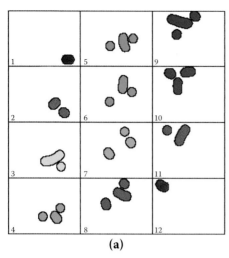

(a)

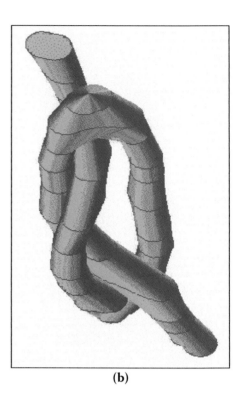

(b)

Figure 9.24

(a) *Multiple sections through a tubular structure, from which the volume, surface area, and length can be determined.*

(b) *Only by arranging them in order, aligning them, and reconstructing the volume can the presence of a single string arranged in a right-handed knot be recognized.*

tubular structure (**Equation 9.1**) from the areas of the intersections or by using a point count with a grid. From the length of the boundary line, or by using intercept counts of the boundary with a suitable line grid, the total surface area of the structure can be determined (**Equation 9.3** and **Equation 9.4**). From the number of separate features produced by the intersection of the object with the planes, the length of the tube can be estimated (**Equation 9.7**). But there is nothing in the individual section planes that reveals whether this is one object or many, and if it is one object whether the tube is branched or not. The fact that the single tube is actually tied into a knot is of course entirely hidden. It is only by connecting the information in the planes together, by interpolating surfaces between closely spaced planes and creating a reconstruction of the three-dimensional object, that these topological properties can be assessed.

Volume, surface area, and length are metric properties. The plane surfaces cut through the structure, and the grids of lines and points placed on them represent probes that sample the structure and provide numerical information that can be used to calculate these metric properties, subject to the precision of the measurement and to the need for uniform, random, and (except for volume measurement) isotropic sampling. Topological properties of number and connectedness cannot be measured using plane, line, or point probes. It is necessary to actually examine a volume of the sample.

In the limit, of course, this could be a complete volumetric imaging of the entire structure. Nondestructive techniques such as confocal light microscopy, medical CT, MRI or sonic scans, or stereoscopic viewing through transparent volumes, can be used in some instances. They produce dramatic visual results when coupled with computer graphics techniques (which are shown in **Chapters 12** and **13**). However, these are costly and time-consuming methods that cannot easily be applied to many types of samples. Serial-sectioning methods, in which many sequential thin sections are cut or many sequential planes of polish are prepared and examined, are even more difficult and costly because of the problems of aligning the images and compensating for distortion or variation in spacing or lack or parallel orientation.

It is a very common mistake to count the number of features visible on a section plane and from that try to infer the number of objects in the three-dimensional volume. The fact that the units are wrong is an early indication of trouble. The number of features imaged per unit area does not correspond to the number per unit volume. In fact, the section plane is more likely to strike a large object than a small one, so the size of the objects strongly influences the numbers that are observed to intersect the sectioning plane, as shown in **Figure 9.25**.

There is a relationship between number per unit area and number per unit volume based on the concept of a mean diameter for the features. For spheres, the mean diameter has a simple meaning. The number per unit volume N_V can be determined from the number per unit area N_A as

$$N_V = \frac{N_A}{D_{mean}}$$

(9.8)

More precisely, the expected value of N_A is the product of $N_V \cdot D_{mean}$. **Figure 9.26** illustrates a case in which this method can be applied. The image is a section through a foam. The bubble size is controlled by the air pressure and nozzle size, and is known. If it were not known, but the bubbles could be assumed to be uniform in size, a good estimate could be obtained by using the largest diameter bubble observed, which would correspond to a cut near the equator. Counting the number of bubbles per unit area can thus be used to determine the number of bubbles per unit volume using **Equation 9.8**. The correct technique for counting and correcting for edge-touching features will be discussed below.

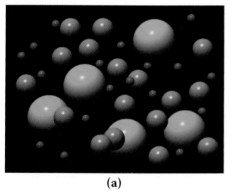

(a)

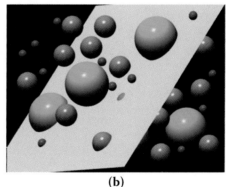

(b)

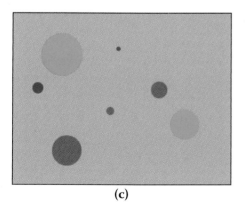

(c)

Figure 9.25

(a) A volume contains large (green), medium (orange), and small (purple) objects.

(b) An arbitrary section can be cut through the volume.

(c) The appearance of the objects in the plane shows that the sizes of the intersections are not the size of the objects, and the number of intersections with each does not correspond to the number per unit volume, because large objects are more likely to be intersected by the plane.

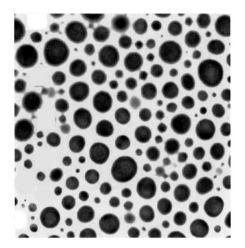

Figure 9.26 *Section through a foam. Counting the number of bubbles per unit area can be used to determine the number per unit volume in this case, because the mean bubble size is known.*

For convex but not spherical shapes, the mean diameter is the mean caliper or tangent diameter averaged over all orientations. This can be calculated for various regular or known shapes, but it is not something that is known *a priori* for most structures. So determining something like the number of grains or cells or nuclei per unit volume (whose inverse would give the mean volume of each object) is in fact rarely practical.

For objects that are not convex, or that have protrusions or internal voids, or holes and bridges (multiply connected shapes), the concept of a mean diameter becomes even more nebulous and less useful. It turns out that the integral of the mean surface curvature over the entire surface of the object is related to this mean diameter. As noted below, the surface curvature is defined by two principal radii. Defining the mean local curvature as

$$H = \frac{1}{2}\left(\frac{1}{r_1} + \frac{1}{r_2}\right)$$

(9.9)

and integrating over the entire surface gives a value called the integral mean curvature M, which equals $2\pi \cdot D_{mean}$. In other words, the feature count N_A on a section plane is actually a measure of the mean curvature of the particles and hence the mean diameter as it has been defined above. If the number per unit volume can be independently determined, for instance using the Disector method below, it can be combined with N_A to calculate the mean diameter, if that is of interest for characterizing the objects.

Curvature, connectivity, and the Disector

Surfaces and lines in three-dimensional structures are rarely flat or straight, and in addition to the relationship to mean diameter introduced above, their curvature may hold important information about the evolution of the structure or about chemical and pressure gradients. For grain structures in equilibrium, the contact surfaces are ideally flat, but the edges still represent localized curvature. This curvature can be measured by stereology.

Surface curvature is defined by two radii (maximum and minimum). If both are positive as viewed from "inside" the object bounded by the surface, the surface is convex. If both are negative, the surface is concave, and if they have opposite signs, the surface has saddle curvature (**Figure 9.27**). The total integrated curvature for any closed surface around a simply connected object (no holes, bridges, etc.) is always 4π. For a set of more complicated shapes, the total curvature is $4\pi(N - C)$, where N is the number of separate objects and C is the connectivity.

For a simple array of separate objects, regardless of the details of their shape, C is zero (they are not connected) and the total integrated curvature of the structure gives a measure of how many objects are present. To measure this topological quantity, a simple plane surface is not adequate, as explained above. The total curvature can be measured by considering a sweeping plane probe moving through the sample (this can be physically realized by moving the plane of focus of a confocal microscope through the sample, or by using a medical imaging device)

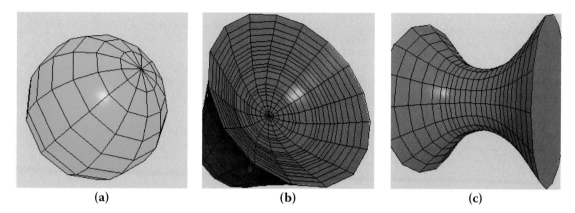

Figure 9.27 *Surface curvature:* **(a)** *convex;* **(b)** *concave;* **(c)** *saddle.*

and counting the events when the plane probe is tangent to the surface of interest. Convex and concave tangent points (T^{++} and T^{--}, respectively) are counted separately from saddle tangencies (T^{+-}). The net tangent count is ($T^{++} + T^{--} - T^{+-}$) and gives the quantity ($N - C$), also called the Euler characteristic of the structure, as

$$(N - C) = \tfrac{1}{2}\left(T^{++} + T^{--} - T^{+-}\right) = \tfrac{1}{2}T_{net}$$

(9.10)

There are two extreme cases in which this is useful. One is the case of separate (but arbitrarily and complexly shaped) objects, in which C is zero and N is one-half the net tangent count. This provides a straightforward way to determine the number of objects in the measured volume. The other situation of interest is the case of a single object, typically an extended complex network with many branchings such as neurons, capillaries, textiles used as reinforcement in composites, etc. In this case N is 1 and the connectivity can be measured. Connectivity is the minimum number of cuts that would be needed to separate the network. For flow or communication through a network, it is the number of alternate paths, or the number of blockages, that would be required to stop the flow or transmission.

In many situations, such as the case of an opaque matrix, it is not practical to implement a sweeping tangent plane. The simplest practical implementation of a volume probe that can reveal the important topological properties of the structure is the Disector (Geuna 2005; Sterio 1984). This consists of two parallel planes of examination, which can be two sequential or closely spaced thin sections examined in transmission. For many materials samples, it is implemented by polishing an examination plane, which is imaged and recorded and then polished down an additional small distance (usually using hardness indentations or scratches to gauge the distance and also to facilitate aligning the images) before acquiring a second image.

The Disector logic compares the images in the two parallel planes and ignores any feature that continues through both planes, even if the position and shape have changed somewhat. The planes must of course be close enough together that this determination can be made unequivocally. Usually this means that the spacing must be significantly less than any characteristic dimension of the features or structure of interest, and so most features that intersect one plane will intersect both. **Figure 9.28** shows the possible combinations of events that may be found.

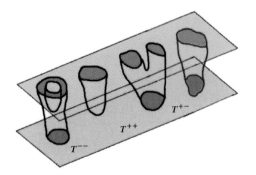

Figure 9.28 Possible combinations of features in the two planes of the Disector. Features that continue through with no topological change are ignored. Feature ends are counted as convex (T^{++}) events and void ends are counted as concave (T^{--}) ones. Branching indicates the presence of a saddle surface with T^{+-} curvature.

Any features that are present in one plane and not the other imply that the three-dimensional structure had an endpoint somewhere between the two planes. This represents a convex curvature and is counted as a T^{++} event. For a set of convex, discrete objects, only these ends will be present. Typically rare is the case in which a hollow feature in one plane becomes solid in the other plane. This represents the end of a void or, more generally, a hollow with concave curvature, and is counted as a T^{--} event. Any branching in the structure, in which one feature in one of the two planes can be presumed to connect to two features in the other, represents a saddle surface and is counted as a T^{+-} event. The tangent events from the Disector are summed in the same way shown in **Equation 9.10** to determine the net tangent count and the Euler characteristic of the structure.

Because most of the features seen in the Disector images continue through both sections, and thus contribute no new information, it is necessary to examine many pairs of sections, which of course must be aligned to compare intersections with the features. When the matrix is transparent and viewed in a confocal microscope, examining and comparing the parallel section planes is straightforward. **Figure 8.33** in **Chapter 8** showed an example. When conventional serial sections are used, it is attractive to use computer processing to align and compare the images. In this regard, the marker selection (Feature-AND) logic described in **Chapter 8** is particularly useful in finding new features and ignoring those that continue through both sections. It is also necessary to sample a large image area, well distributed to meet the usual criteria of random, uniform sampling. Since the Disector is a volume probe, isotropy is not a concern.

Figure 9.29 shows an example using sections obtained by nondestructive imaging of bubbles in a candy bar. The area of each circular image is 1.54 cm², and the spacing between the section planes is 6.3 μm. After thresholding the images and applying the Boolean logic, there are 65 ends counted. Applying **Equation 9.10** calculates a value of 3.35 bubbles per cubic millimeter. Since the volume fraction of the voids can also be determined from the images (6.1%), the mean volume of a bubble can be calculated as 0.0018 mm³.

For opaque matrices that must be physically sectioned, the problems are more severe. Generally it is necessary to prepare a polished section, image it, place some fiducial marks on it for reference, and then polish down to some greater depth in the sample and repeat the process. If the fiducial marks are small pyramidal hardness indentations (commonly used to measure hardness of materials), the reduction in their size provides a measure of the distance between the two planes. Aligning and comparing the two images to locate new features can be quite tedious. Focused ion beam (FIB) machining of the surface presents another way to prepare closely spaced parallel planes for imaging, which can be very useful for this purpose.

Figure 9.30 shows an example. The specimen is a titanium alloy in which the size of colonies of Widmanstatten laths is of interest. Each colony is identified by its lath orientation. After one

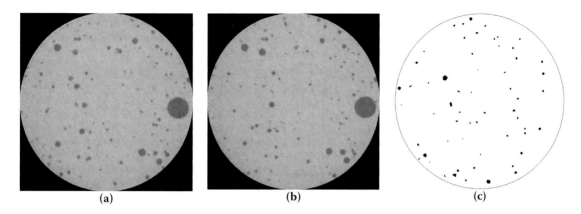

(a)   (b)   (c)

Figure 9.29 *Two sections through a candy bar (**a, b**) imaged by CT, and the intersections (**c**) that are unique to one or the other of the section planes, obtained using the same procedures shown in **Chapter 8, Figure 8.33**. (Courtesy of Dr. G. Ziegler, Pennsylvania State University, State College.)*

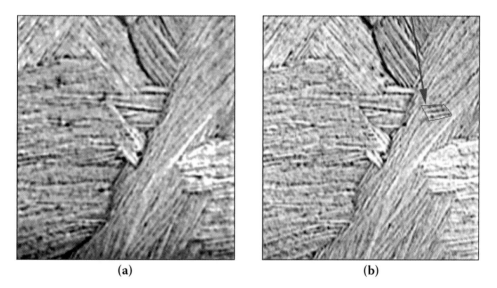

(a)   (b)

Figure 9.30 *EMs of colonies of laths in a titanium alloy. The two images represent parallel planes with a measured spacing of 5 µm. A new colony (red arrow and outline) appears in image (**b**), producing a single positive tangent count (T^{++}). (Courtesy of Dr. H. Fraser, Dept. of Materials Science and Engineering, The Ohio State University, Columbus.)*

set of images was acquired on a metallographically polished plane, the material was polished down a further 5 µm (as measured from the size change of a microhardness indentation) and additional corresponding images acquired. In the example, another colony (identified by the red arrow) has appeared. From the total number of such positive tangent events and the volume sampled by the Disector, the mean colony volume was determined.

Anisotropy and gradients

The previous discussion has emphasized methods for performing sectioning and applying grids that eliminate bias in structures that may not be isotropic, uniform, and random (IUR). Of course, when the specimen meets those criteria, then any sampling method and grid can be used, but in most cases it is not possible to assume an IUR structure. Hence, techniques such as vertical sectioning and cycloid grids are used, since they will provide unbiased results whether the specimen is IUR or not, at the cost of somewhat more effort in preparation and measurement.

In some situations, it may be important to actually measure the anisotropy (preferred orientation) in the specimen, or to characterize the nonuniformity (gradients) present in the structure. This requires more effort. First, it is usually very important to decide beforehand what kind of anisotropy or gradient is of interest. Sometimes this is known *a priori* based on the physics of the situation. For example, deformation of materials in fabrication and the growth of plants typically produce grains or cells that are elongated in a known direction. Many physical materials and biological tissues have structures that vary significantly near surfaces and outer boundaries, so a gradient in that direction can be anticipated. Anisotropy can be qualitatively determined visually by examining images of planes cut in orthogonal directions, as shown in **Figure 9.31** and **Figure 9.32**. It is usually necessary to examine at least two planes to distinguish the nature of the anisotropy, as shown in **Figure 9.33**.

When there is expectation that directionality is present in the structure, the classic approach is to use grids to measure selectively in different directions. For example, in the case shown in **Figure 9.34**, the number of intercepts per unit line length (which measures the surface area per unit volume) can be measured in different directions by using a rotated grid of parallel lines. Since each set of lines measures the projected surface area normal to the line direction, the result shows the anisotropy of surface orientation. Plotting the reciprocal of number of intersections per unit line length (called the intercept length) as a function of orientation produces a polar (or rose) plot as shown in the figure, which characterizes the mean shape of the grains or cells.

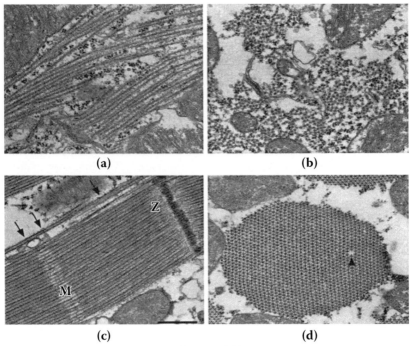

(a)　　　　(b)

(c)　　　　(d)

Figure 9.31 *Anisotropy in muscle tissue, visible as a difference in structure in transverse (b, d) and longitudinal (a, c) sections.*

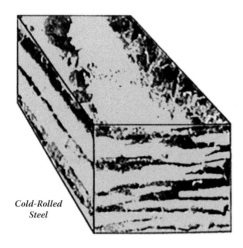

Cold-Rolled
Steel

Figure 9.32 Anisotropy in rolled steel,
shown by microscopic examination of
three orthogonal polished surfaces.

Gradients can sometimes be observed by comparing images from different parts of a specimen, but because visual judgment of metric properties such as length of boundary lines and area fraction of a phase is not very reliable, it is usually safest to actually perform measurements and compare the data statistically to find variations. The major problem with characterizing gradients is that they are rarely simple. An apparent change in the number of features per unit area or volume may hide a more significant change in feature size or shape, for example. **Figure 9.35** shows some examples in which gradients of size, number, shape, and orientation are present. A secondary problem is that, once the suspected gradient has been identified, a great many samples and fields of view may be required to obtain adequate statistical precision to properly characterize it.

Figure 9.36 shows a simple example representing the distribution of cell colonies in a petri dish. Are they preferentially clustered near the center, or uniformly distributed across the area? By using the method shown in **Chapter 8** to assign a value from the Euclidean distance map (of the area inside the petri dish) to each feature, and then plotting the number of features as a function of that value, the plot of count vs. radial distance shown in the figure is obtained. This might appear to show an increase in the number of features away from the center of the dish. But that does not correctly represent the actual situation, because it is not the number but the number per unit area that is important, and there is much more area near the periphery of the dish than near the center. If the distribution of number of features as a function of radius from the center is divided by the number of pixels as a function of radius (which is simply the histogram of the Euclidean distance map), the true variation of number per unit area is obtained, as shown in the figure.

Size distributions

As noted previously, much of the contemporary effort in stereological development and research has been concerned with improved sampling strategies to eliminate bias in cases of non-IUR specimens. There have also been interesting developments in so-called second-order

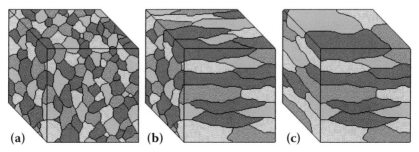

(a)   (b)   (c)

Figure 9.33 It is necessary to examine at least two orthogonal surfaces to reveal the nature of anisotropy. In the diagrams, the same appearance on one face can result from different three-dimensional structures: **(a)** equiaxial structure; **(b)** needlelike structure; **(c)** platelike structure.

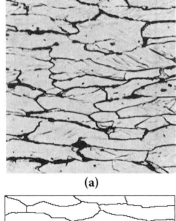

(a)

Figure 9.34 *Characterizing anisotropy:*
   (a) *an anisotropic metal grain structure;*
   (b) *the idealized grain boundaries produced by thresholding and skeletonization;*
   (c) *measuring the number of intercepts per unit line length in different orientations by rotating a grid of parallel lines;*
   (d) *the results shown as a polar plot of mean intercept length vs. angle.*

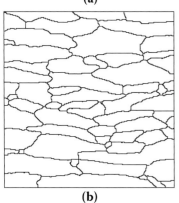

(b)

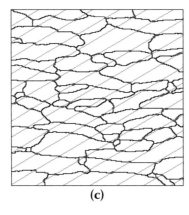

(c)

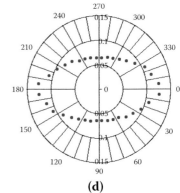

(d)

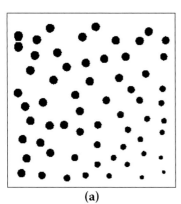

(a)

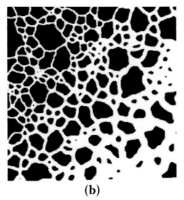

(b)

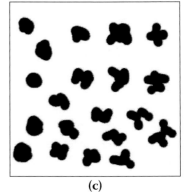

(c)

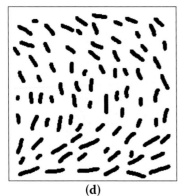

(d)

Figure 9.35 *Schematic diagrams of gradients in*
   (a) *size,*
   (b) *area fraction,*
   (c) *shape, and*
   (d) *orientation.*

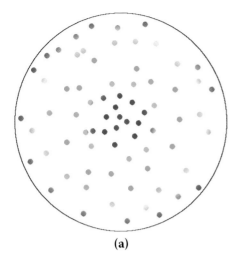

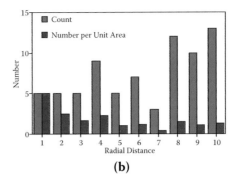

(b)

Figure 9.36 *Distribution of features within an area (e.g., cell colonies in a petri dish):*

(a) *each feature labeled according to distance from the periphery;*

(b) *plot of number and number per unit area as a function of distance.*

(a)

stereology that combine results from different types of measurements, such as using two different types of grids to probe a structure or two different and independent measurements. One example is to use a point grid to select features for measurement in proportion to their volume (points are more likely to hit large than small particles). For each particle that is thus selected, a line is drawn in a random direction from the selection point to measure the radius from that point to the boundary of the particle.

Figure 9.37 shows this procedure applied to the white dendritic phase in the image used in **Figure 9.3**. The grid of points selects locations. For each point that falls onto the phase of interest, a radial line in uniformly randomized directions is drawn to the feature boundary. For nonconvex shapes, the length of this line may consist of multiple segments that must be added together. For isotropic structures or isotropic section planes, the line angles uniformly sample directions. For vertical sections through potentially anisotropic structures, a set of sine-weighted angles should be used. The length of each line gives an estimate of particle volume:

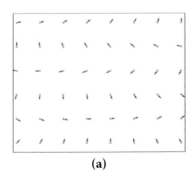

(a)

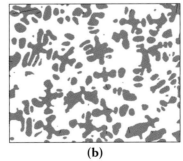

(b)

Figure 9.37 *Measuring point-sampled intercepts:* *(a)* *an array of grid points, each having a direction associated with it;* *(b)* *applying the grid to the image from* *Figure 9.3* *and measuring the radial distance from those grid points that fall on the phase of interest to the boundary in the chosen direction. Note that for nonconvex shapes, the radial distance is the sum of all portions of the intercept line.*

$$V = \tfrac{4}{3}\pi r^3$$

(9.11)

which is independent of particle shape. Averaging this measurement over a surprisingly small number of particles and radius measurements gives a robust estimate of the volume-weighted mean volume (in other words, the volume-weighted average counts large particles more often than small ones, in proportion to their volume).

A more familiar way to define a mean volume is on a number-weighted basis, where each particle counts equally. This can be determined by dividing the total volume of the phase by the number of particles. We have already seen how to determine the total volume fraction using a point count and the number of particles per unit volume using the Disector. Dividing the total by the number gives the number-weighted mean volume.

Once both the mean volumes have been determined, they can be combined to determine the standard deviation of the distribution of particle sizes, independent of particle shape, since the variance for the conventional number-weighted distribution is given by the difference between the square of the volume-weighted mean volume and the square of the number-weighted mean volume

$$\sigma^2 = V_V^2 - V_N^2$$

(9.12)

Although this may seem to be a rather esoteric measurement, in fact it gives an important characterization of the size distribution of particles or other features that may be present in a solid, which as we have seen are not directly measurable from the size distribution of their intersections with a plane section.

Classical stereology (unfolding)

Historically, much of classical stereology was concerned with determining the size distribution of three-dimensional features when only two-dimensional sections through them were measurable (Cruz-Orive 1976, 1983; Weibel 1979). The classical method used was to assume a shape for the particles (i.e., that all of the particles were the same shape, which did not vary with size). The most convenient shape to assume is, of course, a sphere. The distribution of the sizes of circles produced by random sectioning of a sphere can be calculated as shown in **Figure 9.38**. Knowing the sizes of circles that should be produced if all of the spheres were of the same size makes it possible to calculate a matrix of α values to be used in **Equation 9.13**

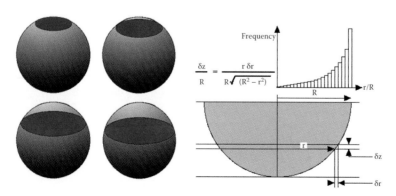

Figure 9.38 Sectioning a sphere randomly produces a distribution of circle sizes.

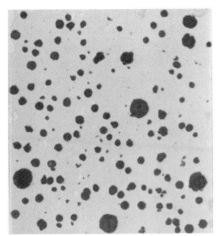

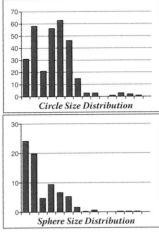

Circle Size Distribution

Sphere Size Distribution

Figure 9.39 *Unfolding the size distribution of spheres that must have been present to produce an observed distribution of circle sizes. The sample is a cast iron containing graphite nodules; note that the features are not perfectly circular, even though a sphere model has been used in the unfolding.*

to solve for the distribution of sphere sizes that must have been present in the three-dimensional structure to produce the observed distribution of circle sizes, as shown in **Figure 9.39**.

$$N_{V_{sphere,i}} = \sum \alpha_{i,j} \cdot N_{A_{circle,j}}$$

(9.13)

Other shapes have also been proposed, as a compromise between mathematical ease of calculation and possible realistic modeling of real-world shapes. These have included ellipsoids of revolution (both oblate and prolate), disks, cylinders (Kok 1990), and a wide variety of polyhedra (Wasen and Warren 1990), some of which can be assembled to fill space (as real cells and grains do). Tables of alpha coefficients for all of these exist and can be rather straightforwardly applied to a measured distribution of the size of two-dimensional features viewed on the section plane.

However, there are several critical drawbacks to this approach. First, the ideal shapes do not usually exist. Nuclei are not ideal spheres, cells and grains are not all the same polyhedral shape (in fact, the larger ones usually have more faces and edges than smaller ones), precipitate particles in metals are rarely perfect disks or rods, etc. Knowledge of the shape of the three-dimensional object is critical to the success of the unfolding method, since the distribution of intersection sizes varies considerably with shape (**Figure 9.40** shows an example of cubes vs. spheres). It is very common to find that size varies with shape, which strongly biases the results. Small errors in the shape assumption produce very large errors in the results. For example, the presence of a few irregularities or protrusions on spheres results in many smaller intersection features, which are misinterpreted as many small spherical particles.

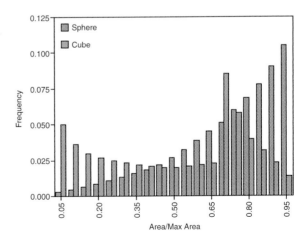

Figure 9.40 *Size distribution of intercept areas produced by random sectioning of a sphere and a cube.*

The second problem is that, from a mathematical point of view, the unfolding calculation is ill-posed and unstable. Variations in the distribution of the number of two-dimensional features as a function of size result from counting statistics. The variations are typically greatest at the end of the distribution, for the few largest features that are rarely encountered. But in the unfolding process, these errors are magnified and propagated down to smaller sizes, often resulting in negative numbers of features in some size classes and greatly amplifying the statistical uncertainty.

For these reasons, although unfolding was a widely used classical stereological method for decades, it has fallen out of favor in the last 20 years. Instead, there has been increased emphasis on finding unbiased ways to measure structural parameters using more-robust tools. Nevertheless, despite these limitations (or perhaps because their magnitude and effect are not sufficiently appreciated), unfolding of size distributions is still often performed. When the shape of the three-dimensional objects is not known, it is common to assume they are simple spheres, even when the observed section features are clearly not circles. The argument that this gives some data that can be compared from one sample to another, even if it is not really accurate, is actually quite wrong and simply betrays the general level of ignorance about the rules and application of stereological procedures.

10

Feature-Specific Measurements

Measurements that can be performed on each of the individual features in images can be grouped into four classes: brightness (including color values and parameters such as density that are related to brightness), location (both absolute position and relative to other features present), size, and shape. For each class, quite a variety of different specific measurements can be made, and there are also a variety of different ways to perform the operations. Most image-analysis systems offer at least a few measures in each class. Users find themselves at some time or another having to select from several different measurement parameters. The problem is frequently to decide which of the measured parameters is most useful or appropriate for solving a particular problem.

These measurements usually produce a numeric output suitable for statistical analysis, feature selection, or presentation graphics. Frequently, the interpretation of the data is left to a separate program, either a simple spreadsheet relying on the user's programming ability, or a dedicated statistics package. In a few cases, the numbers are converted to go/no-go decisions or become the basis for classification, discussed in the next chapter. Examples might include quality control testing of the size and placement of holes in a part, medical pathology decisions based on the identification of the presence of precancerous cells, or recognition of different objects in the field of view.

Brightness measurements

Normally in the kinds of images discussed here, each pixel records a numeric value that represents the brightness of the corresponding point in the original scene. Several such values can be combined to represent color information. The most typical range of brightness values is from 0 to 255 (8-bit range), but depending on the type of camera, scanner, or other acquisition device, a larger dynamic range of 10 or more bits, up to perhaps 16 (0 to 65,535), may be encountered. Most programs that accept images from sources such as cooled cameras and scanners having more than 8 bits of depth store them as 16-bit images (occupying 2 bytes per pixel for gray-scale images, or 6 bytes per pixel of red, green, and blue values for color images), even if the actual gray-scale or tonal resolution is less than 16 bits. Some systems use the 0- to 255-value range for all bit depths but report decimal values rather than integers for images having more than 8 bits of depth. This has the advantage of permitting easy comparisons between images acquired with different depths, and is the convention adopted here. Rarely, the stored values are real numbers rather than integers (for instance, elevation data). However, in most cases these images are still stored with a set of discrete integer "gray" values because it is easier to manipulate such arrays and convert them to displays. In many cases a calibration table or function is maintained to convert the pixel values to meaningful real numbers when needed.

The process of creating such a calibration function for a particular imaging device, or indeed for a particular image, is far from trivial (Boddeke 1998; Chieco et al. 1994; Inoué 1986; Ortiz and O'Connell 2004; Swing 1997). Many of the cameras and other devices that have been mentioned for acquiring images are neither perfectly linear nor exactly logarithmic, nor are they completely consistent in the relationship between the pixel's numeric value and the input signal (e.g., photon intensity). Many video cameras have an output function that varies in response with the overall illumination level. The presence of automatic gain circuits, or user-adjustable gamma controls, makes it more difficult to establish and maintain any kind of calibration. In general, any kind of automatic gain or dark-level circuitry, automatic color balancing, etc., will frustrate efforts to calibrate the camera. With consumer-level video and still cameras, it is not always possible to turn such "features" off.

For color imaging, cameras may incorporate automatic white-balance adjustments (which are intended for a type of scene much different from the majority of scientific images). Control of the color temperature of the light source and maintaining consistency of the camera response to perform meaningful color measurement is rarely possible with consumer-grade still or video cameras. **Chapter 1** showed examples of correcting color values using measured RGB (red, green, blue) intensities from a standard color chart. It is important to note that the typical color camera has RGB sensors that respond to a relatively broad range of wavelengths, and that many different combinations of actual wavelengths and intensities can produce identical stored RGB values. In general, it is not practical to attempt to perform colorimetry (the measurement of color) using such cameras, and of course complications arising from light sources, viewing geometry, optics, etc., make the problem even more difficult. The color-correction procedures described in **Chapter 1** produce visual color matching, not spectrophotometric measurements.

Even when the use of a stable light source and consistent camera settings can be assured, the problem of gray-scale calibration remains. Some standards are reasonably accessible, for example, density standards in the form of a step-wedge of film. Measurement of the brightness of regions in such a standard can be performed as often as needed to keep a system in calibration. In scanning large-area samples such as electrophoresis gels or X-ray films, it is practical to incorporate some density standards into every scan so that calibration can be performed directly. In other cases, separate standard samples can be introduced periodically to check calibration.

Optical density is defined as

$$O.D. = -\log_{10}\left(\frac{I}{I_0}\right)$$

(10.1)

where I/I_0 is the fraction of the incident light that penetrates through the sample without being absorbed or scattered. If a camera or scanner and its light source are carefully adjusted so that the full range of linear brightness values covers the range of optical density from 0.1 (a typical value for the fog level of unexposed film) to 2.5 (a moderately dense exposed film), the resulting calibration of brightness vs. optical density would be as shown in **Figure 10.1**. The shape of the curve is logarithmic.

At relatively low-density/bright pixel values the sensitivity is quite good. A difference of 1 pixel brightness value at the bright end of the scale corresponds to less than 0.01 in optical density. But at the high-density/dark pixel end of the scale, a difference of one pixel brightness value corresponds to an optical-density change of 0.3, which is very large. This is an indication that when trying to apply a linear camera or scanner to optical-density reading, more than 8 bits of gray scale are needed. An input device with more precision can be used with a lookup table that converts the values to the logarithmic optical-density scale and then stores that in an 8-bit image. This problem becomes more severe as higher density values are encountered. Films containing large amounts of silver, such as X-ray film or TEM (transmission electron microscope) film, can easily reach densities of 3.5 to 4.0. To be satisfactorily digitized, such films require the use of scanners with a precision of at least 12, and preferably 14, bits per channel. It is always preferable to scan negatives rather than prints, but sometimes these are inaccessible and prints must be used. Ortiz and O'Connell (2004) discuss the difficulties these create, in terms of nonlinearities and loss of dynamic range.

It is not uncommon to include a gray wedge in a film to be scanned for one- or two-dimensional separation of organic molecules. **Figure 10.2** shows an example. The gray wedge of known density values allows the construction of a calibration scale (**Figure 10.3**) that can then be used to measure the optical density of each object (**Figure 10.4**). In this application, the total amount of protein in each spot is proportional to the integrated optical density, which is the product of the average density and the area. There are few sources of densitometric standards suitable for microscopy, and even fewer sources of color standards, although it is sometimes practical to prepare ones using dyes (Hoffmann et al. 2005).

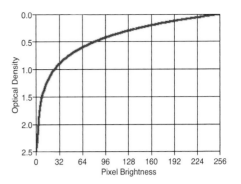

Figure 10.1 Calibration of optical density vs. pixel brightness if the latter is adjusted linearly to span the range from 0.1 (fog level) to 2.5 (typical exposed film).

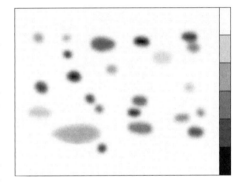

Figure 10.2 Scanned image of a two-dimensional electrophoresis separation, with a gray-scale calibration wedge.

The use of a calibration scale raises another point. It is common for features in an image to contain some variation in pixel brightness. The average density (or whatever other quantity is calibrated against pixel brightness) is not usually recorded linearly. It thus becomes important to take this into account when determining an average value for the density, or for an integrated total dose, or for any other calibrated quantity. If all of the pixels within the feature are simply averaged in brightness, and then that value is converted using the calibration scale, the wrong answer will be obtained. It is instead proper to convert the value from each pixel to the calibrated values, and then sum or average those. It is also important not to include adjacent

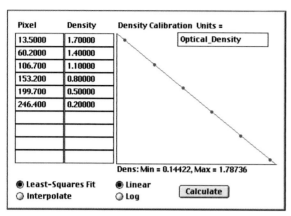

Pixel	Density
13.5000	1.70000
60.2000	1.40000
106.700	1.10000
153.200	0.80000
199.700	0.50000
246.400	0.20000

Density Calibration Units =
Optical_Density

Dens: Min = 0.14422, Max = 1.78736

◉ Least-Squares Fit   ◉ Linear
○ Interpolate   ○ Log   [Calculate]

Figure 10.3 Calibration plot from the gray-scale wedge in *Figure 10.2*, showing the relationship between optical density and pixel brightness for this particular scanner (on a particular day).

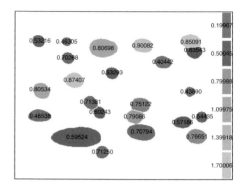

Figure 10.4 Measured data from *Figure 10.2*, using the calibration plot from *Figure 10.3* to compute the optical density of each spot.

background pixels that are not part of the feature, which means that the delineation should be exact and not some arbitrary shape (a circle or square) drawn around the features. Reliance on manual outlining is not usually acceptable, since humans often draw outlines larger than the boundaries around features. The solution is to use the same routines that threshold and segment the image into discrete features. The pixels in that binary image define the features and can be used as a mask to define the pixels in the gray-scale array.

For one-dimensional measurements of density, the procedure is the same. **Figure 10.5** shows an example of a film exposed in a Debye-Scherer X-ray camera. The total density of each line, and its position, are used to measure the crystal structure of materials. Knowing that the lines extend vertically, it is reasonable to average the values in the vertical direction to reduce noise and obtain a more precise plot of the density variations along the film (**Figure 10.6**). Converting the individual pixel values to density before summing them is the correct procedure that gives the proper values for the relative line intensities. The linear plots of intensity values can be subtracted to find differences or used with spectrum-processing routines to detect peaks. Similar procedures are appropriate for measuring a variety of samples, including growth rings in plants and varves in lake sediments, that have essentially one-dimensional variations. Some

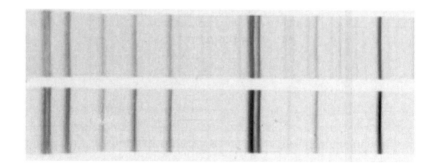

Figure 10.5 Two Debye-Scherer X-ray films. The vertical lines occur at positions (angles) that are related to the atomic spacing in the lattice structure of the target material. Small differences in intensity and the presence of additional lines indicate the presence of trace amounts of additional compounds.

of these may not require intensity calibration, as it is only the spatial location of peaks and valleys that is of interest.

Figure 10.7 shows a similar procedure for tracks or columns in an electrophoresis separation. Using the brightness profile measured between the tracks allows a simple correction to be made for background variations due to nonuniformities in thickness or illumination. The brightness values are averaged across the center of the columns, avoiding the edges. Calibration of the position of bands within the columns is usually done with respect to markers of known molecular weight that are placed in adjacent columns. This is necessary because the distance scale is generally not linear or constant in such specimens.

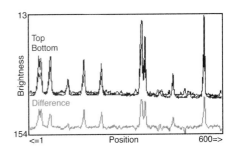

Figure 10.6 Integrated intensity plots along the films from Figure 10.5, with the difference between them.

Profile plots also offer a convenient alternative to the method of applying grid lines for the measurement of dimensions such as coating thickness. **Figure 10.8** shows the same cross section of paint layers as **Figure 8.19** in **Chapter 8**, with a plot of the variation along a vertical direction of the mean pixel values (averaged horizontally). The blue profile shows well-defined transitions at the top and bottom of the red pigment layer that can be used to determine the mean thickness, and the breadth of the transition zone in the plot offers a measure of the variation in the thickness. Plots for hue and saturation also delineate the layers well in this example.

Of course, not all images have this convenient relationship between recorded pixel intensity and a property of the sample being imaged, such as density. In microscope images, compositional or structural differences can also produce contrast, and diffraction or polarization effects may also be present. In real-world images of surfaces, the local surface orientation and texture influence the brightness, as does the interplay between the light-source color and the surface color. In most of these cases, the brightness cannot be measured to provide information about the sample. The goal is generally to use the relative channel brightness values to delineate regions that are to be grouped together or separated from each other.

When color images are digitized, the problem of having enough bits to give enough precision for each of the color planes is amplified. Many of the higher-end scanners acquire more than 8 bits, often at least 12, for each of the RGB channels, use these to determine the color information, and then may create an optimized 8-bit representation to send to the computer. But even with this increase in precision, it is difficult to achieve accurate color representation.

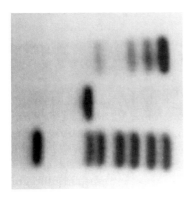

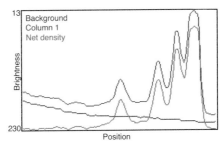

Figure 10.7 A one-dimensional protein separation. Intensity scans along the center of each track are leveled by subtracting scans between the tracks (the example shows the top track).

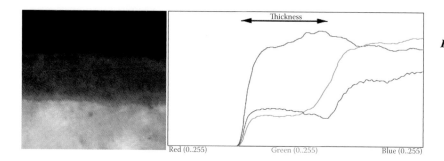

Figure 10.8
Measurement of
layer thickness
from a profile plot
(same image as
Figure 8.19 in
Chapter 8).

As pointed out in **Chapter 1**, the digitization of color requires far greater control of camera settings and lighting than can normally be achieved with a video camera. Even a flatbed scanner, which offers greater consistency of illumination and typically uses a single CCD (charge-coupled device) linear array with various filters to obtain the RGB information, is not a good choice for measurement of actual color information. However, such scanners can be calibrated to reproduce colors adequately on the computer monitor and on printed output.

The pixel brightness value need not be optical-density or color-component information, of course. Images are so useful in communicating information to humans that they are used for all kinds of data. Even within the most conventional expression of the idea of imaging, pixel values can be related to the concentration of dyes and stains introduced into a specimen. In an X-ray image from the SEM (scanning electron microscope), the brightness values are approximately proportional to elemental concentration. These relationships are not necessarily linear nor easy to calibrate. X-ray emission intensities are affected by the presence of other elements. Fluorescence intensities depend not only on staining techniques and tissue characteristics, but also on time, since bleaching is a common phenomenon. Zwier et al. (2004) review the calibration procedures and corrections appropriate for fluorescence microscopy.

In infrared imaging, brightness can be a measure of temperature. Backscattered electron images from the SEM have brightness values that increase with the average atomic number, so that they can be used to determine chemical composition of small regions on the sample. In a range image (discussed further in **Chapter 14**), the pixel brightness values represent the elevation of points on the surface and are often calibrated in appropriate units.

To support this range of applications, it is generally useful to be able to measure the mean intensity or a calibrated "density" value, as well as to find the brightest or darkest pixel values in each region or feature, and perhaps the standard deviation of the brightness values as a measure of variation or texture. For color images, it may be useful to report the RGB components (usually as values ranging from 0 to 255), but in most cases the hue, saturation, and intensity (HSI) are more directly useful. The saturation and intensity are generally measured on either the 0 to 255 scale or reported as percentages, but the hue may be reported as an angle from 0 to 360°, as is shown in **Figure 10.9**. Note that there are several different HSI spaces, as discussed in **Chapter 1**, and it is important to know which one is being used to convert the stored RGB pixel values, particularly for the saturation values.

These examples are at best a tiny sample of the possible uses of pixel values. But the measurement of the stored values and conversion to some calibrated scale is a broadly useful technique. Statistical analysis of the data provides mean values and standard deviations, trends with position, comparisons between locations, comparisons within or between images, and so forth. For such procedures to work, it is important to establish useful calibration curves, which requires standards and/or fundamental knowledge and is a subject beyond the scope of this text.

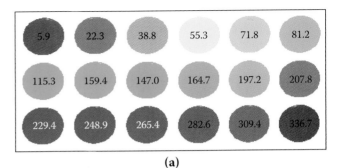

(a)

Figure 10.9 Mean color values for a series of color spots:
  (a) hue, labeled as angles from 0 to 360°, for features with full saturation;
  (b) saturation, labeled as percent, for features with constant hue and intensity;
  (c) intensity, labeled as percent, for features with constant hue and saturation.

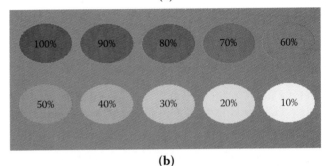

(b)

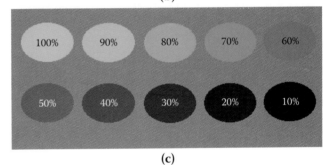

(c)

Determining location

In several of the examples for measuring brightness values, the location of features was also needed for interpretation of the results. For a typical irregular feature extending over several pixels, there can be several different definitions of location, some easier to calculate than others. For instance, the *x,y* coordinates of the midpoint of a feature can be determined simply as halfway between the minimum and maximum limits of the pixels comprising the feature. Normally, the pixel addresses themselves are just integer counts of position, most often starting from the top left corner of the array. This convention arises from the way that most computer displays work, using a raster scan from the top left corner. There may be some global coordinate system of which the individual image is just a part, and these values may also be integers, or real number values that calibrate the pixel dimensions to some real-world units such as latitude and longitude, or millimeters from the edge of a microscope slide or workpiece.

Establishing a real-world calibration for pixel dimensions is often quite difficult, and maintaining them while shifting the specimen or the camera (by moving the microscope stage or the satellite, for instance) presents a variety of challenges. The technology used to produce the first-down line and other graphics that are superimposed on a football field during TV broadcasts of games requires careful surveying measurement of camera locations beforehand, as well as encoders for camera orientation as they are turned to follow action, and sophisticated computer software. Generation of political boundary lines superimposed on weather maps is a time-consuming process that fortunately has to be done only a few times a year (when the satellite positions are changed).

Often, locating a few known features in the image itself can serve to establish fiduciary marks that allow calibration, so that all of the other features in the image can be accurately located. Shifting the sample, stage, or camera so that successive viewing frames overlap allows position calibration to be transferred from one field to the next, but the errors are cumulative and can grow rapidly due to the difficulty of accurately locating the same feature(s) in each field to a fraction of a pixel. This also assumes that there are no distortions or scan nonlinearities in the images. Relying on the stage motion for position information depends upon the precision of that mechanism (which may be much worse if the direction of motion is reversed, due to backlash), and the fidelity with which the sample motion corresponds to that of the stage. Real-world imaging is facilitated in some applications by the incorporation of GPS (Global Positioning System) receivers into some cameras to automatically record information in image files.

A feature's minimum and maximum limits are easy to determine by finding the pixels with the largest and smallest coordinates in the horizontal and vertical directions. These limiting coordinates define a bounding rectangle around the feature, and the midpoint of the box can then be used as a location for the feature. However, the midpoint is not usually the preferred representation of location, because it is too easily biased by just a few pixels (for instance a whisker sticking out from the rest of the feature). One application in which these box coordinates are used, however, is in computer drawing programs. Many such programs allow the user to select a number of drawn objects and then move them into alignment automatically. The options are typically to align the objects vertically by their top, center, or bottom edges and horizontally by their left, center, or right edges. These are exactly the box coordinates and midpoint.

The center of the so-called bounding box is useful in a few situations such as the gel scan, because the x and y coordinates have meaning in terms of how the sample was created. For most real images, this is not the case. When the x- and y-axes are arbitrary, the bounding box is very biased and sensitive to object orientation, as shown in **Figure 10.10**. More representative of the geometric center of a feature is the location of the center of a bounding or circumscribed circle (illustrated **Figure 10.11**). Fitting such a circle to the points on the object periphery is straightforward, and made more efficient by using only those points that represent the vertices of a bounding polygon, fitted as described later in this chapter by rotating axes to a limited number of directions (typically about every 10°) and finding the bounding-box limits for each orientation. Of course, the size and center location of the bounding circle is not sensitive to changes in the orientation of the axes or the feature.

For a nonconvex feature or one containing internal holes, the geometric center may not lie within the feature bounds. Nor is it sensitive to changes in the interior of the actual feature shape. For irregularly shaped features, it is usually preferable to take into account the feature shape and the location of all the pixels present. This approach defines the centroid of the feature, a unique x,y point that would serve to balance the feature on a pinpoint if it were cut out of a rigid, uniform sheet of cardboard. The coordinates of this point can be determined by averaging the coordinates of each pixel in the object:

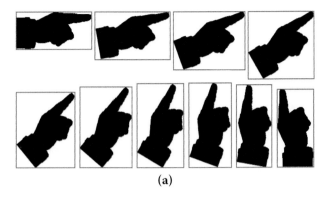

(a)

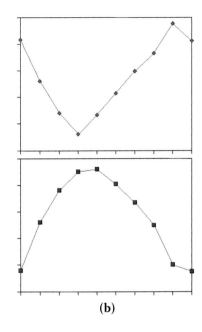

(b)

Figure 10.10
   (a) Rotation of a feature and
   (b) the changes in the size and shape of the
       bounding box.

$$C.G._x = \frac{\sum_i x_i}{Area}$$

$$C.G._y = \frac{\sum_i y_i}{Area} \qquad (10.2)$$

where the area is just the total number of pixels present. Notice that this equation provides a set of coordinates that are not, in general, integers. The center of gravity or centroid of an object can be determined to subpixel accuracy, which can be very important for locating features accurately in a scene. **Figure 10.11** compares the geometric center and the centroid for an irregular feature.

If the centroid is calculated according to **Equation 10.2** using only the boundary pixels, as is sometimes done (especially if features are encoded with boundary representation, as described in **Chapter 8**), the result is incorrect. The calculated point will be biased toward whichever part of the boundary is most complex and contains the most pixels (**Figure 10.12**). This bias will also vary with the orientation of the boundary with respect to the pixel array because square pixels are larger in the diagonal direction than in their horizontal and vertical dimension.

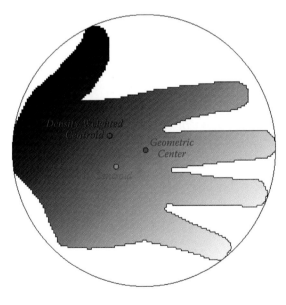

Figure 10.11 *Centroid (green), density-weighted centroid (red) using the pixel density values, and geometric center (blue) determined as the center of the bounding circle, for an irregular feature.*

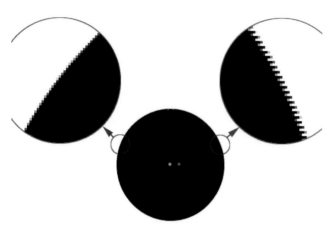

The centroid location, also called the center of gravity (C.G.), can be calculated correctly from a boundary representation such as chain code. The correct calculation uses the pairs of coordinates x_i, y_i for each point in the boundary, where x_0, y_0 and x_n, y_n are the same point (i.e., the boundary representation is a closed loop with the two ends at the same place).

$$C.G._x = \frac{\sum_i (x_i + x_{i-1})^2 \cdot (y_i - y_{i-1})}{Area}$$

$$C.G._y = \frac{\sum_i (y_i + y_{i-1})^2 \cdot (x_i - x_{i-1})}{Area} \quad (10.3)$$

Figure 10.12 *Effect of boundary irregularities on centroid determination. The right-hand side of the circle is irregular, while the left-hand side is smooth. The centroid location determined by using just the boundary pixels (magenta) is shifted to the right, as compared with the location determined using all of the pixels in the feature (green).*

and it is now necessary to calculate the area as

$$Area = \frac{\sum_i (x_i + x_{i-1}) \cdot (y_i - y_{i-1})}{2} \quad (10.4)$$

Parenthetically, it is worth noting here that some of the attractiveness of chain code or boundary representation as a compact way to describe a feature is lost when using that data to calculate things like the area or centroid of the feature.

The definition of the centroid or C.G. just given treats each pixel within the feature equally. For some purposes, the pixel brightness, or a value calculated from it using a calibration curve, makes some pixels more important than others. For example, the accurate location of the spots and lines in the densitometric examples shown earlier would benefit from this kind of weighting. That modification is quite easy to introduce by including the brightness-derived value in the summations in **Equation 10.5**. **Figure 10.11** shows the density-weighted centroid in comparison with the conventional centroid in which all pixels are treated as equal.

$$C.G._x = \frac{\sum_i Value_i \cdot x_i}{\sum_i Value_i}$$

$$\quad (10.5)$$

$$C.G._y = \frac{\sum_i Value_i \cdot y_i}{\sum_i Value_i}$$

The denominator is now the integrated density (or whatever the parameter related to brightness may be). Of course, this kind of calculation requires access to the individual pixel brightness values, and so cannot be used with a boundary representation of the feature.

For a nonconvex shape, the centroid may not lie within the bounds of the feature. When a unique representative point that always lies within the bounds of a potentially irregular shape is required, the ultimate eroded point or UEP determined from the Euclidean distance map (**Chapter 8**) is the center of the largest inscribed circle in the feature and can often be used.

Orientation

Closely related to the location of the centroid of a feature is the idea of determining its orientation. There are a number of different parameters that are used, including the orientation of the longest dimension in the feature (the line between the two points on the periphery that are farthest apart, also known as the maximum Feret's diameter or maximum caliper dimension) and the orientation of the major axis of an ellipse fitted to the feature boundary. But just as the centroid is a more robust descriptor of the feature's location than is the midpoint, an orientation defined by all of the pixels in the image is often better than any of these because it is less influenced by the presence or absence of a single pixel around the periphery, where accidents of acquisition or noise may make slight alterations in the boundary.

The moment axis of a feature is the line around which the feature, if it were cut from rigid, uniform cardboard, would have the lowest moment of rotation. It can also be described as the axis that best fits all of the pixels, in the sense that the sum of the squares of their individual distances from the axis is minimized. This is the same criterion that can be used to fit lines to data points when constructing graphs. Determining this axis and its orientation angle is straightforward, and just involves summing pixel coordinates and the products of pixel coordinates for all of the pixels in the image. As for the example in **Equation 10.5**, it is possible to weight each pixel with some value, such as the density, instead of letting each one vote equally. The most convenient procedure for the calculation is to add up a set of summations as listed in **Equation 10.6**.

$$S_x = \sum x_i$$
$$S_y = \sum y_i$$
$$S_{xx} = \sum x_i^2 \qquad (10.6)$$
$$S_{yy} = \sum y_i^2$$
$$S_{xy} = \sum x_i y_i$$

Once these sums have been accumulated for the feature, the net moments about the x- and y-axes and the angle of the minimum moment are calculated as shown in **Equation 10.7**.

$$M_x = S_{xx} - \frac{S_x^2}{Area}$$

$$M_y = S_{yy} - \frac{S_y^2}{Area}$$

$$M_{xy} = S_{xy} - \frac{S_x \cdot S_y}{Area} \qquad\qquad (10.7)$$

$$\Theta = \tan^{-1}\left\{ \frac{M_{xx} - M_{yy} + \sqrt{(M_{xx} - M_{yy})^2 + 4 \cdot M_{xy}^2}}{2 \cdot M_{xy}} \right\}$$

Figure 10.13 shows an example of the measurement of orientation angle on features. Notice that features that intersect the edges of the image field are not measured, as will be discussed below. The measurement can also be applied to lines, as shown in **Figure 10.14.** In this case the axons were thresholded and skeletonized, and the nodes were removed, leaving line segments. To characterize the distribution of orientations for the axons, it was more meaningful to plot the total length of segments as a function of angle rather than the number. **Figure 10.15** shows an example combining position and angle. The orientation of the cells in the tissue varies with vertical position. This is an example of a gradient, as discussed in **Chapter 9**, but characterized by the measurement of individual features within the image.

Neighbor relationships

The location of individual features can be less important in some applications than the relationships between neighboring features. For instance, **Figure 10.16** shows several distributions of features. How can such distributions be compactly described to reveal the extent to which they are random, spaced apart ("self-avoiding"), or clustered?

Schwarz and Exner (1983) showed that a histogram of the distribution of the distances between nearest neighbors can provide an answer. Actually, the distance between any pair of neighbors, second nearest, etc., can be used as well, but in most cases the nearest-neighbor pairs are the easiest to identify. Once the coordinates of the centroid points representing each feature have been determined, sorting through the resulting table to locate the nearest neighbor for each

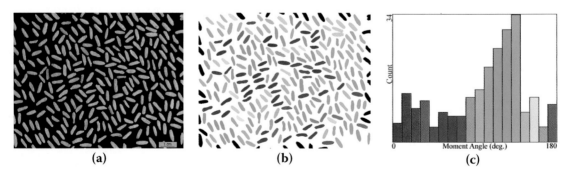

(a)   (b)   (c)

Figure 10.13 Measurement of feature orientation: (a) rice grains; (b) color (hue) coded according to angle; (c) distribution of grains according to angle.

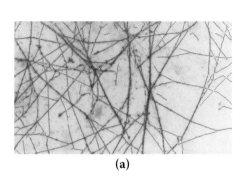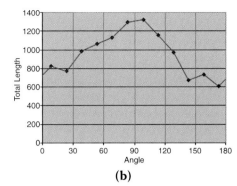

(a)   (b)

Figure 10.14 *Measurement of fiber orientation:* *(a)* *image of axons, with skeleton segments superimposed (nodes removed as described in* *Chapter 8)*; *(b)* *cumulative length of fibers as a function of their angle, showing preferred orientation.*

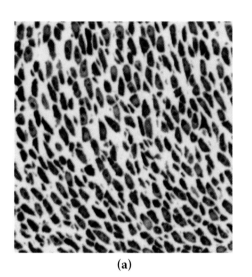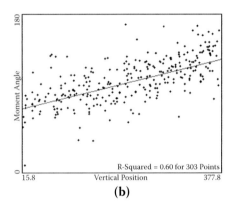

(b)

Figure 10.15 *Cells in tissue* *(a)*, *showing a gradient of moment angle with vertical position* *(b)*.

(a)

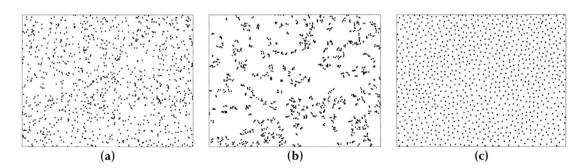

(a)   (b)   (c)

Figure 10.16 *Feature distributions illustrating* *(a)* *random;* *(b)* *clustered, and* *(c)* *spaced or self-avoiding arrangements.*

point is a straightforward task (best left to the computer). The straight-line distances between these points are calculated and used to construct the histogram. This in turn can be characterized by the mean and variance (or standard deviation) of the distribution. A word of caution is needed in dealing with feature points located adjacent to the edge of the field of view (Howard and Reed 1998): if the distance to the edge is less than the distance found to the nearest neighbor within the field of view, the distance should not be used in the distribution because it may cause bias. It is possible that another feature outside the field of view would actually be closer. For large images (fields of view) containing many features, this problem is only a minor concern. The nearest-neighbor distance method also generalizes to three dimensions, in the case of 3-D imaging; the method has been used with a confocal microscope (Baddeley et al. 1987; Reed et al. 1997; Russ et al. 1989). A related statistical test on all neighbor pairs can also be used (Mattfeldt 2005; Shapiro and Haralick 1985).

Consider now the particular distributions shown in **Figure 10.16**. The image in **Figure 10.16a** is actually a random distribution of points, often called a Poisson random distribution because the histogram of nearest-neighbor distances is in fact a Poisson distribution. This is the sort of point distribution you might observe if you just sprinkled salt on the table. Each point is entirely independent of the others, hence "random." For such a distribution, the mean distance between nearest neighbors is just

$$Mean = \frac{0.5}{\sqrt{\frac{N}{Area}}}$$

(10.8)

where N is the number of points within the area of the field of view. For a Poisson distribution, the variance is equal to the mean (the standard deviation is equal to the square root of the mean). The consequence is that for a random distribution of points, the number of points per unit area of the surface is all that is needed to determine the mean and variance of the histogram of nearest-neighbor distances.

When clustering is present in the point distribution, most points have at least one neighbor that is quite close by. Consequently, the mean nearest-neighbor distance is reduced. In most cases, the variance also becomes less, as a measure of the uniformity of the spacing between the clustered points. As shown in the image in **Figure 10.16b**, this clustering produces a histogram of nearest-neighbor distances (**Figure 10.17**) that is much narrower and has a much smaller mean value than the Poisson distribution obtained for the random case. Examination of stars in the heavens indicates that they strongly cluster (into galaxies and clusters of galaxies). People also cluster, gathering together in towns and cities.

When the points are self-avoiding, as shown in **Figure 10.16c**, the nearest-neighbor distances are also affected. The mean value of the histogram increases to a larger value than for the random case. The variance also usually drops, as a measure of the uniformity of the spacings between points. Self-avoiding or regular distributions are common in nature, whether you look at the arrangement of mitochondria in muscle tissue or precipitate particles in metals, because the physics of diffusion plays a role in determining the arrange-

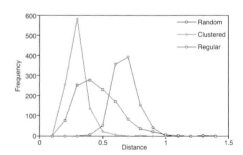

*Figure 10.17 Histogram of nearest-neighbor distances for each of the point distributions in **Figure 10.16**. The mean value of the clustered distribution is less than that for the random one, while the mean for the self-avoiding distribution is greater.*

ment. The mitochondria are distributed to provide energy as uniformly as practical to the fibers. Forming one precipitate particle depletes the surrounding matrix of that element. The same effect occurs in the growth of cacti in the desert. Even the location of shopping centers is to some degree self-avoiding to attract a fresh market of customers (but they tend to cluster in towns where the people live).

The ratio of the mean value of the nearest-neighbor distance distribution to that which would be obtained if the same number of points were randomly distributed in the same area provides a useful measure of the tendency toward clustering or self-avoidance for the features, and the variance of the distribution provides a measure of the uniformity of the tendency. Because the mean and variance for the random case depend only upon the number of features present in the image area, this comparison is easily made.

Finding nearest-neighbor pairs using the centroid coordinates of features can also be used to characterize anisotropy in feature distributions. Instead of the distance between nearest neighbors, we can measure the direction from each feature to its nearest neighbor. For an isotropic arrangement of features, the nearest-neighbor directions should be a uniform function of angle. Plotting the histogram as a rose plot shows any deviations from this uniform function and indicates the degree of anisotropy.

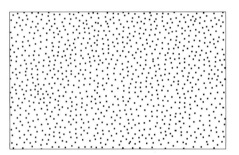

For instance, if the regularly spaced distribution of feature points in **Figure 10.16c** is measured, the rose plot is reasonably circular and indicates that the distribution is isotropic. If the image is stretched 10% in the horizontal direction and shrunk 10% in the vertical direction, the total number of features per unit area is unchanged. The visual appearance of the image (**Figure 10.18**) does not reveal the anisotropy to a casual observer. But a plot of the rose of nearest-neighbor directions (**Figure 10.19**) shows that most of the features now have a nearest neighbor that is situated above or below rather than being approximately uniform in all directions. The shape of the rose plot is a sensitive indicator of this type of anisotropy.

*Figure 10.18 Stretching the point distribution in **Figure 10.16c** horizontally and compressing it vertically introduces nonuniformity in the nearest-neighbor directions.*

Measuring nearest-neighbor distances using the feature centroids is fine when the features are small compared with the distances between them. When features are large compared with the distances that separate them, and particularly when they are irregular in shape, vary in size, and have different orientations, it may be more appropriate to measure the distance from edge to edge rather than between centroids. Yang et al. (2001) suggest that it is the variance of the distribution of these distances that is most sensitive to inhomogeneity and to anisotropic clustering. The minimum separation distance is the shortest edge-to-edge distance between a point on one feature and that on its neighbor. As shown in **Figure 10.20**, this may be much different from the centroid-to-centroid distance, and in fact may involve a different neighbor.

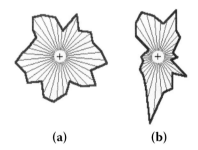

(a)   (b)

Figure 10.19 Rose plots of the number of features as a function of nearest-neighbor direction:
(a) Figure 10.16c;
(b) Figure 10.18.

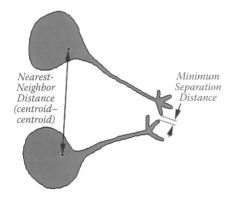

Nearest-
Neighbor
Distance
(centroid–
centroid)

The Euclidean distance map (EDM) introduced in **Chapter 8** can be used to determine those edge-to-edge distances, as shown in **Figure 10.21**. The skiz, or skeleton of the background between features, is a Voronoi tessellation of the image with one feature in each cell. The EDM of the cells in this tessellation measures the distance of every pixel from the lines in the skiz. Assigning these EDM values to the features (the masking operation used in **Chapter 8**) gives each feature a minimum brightness or distance value that is exactly half the distance to the feature with the closest boundary point, because the skiz passes halfway between features.

Figure 10.20 Centroid-to-centroid distance and minimum separation distance for two features.

A second method for measuring minimum separation distance is to construct the EDM of the background and find the local minima along the points in the skiz. These are midway between points of closest approach and provide another measurement of minimum separation distance between features. With this technique, it is possible to measure multiple minimum separations between different points on one feature and those on one or several neighbors.

In the case of a space-filling structure such as cells in tissue, grains in a metal, or fields in an aerial survey, the number of adjacent neighbors is also of interest. Since the features are separate, there must be a line of background pixels that separate them. In many cases, this line is produced by skeletonizing the original thresholded image of the boundaries and then inverting it to define the pixels. Counting the number of neighbors for each feature can be accomplished by checking the feature identification number of pixels that touch each of the background pixels in the boundaries. Building a table of the features that abut each other feature allows counting the number of such neighbors.

Labeling the features according to the number of neighbors can reveal some interesting properties of the structure. **Figure 10.22** shows the labeling of the number of neighbors in a dia-

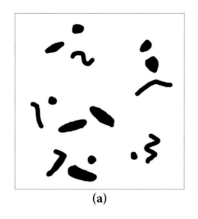 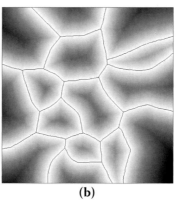 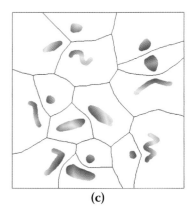

| (a) | (b) | (c) |

***Figure 10.21** Determining minimum separation distance: **(a)** features; **(b)** the skiz of the features and the EDM of the cells in the resulting Voronoi tessellation; **(c)** EDM values assigned to pixels in the features (shown in false color). The minimum value for each feature is half the edge-to-edge distance to its nearest neighbor.*

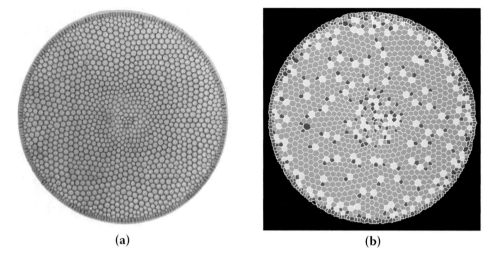

(a)   (b)

Figure 10.22 An image of a diatom **(a)** with the holes in the structure color-coded according to the number of sides **(b)**. The predominant shape is six-sided, but there are some five- and seven-sided holes that generally lie adjacent to each other.

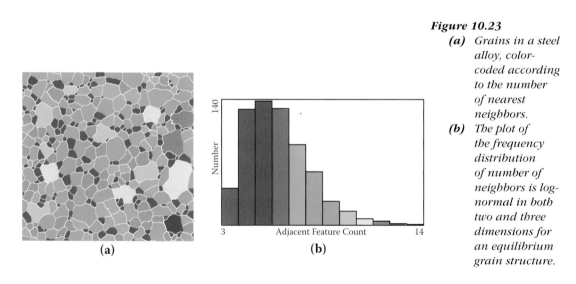

(a)   (b)

Figure 10.23
(a) *Grains in a steel alloy, color-coded according to the number of nearest neighbors.*
(b) *The plot of the frequency distribution of number of neighbors is log-normal in both two and three dimensions for an equilibrium grain structure.*

tom, an essentially two-dimensional structure. The pairing of the five- and seven-neighbor cells is apparent in the colored image, but might go unnoticed in the original. **Figure 10.23** shows a similar labeling for grains in a three-dimensional metal structure, as revealed on a two-dimensional section. For the equilibrium structure in a fully recrystallized metal, the distribution of nearest neighbors should be log normal (as it is for the example shown).

Alignment

One thing that people are very good at finding visually in images, but that requires a special computer algorithm, is the alignment and arrangement of features. We are so good at it that we sometimes find such alignments and arrangements when they do not really exist.

Chapter 2 illustrated constellations in the sky as a good example of this tendency to bring order to disorder.

There are many image-analysis situations in which an algorithmic procedure for determining an alignment or arrangement is needed. One of the most common is completing broken lines or fitting a line through a series of points, especially straight lines. Such a procedure is useful at all magnifications, from trying to locate electric transmission lines in reconnaissance photos (which show the towers but do not resolve the wires) to trying to delineate atomic lattices in transmission electron microscopy. In general, the points along the line are not spaced with perfect regularity and may not lie precisely on the line. This irregularity, and the sensitivity to noise in the form of other points or features in the field of view that are not part of the line, presents challenges.

Transforming the image into a different space provides the key. The use of Fourier space was shown in **Chapter 6**, but it is not generally a good choice for this purpose because of the irregularity of the point spacings. However, there are many other transform spaces that are less familiar. Converting the image data into Hough space can be used to find alignments (Ballard 1981; Duda and Hart 1972; Hough 1962). Different Hough spaces are used to fit different kinds of shapes, and it is necessary in most cases to have a pretty good idea of the type of line or other arrangement that is to be fit to the data. The following example shows the case of a straight line, since it is the simplest case as well as one of the most widely used.

The conventional way to fit a line to data points on a graph is the so-called "least squares" method, where the sum of the squares of the deviations of each point from the line is minimized. The Hough method accomplishes this automatically because it minimizes the deviations of points from the line and deals correctly with the case of the points not being uniformly distributed along the line.

Two parameters are required to define a straight line. In Cartesian coordinates, the equation of a straight line is

$$y = m \cdot x + b \tag{10.9}$$

where m is the slope and b the intercept. Because m becomes infinitely large for lines that are nearly parallel to the y-axis, this representation is not usually employed in the Hough transform. Instead, the polar-coordinate representation of a line is used. The radius ρ and angle ϕ (the length and angle of a normal to the line from the origin) define the line. It is possible either to allow the angle to vary from 0 to 2π and to keep ρ positive, or to allow ρ to be either positive or negative and to restrict the angle ϕ to a range of 0 to π. The latter convention is used in the examples that follow. The single black point in real (or pixel) space shown in **Figure 10.24a** generates the sinusoid in Hough space shown in **Figure 10.24b**. Each point along this sinusoid corresponds to the ρ-ϕ values for a single line passing through the original point. Several of these are shown in color, where the color of the point in Hough space matches the corresponding line in real space.

Hough space is an accumulator space. This means that it sums up the votes of many pixels in the image, and points in Hough space that have a large total vote are then interpreted as indicating the corresponding alignment in the real-space image. For the linear Hough transform, used to fit straight lines to data, the space is an array of cells (pixels, since this is another image) with coordinates of angle and radius. Every point in Hough space defines a single straight line with the corresponding angle ϕ and radius ρ that can be drawn in the real-space image. Although Hough space and its construction and use are described here in terms of finding alignments, the reader may recognize that the sinusoidal (polar coordinate) version of Hough

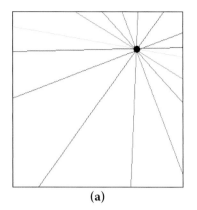

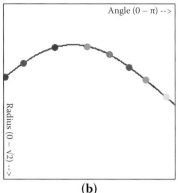

(a)   (b)

Figure 10.24 *Principle of the Hough transform. Each point in the real-space image produces*
(a) a sinusoidal line in Hough space representing all possible lines that can be drawn through it.
(b) Each point in Hough space corresponds to a line in real space. The real-space lines corresponding to a few of the points along the sinusoid are shown, with color coding to match them to the points.

space is identical to the Radon transform used in tomography and illustrated in **Chapter 12**.

To construct the Hough transform, every point present in the real-space image casts its votes into the Hough space for each of the lines that can possibly pass through it. As shown in **Figure 10.24**, this means that each point in the real-space image generates a sinusoid in Hough space. Each point along the sinusoid in Hough space gets one vote added to it for each point in the real-space image, or possibly a fractional vote based on the intensity associated with the point in real space. The superposition of the sinusoids from several points in real space causes the votes to add together where they cross. These crossing points in Hough space occur at values of ρ and ϕ that identify the lines that go through multiple points in the real-space image, as shown in **Figure 10.25**.

In this example, the duality of lines and points in real and Hough space is emphasized. Each of the five original points (labeled A, B, C, D, E) in real space produces a sinusoid (similarly labeled) in Hough space. Where these sinusoids cross, they identify points in Hough space (labeled 1, 2, 3, 4, 5, 6). These points correspond to straight lines back in real space (similarly labeled) that pass through the same points. Notice for instance that three lines pass through

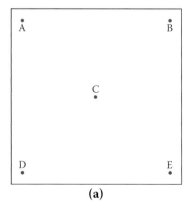

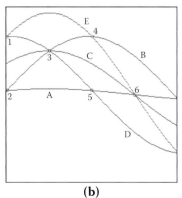

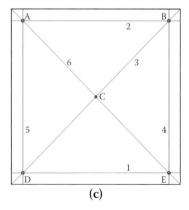

(a)   (b)   (c)

Figure 10.25 *Duality of lines and points in Hough and real space. Each of the labeled points in the real-space image (a) generates a sinusoidal line in the Hough-space image (b). The numbered crossing points in this space generate the lines in the real-space image (c).*

point A in real space and that the sinusoid labeled A in Hough space passes through the points for each of those three lines.

If there are several such alignments of points in the real-space image, then there will be several locations in the Hough transform that receive numerous votes. It is possible to find these points either by thresholding (which is equivalent to finding lines that pass through a selected minimum number of points) or by looking for local maxima (peaks in the Hough transform), for example by using a top-hat filter.

If the original real-space image contains a step in brightness, and an image processing operation such as a gradient (e.g., Sobel filter) has been applied, then an improved detection and fit of a line to the edge can be achieved by letting each point in the image vote according to the magnitude of the gradient. This means that some points have more votes than others, according to how probable it is that they lie on the line. The only drawback to this approach is that the accumulator space must be able to handle much larger integer values or real numbers when this type of voting is used, as compared with the simpler case where pixels in a binary image of feature points either have one vote or none. **Figure 10.26** shows an example of fitting a line to a noisy edge using a gradient operator and the Hough transform. Notice that the location of the maximum point in Hough space can take advantage of the same techniques for using the pixel values to interpolate a location to subpixel dimensions, as discussed at the start of this chapter. It is also possible to make the Hough space image as large as desired to achieve improved accuracy for the ρ, ϕ values.

For measurement of the spacings of parallel lines, Hough space reduces the problem to measuring the vertical distance between peaks in the transform. As shown in **Figure 10.27**, the application of a derivative to an SEM image of a line on an integrated circuit produces peaks

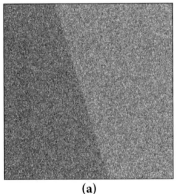

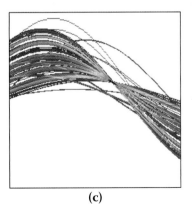
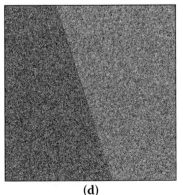
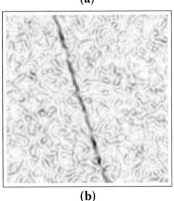

Figure 10.26 Fitting a line to a noisy edge using the Hough transform:
    (a) the original noisy image;
    (b) smoothing to reduce the noise and application of a Sobel gradient filter;
    (c) Hough transform produced from the gradient image;
    (d) line defined by the maximum point in the Hough transform.

(a)

(b)   (c)   (d)

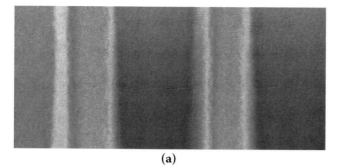

(a)

Figure 10.27 *Measuring line width and spacing on an integrated circuit:*
(a) *original SEM image,*
(b) *horizontal derivative applied;*
(c) *Hough transform, showing peaks corresponding to line edges and the distances that measure width and spacing.*

(b)

at the same ϕ value (corresponding to the line orientation), and measuring the distance in ρ provides direct measures of the width and spacing of the lines. Similarly, to measure the angular orientation of lines, it is straightforward to determine the ϕ values by position on the horizontal axis in the transform.

This proportional voting system is useful when there are many points to be fit, with some points being more important than others. Summing the votes according to brightness (or

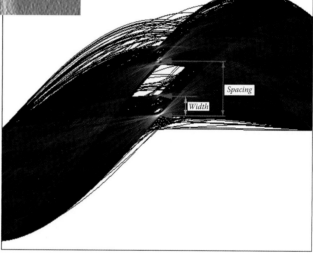

(c)

some value obtained from brightness) allows some points to be weighted more and produces an improved fit. **Figure 10.28** shows a Hough transform of a convergent beam electron diffraction pattern. The most intense spots in the Hough transform identify the spot alignments in the pattern.

The Hough transform can be adapted straightforwardly to other shapes, but the size and dimensionality of the Hough space used to accumulate the votes increases with the complexity of the shape. Fitting a circle to a series of points is used to measure electron diffraction patterns and to locate drilled holes in machined parts. The circular Hough transform requires a three-dimensional space, since three parameters are required to define a circle (the x,y coordinates of the center and the radius). Each point in the real-space image produces a cone of votes into this Hough space, corresponding to all of the circles of various radii and center positions that could be drawn through the point.

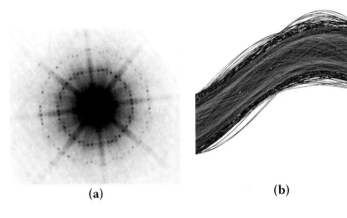

(a)   **(b)**

Figure 10.28
  (a) *Convergent beam*
      electron diffraction
      pattern and
  (b) *its Hough transform.*
      Each peak (several
      are marked) in the
      transform space
      identifies an alignment
      of points in the original
      pattern.

But if one or two of these values are known (for instance, the center of the electron diffraction pattern, or the radius of the drilled hole), or at least can vary over only a small range of possible values, then the dimensionality or size of the Hough space is reduced and the entire procedure becomes quite efficient. Accurately fitting a circle to an irregularly spaced set of points of varying brightness is a good example of the power that the Hough approach brings to image measurement. Since the brightness of the point resulting from multiple votes in Hough space that defines the circle is also the summation of those votes from all of the points on the corresponding circle in real space, this approach offers a useful way to integrate the total brightness of points in the electron diffraction pattern as well.

Figure 10.29 shows an example of using a circular Hough transform to locate the "best fit" circles in a selected area diffraction pattern. The pattern itself has bright spots with irregular locations around each circle. A human has little difficulty in estimating where the circles lie,

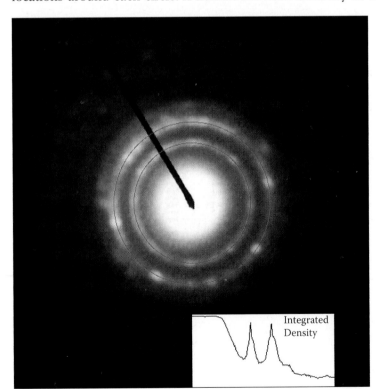

Figure 10.29 Selected area electron diffraction pattern with principal circles located by a circular Hough transform, and the integrated circular density of the pattern.

but this is generally a difficult thing for computer algorithms that examine only local pixel regions to accomplish. The Hough transform locates the circles and also provides a way to easily measure the integrated brightness around each circle. The values along the line located at the center of the pattern and parallel to the radius axis in Hough space gives the integrated radial intensity plot for the pattern. This approach has been used to identify asbestos fibers from the very spotty electron diffraction patterns obtained from a few fibers (Russ et al. 1989).

Figure 10.30 shows an example from machine vision in which the linear and circular Hough transforms are used to locate edges and holes accurately for quality control purposes or robotics guidance. Despite the overall noise in the image, the fit is quite rapid and robust. A separate region of interest (ROI) is set up covering the area where each feature is expected. In each ROI, a gradient operator is applied to identify pixels along the edge. These are then used to perform a Hough transform, one for a straight line and one

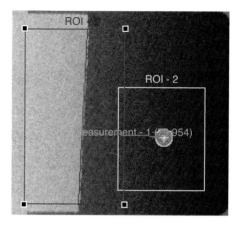

Figure 10.30 Use of the Hough transform to locate an edge and a circle in a machined part to measure the distance between them to subpixel accuracy.

for a circle. The resulting feature boundaries are shown, along with the measured distance between them. Since many pixels have contributed to each feature, the accuracy of location is much better than the pixel dimensions.

The Hough transform approach can be used to fit other alignment models to data as well. The limitation is that as the algebraic form of the model changes, each of the adjustable constants requires another dimension in Hough space. Constructing the transform and finding the maximum points becomes quite memory-intensive.

Counting features

Counting the number of features present in an image or field of view is one of the most common procedures in image analysis. The concept seems entirely straightforward, and it is surprising how many systems get it wrong. The problem has to do with the finite bounds of the field of view. In the case in which the entire field of interest is within the image, there is little difficulty. Each feature has simply to be defined by some unique point, and those points counted. Depending on how features are recognized, some algorithms may ignore features that are entirely contained within holes in other features. This problem most often arises when boundary representation is used to define the feature boundaries in the binary image. Determining whether or not it is appropriate to count features that lie inside other features is a function of the application, and consequently must be left up to the user.

When the field of view is a sample of the entire structure or universe, the result for the number of features is generally given as a number per unit area. When features intersect the edge of the field of view, it is not proper to count all features that can be seen. The most common solution to produce an unbiased result is to count those features that touch two adjacent edges, for instance the top and left, and to ignore those that touch the other two edges, for instance the right and bottom. This is equivalent to counting each feature by its lower right corner. Since

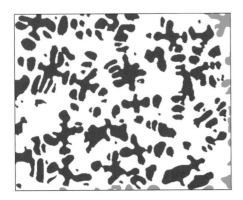

Figure 10.31 Counting features by a unique point. The red dots mark the right end of the lowest line of pixels in each feature. Features that touch the upper and left boundaries are counted, but those that touch the bottom and right edges are not.

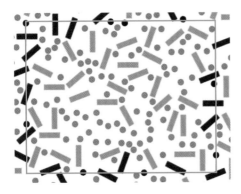

Figure 10.32 When an image area (shown by the green frame) lies within a larger field of objects to be measured, some will be intersected by the edge. These cannot be measured because their extent outside the image area is unknown. In the example shown, although there are three times as many small red features as long blue ones, the frame intersects (and removes from the measurement) twice as many blue ones, biasing the result.

each feature has one and only one lower right corner, counting those points is equivalent to counting the features (**Figure 10.31**). An alternative method counts features that intersect any edge as one-half. Both methods are equivalent for convex features, but can be fooled if the features have nonconvex shapes that produce more than a single intersection with the edge.

The "lower right corner" method is the same as determining the number of people in a room by counting noses. Since each person has one nose, the nose count is the same as the people count. If a smaller region were marked within the room, so that people might happen to straddle the boundary, counting the noses would still work. Anyone whose nose was inside the region would be counted, regardless of how much of the person lay outside the region. Conversely, any person whose nose was outside would not be counted, no matter how much of the person lay inside the region. It is important to note that, in this example, we can see the portions of the people that are outside the region, but in the case of the features in the image, we usually cannot (unless the counting is performed within a reduced area inside the full image, another possible solution). Any part of the feature outside the field of view is by definition not visible, and we cannot know anything about the amount or shape of the feature outside the field of view. That is why it is important to define a unique point for each feature to use in counting.

The convention of counting features that touch two edges only is not implemented in all systems. Some software packages offer a choice of counting all features regardless of edge touching, or counting only those features that do not touch any edge. Both are incorrect. Note that when measuring features, as opposed to counting them, a more complicated procedure will be needed. A feature that intersects any edge cannot be measured because it is not all imaged, and therefore no size, shape, or position information can be correctly obtained. If only the features in **Figure 10.32** that did not touch any edge were counted, the proportions of large and small features would be wrong. It is more likely that a large feature will touch an edge, and so a disproportionate fraction of the large features intersect an edge of the field of view and would not be measured.

There are two ways to correct for this bias. They produce the same result, but are implemented differently. The older method, which was used originally for manual measurements on photographic prints, is to set up a "guard frame" within the image, as shown in **Figure 10.33**. In this case, features that touch the lower and right edges of the field of view are not counted or measured, as before. Features that cross the top and left edges of the guard frame are counted and measured in their entirety. Features that lie only within the guard region are not counted, whether they touch the actual edge of the field of view or not. The number of features counted is then an accurate and unbiased measure of the number per unit area, but the area reported for the measurement is the area within the guard frame, not the entire area of the image. Since it is necessary for the guard region to be wide enough so that no feature can extend from within the active region across the guard region to the edge of the field, the active region can be reduced to a fraction of the total image area.

The second method uses the entire image area and measures all of those features that do not touch any

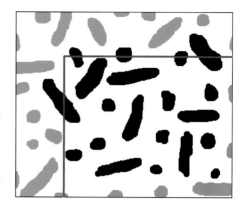

Figure 10.33 Measurement using a guard frame (shown in red). Features that lie partially or entirely within the inner region (black) are counted. Features that touch the outer edge of the image or lie entirely within the guard frame (blue or green) are not. The width of the guard region must be large enough that no feature can span it.

of the edges. To compensate for the bias arising from the fact that larger features are more likely to touch the edge and be bypassed in the measurement process, features are counted in proportion to the likelihood that a feature of that particular size and shape would be likely to touch the edge of a randomly placed image frame. The so-called adjusted count for each feature is calculated as shown in **Figure 10.34** as:

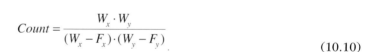

$$Count = \frac{W_x \cdot W_y}{(W_x - F_x) \cdot (W_y - F_y)}$$

$$(10.10)$$

where W_x and W_y are the dimensions of the image in the x and y directions (in pixels), and F_x and F_y are the maximum projected dimensions of the feature in those directions. These are simply the same bounding-box coordinates as discussed previously in connection with finding a feature's location. When the feature dimensions are small compared with the dimensions of the field of view, the fraction is nearly 1.0, and counting is little affected. When the feature extends across a larger fraction of the field of view in either direction, it is more likely that a random placement of the field of view on the sample would cause it to intersect an edge; thus the features that can be measured must be counted as more than one to correct for those that have been overlooked. The adjusted count factor makes that compensation.

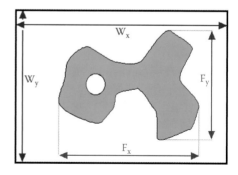

*Figure 10.34 Dimensions of the image and the feature used to adjust the count for correct results in **Equation 10.10**.*

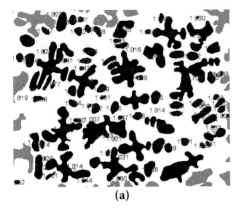

(a)

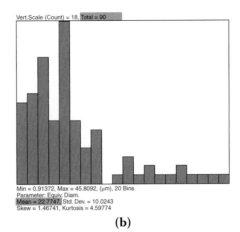

Vert.Scale (Count) = 18, Total = 90

Min = 0.91372, Max = 45.8092, (μm), 20 Bins
Parameter: Equiv. Diam.
Mean = 22.7747, Std. Dev. = 10.0243
Skew = 1.46741, Kurtosis = 4.59774

(b)

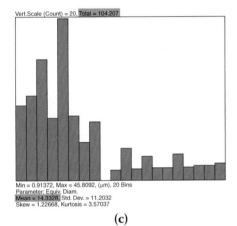

Vert.Scale (Count) = 20, Total = 104.207

Min = 0.91372, Max = 45.8092, (μm), 20 Bins
Parameter: Equiv. Diam.
Mean = 14.3328, Std. Dev. = 11.2032
Skew = 1.22668, Kurtosis = 3.57037

(c)

Figure 10.35 *Example of the adjusted count for features that vary in size:*

   (a) *adjusted count for each feature;*

   (b) *size distribution data with no adjustment to correct for bias due to features intersecting the edge;*

   (c) *using the adjusted count. Note the difference in the total number of features (90 vs. 104.2) and mean feature size (12.8 vs. 14.3 μm).*

Figure 10.35 shows an example of an image containing features of varying sizes and shapes, with the adjusted count for each. A plot of the size distribution shows that using the adjusted count significantly affects the mean size, the shape of the distribution, and the total number of features.

Special counting procedures

The examples of counting in the previous section make the tacit assumption that the features are separate and distinct. In earlier chapters, general procedures for processing images in either color or gray scale or the binary format resulting from thresholding were shown, whose goal was to accomplish the separate delineation of features to permit counting and measurement (for example, watershed segmentation). However, there are many specific situations in which these methods are not successful or, at best, are very difficult. Sometimes, if there is enough independent knowledge about the specimen, counting can be accomplished even in these difficult cases.

As an example, **Figure 8.77** in **Chapter 8** shows a collection of crossing fibers. Such structures are common in biological samples, wood fibers used in paper production, food technology, textiles, and many more situations. Since the fibers cross, from the point of view of the image-analysis algorithms, there is only a single feature present, and furthermore it touches all sides of the field of view. However, it is possible to estimate the number of fibers per unit area and the average fiber length. By thresholding the fibers and skeletonizing the resulting binary image, a series of crossing midlines is revealed. As discussed in **Chapter 8**, the endpoints of fibers can be counted as those pixels in the skeleton that have exactly one touching neighbor. This is not a perfect method, as there may be some ends of real fibers that are hidden because they lie exactly on another fiber, but in principle it is possible to detect these occurrences as well because they produce pixels with exactly three neighbors, and one of the angles at the junction will be about 180°. However, even without this refinement, half of the endpoint count gives a useful approximation for the number of fibers.

Recall that in the preceding section we decided to count each feature by one unique point. Counting the endpoints of fibers uses two unique points per fiber. If a fiber has one end in the field of view and the other end out, it is counted (correctly) as half a fiber, because the other end would be counted in a different field of view. Dividing by the image area gives the number of fibers per unit area. If the total length of fiber (the total length of the skeletonized midline) is divided by the number of fibers (one-half the number of ends), the result is the average fiber length. If the fibers are much longer than the field of view so that there are no endpoints present in most fields of view, it then becomes necessary to combine the data from many fields of view to obtain a statistically meaningful result.

Chapter 8, on binary image processing, presented several techniques for separating touching features. One of the more powerful, watershed segmentation, utilizes the Euclidean distance map (EDM). This operation assigns a gray-scale value to each pixel within a feature proportional to the distance from that pixel to the nearest background point. The valleys, or points that lie between two higher pixels in this distance map, are then used to locate boundaries that are ultimately drawn between features to separate them. Because there is a built-in assumption in this method that any indentation around the periphery of the feature cluster indicates a separation point, this technique is also known as convex segmentation.

If the purpose of the processing and segmentation is to count the features, there is a shortcut method that saves much of the computation. In the EDM, every local maximum point (pixels equal to or greater than all eight of their neighbors) is a unique point that represents one feature that will eventually be separated from its touching companions. Finding these so-called ultimate eroded points (UEPs) provides another rapid way to count the features present. In addition, the gray-scale value of that point in the EDM is a measure of the size of the feature, since it corresponds to the radius of the circle that can be drawn within it. **Figure 10.36** shows a simple example of some touching circles, with the ultimate points found from the EDM.

Counting touching particles presents many difficulties for image-analysis algorithms. If the particles are not simple convex shapes that lie in a single plane and happen to touch at their boundaries, watershed segmentation is not usually able to separate them successfully. A typical example of a more difficult problem is shown in **Figure 10.37**. The clay particles that coat this paper sample form a layer that is essentially one particle thick, but the overlaps are quite extensive. To obtain a useful estimate of the number of particles per unit area of the paper, it is again necessary to use the idea of finding one unique point per particle.

In this case, the way the image is formed by the scanning electron microscope provides an answer. Most of the particles are somewhat angular and have a single highest point that appears bright in the secondary electron image. These points (shown in the figure) can be isolated using a top-hat filter, as discussed in **Chapter 5**. In the example, the top-hat filter finds one unique point with a local maximum in brightness for most of the clay particles. A few are missed altogether because they have a shape or orientation that does not produce a character-

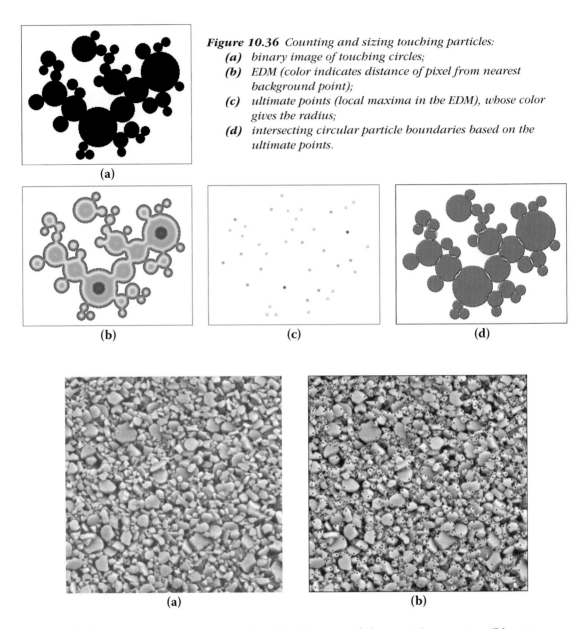

Figure 10.36 *Counting and sizing touching particles:*
(a) *binary image of touching circles;*
(b) *EDM (color indicates distance of pixel from nearest background point);*
(c) *ultimate points (local maxima in the EDM), whose color gives the radius;*
(d) *intersecting circular particle boundaries based on the ultimate points.*

(a)

(b)   (c)   (d)

(a)   (b)

Figure 10.37 *Counting overlapping particles:* *(a)* *SEM image of clay particles on paper;* *(b)* *superimposed points from a top-hat filter used to locate a local brightest point, which can be used to estimate the number of particles.*

istic bright point, and a few particles have sufficiently irregular shapes that they produce more than a single characteristic point. This means that counting the points gives only an estimate of the particle density on the paper, but for many quality control purposes this sort of estimate is sufficient to monitor changes.

The top-hat filter used in the preceding example is a specific case of a feature-matching or template operation that looks throughout the image for a particular pattern of bright and dark pixels. A more general case uses cross-correlation, as discussed in **Chapter 6**. The example in **Figure 10.38** shows an aerial photograph of trees in the forests on Mount Mitchell,

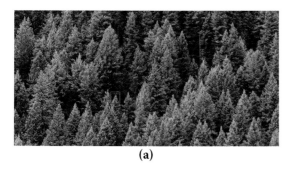 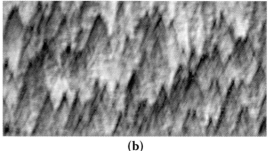

| (a) | (b) |

Figure 10.38 *Counting with cross-correlation: **(a)** aerial photograph of trees, with the red outline marking the treetop selected as the target for matching; **(b)** cross-correlation result, with identified treetops marked.*

North Carolina. It is desired to count the trees to monitor damage from acid rain. A useful shortcut method is to use the image of the pointed top of one tree as a target, cross-correlate with the entire image, and count the resulting spots. Of course, this method is only approximate; it does a good job of finding trees that are partially hidden or in front of another tree, but it will miss trees that do not have the characteristic pointed top of the target example.

Another approach to counting particles in clusters is shown in **Figure 10.39**. This is a TEM image of carbon black particles that are present in the form of clusters of varying sizes. If it can be assumed that the particles in the clusters are similar in size and density to the isolated one, then it becomes possible to estimate the number of particles in a cluster from the integrated density of the cluster. Measuring the average value of the integrated optical density of an isolated particle (or better, getting an average from several such measurements), and dividing that value into the integrated density of each cluster, provides a number that is an estimate of the number of particles present.

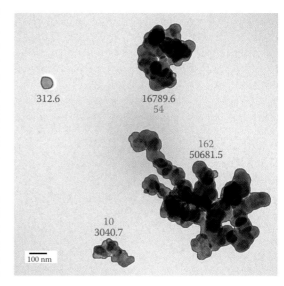

Figure 10.39 *Clusters of carbon black particles viewed in the TEM. Dividing the integrated optical density of each cluster (shown in red) by the integrated density for the single particle provides an estimate of the number of particles in each cluster (shown in blue).*

This method also works well with transmitted light images and with X-ray images. A calibration curve for density can be set up easily using Beer's law (exponential absorption with mass density), setting the background intensity value for the image to correspond to zero density and the darkest value to an arbitrary positive density. Since only ratios are used, no actual calibration standard is needed. Of course, it is assumed that no points in the image are completely black.

Feature size

The most basic measure of the size of features in images is simply the area. For a pixel-based representation, this is the number of pixels within the feature, which is determined simply by counting. For boundary representation, the area can be calculated as discussed previously (**Equation 10.4**). Of course, it must be remembered that the size of a feature in a two-dimensional image may be related to the size of the corresponding object in three-dimensional space in various ways, depending on how the image was obtained. The most common types of images are projections, in which the features show the outer dimensions of the objects, or planar sections, in which the features are slices across the objects. In the latter case, it is possible to estimate the volume of the objects using stereological methods, as discussed in **Chapter 9**. This chapter deals with measuring the feature size as represented in the image.

Figure 10.40 shows an image of spherical particles dispersed on a flat substrate. The diameters can be measured straightforwardly from such an image, subject to the usual restriction that there must be enough pixels in each feature to give a precise measure of its size. When the particles cover a large size range, as they do in this image, this creates a problem. The smallest features are only one or a few pixels in size, and are not well defined (in fact many are not even thresholded). A high-resolution camera or the combination of multiple images is needed to image both the large and small features at the same time. Even the higher-resolution camera does not provide enough pixels to accurately measure the smaller particles in this case. A solution would be to increase the optical magnification to enlarge the small particles, but then the large ones would be likely to intersect the edges of the screen and could not be measured.

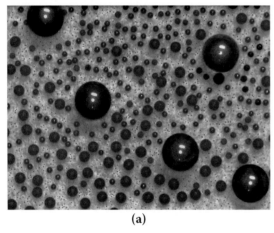

(a)

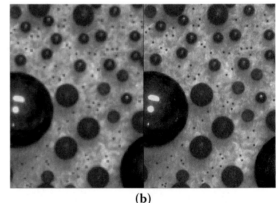

(b)

Figure 10.40 *Effect of resolution on feature measurement:*
- *(a)* *image of spherical particles dispersed on a flat surface;*
- *(b)* *enlarged portions of images obtained at video camera resolution and digital camera resolution;*
- *(c)* *same regions after thresholding, hole filling, and watershed segmentation. The smallest particles are all the same size, but because of limited resolution the image representations vary and do not adequately represent them.*

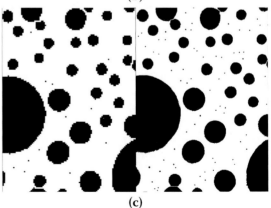

(c)

Multiple sets of data taken at several magnifications would be required.

Even for such a simple idea as counting pixels to determine feature area, some decisions must be made. For instance, consider the feature shown diagrammatically in **Figure 10.41**. Should the pixels within internal holes be included in the area or not? Of course, this depends on the intended use of the data. If the hole is a section through an internal void in an object, then it should be included if the area of the feature is to be related to the object volume, but not if the area is to be related to the object mass. But it is hard to know whether the hole is a section through a surface indentation in that object, in which case it would be more consistent to also include in the area those pixels in indentations around the feature boundary. As shown in the figure, this produces three different possible area measurements, the net area, the filled area, and the convex area.

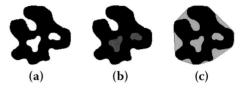

(a)   (b)   (c)

Figure 10.41 Three possible measures for feature area:
(a) net (8,529 pixels);
(b) filled (9,376 pixels);
(c) convex (11,227 pixels).

Measuring the first two can be accomplished as a simple pixel-counting exercise. In the process of labeling the pixels that touch each other and compose the feature, the presence of internal holes can be detected and the pixels within them counted. These pixels can be added back to the original image to fill in the holes, if desired. Determining whether to include those pixels in the area then becomes a user decision based on other knowledge.

The convex area is a slightly more difficult proposition. In some cases, a combination of dilation and erosion steps can be used to construct a convex hull for the feature and fill any boundary irregularities, so that pixel counting can be used to determine the area. However, on a square-pixel grid these methods can cause some distortions of the feature shape, as was shown in **Chapter 8**. Another approach that constructs an n-sided polygon around the feature is sometimes called the taut-string or rubber-band boundary of the feature, since it effectively defines the minimum area for a convex shape that will cover the original feature pixels.

By rotating the pixel coordinate axes, it is possible to locate the minimum and maximum points in any direction. The procedure of rotating the coordinate system, calculating new x',y' values for the points along the feature boundary, and searching for the minimum and maximum values is simple and efficient. For any particular angle of rotation α, the sine and cosine values are needed. In most cases these are simply stored in a short table corresponding to the specific angles used in the program. Then the new coordinates are calculated as

$$x' = x \cdot \cos\alpha + y \cdot \sin\alpha$$

$$y' = y \cdot \sin\alpha - x \cdot \cos\alpha \tag{10.11}$$

When this process is carried out at a series of rotational angles, the points with the largest difference in each rotated coordinate system form the vertices of the bounding polygon discussed above. For purposes of constructing the convex or taut-string outline, using a modest number of rotation steps will produce a useful result. For instance, with 18 steps (rotating the axes in 10° steps), a bounding polygon with 36 vertices and sides is obtained. **Figure 10.42** shows an example, comparing the bounding polygon to the equivalent circle and longest dimension for various feature shapes. It is only for extremely long and narrow features that more sides might be required to produce a bounding polygon that is a good approximation to the outer boundary.

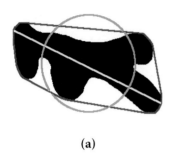 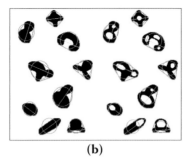

Figure 10.42 *Comparison of the bounding polygon (red), the longest chord (yellow), and equivalent circle (green, the circle centered at the feature centroid having the same area as the feature) for* **(a)** *an irregular feature and* **(b)** *an assortment of features.*

(a)

(b)

However the area is defined and determined, it of course requires that a conversion factor between the size of the pixels and the dimensions of the real-world structures be established. Calibration of dimension is usually done by capturing an image of a known standard feature and measuring it with the same algorithms, as used later for unknown features. For macroscopic or microscopic images, a measurement scale can be used. Of course, it is assumed that the imaging geometry and optics will not vary; this is a good assumption for glass lenses in light microscopes, but not necessarily for electron lenses used in electron microscopes. For some remote-sensing operations, the position and characteristics of the camera are known and the magnification is calculated geometrically. If the magnification scale varies from place to place in the image or in different directions, either because of the scene geometry (e.g., an oblique viewing angle) or instrumental variability (e.g., rate-dependent distortions in the scan of an atomic force microscope, see Nederbracht et al. 2004), severe problems in obtaining useful measurements may result.

Most modern systems use square pixels that have the same vertical and horizontal dimensions, but for distances to be the same in any direction on the image, it is also necessary that the viewing direction be normal to the surface. If it is not, then image warping, as discussed in **Chapter 4**, is required. Some systems, particularly those that do not have square pixels, allow different spatial calibrations to be established for the horizontal and vertical directions. For area measurements based on pixel counting, this is easy to handle. But for area calculation from boundary representation, or for length measurements and the shape parameters discussed below, this discrepancy can create serious difficulties.

Circles and ellipses

Once the area has been determined, it is often convenient to express it as the equivalent circular diameter. This is a linear size measure, calculated simply from the area as

$$Eq.\ Diam. = \sqrt{\frac{4}{\pi}\ Area}$$

(10.12)

Figure 10.42b shows several features of different sizes and shapes with the equivalent circle diameter shown based on the net feature area (pixel count). Features of different shape or orientation can fool the eye and make it difficult to judge relative size. The equivalent-diameter values offer a simple and easily compared parameter to characterize size.

Circles are widely used as size measures. Besides the equivalent circle with the same area as the feature, the inscribed or circumscribed circle can be used (**Figure 10.43**). The circumscribed circle is determined by using the corners of the bounding polygon, sorting through them to find the two or three that define the circle that encloses all of the others (see Arvo 1991 for a concise algorithm for finding the circle). The inscribed circle is easily found as the maximum value of the Euclidean distance map of the feature; the maximum pixel marks the center and its value gives the radius.

Since most real features have quite irregular shapes, it is not easy to find size measures that compactly and robustly describe them and allow for their classification and comparison. The use of an equivalent circular diameter is one attempt. Recognizing that not all features are equiaxial or even approximately round, some systems also provide for the use of an ellipse to describe the feature. The fact that the ellipse has two axes seems to allow describing both a size, a degree of departure from circularity, and even an orientation.

The major and minor axes of the ellipse can be determined in several different ways, however. These actually represent some quite different aspects of the feature size and shape, and they may be more misleading than helpful unless the user is fully aware of (and careful with) their various biases.

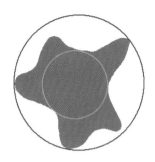

Figure 10.43 *Circumscribed and inscribed circles for an irregular feature. The centers of these circles do not generally coincide with each other or with the feature centroid.*

One definition of the ellipse axes can be taken from the minimum and maximum caliper dimensions of the feature, discussed above. The maximum caliper dimension does a good job of representing a maximum dimension and indicates the feature orientation, at least within the step size of the search (e.g., 10°). If this is taken as the major dimension of the ellipse, then the minor axis could be assigned to the minimum caliper dimension. This approach can lead to several difficulties. First, as pointed out above, this value can seriously overestimate the actual minimum dimension for a long, narrow feature. Second, the direction of the minimum dimension is not, in general, perpendicular to the maximum dimension. Third, the area of the resulting ellipse is not the same as the area of the feature.

Since basing the ellipse breadth on the minimum caliper dimension is suspect, a modification of this approach uses the maximum caliper dimension as the ellipse major axis, and then determines the minor axis to make the ellipse area agree with the feature area. Since the area of an ellipse is $(\pi/4) \cdot a \cdot b$, where a and b are the axes, once the major axis has been determined, the minor axis can be adjusted to agree with the feature area. The orientation angle can be either the approximate value determined from the steps used in the maximum-caliper-dimension search or the orientation angle determined from the moment calculation shown earlier (**Equation 10.7**). This tends to produce ellipses that have a longer and narrower shape than our visual perception of the feature.

The moments from **Equation 10.7** can also be used to produce a fitted ellipse. This is perhaps the most robust measure, although it requires the most calculation. Surprisingly, it seems to be little used. Instead, many systems fit an ellipse not to all of the pixels in the feature area, but instead to the pixels along the feature boundary. This procedure is computationally simple but very hard to justify analytically, and irregularities along any portion of the feature's boundary will significantly bias the ellipse.

Caliper dimensions

Caliper dimensions represent another description of feature size. The maximum caliper or maximum Feret's diameter is sometimes called the feature length, since it is the longest distance between any two points on the periphery. A projected or shadow dimension in the horizontal or vertical direction can be determined simply by sorting through the pixels or the boundary points to find the minimum and maximum coordinate values, and then taking the difference. These dimensions were introduced previously in terms of the bounding box around the feature, used to correct for its probability of intersecting the edge of a randomly placed image field.

The extreme points determined in a variety of directions were used to construct the bounding polygon described above. With such a polygon, the minimum and maximum caliper diameters can be found simply by sorting through the pairs of corner points. The pair of vertices with the greatest separation distance is a close approximation to the actual maximum dimension of the feature. The worst-case error occurs when the actual maximum chord is exactly halfway between the angle steps, and in that case the measured length is short by

$$Meas.Value = True\ Value \cdot \cos\left(\frac{\alpha}{2}\right)$$

(10.13)

For the previously mentioned example of 10° steps, the cosine of 5° is 0.996. This means that the measurement is less than 0.5% low. For a feature whose actual maximum dimension is 250 pixels, the value obtained by the rotation of coordinate axes would be 1 pixel short in the worst-case orientation.

If the same method is used to determine a minimum caliper dimension for the feature (sometimes called the breadth), this is equivalent to finding the pair of opposite vertices on the bounding polygon that are closest together. The error here can be much greater than for the maximum caliper dimension, because it depends on the sine of the angle and on the length of the feature rather than on its actual breadth. A narrow feature of length L and actual width W oriented at an angle the same 5° away from the nearest rotation step would have its breadth estimated as $L \cdot \sin(5) = 0.087 \cdot L$. This does not even depend on the width W, and if the actual length L is large and the width W is small, the potential error is very great.

Figure 10.44 shows a case in which the length is the appropriate measure and also easily determined as described. The sample is grains of rice (imaged by spreading them on a flatbed scanner and separating them by briefly holding a vibrator against the unit). USDA standards for long-grain rice specify the maximum fraction of grains that can be shorter than 6 mm. Measuring the distribution of lengths for these grains provides a fast and conclusive determination.

Of course, it is also possible to search directly for the maximum chord by sorting through the boundary points to find the two with maximum separation. There are various ways to speed up this search, which would otherwise have to calculate the sum of squares of the x- and y-coordinate differences between all pairs of boundary points. One is to consider only those points that lie outside the equivalent circle. Determining the area (in this case, the area including any internal holes) and converting it to the equivalent diameter with **Equation 10.12** provides a circle size. Locating that circle with its center on the feature centroid will cover any points inside the circle and leave just those points that lie farther away. These are candidates for the most widely separated pair.

An even more restrictive selection of the points to be searched can be obtained from the dimensions of the bounding rectangle. As shown in **Figure 10.45**, arcs drawn tangent to each

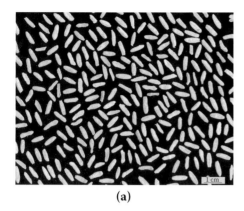 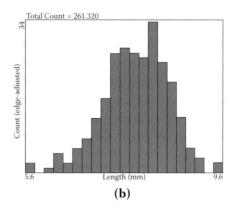

(a)　　　　　　　　　　　　　　　(b)

Figure 10.44 *Measurement of feature length:* **(a)** *original image (rice grains);* **(b)** *distribution plot for individual grain lengths.*

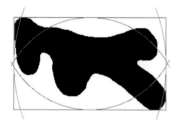

Figure 10.45 *Construction used to limit the search for boundary points giving the maximum chord. The blue arcs are drawn with centers in the middle of the horizontal edges of the bounding box, and the green arcs are drawn with centers in the middle of the vertical edges. Only the red points along the perimeter, which lie outside those arcs, are candidates for endpoints of the longest chord (shown in* **Figure 10.42a***).*

side with their center in the middle of the opposite side will enclose most of the boundary of the feature. Only points that lie on or outside the arcs need to be used in the search, and points lying outside one arc need only to be combined with those that lie outside the opposite arc. For a reasonably complex feature whose boundary may contain thousands of points, these selection algorithms offer enough advantage to be worth their computational overhead when the exact maximum dimension is needed.

Consider a feature shaped like the letter *S* shown in **Figure 10.46**. If this is a rigid body, say a cast-iron hook for use in a chain, the length and breadth as defined by the minimum and maximum caliper dimensions may have a useful meaning. On the other hand, if the object is really a worm or fiber that is flexible, and the overall shape is an accident of placement, it would be much more meaningful to measure the length along the fiber axis and the width across it. To distinguish these from the maximum and minimum caliper dimensions, often called length and breadth, these are sometimes called the fiber length and fiber width.

There are two quite different approaches to measuring these dimensions. Of course, it is still up to the user to determine which set of

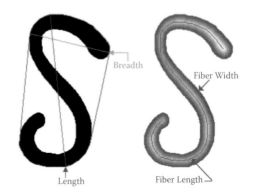

Figure 10.46 *Comparison of caliper dimensions (length and breadth) with values determined from the skeleton and EDM (fiber length and fiber width).*

parameters offers the most useful values for describing the features in a particular situation. One approach goes back to the binary image processing discussed in **Chapter 8**. If the feature is skeletonized, the length of the skeleton offers a measure of the length of the fiber. The skeleton is shorter than the actual length of the fiber, but this can be corrected by adding the value of the Euclidean distance map at each endpoint of the skeleton.

The length of the skeleton itself can be estimated by counting the pixel pairs that are present, keeping track of those that touch along their edges and their corners (because on a square-pixel grid the distance between pixels that touch diagonally is greater by $\sqrt{2}$ than the distance orthogonally). This produces a slight overestimate of the length. Instead of using the strictly geometric distances of 1.0 and 1.414, Beckers and Smeulders (1989) have shown that calculating the length as

$$Length = 0.948 \cdot (num.orthogonal\ nbors)$$

$$+ 1.340 \cdot (num.diagonal\ nbors) \qquad (10.14)$$

gives a mean error of only 2.5% for straight lines that run in all directions across the square-pixel grid, but of course larger errors can be encountered for specific worst-case orientations.

A more accurate measurement can be performed by fitting a smooth curve to the pixels. There are several ways to accomplish this, including polynomial and Bezier curves. The most efficient and robust method is to use the same technique described below for perimeter measurement, in which the image is smoothed and a superresolution line interpolated through the pixels.

As described in **Chapter 8**, combining the skeleton with the Euclidean distance map also provides a tool to measure the fiber width. Assigning the gray-scale values from the EDM to the skeleton pixels along the midline represents the radius of the inscribed circle centered at each point. Averaging these values for all of the points in the midline gives the mean fiber width, and it is also possible to measure the variation in width.

An older and less accurate (but still used) approach to estimating values for the length and width of a fiber is based on making a geometric assumption about the fiber shape. If the feature is assumed to be a uniform-width ribbon of dimensions F (fiber length) and W (fiber width), then the area (A) and perimeter (P) of the feature will be $A = F \cdot W$ and $P = 2 \cdot (F + W)$. The area and perimeter parameters can both be measured directly. As we will see below, the perimeter is one of the more troublesome values to determine. But for a ribbon with smooth boundaries, as assumed here, the perimeter can be measured with reasonable accuracy. Then the fiber length and width can be calculated from the measured perimeter and area as

$$F = \frac{P - \sqrt{P^2 - 16 \cdot A}}{4}$$

$$W = \frac{A}{F} \qquad (10.15)$$

Minor modifications to this model can be made, for example by assuming that the ends of the ribbon are rounded instead of square, but the principle remains the same. The difficulties with this approach are its sensitivity to the shape model used and the problems associated with perimeter measurement. If the feature is not of uniform width or is branched, for instance, the average width obtained from the skeleton and EDM still produces a consistent and meaningful result, while the calculation in **Equation 10.15** may not.

Perimeter

The perimeter of a feature seems to be a well-defined and familiar geometrical parameter. Measuring a numerical value that really describes the object turns out to be less than simple, however. Some systems estimate the length of the boundary around the object by counting the pixels that touch the background. Of course, this underestimates the actual perimeter because, as noted above for the measurement of skeleton length, the distance between corner-touching pixels is greater than it is for edge-touching pixels. Furthermore, this error depends on orientation, and the perimeter of a simple object like a square will change as it is rotated under the camera. **Figure 10.47** compares the variation in perimeter as a square is rotated, obtained by counting the edges of pixels with the more accurate value obtained from the chain code. The sensitivity of measurement values to orientation is often used as a test of system performance.

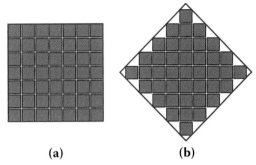

(a)   **(b)**

Figure 10.47 Comparison of perimeter estimation by chain code vs. summation of pixel edge lengths, as a function of orientation:
(a) sum of edges = 28 units, chain code perimeter = 28.0 units;
(b) sum of edges = 36 units, chain code perimeter = 20·2 = 28.28 units.

If boundary representation is used to represent the feature, then the Pythagorean distance between successive points can be summed to estimate the perimeter as

$$Perim. = \sum_i \sqrt{\left(x_i - x_{i-1}\right)^2 + \left(y_i - y_{i-1}\right)^2}$$

(10.16)

In the limiting case of chain code, the links in the chain used for boundary representation are either 1.0 or 1.4142 pixels long, and these can be used to estimate the perimeter. It is only necessary to count the number of odd chain code values and the number of even chain code values, since these distinguish the orthogonal or diagonal directions. The same argument as used above for the irregularity of the pixel representation of the midline applies to the boundary line, and the modified values from **Equation 10.14** can be applied to reduce bias.

The most accurate perimeter measurements, with the least sensitivity to the orientation of feature edges, are obtained by fitting smooth curves to the feature boundaries. The easiest way to do this is by antialiasing the edge so that the pixels near the edge have gray values that fill in the steps (Neal et al. 1998), as shown in **Figure 10.48**. The process uses the Laplacian of a Gaussian (LoG) filter, which is also used in operators such as the Canny edge locator discussed

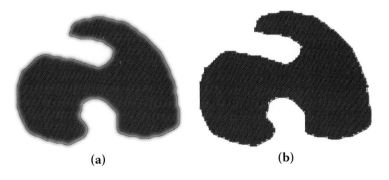

(a)   **(b)**

Figure 10.48 Fitting a smooth boundary for perimeter measurement:
(a) contour line on a smoothed (antialiased) feature;
(b) the contour line superimposed on the original pixels.

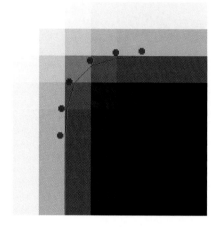

Figure 10.49 Interpolating the
boundary between points on
the edges of the smoothed pixels,
showing how an abrupt corner is
smoothly rounded.

in **Chapter 5**, to define the location of feature boundaries most accurately.

The actual boundary is constructed by drawing and measuring straight-line segments across the antialiased pixels. These line segments are drawn between points along the pixel edges that are linearly interpolated based on the gray-scale values. The points correspond to the location where the midpoint value would lie, treating the pixels as spaced points. This is functionally equivalent to enlarging the image using superresolution and bilinear interpolation to fill in the new, tiny pixels, as shown in **Figure 10.49**.

While the superresolution boundary measurement technique is very accurate and extremely robust to feature rotation, the basic difficulty with perimeter measurements is that, for most objects, the perimeter itself is very magnification dependent. Higher image magnification reveals more boundary irregularities and hence a larger value for the perimeter. This is not the case for area, length, or the other size dimensions discussed previously. As the imaging scale is changed so that the size of individual pixels becomes smaller compared with the size of the features, measurement of these other parameters will of course change, but the results will tend to converge toward a single best estimate. For perimeter, the value usually increases.

In many cases, plotting the measured perimeter against the size of the pixels, or a similar index of the resolution of the measurement, produces a plot that is linear on logarithmic axes. This kind of self-similarity is an indication of fractal behavior, and the slope of the line gives the fractal dimension of the boundary. This will be used below as a measure of feature shape.

Even if the feature boundary is not strictly fractal (implying the self-similarity expressed by the linear log-log plot of perimeter vs. measurement scale), there is still often some increase in measured perimeter with increased imaging magnification. The only exceptions are smooth (Euclidean) objects such as membranes or surfaces in which tension or an energy term enforces local smoothness for physical reasons. This dependency on resolution makes the perimeter values suspect as real descriptors of the object, and at least partially an artifact of the imaging method and scale used. Further, any noise in the image can be expected to cause a roughening of the boundary and increase the apparent perimeter.

Figure 10.50 shows a simple example. Random gray-scale noise is superimposed on six circles. The original circles were drawn with a diameter of 80 pixels, and had a measured area of 5024 pixels and perimeter of 254 pixels (close to the ideal values of 5026.5 and 251.3, respectively). Measuring a series of noisy images will produce a value for the area that averages to the correct mean as pixels are added to or removed from the feature. But the perimeter is always increased, as shown by the results in **Table 10.1**. The variation in area measurements is only 0.5%, while that for the perimeter measurements is 8%, and the mean value is far too high. This bias introduced by noise in the imaging procedure is another cause for concern in perimeter measurements. Smoothing the boundary with a morphological opening or closing would reduce the perimeter values and their variation, but this assumes independent knowledge that the boundaries should be smooth.

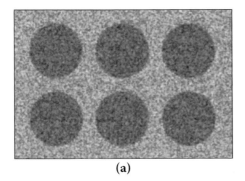 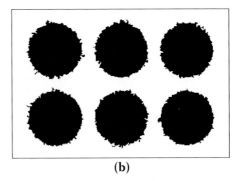

(a)   (b)

Figure 10.50 *Six identical circles superimposed on gray-scale noise* *(a)*, *then thresholded, internal holes filled* *(b)*, *and measured. The results are shown in* *Table 10.1*.

Table 10.1. Results from Circle Measurements in Figure 10.50

Circle	Area	Perimeter
1	5027	358
2	5042	338
3	4988	343
4	5065	391
5	5020	372
6	5030	313
Average	5028.7	352.5
Std. dev.	25.4 (0.5%)	27.4 (8%)
Original	5024	254

If perimeter is measured, there is still the need to choose among the same three alternatives discussed for area measurements. The total perimeter includes the length of boundaries around any internal holes in the feature. The net or filled perimeter excludes internal holes and just measures the exterior perimeter. The convex perimeter is the length of the convex hull or bounding polygon, and bridges over indentations around the periphery of the feature. The same considerations as mentioned in connection with area measurement apply to selecting whichever of these measures describes the aspect of the feature that is important in any particular application.

Describing shape

Shape is not something that human languages are well equipped to deal with. We have few adjectives that describe shape, even in an approximate way (e.g., rough vs. smooth, or fat vs. skinny). In most conversational discussions of shapes, it is common to use a prototypical object instead ("shaped like a …"). Of course, this assumes we all agree about the important aspects of shape found in the selected prototype. Finding numerical descriptors of shape is difficult because the correspondence between them and our everyday experience is slight, and the parameters all have a "made-up" character. When adjectival descriptors for classes of shapes are assigned based on subjective human examination, it can be difficult to find any measurement procedure that yields results that are in agreement with those labels and that would permit automatic (and consistent) computer-based measurement. For instance Les and Les (2005) propose classes such as "thin, convex, cyclic, complex" and so forth, but do not indicate how these groups are defined except by example.

The oldest class of numeric shape descriptors are simply combinations of size parameters, arranged so that the dimensions cancel out. Length/breadth, for example, gives us aspect ratio, and changing the size of the feature does not change the numerical value of aspect ratio. Of course, this assumes we have correctly measured a meaningful value for length and breadth, as discussed previously.

Since there are dozens of possible size parameters, there are hundreds of ways that these can be combined into a formally dimensionless expression that might be used as a shape descriptor. In fact, there are only a few relatively common combinations, but even these are plagued by inconsistency in naming conventions. **Table 10.2** summarizes some of the most widely used

Table 10.2. Representative Shape Descriptors

$$Formfactor = \frac{4\pi \cdot Area}{Perimeter^2}$$

$$Roundness = \frac{4 \cdot Area}{\pi \cdot Maximum\ Diameter^2}$$

$$Aspect\ Ratio = \frac{Maximum\ Diameter}{Minimum\ Diameter}$$

$$Elongation = \frac{Fiber\ Length}{Fiber\ Width}$$

$$Curl = \frac{Length}{Fiber\ Length}$$

$$Convexity = \frac{Convex\ Perimeter}{Perimeter}$$

$$Solidity = \frac{Area}{Convex\ Area}$$

$$Compactness = \frac{\sqrt{\left(\frac{4}{\pi}\right)Area}}{Maximum\ Diameter}$$

$$Modification\ Ratio = \frac{Inscribed\ Diameter}{Maximum\ Diameter}$$

$$Extent = \frac{Net\ Area}{Bounding\ Rectangle}$$

shape parameters calculated as combinations of size measurements, with the names used in this text. It is important to be aware that some systems define the parameters as the inverse of the formula shown or that they may omit constant multipliers such as π. Also, in any particular instrument, the same calculation may be called by some quite different name or use the name shown for a different relationship in the table. Some of the descriptors have a history of successful use in particular fields of application. For example, the modification ratio (ratio of inscribed to circumscribed circle, also called the radius ratio) is used to measure the cross section of extruded fibers, such as those used in making carpeting. The increase in the inscribed diameter of these "star-shaped" cross sections indicates wear on the spinnerets and corresponds to less flexibility in the fibers and an increase in their weight. Before the advent of computer measurement, this ratio was determined by visually fitting circle templates to the cross sections.

The burden placed on the user, of course, is to be sure that the meaning of any particular shape descriptor is clearly understood and that it is selected because it bears some relationship to the observed changes in the shape of features, since it is presumably being measured to facilitate or quantify some comparison. **Figure 10.51**, **Figure 10.52**, **Figure 10.53**, and **Figure 10.54** illustrate several of these parameters that distinguish between features. In general, each of them captures some aspect of shape, but of course none of them is unique. An unlimited number of visually quite different shapes can be created with identical values for any of these dimensionless shape parameters (**Figure 10.55**).

Figure 10.51 shows four variations on one basic shape, which is stretched and smoothed by erosion and dilation. Notice that *formfactor* varies with surface irregularities, but not with overall elongation, while *aspect ratio* has the opposite behavior. **Figure 10.52** shows four variations on one basic shape with the values of several shape parameters. Examination of the values shows that the parameters vary quite differently from one shape to another. **Figure 10.53** shows several shapes with the values of their *curl*.

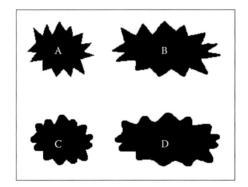

Shape	Formfactor	Aspect Ratio
A	0.257	1.339
B	0.256	2.005
C	0.459	1.294
D	0.457	2.017

Figure 10.51 *Variations on a shape produced by erosion/dilation and by horizontal stretching. The numeric values for formfactor and aspect ratio (listed below) show that stretching changes the aspect ratio and not the formfactor, and vice versa for smoothing the boundary.*

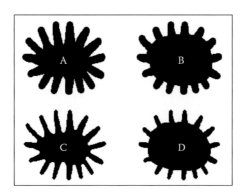

Shape	Roundness	Convexity	Solidity	Compactness
A	0.587	0.351	0.731	0.766
B	0.584	0.483	0.782	0.764
C	0.447	0.349	0.592	0.668
D	0.589	0.497	0.714	0.768

Figure 10.52 *Another set of four related shapes with the numeric values for their measured shape parameters.*

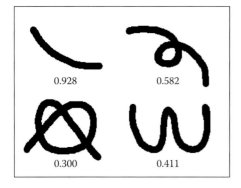

Figure 10.53 *Four features with different values of curl, indicating the degree to which they are "curled up."*

Figure 10.54 illustrates the differences between these parameters in a different way. The "features" are simply the 26 capital letters, printed in a font with a serif (Times Roman). In each horizontal row, the colors code the value of a different measured shape parameter. The variation in each set is from red (largest numeric value) to magenta (smallest numeric value). The independent variation of each of the shape factors is remarkable. This suggests on the one hand that shape factors can be a powerful tool for feature identification. However, the large variety of such factors, and the inability of human vision to categorize or estimate them, reminds us that people do not use these parameters for recognition. The relative values measured for the various shapes would be different if another font was substituted.

Another group of simple dimensionless shape parameters can be calculated based on the various definitions of location introduced above. For a perfectly symmetrical feature, such as a circle, the centroid and geometric center (the center of the bounding circle) will coincide. If the feature is not symmetric, the distance between these two points, normalized by dividing by the radius of the bounding circle, produces a value between 0 and 1 that measures the asymmetry. The distance between the unweighted centroid (in which all pixels in the feature are counted equally) and the weighted centroid (in which pixels are counted according to some calibrated density function) can be used in the same way.

Similar ratios using other location measures are less useful. For example, the center determined as an average of the location of perimeter pixels is very resolution-sensitive. As shown

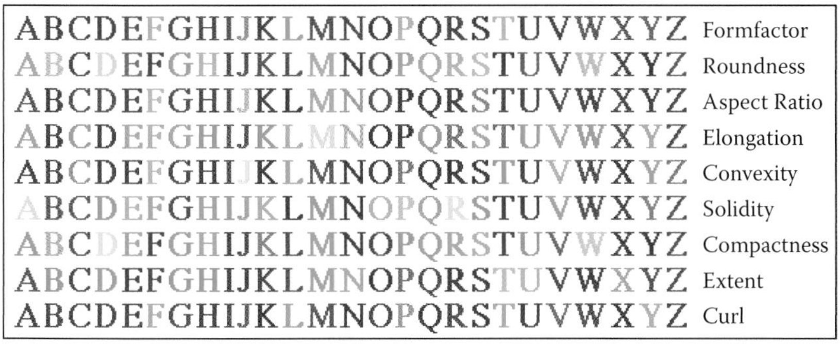

ABCDEFGHIJKLMNOPQRSTUVWXYZ	Formfactor
ABCDEFGHIJKLMNOPQRSTUVWXYZ	Roundness
ABCDEFGHIJKLMNOPQRSTUVWXYZ	Aspect Ratio
ABCDEFGHIJKLMNOPQRSTUVWXYZ	Elongation
ABCDEFGHIJKLMNOPQRSTUVWXYZ	Convexity
ABCDEFGHIJKLMNOPQRSTUVWXYZ	Solidity
ABCDEFGHIJKLMNOPQRSTUVWXYZ	Compactness
ABCDEFGHIJKLMNOPQRSTUVWXYZ	Extent
ABCDEFGHIJKLMNOPQRSTUVWXYZ	Curl

Figure 10.54 *Measurement of a series of shapes (letters of the alphabet). In each row, the colors of the features code the relative numeric value (red = high, magenta = low) of a different shape parameter corresponding to the labels.*

previously in **Figure 10.12**, the roughness on the right side of the circle becomes visible only at high magnification, but would shift the apparent center of this visually symmetrical feature.

Likewise, the center of the largest inscribed circle in the feature also creates difficulties. Many nonconvex features have more than one maximum in their Euclidean distance map. Each local maximum is the center of an inscribed circle (tangent to at least three points on the feature boundary). Using the largest as a measure of size is meaningful in some circumstances, but the location is rarely useful. As shown in **Figure 10.56**, the inscribed circle center is undefined when the feature has more than one equal maximum in the EDM, and even when it does not, the location is insensitive to many aspects of feature shape.

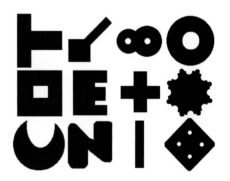

Figure 10.55 *A set of features that are visually distinct but have identical values for the formfactor (= 0.44). This is a reminder that dimensionless ratios capture only a single and very limited piece of information about "shape."*

Fractal dimension

Quite a few of the shape parameters discussed above and summarized in **Table 10.2** include the perimeter of the feature. As noted previously, this is often a problematic size parameter to measure, with a value that is an artifact of image resolution and magnification. In fact, the concept of perimeter may be fundamentally flawed when it is applied to many real objects. If a real-world object is actually fractal in shape, the perimeter is undefined. Measuring the object boundary at higher magnification will always produce a larger value of perimeter. Consider a cloud, for example: what is the length of the boundary around the projected image of the cloud? Measurements covering many orders of magnitude, from a single small cloud in the sky observed by visible light, up to entire storm systems viewed by radar or from weather satellites, show that the perimeter of clouds obeys fractal geometry. Presumably this trend would continue at smaller and smaller scales, at least down to the dimensions of the water molecules. What, then, does the perimeter really mean?

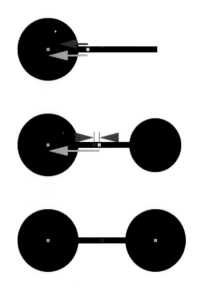

Figure 10.56 *Location of the geometric center (yellow), center of the inscribed circle (cyan), and centroid (red), showing the effects of asymmetry and shape.*

Objects that are fractal seem to be the norm rather than the exception in nature. Euclidean geometry, with its well-defined and mathematically tractable planes and surfaces, is usually only found as an approximation over a narrow range of dimensions where mankind has imposed it, or in limited situations where a single energy or force term dominates (e.g., surface tension). Roads, buildings, and the surface of the paper on which this book is printed are flat, straight, and Euclidean, but only in the dimension or scale that humans perceive and control. Magnify the paper surface and it becomes rough. Look at the roads from space and they cease to be straight. The use of fractal dimensions to describe these departures from Euclidean lines and planes is a relatively recent conceptual breakthrough that promises a new tool for describing roughness, and also shape.

Briefly, the fractal dimension is the rate at which the perimeter (or surface area in three dimensions) of an object increases as the measurement scale is reduced. There are a variety of ways to measure it. Some are physical, such as the number of gas molecules that can adhere to the surface in a monolayer, as a function of the size of the molecule (smaller molecules probe more of the small surface irregularities and indicate a larger surface area). Some are most easily applied in frequency space by examining the power spectrum from a two-dimensional Fourier transform, as discussed in **Chapter 14**. Others can be measured on a thresholded binary image of features.

Perhaps the most widely known fractal measurement tool is the so-called Richardson plot. This was originally introduced as a procedure applied manually to the measurement of maps. Setting a pair of dividers to a known distance, the user starts at some point on the boundary and strides around the perimeter. The number of steps multiplied by the stride length produces a perimeter measurement. As the stride length is reduced, the path follows more of the local irregularities of the boundary, and the measured perimeter increases. The result, plotted on log-log axes, is a straight line whose slope gives the fractal dimension. Deviations from linearity occur at each end: at long stride lengths, the step may miss the boundary altogether, while at short stride lengths the finite resolution of the map limits the measurement.

When boundary representation is used for a feature, a Richardson plot can be constructed from the points by calculating the perimeter using the expression in **Equation 10.16**, and then repeating the same procedure using every second point in the list, every third point, and so forth. As points are skipped, the average stride length increases and the perimeter decreases, and a Richardson plot can be constructed. When every nth point in the list is used to estimate the perimeter, there are n possible starting positions. Calculating the perimeter using each of them, and averaging the result, gives the best estimate. The stride length for a particular value of n is usually obtained by dividing the total perimeter length by the number of strides. In all these procedures, it is recognized that there may be a partial stride needed at the end of the circuit, and this is included in the process.

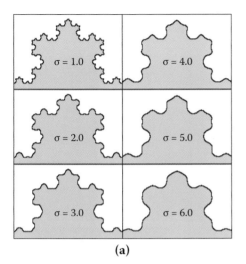

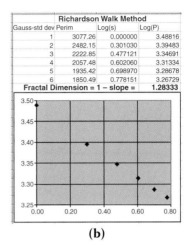

The table in image 2 contains:

Richardson Walk Method			
Gauss-std dev Perim		Log(s)	Log(P)
1	3077.26	0.000000	3.48816
2	2482.15	0.301030	3.39483
3	2222.85	0.477121	3.34691
4	2057.48	0.602060	3.31334
5	1935.42	0.698970	3.28678
6	1850.49	0.778151	3.26729
Fractal Dimension = 1 – slope =			1.28333

(a) (b)

Figure 10.57 *Progressive Gaussian smoothing of the outline **(a)** of a Koch snowflake (theoretical fractal dimension = 1.262) and plotting the perimeter measurement **(b)** produces a Richardson measurement of the fractal dimension.*

When the x,y coordinates of the boundary points are digitized in a grid, a variability in the stride length is introduced. Unlike the manual process of walking along a map boundary, there may not be a point recorded at the location one stride length away from the last point, and so it is necessary either to interpolate from the actual data or to use some other point and alter the stride length. Interpolation makes the tacit assumption that the boundary is locally straight, which is in conflict with the entire fractal model. Altering the stride length may bias the plot. Combined with the general difficulties inherent in the perimeter measurement procedure, the classical stride length method is usually a poor choice for measuring digitized pixel images.

However, using the superresolution perimeter measurement approach, another method closely related to the Richardson technique can be employed. By applying smoothing kernels with progressively larger Gaussian standard deviations to blur the boundary, small irregularities are removed and the perimeter decreases. Plotting the measured perimeter vs. the standard deviation of the smoothing kernel, on log-log axes, produces a straight line whose slope gives the feature fractal dimension, as shown in **Figure 10.57**. The dimension is a value greater than 1 (the topological or Euclidean dimension of a line) and less than 2 (the dimension of a plane), and can be thought of as the degree to which the line spreads out into the plane.

A second measurement technique was shown in **Chapter 7** on binary image processing. Dilating the boundary line by various amounts is equivalent to sweeping a circle along it. The area of the band swept over by the circle does not increase directly with the radius because of the irregularities of the boundary. Plotting the area swept out by the circle (sometimes called the sausage) vs. the radius (again on log-log axes) produces a line whose slope gives the fractal dimension. This Minkowski technique is actually older than the Richardson method. It works well on pixel-based images, particularly when the Euclidean distance map is used to perform the dilation. Using the cumulative histogram of the Euclidean distance map of the region on either side of the feature outline to construct the log-log plot is quite insensitive to feature orientation and much faster than iterative dilation, since it assigns to each pixel a gray-scale value equal to the distance from the boundary. Examples of this method were shown in **Chapter 8**; **Figure 10.58** shows the measurement of the same Koch snowflake.

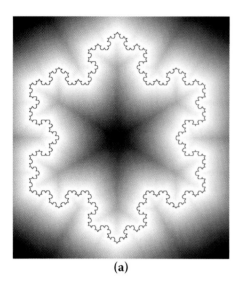

(a)

Minkowski Sausage Method				
EDM Value	Pixel Count	Cumulative	Log(R)	Log(A)
1	9330	9330	0.00000	3.96988
2	5956	15286	0.30103	4.18429
3	5198	20484	0.47712	4.31141
4	4052	24536	0.60206	4.38980
5	4448	28984	0.69897	4.46216
6	4008	32992	0.77815	4.51841
7	4070	37062	0.84510	4.56893
8	3416	40478	0.90309	4.60722
9	3580	44058	0.95424	4.64402
10	3620	47678	1.00000	4.67832
11	3640	51318	1.04139	4.71027
12	3796	55114	1.07918	4.74126
13	3096	58210	1.11394	4.76500
14	3260	61470	1.14613	4.78866
15	3074	64544	1.17609	4.80986
16	3114	67658	1.20412	4.83032
17	2978	70636	1.23045	4.84903
18	3082	73718	1.25527	4.86757
19	3072	76790	1.27875	4.88530
20	3000	79790	1.30103	4.90195
Fractal Dimension = 2 – Slope =			1.28257	

(b)

Figure 10.58 The cumulative histogram of the EDM around the
  (a) outline of the Koch snowflake
  (b) produces a Minkowski measurement of the fractal dimension.

The Minkowski method produces a dimension that is not necessarily identical to the Richardson method (or to other fractal dimension procedures), and so it is important when comparing values obtained from different specimens to use only one of these methods. Neither method gives the exact result expected theoretically for the Koch snowflake fractal, due to the finite resolution available in the pixel image, but both are reasonably close.

A third approach to fractal dimension measurement produces another dimension, similar in meaning but generally quite different in value to the others discussed. The Kolmogorov dimension is determined by grid counting. A mesh of lines is drawn on the image, and the number of grid squares through which the boundary passes is counted. When this number is plotted on log-log axes vs. the size of the grid, the slope of the line again gives a dimension, as shown in **Figure 10.59**. Automatic implementation and application to a pixel image can be performed by progressively coarsening the image into 2 × 2, 3 × 3, etc., blocks of pixels, and is sometimes called mosaic amalgamation. This is perhaps the fastest method but has both the poorest accuracy and the least numeric precision because it has the fewest steps and hence the fewest points to establish the line.

However it is determined, the fractal dimension produces a single numeric value that summarizes the irregularity or "roughness" of the feature boundary. This is one of the aspects of feature "shape" that humans notice and use in a qualitative way for classifying or comparing features. **Figure 10.60** shows examples of several natural fractals. The relationship between this boundary and what it may represent in three dimensions is not simple. For the case of a section through an isotropic surface, the boundary fractal dimension is smaller than the surface fractal dimension by exactly 1.0, the difference between the topological dimension of the sectioning plane and the volume in which the object resides. However, few real surfaces are

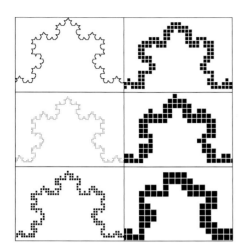

Kolmogorov Box Count Method			
Cell Width	Count	Log(w)	Log(N)
1	4020	0	3.60422605
2	1985	0.30103	3.29776051
3	1294	0.47712125	3.11193428
4	928	0.60205999	2.96754798
5	713	0.69897	2.85308953
6	603	0.77815125	2.78031731
7	521	0.84509804	2.71683772
8	432	0.90308999	2.63548375
9	363	0.954242251	2.55990663
10	322	1	2.50785587
Fractal Dimension = − Slope =			1.093811

Figure 10.59 Counting the boxes of increasing size through which the boundary of the Koch snowflake passes, and the log-log plot. The plot is a straight line, but the slope does not give an accurate fractal dimension for the shape.

perfectly isotropic, and in the presence of preferred orientation this simple relationship breaks down. Even more serious, if the boundary measured is a projected outline of a particle, the boundary irregularities will be partially hidden by other surface protrusions, and the measured fractal dimension will be too small by an amount that depends on the size of the particle and on its roughness. There is no general correction for this, and despite the fact that this procedure is very commonly used, the data obtained (and their subsequent interpretation) remain very open to question. **Chapter 14** discusses the meaning and method of measurement for fractal surfaces that have dimensions between 2 and 3.

Harmonic analysis

The fractal dimension attempts to condense all of the details of the boundary shape into a single number that describes the roughness in one particular way. There can, of course, be an unlimited number of visually or topologically different boundary shapes with the same fractal dimension or local roughness. At the other extreme it is possible to use a few numbers to preserve all of the boundary information in enough detail to effectively reconstruct the details of its appearance.

Harmonic analysis is also known as spectral analysis, Fourier descriptors, or shape unrolling (Barth and Sun 1985; Beddow et al. 1977; Bird et al. 1986; Diaz et al. 1989; Diaz et al. 1990; Ehrlich and Weinberg 1970; Ferson et al. 1985; Flook 1982; Granlund 1972; Kaye et al. 1983; Kuhl and Giardina 1982; Lestrel 1997; Persoon and Fu 1977; Rohlf 1990; Rohlf and Archie 1984; Schwartz and Shane 1969; Verschueren et al. 1993; Zahn and Roskies 1972). It begins by converting the boundary to a function of the form radius (angle) or $\rho(\phi)$. As shown in **Figure 10.61**, a radius drawn from the feature centroid is drawn as a function of angle and plotted to unroll the shape. This plot obviously repeats every 2π, and as a periodic or repeat-

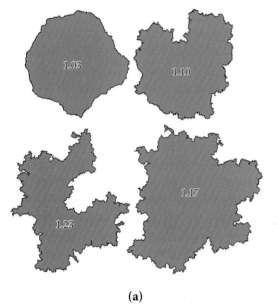

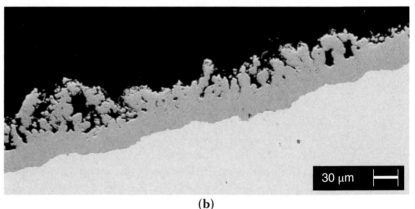

Figure 10.60 *Several fractal outlines with varying fractal dimensions:*
(a) *shapes of dust particles sampled at different altitudes;*
(b) *cross section of oxide coating on a metal (fractal dimension = 1.505).*

(a)

30 μm

(b)

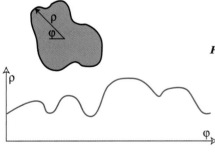

Figure 10.61 *Illustration of the procedure for unrolling a feature profile.*

ing function is straightforwardly subjected to Fourier analysis. This allows the determination of the *a* and *b* terms in the series expansion

$$\rho(\varphi) = a_0 + a_1 \cos(\varphi) + b_1 \sin(\varphi) + a_2 \cos(2\varphi) + b_2 \sin(2\varphi) + \dots \qquad (10.17)$$

It is often more convenient to represent the values as amplitude *c* and phase δ for each sinusoid:

Figure 10.62 *Reconstruction of a real feature outline (an extraterrestrial dust particle) from the first 5, 10, and 25 terms in the Fourier expansion. (From Kaye, B.H. 1989. Courtesy of B. Kaye, Laurentian University.)*

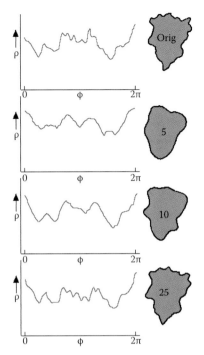

$$c_i = \sqrt{a_i^2 + b_i^2}$$

$$\rho(\varphi) = \sum c_i \cdot \sin(2\pi i \varphi - \delta_i)$$

(10.18)

This series continues up to an *n*th term equal to half the number of points along the periphery. However, it is a characteristic of Fourier analysis that only the first few terms are needed to preserve most of the details of feature shape. As shown in **Figure 10.62**, with only one or two dozen terms in the series, the original shape can be redrawn to as good a precision as the original pixel representation. In many cases, the phase information δ_i for each term in the series can be discarded without much effect on the shape characterization (although of course the phase is essential for actually reconstructing the original shape), and a single coefficient c_i can be used for each frequency. The first few values of c in the harmonic or Fourier expansion of the unrolled boundary thus contain a great deal of information about the feature shape.

Of course, this method has serious problems if the shape is reentrant such that the radial vector is multivalued. To avoid that problem, an alternative approach to shape unrolling plots, instead, the slope of the line as a function of the distance along the line. This plot is also a repeating function and can be analyzed in exactly the same way, but it has the problem that the slope may be infinite at some points. Plotting the change in slope as a function of position overcomes that limitation.

The chain code boundary representation of a feature already contains the slope-vs.-position information along the boundary, but with the problem that the data are not uniformly spaced (the diagonal links being longer than the horizontal and vertical ones). An effective way to deal with this is to replace each horizontal link with five shorter conceptual sublinks, each in the same direction, and each diagonal line with seven shorter sublinks. The ratio of 7:5 is close enough to $\sqrt{2}$ for practical purposes, and the total number of sublinks along the boundary is still reasonably short. A plot of the link value (which indicates direction) vs. position now gives the unrolled feature shape. Performing a Fourier analysis of the sequence of values along the chain code for the feature produces a list of c_i values that contain the shape information. The interpretation of these values is hampered because of the discontinuity in the direction numbers.

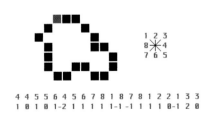

4 4 5 5 6 4 5 6 7 8 1 8 7 8 1 2 2 1 3 3
1 0 1 0 1-2 1 1 1 1 1 1-1 -1 1 1 1 0-1 2 0

Figure 10.63 *Chain code representations for a feature outline starting at the blue pixel, showing the conventional direction codes and below them the differential chain code.*

Chain code need not be recorded as a set of values corresponding to each of the eight possible pixel neighbor directions. The difficulty in analysis that results from the discontinuity between directions 8 and 1 can be overcome by converting to the "first difference chain code" (or differential chain code), as shown in **Figure 10.63**.

This is just the differences between values using modulo arithmetic, so that a zero indicates the edge proceeding straight ahead in whatever direction it was already, positive values indicate bends of increasing angle in one direction and negative values indicate the opposite direction. In this form, the shape is rotation-invariant (at least in 45° steps), except for the fact that the links in the original chain were not all of the same length. It is also easier to find corners by defining them as a minimum absolute magnitude for the net change in value over some distance (Freeman and Davis 1977).

The most general of the harmonic analysis techniques is to plot the x- and y-projections of the feature outline, treat them as real and imaginary parts of a complex number, and perform a Fourier transform on the resulting values as a function of position along the boundary, as shown in **Figure 10.64**. Again, this results in a set of c_i values that summarize the feature shape.

These can be compared among classes of objects, using standard statistical tests such as stepwise regression or principal-components analysis, to determine which of the terms may be useful for feature classification or recognition. In a surprising number of cases, this approach proves to be successful. The identification of particles in sediments with the rivers that deposited them, the correlation of the shape of foraminifera with the water temperature in which they grew, distinguishing the seeds from various closely related plant species, and the discrimination of healthy from cancerous cells in Pap smears are but a few of the successes of this approach.

Despite its successes, the harmonic analysis approach has been little used outside of the field of sedimentation studies and some paleontological applications. In part this neglect is due to the rather significant amount of computing needed to determine the parameters, and the need to apply extensive statistical analysis to interpret them. However, as computer power has continued to increase and cost to decrease, this cannot be the major reason any longer. The probable cause is that the frequency terms are unfamiliar and have no obvious counterpart in human vision. The shape information that we extract visually from images does not reveal these numeric factors. The distinction between two sediments based on the seventh harmonic coefficient can be understood intellectually to somehow represent a difference in the amplitude of that frequency in the boundary irregularities of the object, but to a human observer that is masked by other variables. The success of the approach illustrates the power of computer-based measurement algorithms to surpass human skills not only quantitatively (in terms of accuracy and precision), but even qualitatively (in terms of the types of things that can be measured). But that does not mean that humans feel comfortable using such tools.

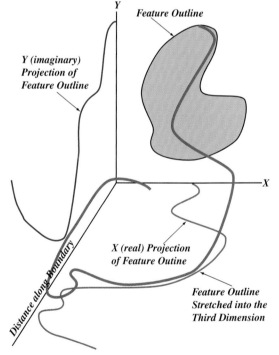

Figure 10.64 Unrolling a feature shape by plotting the x- and y-coordinates of boundary points as a function of position along the boundary (the red and blue graphs), and combining them as real and imaginary parts of complex numbers (the magenta line).

Topology

Harmonic analysis uses characteristics of feature shape that are quite different from those that human vision selects. On the other hand, topological parameters are those that seem most obvious to most observers. When asked to differentiate the stars on the U.S., Australian, and Israeli flags, we do not use color, dimension, or angles; we use the number of points. The most obvious difference between a disk and the letter "O" is not the slight ellipticity of the latter, but the presence of the central hole. Topological properties are quite different from metric ones. If the feature were drawn onto a sheet of rubber, stretching it to any size and with any distortion will not change the topology. Smoothing an irregular outline does not alter the topological information.

Some topological properties of features can be determined directly from the pixel array, such as the number of internal holes. Other properties, such as the number of points on the stars shown in **Chapter 8**, are most readily determined using the skeleton. The skeleton consists of pixels along the midline of the features. Pixels with only a single touching neighbor are endpoints, while those with more than two neighbors are branch points. Counting the branch and endpoints, and the number of loops (holes), provides a compact topological representation of feature characteristics. **Figure 8.74a** in **Chapter 8** showed an example of using the skeleton endpoints to characterize shape.

These characteristics of features are important to visual classification and recognition, as can be easily shown by considering our ability to recognize the printed letters in the alphabet regardless of size and modest changes in font or style. Many character-recognition programs that convert images of text to letters stored in a file make heavy use of topological rules.

Chapter 8 (**Figure 8.71**) illustrates the various components of the skeleton that can be distinguished and may be useful for topological shape characterization. Some, like the number of endpoints, number of loops or holes, and number of nodes, are determined simply by counting. Others, such as the relative length of external branches (which terminate at an endpoint) and internal branches (which extend from one node to another) can be used in dimensionless ratios like those introduced above, and require measurement and calculation. It is also useful (as described in **Chapter 8**) to combine the skeleton with the Euclidean distance map to determine properties such as the width of irregular structures.

Figure 10.65 illustrates this with several features that vary in the number, length, and breadth of their arms. The features are sufficiently complex that immediate visual recognition and labeling does not occur, so trying to find the single pair of features that share the same values for all three parameters is difficult. Measuring each feature's shape parameters using the skeleton (and EDM) indicates which two features are the pair (the ones with five long, thick arms), but they have intentionally not been labeled in the illustration.

Another topological property of a feature is its number of sides. In the case of a space-filling structure such as cells in tissue, grains in a metal, or fields in an aerial survey, the number of sides that each feature has is the number of other features it adjoins. This

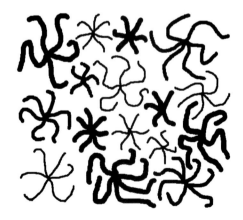

Figure 10.65 Complex branched features with combinations of three levels of external branch length, line width, and number or branches. Which two share the same values for all three parameters?

was discussed previously in its relation to relative feature position. Labeling the features according to the number of neighbors can reveal some interesting properties of the structure, as was shown in **Figure 10.22** and **Figure 10.23**.

The number of sides that a feature has can also be described in another way. If corner points are defined as arbitrarily abrupt changes in boundary direction, then counting the number of sides can be accomplished directly from the chain code. A second approach that is less sensitive to minor irregularities in the boundary pixels uses the convex or bounding polygon. As described above, this polygon is usually constructed with some fixed and relatively large number of sides. For instance, performing rotation of axes in 10° steps would form a 36-sided polygon. Several of the vertices in this polygon may coincide or lie close together if the feature shape has a relatively sharp corner. Setting an arbitrary limit on the distance between vertices that can be merged (usually expressed as a percentage of the total polygon perimeter) allows collecting nearby vertices together. Of course, counting the vertices is equivalent to counting the sides. Setting a threshold for the minimum length of the polygon side (again, usually as a percentage of the total perimeter) to consider it as a representation of a side of the feature can also be used to count sides.

None of the four types of shape characterization (dimensionless ratios, fractal dimension, harmonic analysis, and topology) is completely satisfactory. One (harmonic analysis) is too unfamiliar and different from the human interpretation of shape. One (dimensionless ratios) is convenient for calculation but not very specific. One (fractal dimension) corresponds well with the human idea of boundary roughness but does not capture more macroscopic aspects of shape. And one (topology) is just the opposite in that it represents the gross aspects of feature shape but not the fine details. In real situations, several complementary techniques may be needed.

Three-dimensional measurements

Many of the previously discussed measurement procedures for two-dimensional images generalize directly into three dimensions. Images acquired by confocal light microscopy, seismic imaging, medical or industrial tomography, and even in some cases serial sectioning can be represented in many different ways, as discussed in **Chapter 13**. But for image processing and measurement purposes, an array of cubic voxels (volume elements, the three-dimensional [3-D] analog to pixels or picture elements) is the most useful. Image processing in these arrays uses neighborhoods just as in two dimensions, although these contain many more neighbors and consequently take longer to apply (in addition to the fact that there are many more voxels present in the 3-D image).

Image measurements still require identifying those pixels that are connected to each other. In two dimensions, it is necessary to decide between an eight-connected and a four-connected interpretation of touching pixels. In three dimensions, voxels can touch on a face, edge, or corner (6-, 18-, or 26-connectedness), and again the rules for features and background cannot be the same. It is more difficult to identify internal holes in features, since the entire array must be tested to see if there is any connection to the outside. However, the logic remains the same.

This consistency of principle applies to most of the measurements discussed in this chapter. Summing up the numeric values of voxels in a CT (computed tomography) or MRI (magnetic resonance imaging) data set, or a series of confocal microscope images (or some property calculated from the voxel values) to obtain the total density, or water content, or whatever property has been calibrated, is straightforward. So are location measurements using the voxel moments. Orientations in three-dimensional space require two angles instead of one. Neighbor relationships (distance and direction) have the same meaning and interpretation as in two dimensions.

The three-dimensional analog to feature area is feature volume, obtained by counting voxels. The caliper dimensions in many directions and the bounding polyhedron can be determined by rotation of coordinate axes and searching for minimum and maximum points. Of course, getting enough rotations in three dimensions to fit the polyhedron adequately to the sample is much more work than in two dimensions. In fact, everything done in three-dimensional voxel arrays taxes the current limits of small computers: their speed, memory (to hold all of the voxels), displays (to present the data using volumetric or surface rendering), and the human interface. For instance, with a mouse, trackball, or other pointing device it is easy to select a location in a two-dimensional image. How do you accomplish this in three dimensions? Various schemes have been tried (some requiring a real-time stereo display), none with wide acceptance. The development of gaming consoles may offer some techniques for the future.

It was noted previously that perimeter is a somewhat troublesome concept and a difficult measurement in two dimensions. The analog to perimeter in three dimensions is the surface area of the feature, and it has all of the problems of perimeter plus some more. The idea that the surface area may be an artifact of voxel resolution remains, and this is exacerbated by the somewhat coarser resolution usually available in three-dimensional images. If the voxels are not cubic, the problem gets harder. Measuring the length of the perimeter accurately is difficult in two dimensions. For a three-dimensional surface, the boundary representation is the list of coordinates of vertices of a polyhedron with triangular facets. Calculating the area of a triangle from its three corners is straightforward, but knowing which three points to use for any particular triangle is not. As a very simple example, consider four points as shown in **Figure 10.66**. There are two different ways the surface can be constructed between them, each with different surface areas (sometimes both are calculated and the average used).

Boundary representation in two dimensions relies on the fact that there is only one path around any feature, no matter how complicated. This is not true in three dimensions. There is no unique order in which triangular facets between boundary voxels must or can be followed. In fact, for objects that are topologically shaped like a torus (have at least one open hole through them), there is no guarantee that a continuous surface path will completely cover the surface and reach all points on it. This means that there is no convenient analog to chain code, and many of the two-dimensional measurements that were based on it become difficult to perform in three dimensions.

Likewise, the three-dimensional skeleton is harder to obtain. There are actually two "kinds" of skeleton that can be calculated for voxel arrays. One is the set of midlines, and the other is a set of midplanes. The latter is formed by connecting the skeleton lines in each plane section, while the former is a connection between the junction points

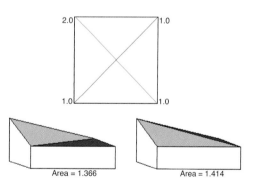

Figure 10.66 *Tiling a surface with triangular facets has two different solutions. In this simple example, the elevation of the four corners of a square are shown. Triangles can be constructed using either diagonal as the common line. As shown, this produces a surface that is either convex or concave, with a surface area of either 1.366 or 1.414 square units.*

or nodes of the skeletons in each plane section. This set of midlines can also be obtained as a medial-axis transform (MAT) by using the three-dimensional analog of the Euclidean distance map to find the centers of inscribed spheres. Neither type of skeleton by itself captures all of the topological properties of the feature. The planes can show twists and protrusions not visible in the line skeleton, for example.

Measuring the length of a voxel line is similar to a pixel line. Since there are three ways the voxels can touch, the rule shown earlier in **Equation 10.14** must be extended, to become:

$$Length = 0.877 \cdot (num.\ of\ face\text{-}touching\ neighbors)$$
$$+\, 1.342 \cdot (num.\ of\ edge\text{-}touching\ neighbors) \qquad (10.19)$$
$$+\, 1.647 \cdot (num.\ of\ corner\text{-}touching\ neighbors)$$

Euler's relationship (**Equation 8.3** in **Chapter 8**) still holds, but deciding what voxel patterns to count to identify the important topological properties of the structure is not entirely clear.

Most of the shape parameters calculated as ratios of dimensions have simple (although equally limited) generalizations to three dimensions. Harmonic analysis can also be performed in three dimensions by expressing the radius as a function of two angles and performing the Fourier expansion in two dimensions. Since there is no analog to chain code or the description of slope as a function of position, the method is restricted to shapes that are not reentrant or otherwise multiple-valued (only one radius value at each angle). Fractal dimensions are very important for dealing with three-dimensional surfaces and networks, although in most cases it remains easier to measure them in two-dimensional sections.

In fact, this generalization holds for most image-measurement tasks. The practical difficulties of working with three-dimensional voxel arrays are considerable. The size of the array and the amount of computing needed to obtain results are significant. Because of memory restriction, or limitations in the resolution of the 3-D imaging techniques, the voxel resolution is usually much poorer than the attainable pixel resolution in a two-dimensional image of the structure. Consequently, to the extent that the needed information can be obtained from two-dimensional images and related by stereology to the three-dimensional structure, that is the preferred technique. It is faster and often more precise.

This approach does not work for all purposes. Strongly anisotropic materials require so much effort to section in enough carefully controlled orientations, and are still so difficult to describe quantitatively, that three-dimensional imaging may be preferred. And above all, topological properties of the structure such as the number of objects per unit volume, or the connectivity of a network, are simply not accessible on two-dimensional sections (although the Disector technique using two such parallel planes to sample three-dimensional topology was presented in **Chapter 9**). Many aspects of three-dimensional topology can only be studied in three dimensions, and consequently require three-dimensional imaging, processing, and measurement.

The discussion of two-dimensional images was based on an array of pixels, and so far all of the discussion of 3-D images has assumed they consist of voxels. But as will be discussed in **Chapter 13**, many three-dimensional structures are studied by obtaining a set of parallel section planes that are relatively widely spaced. This is generally described as a "serial section" technique, although physical sectioning is not always required. Constructing the object(s) from the sections is discussed in that chapter as well.

Measuring the features from the sections is computationally straightforward. The volume is estimated as the summation of section area times section spacing, and the surface area can be estimated as the summation of the section perimeter times section spacing. But few objects have perfectly smooth surfaces. The section perimeter will reveal the roughness in the plane of the section. However, the reconstruction technique generally connects the section profiles together with planes that are perfectly smooth, which underestimates the surface area. Even if the surface is smooth, the volume and surface area will be underestimated if it is curved.

Aligning the sections correctly is vital both to correctly understand the topology of the structure and to measure the volume and surface. **Chapter 13** illustrates some of the potential difficulties. When the sections are very closely spaced, these problems are reduced. In the limit when the section spacing is the same as the resolution within the individual section images, it is equivalent to a cubic voxel array. This is generally preferred for measurement purposes.

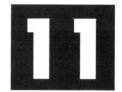

Feature Recognition and Classification

Template matching and cross-correlation

Recognition and classification are essentially complementary functions that lie at the "high end" (i.e., that require the most complicated algorithms) in the field of image analysis (Duda and Hart 1973). Classification is concerned with establishing criteria that can be used to identify or distinguish different populations of objects that appear in images. These criteria can vary widely in form and sophistication, ranging from example images of prototypical representatives of each class, to numeric parameters for measurement, to syntactical descriptions of key features. Recognition is the process by which these tools are subsequently used to find a particular feature within an image. It functions at many different levels, including such different processes as finding a face in an image, or matching that face to a specific individual.

Generally, computers tend to be better than humans at classification because they are not distracted by random variations in noncritical parameters and can extract meaningful statistical behavior to isolate groups. Sometimes these groups are meaningful, but in other cases they may not correspond to the intended classes. On the other hand, people are generally much better (or at least faster) at recognition than are computers, because they can detect the few critical factors that provide identification of familiar objects. But humans do not fare well with unfamiliar objects or even with unfamiliar views of common ones.

Various recognition and classification techniques involve an extremely broad range of complexities. At the low end, operations such as scanning UPC bar codes (Universal Product Code) on supermarket packaging or automatic sorting and routing of mail to the proper zip code are based on careful design of the target to facilitate the reading function. These are normally detected by linear scans rather than acquiring full images as used elsewhere in this text, and UPC codes are symmetric (with black-and-white reversal) so that the scan can be used in either direction.

The basic statistical processing behind classification is independent of image analysis, since the parameters used for classification and identification can come from any source. A good introduction to the statistics can be found in textbooks (Devijver and Kittler 1980; Hand 1981; Haykin 1993; Pao 1989; Schalkoff 1992; Stefik 1995, and many others).

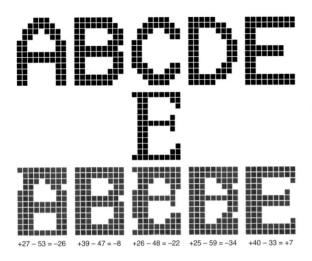

+27 − 53 = −26   +39 − 47 = −8   +26 − 48 = −22   +25 − 59 = −34   +40 − 33 = +7

Figure 11.1 Matching each of the five letter templates (top row) with a target letter (center) produces a net score (sum of red matched pixels minus blue unmatched pixels) that is greatest for the correct match.

Probably the lowest level functionality that utilizes two-dimensional pixel images is the restricted optical character recognition (OCR) of the type applied to processing checks. The characters printed on bank checks are restricted to numerals 0 to 9 and a few punctuation marks. Furthermore, the characters are in a fixed size, location, and orientation, and are printed in a special font designed to make them easily distinguishable. In such highly constrained situations, a technique known as template matching provides fast results with minimum computation.

The example in **Figure 11.1** shows the application of template matching to the letters A through E. A template consisting of black pixels that cover the shape of each target character is stored in memory. Each letter to be recognized is combined with all of the stored templates using an exclusive-OR function to count the number of pixels that match and those that do not. The template that gives the highest net score (number of matches minus number of misses) is selected as the identification of the character. In some implementations, the net score can be normalized by dividing by the number of black pixels in the template, if this varies substantially for the various characters.

In the example, the templates are not exact and have enough width and extra pixels to cover a modest range of variation in the target character, but obviously cannot handle widely divergent fonts or styles. The similarities in shape between several letters (e.g., B and E) do not create a serious problem, and the error rate for this approach is very low, provided that the characters meet the assumptions of size, orientation, font, etc., that are built into the templates. The presence of small amounts of noise due to dirt, etc., is tolerated as well.

This type of template matching is a rather specialized and restricted case of cross-correlation, which can be used for gray-scale or color images as well as binary pixel arrays. **Chapter 6**, on image processing in Fourier space, introduced the cross-correlation procedure as a technique for matching a target image with a second image to locate brightness patterns. This method can be applied to images of text or any other features, provided that a set of representative target images can be established.

It is not necessary to perform cross-correlation using a Fourier transform. When the target is relatively small, it may be efficient to perform the mathematics in the spatial domain. The target pattern is moved to every possible position in the image, and at each location i,j, the cross-correlation value is summed according to **Equation 11.1** to produce a result, as shown in **Figure 11.2**.

$$\frac{\displaystyle\sum_{x=0}^{s}\sum_{y=0}^{s} B_{x+i,y+j}\cdot T_{x,y}}{\sqrt{\displaystyle\sum_{x=0}^{s}\sum_{y=0}^{s} B^2_{x+i,y+j}\cdot \sum_{x=0}^{s}\sum_{y=0}^{s} T^2_{x,y}}} \qquad (11.1)$$

where B and T are the pixel brightness values for the image and target, respectively, and the summations are carried out over the size s of the target. This value is very high where bright pixels in the target and image align, and the denominator normalizes the result for variations in overall brightness of the target or the image. In addition to providing a quantitative measure of the degree of match, the correlation score can be scaled appropriately to produce another gray-scale image in which brightness is a measure of how well the target matches each location in the image, and this image can be processed with a top-hat filter, or thresholded, to detect matches.

```
273988999347777
169777226863788
884344924776533
595654879169484
947178683495148
555859563987931              357
251725634726494              595
836369422783746              753
455884199783686
755415676823233
533566267995831
596523999583624
884745817766595
454864279724597
737488293735571
      Image                  Target
```

```
5866533257677
7646343663764
6463665725833
5435877118434
4356666277253
5352565354634
3535910457555
6677104776356
7642366563354
4557436765473
7675167666540
7455751576536
4475613854567
    Result
```

Figure 11.2 *Cross-correlation using pixels with single-digit values. The best match is marked in red (note that it is not an exact match).*

Figure 11.3 shows an example image in which several different fonts have been used for the letters A through E. Each of the letters in the first set (which is repeated in sets 6 and 9) was used as the target. The cross-correlation results are marked with red dots showing the maximum values of cross-correlation. The letter is found where it recurs in the same font, but most of the other fonts are not matched at all. The exception, font number 4, shows that the characters are similar enough to be matched but that they also generate false matches.

Cross-correlation looks for very specific details of feature shape and brightness, and while it is reasonably robust when a feature is partially obscured (by noise or camouflage), it is not very tolerant of changes in size or orientation. **Figure 11.4** shows an example of one of the major uses of the technique, the identification of military targets. The target image (an F-15) produces a cross-correlation value that drops to 84% with a 10° rotation, and 80% for a 20° rotation. Both values are still higher than the correlations with different airplanes, which are 72% for an F-14 and 47% for a B-1. Of course, the images must be scaled to the same approximate size before the calculation is performed. In practice, it would be necessary to have target images at many different orientations, for instance rotated in 15° steps. Views in other directions (from the side, front, oblique views, etc.) would also be required.

Parametric description

Recognition of features in images covers an extremely wide range of applications. In some cases the targets are fully known and can be completely represented by one or several images, so that cross-correlation is an appropriate method. In others, the goal is to have the computer

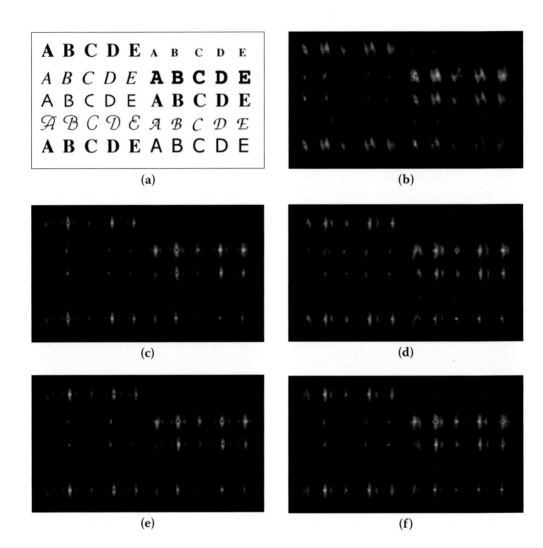

Figure 11.3 *Cross-correlation with letters in different fonts. The letters in the first set (repeated in sets 6 and 9) are matched one by one in images **b, c, d, e, f,** as discussed in the text.*

"understand" natural three-dimensional scenes in which objects may appear in a wide variety of presentations. Applications such as automatic navigation or robotics require that the computer be able to extract surfaces and connect them hierarchically to construct three-dimensional objects, which are then recognized (see, for example, Ballard and Brown 1982; Ballard et al. 1984; Roberts 1982). The topics and goals discussed here are much more limited: to allow the image-analysis system to be able to recognize discrete features in essentially two-dimensional scenes. If the objects are three-dimensional and can appear in different orientations, then each different two-dimensional view can be considered as a different target object.

One application that has become important is facial recognition, used for example to screen surveillance videos for the faces of known individuals. One successful approach uses ratios of vertical and horizontal distances between selected landmarks, as indicated in **Figure 11.5**. By using the ratios of distances, the method becomes relatively insensitive to the orientation of the face with respect to the camera. The use of multiple combinations of dimensions

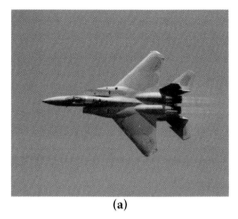

(a)

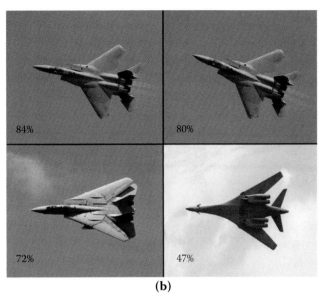

84%   80%

72%   47%

(b)

Figure 11.4 *Cross-correlation for aircraft:*
(a) target image (F-15);
(b) matching scores for four other images showing the effects of shape and orientation. The top two images are the same as the target except for rotation; the bottom two are different aircraft types (F-14 and B-1).

compensates for the fact that some of the landmarks may be obscured in any particular view. The goal of this method is not fully automatic identification, but rather to create a vector in a high-dimensionality space using the various ratios that select a fixed but small number of the most similar faces on file, which are then presented to a human for comparison and matching. This is the same screening approach used in many other applications, some of which are described below. Fingerprint identification, for example, uses a small number of "minutiae" (the location and orientation of details such as branches or ends in the friction-ridge pattern, which can be located either manually or by image processing) as a vector to select a group of the most similar stored prints, which a human then views. The method works for faces, assuming that a suitable database of images has been established, because it is very fast and the dimensional ratios are chosen so that they are resistant to disguise. As

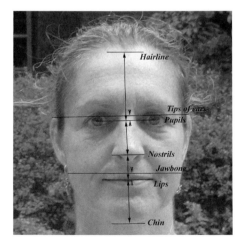

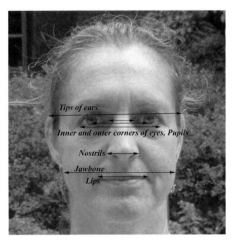

Figure 11.5 *A human face labeled with the principal vertical and horizontal dimensions used in facial identification.*

shown in **Figure 2.43** in **Chapter 2**, slight changes in dimension alter the appearance entirely. But while both the facial recognition and fingerprint recognition methods use computers as an essential part of the process, the ultimate decision step is made by a human.

The simplest situation for feature classification in two-dimensional images, but one that satisfies a very large percentage of practical applications, uses the feature-specific measurement parameters introduced in **Chapter 10**. These methods are called parametric descriptions. **Figure 11.6** shows a simple example, in which the features can be grouped into two classes based on their shape. Several of the shape descriptors introduced before can be used here; the example shows the formfactor (4π area/perimeter^2). A distribution of formfactor values for the features in the image shows two well-separated populations. Setting a limit between the two groups can separate them into the respective classes. In the figure, the "round" features have been identified with a red mark.

Note that other measurement parameters such as area (**Figure 11.6c**) do not distinguish between the groups. Finding a single parameter that can be successfully used to separate classes is not always possible, and when it is, selecting the best one from the many possible candidates by trial and error can be a time-consuming process.

In most cases, a combination of parameters is needed for successful classification, and statistical methods are used to find the best ones. As a simple thought experiment (from Castleman 1996), consider a system to sort fruit, where the target classes are apples, lemons, grapefruit, and cherries. Apples and cherries can be distinguished on the basis of size (e.g., diameter), as can lemons and grapefruit. But apples have a range of sizes that overlap lemons and grapefruit, so a second parameter is needed to distinguish them, for instance the average hue, distinguishing between red and yellow (at least, this will work if green and golden apples are excluded from the process). This can best be shown as a two-dimensional plot of parameter space, as shown in **Figure 11.7**.

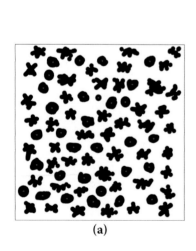

(a)

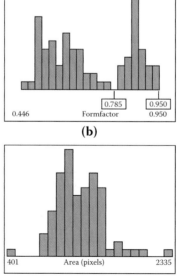

0.446   Formfactor   0.785   0.950   0.950

(b)

401   Area (pixels)   2335

(c)

Figure 11.6
(a) Some hand-drawn features,
(b) with their histograms for formfactor and area.
(c) The formfactor histogram shows two separate classes; the features with values greater than 0.785 are marked with red dots and are visually "rounder" than the others. The area histogram shows only a single grouping and does not distinguish between the two types of features.

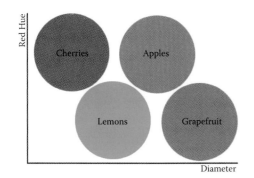

Figure 11.7 Schematic diagram of classes for fruit sorting, as discussed in the text.

Note that the various classes are still distinct in this example, so that drawing "decision lines" between them is straightforward once the range of values for the different classes has been established. This is most typically done by measuring actual samples. Rather than just measuring "typical" specimens, it would be most efficient in this case to intentionally select examples of each fruit that are considered to be extremes (largest, smallest, reddest, yellowest) to map out the boundaries.

The goals in deciding upon the measurement parameters to use are:

1. To be able to discriminate the various classes, preferably with no overlap at all but at least with minimum overlap (handling of situations in which there is overlap is dealt with below)
2. To have the smallest practical number of parameters, which simplifies the training process in which determining extremes in all combinations of parameters is desired
3. To be independent of each other, so that each one measures a very different characteristic of the objects
4. To be reliable, so that the parameter values (a) will not vary over time or due to uncontrolled variables and (b) can be measured consistently if system hardware is modified or replaced

Sometimes these goals conflict with one another. For example, adding more parameters often provides less overlap of classes, but it may complicate the training process. Finding multiple parameters that are truly independent can be difficult. In the case of the apples, one parameter is a measure of size and the other of color, so we can expect them to be independent. But shape parameters, which are often very important for classification, may be quite interrelated to each other and to the size parameters from which they are calculated. It usually requires a statistical procedure to determine which function best in any particular situation (examples are shown below).

Reliability is difficult to predict when a classification scheme is initially established. By definition, changes in object appearance due to unexpected variations cannot be excluded. For instance, if color is being used to distinguish fabricated components and the pigmentation used in the ink being applied is changed by the supplier, or if incandescent lights are replaced by fluorescent ones, or if a different camera is substituted for one that has failed, the RGB (red, green, blue) values and whatever hue or other information is derived from them will change. It may or may not be practical to introduce a calibration step that will adjust the new values to match the old. The alternative is to remeasure a training population using the new ink, lights, or camera and reestablish class limits, which is generally an expensive task.

Three situations are encountered in general classification; each will be dealt with in this chapter:

1. Imposed criteria (the classical expert system). A human expert supplies rules. Software can optimize the order in which they are applied and search for relevant rules, but does not derive them.
2. Supervised classification. A training set of examples that are supposed to be prototypes of the range of classes and class variations are presented to the system, which

then develops a strategy for identifying them. The number of classes and examples identified for each class is specified by a human.

3. Unsupervised classification. The system is presented with a set of examples as above, but not told which class each belongs to, or perhaps even the number of classes. The system attempts to define the class regions to maximize the similarity of objects within each cluster and the differences between groups.

The second approach is one that corresponds to implementation of many existing industry standards, which are based on "type images" that have been selected or created by experts (or committees) to guide identification by technicians. Usually these are presented as proto-typical examples (or idealized drawings of such examples) of various classes, but no specific guidance is given (and no numeric measurement values are provided) on how the matching is to be performed. If the type images are used as the training examples (e.g., Gomes and Paciornik 2005), the system can usually derive the required measurements and limits, but the performance on real samples will depend in large measure on how representative those images actually are.

Medical applications are making increased use of the same approach to automatic feature recognition, at least as a way to select suspicious or comparison images to present to a trained pathologist. For example, to identify mammographic masses, Alto et al. (2005) used the measured values of the shape parameters defined in **Chapter 10** as formfactor (area/perimeter^2) and convexity (convex perimeter/total perimeter), as well as the number and angles of spicules, edge sharpness, texture (entropy), and density as a vector in parameter space that selects a fixed number of the most similar previously stored reference images, which are then presented for visual comparison.

Automatic screening systems for Pap smears use parameters such as the integrated optical density of the nucleus, nuclear texture (standard deviation of the optical density), nuclear formfactor, and the area ratio of nucleus to cytoplasm to select a fixed number of the most suspicious cells on a slide, which are then presented for a human to view (Luck et al. 1993; Rutenberg et al. 2001). The expectation is that if these cells do not include any that indicate a pathological condition, then the slide is "normal" and no further review by a pathologist is warranted.

There are also other situations in which the classification of images is based not on the statistics of individual feature measurement parameters, but on characteristics of the entire scene. The most often cited example of this type of discrimination uses the Brodatz texture images representing various kinds of natural and human-made surfaces (Brodatz 1966). A few are shown in **Figure 11.8**. The Fourier-transform power spectra of these images (**Figure 11.9**) reveal characteristic frequencies and orientations, or ratios of amplitudes at specific frequencies, which can be used to distinguish them. This same logic can be implemented in hardware using a set of filter banks to select the various frequencies and performing identification in real time.

The principal use of this technology seems to be in classification of remote sensing imagery (satellite and aerial photographs). When combined with multiband spectral intensity ratios as discussed below, the textures can be used to identify various types of crops, rocks, and other land-use patterns. However, while they apply to the entire scene rather than a single feature, the various numeric values, such as ratios of amplitudes at various frequencies and orientations, are used in the decision process in the same way as feature-specific measurements in the classification processes described in this chapter.

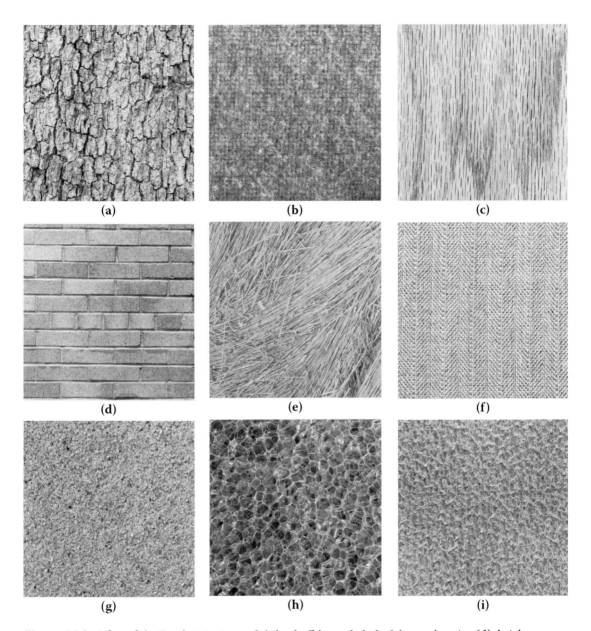

Figure 11.8 *A few of the Brodatz textures:* **(a)** *bark;* **(b)** *wool cloth;* **(c)** *wood grain;* **(d)** *bricks;* **(e)** *straw;* **(f)** *herringbone cloth;* **(g)** *sand;* **(h)** *bubbles; and* **(i)** *pigskin.*

Decision points

In many practical cases, the classes are not as completely distinct as the example shown in **Figure 11.6**. Commonly, when training populations are measured, the histograms of parameter values can overlap, as shown in **Figure 11.10**. Such overlaps usually indicate the need to find other parameters that offer better discrimination, but it is not always possible to avoid some degree of overlap, and in that case it is necessary to establish a decision threshold that produces an acceptably low probability of error.

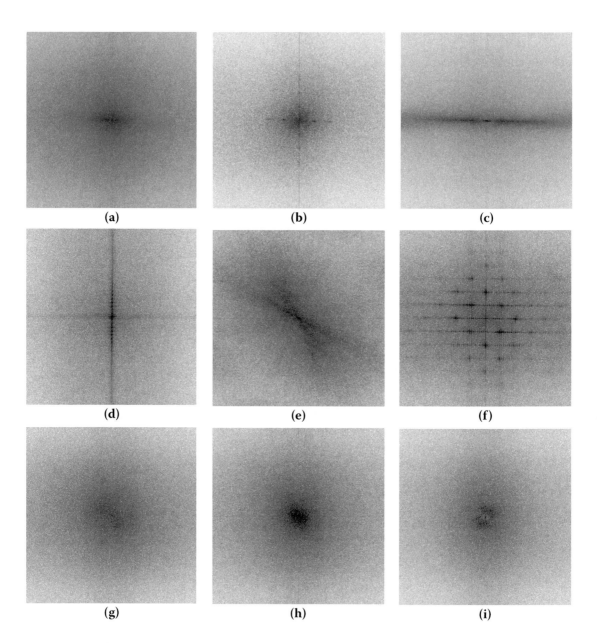

Figure 11.9 *The Fourier-transform power spectra for each of the images in **Figure 11.8**.*

As shown in **Figure 11.11**, the decision threshold combines with the probability distribution function for the measurement parameter to establish the expected error rate. The area of the tail of the distribution function (as a percentage of the total) gives the probability of identifying a member of one population as being in the other class. Sometimes the decision threshold is set to make the two errors (wrongly identifying A as B, or B as A) equal, which minimizes the total error.

In other cases, economic factors must be taken into account. For example, consider the case of two different "O" rings used in engines, one in a tractor engine and the other in a helicopter engine, which are distinguished by an imaging operation that measures thickness or perhaps

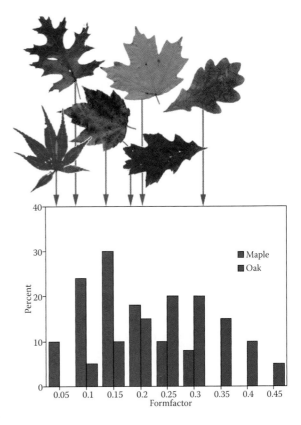

Figure 11.10 Values of formfactor measured on a variety of maple and oak leaves. The histograms are significantly overlapped, indicating that formfactor is not the best parameter to use for identification. Probably a method using the skeleton endpoints and external branches would be more successful.

looks for a colored tag embedded in the polymer. The economic cost of occasionally shipping a part intended for a helicopter to be used in a tractor is probably very small. The part will likely function there, in which case the only extra cost is perhaps the use of a more costly polymer or the loss of the more valuable part. But shipping a tractor part for use in a helicopter would produce much greater liability if the engine failed, and probably a greater likelihood of failure in a more demanding environment. In such a case it would be desirable to set the error rate for mistakenly identifying a tractor part as a helicopter part to something very low (1 in 1 million or less) and accepting a much higher rate (perhaps 1 in 1000) for the opposite error.

Similar considerations arise in biomedical imaging. There is much concern about automated diagnosis, such as the identification using image analysis of cancer cells in Pap smears or lesions in mammograms (Karssemeijer 1998), because of liability issues. The most widely accepted course of action has been to set the decision thresholds for identifying suspicious features very low, accepting many false positives that can subsequently be screened again by an experienced human, but hopefully minimizing false negatives in which disease might be missed.

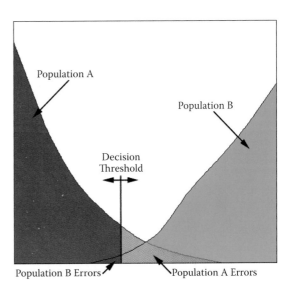

Figure 11.11 Setting a decision point when distributions overlap, as discussed in the text. The probability of misclassifying a feature is measured by the area in the tail of each distribution past the decision threshold.

Multidimensional classification

In the examples shown above, the histogram or probability distribution function has been plotted as a function of a single measurement parameter. In the example of **Figure 11.7**, two parameters (size and color) were used. In such cases, it is often possible to reduce the problem to a single derived parameter by fitting a new axis line through the data, usually called either a linear-discriminant line, principal-components axis, or a context line. As shown in **Figure 11.12**, a distribution of data points measured on a training population and plotted on two parameter axes can have values that overlap in both individual parameters, but these can be much better separated when projected onto another derived axis that is a linear combination of the two. This line can be fit by linear regression through the points or by using principal-components analysis.

Curved lines can be used in principle, but in practice it is difficult to perform robust nonlinear regression unless the form of the functional dependence is known *a priori*, and in that case it is usually better to transform the measurement variables beforehand. For instance, instead of area, it might be better to use equivalent diameter (which varies as the square root of area) to obtain a plot for which a linear regression line provides a better fit, as illustrated in **Figure 11.13**.

Once the new axis has been fit to the data points, a histogram of values projected along the new derived parameter (shown in **Figure 11.12**) can be used for classification just as discussed previously for a directly measured parameter. In fact, the formfactor used above is actually itself a combination of area and perimeter measurements, so this process is simply one more step toward obtaining a derived parameter that most directly distinguishes the classes of interest.

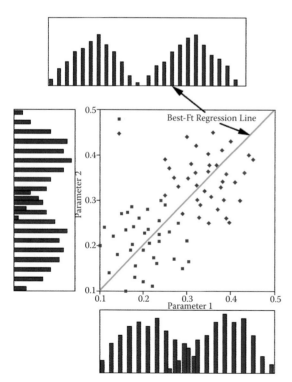

Using a decision point determined along the best-fit line between two populations generates a decision line (or in higher dimension spaces when more than two parameters are used, a decision plane) that separates the two populations. The decision-line method generalizes to more than two classes, as shown in **Figure 11.14**. In this case, two measured parameters (the inscribed radius and the ratio of the inscribed to the circumscribed radius) suffice to distinguish five classes of nuts, as shown on the graph. When applied to the image (produced by placing the nuts on a flatbed scanner), this model successfully labels each object.

Simple decision thresholds work well when the populations are reasonably compact and equiaxial, but, as shown in **Figure 11.15**, they require greater complexity to separate populations that have irregularly shaped regions in parameter space. Techniques that

Figure 11.12 *Two populations of points that overlap on both parameter axes, with a linear-discriminant or context line along which they are best separated.*

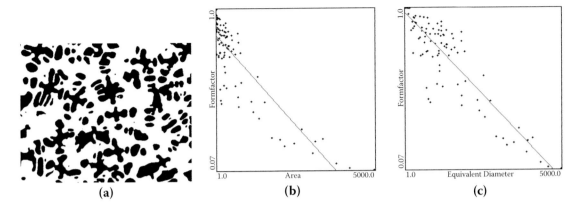

Figure 11.13 *Features from an image of dendrites in a metal alloy **(a)**, showing regression plots for formfactor vs. area **(b)** and formfactor vs. equivalent diameter **(c)**. The latter provides a better fit to the data.*

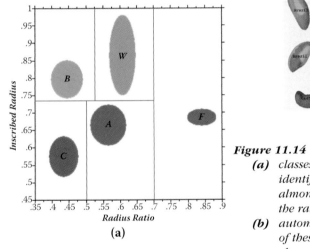

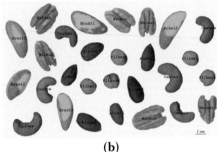

Figure 11.14 *Two-parameter classification:*
    (a) *classes established from a training population that identify Brazil nuts, filberts, cashews, walnuts, and almonds based on the inscribed circle radius and the ratio of the inscribed to circumscribed circle;*
    (b) *automatically coloring and labeling an image of these nuts using the classification scheme. The classes can be described either by the colored regions on the parameter plot or by the red decision lines.*

can locate an optimum decision plane or surface (the Bayes classifier) for such cases are more computationally intensive. It is also possible to distinguish multiple populations by piecewise-linear decision boundaries or by quadratic or higher power boundaries. Fortunately, in most such cases the addition of additional parameters separates the various population classes well enough that simpler linear methods can be used.

Population classes like those shown in **Figure 11.15b**, which are elongated and oriented at an angle to the axes defined by the measurement parameters, reveal a correlation between the parameters. This creates problems for classification, as noted previously, so it is desirable to make the population area more equiaxial, and preferably circular. The covariance of the data set is defined as

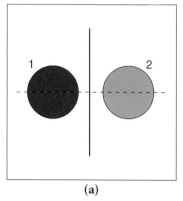 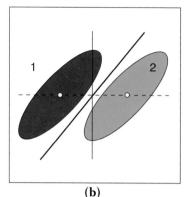 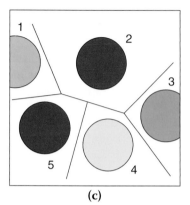

(a)   (b)   (c)

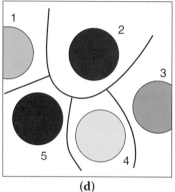

(d)

Figure 11.15 *Classification examples in two dimensions:*
  (a) *separable classes showing the decision boundary perpendicular to the linear-discriminant or regression line;*
  (b) *classes that are not separable by the boundary in diagram **a**, with an optimal Bayes classifier (blue line) that does separate them;*
  (c) *multiple classes separated by piecewise linear decision boundaries;*
  (d) *multiple classes separated by quadratic decision boundaries.*

$$c(i,j) = \frac{\sum_{k=1}^{n} \left(x_{k,i} - \mu_i \right) \cdot \left(x_{k,j} - \mu_j \right)}{n-1}$$

(11.2)

where x is the measurement value, i and j identify the two parameters, μ is the mean values for each parameter, and k runs through the n features in the population. The covariance can vary between $+\sigma_i\sigma_j$ and $-\sigma_i\sigma_j$, where σ represents the standard deviation values for each parameter. A value of zero for $c(i,j)$ indicates no correlation, and the minimum or maximum value indicates perfect correlation, as shown in **Figure 11.16**.

The examples above showed only two measured parameters, but in general there are N axes for a high-dimensionality space. In that case, all of the covariances $c(i,j)$ for the various parameters measured can be collected into a covariance matrix **C**. This matrix can be used to transform an irregular population cluster to an equiaxial, circular one. For each measurement vector x (defined by all of the n measurement parameters), the quantity r calculated as

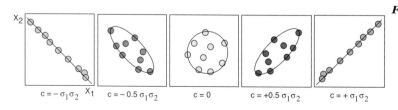

Figure 11.16 *The value of covariance can vary between perfect positive and perfect negative correlation, as discussed in the text. A zero value represents uncorrelated values.*

$$r^2 = (x - \mu)' C^{-1} (x - \mu)$$

(11.3)

is called the Mahalanobis distance from the point representing the feature measurement parameters to the mean of the population μ. This is a generalization of the usual concept of distance, appropriate for measurements in which the axes have different meanings and scales. In the case of an equiaxial population cluster (zero covariance), the Mahalanobis distance is the same as the usual Euclidean or Pythagorean distance.

It is helpful in measuring distances along the various axes to compensate for the different scales of the various measurement parameters by normalizing the distance measurements. This is done by dividing each one by an appropriate scaling constant, ideally the standard deviation of the parameter values. This is called the "standardized Euclidean distance."

Of course, the classification methods can be generalized to more than two dimensions (it just becomes harder to illustrate with simple graphics). **Figure 11.17** shows an example from remote imaging in which the intensities of reflected light detected in different wavelength bands from the Landsat Thematic Mapper satellite are used to classify terrain types (Grasselli 1969; Sabins 1987). Patterns of spectral intensity are associated with particular types of vegetation, minerals, etc. A supervised training program is used in which an operator marks locations and the image-analysis system plots the point in terms of the measured intensities in each

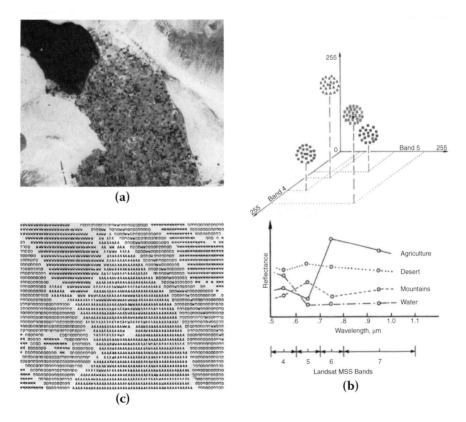

Figure 11.17 *Land-use classification using Landsat Thematic Mapper images: (a) one image showing reflectivity in a single wavelength range; (b) reflectance vs. wavelength plots and cluster diagram for reflectivity values from different terrain types; (c) classification of land use based on these data.*

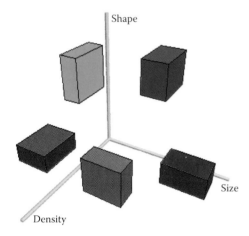

Figure 11.18 Diagram of range limits for class regions in parameter space (illustrating three independent parameters). This is a three-dimensional version of the example shown by the red lines in Figure 11.14a.

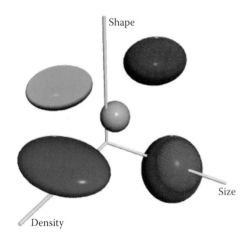

Figure 11.19 Diagram of ellipsoidal class regions calculated from the standard deviation of measured data. This is a three-dimensional version of the example shown by the colored regions in Figure 11.14a.

wavelength band. The clusters of points (which are shown schematically) then mark the various classes, which are used to label the images pixel by pixel.

There is no reason to expect the clusters of points corresponding to each class to form a regular spherical shape in the N-dimensional parameter space, of course, and examples below will show alternative ways of establishing these regions. One of the simplest methods is to establish maximum and minimum limit values for each parameter. This corresponds to a set of rectangular boxes in parameter space (**Figure 11.18**) that define each class. Training such a system is simplified because it is not necessary to find a representative population, but rather to find or predict extreme values.

Another method for establishing region boundaries is to measure a representative training population for each class, and to characterize the distribution of values by the mean and standard deviation for each parameter. Using the mean values as the coordinates of the center and a multiple of each parameter's standard deviation as the lengths of the axes, this generates ellipsoids, as shown in **Figure 11.19**. The surfaces of these ellipsoids can be used as absolute class boundaries, but it is often more useful to measure the distance of each new feature's parameter coordinates from the various classes in terms of the standard deviation.

Figure 11.20 shows a two-dimensional example for the sake of simplicity. The training populations are shown at the top, along with the plots of the points and the 2-σ ellipses for each class. Note that, for the training population and for additional features measured subsequently, some of the points lie outside the 2-σ limit, as would be expected. Note also that some of the classes are much larger (more variation in the parameter values) than others, and that the ellipses can be elongated in some cases because one parameter varies more than another. The standard deviation, shown by the length of each ellipse axis, becomes a scale with which to interpret the rather confusing distances of parameter space. Using the standard deviation normalizes the various axis units, as discussed previously. The concept of a "distance" in parameter space is not immediately obvious and may be distorted in different directions or regions of the plot. Unfortunately, this is often the case when shape factors are used for identification, since they are often not all independent (so the axes are not orthogonal) and are certainly not linear (a change in aspect ratio from 1.1 to 1.5 is far different than a change from 4.1 to 4.5, for instance).

If a new feature is measured, and if its parameter coordinates do not place it inside one of the class boundaries, it may still be identified as being "most like" one class by (a) measuring the distance in parameter space from the feature coordinates to the center of each class (the mean values) and (b) scaling this number by dividing by the standard deviation. Because of the different cluster sizes, this means that a point could actually be closer to one class on the plot but more "like" a different one. In the example, a point close to the compact blue class might be fewer standard deviations away from the large red one, and would be identified accordingly.

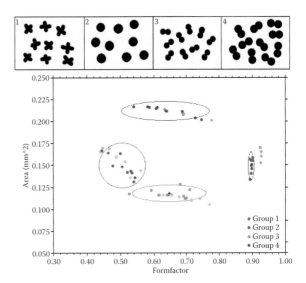

Figure 11.20 *Two-dimensional example of statistical limits. Note that some points lie outside the 2-σ boundaries. Solid points indicate the training populations shown at the top; shaded points represent identification of additional features. Points are identified with the nearest cluster measured, as discussed in the text.*

Learning systems

It can be very difficult to collect a truly representative set of features with which to establish training populations that produce classes that can be applied without alteration to many new features and situations. In particular, the extreme-valued features that lie near the end of the distributions are usually rare. Furthermore, an approach using mean and standard deviation rather than the actual shape of the distribution may oversimplify the measurements, which in many image-analysis situations do not produce Gaussian distributions that are adequately described by just these two statistical parameters.

Figure 11.11 illustrated the ability to estimate the probability of classification error from the shape of the distribution histogram. Using the actual histogram thus extends traditional "hard" classification, in which a feature is assigned to one class or excluded from it, to the "fuzzy" logic situation, in which shades of probability are admitted. Fuzzy logic is an important extension of classical logic in which the various classification rules in the knowledge base contain probabilities. An example would be, "If X can fly, there is a 70% chance that it is a bird; if X cannot fly, there is a 5% chance that it is a bird," which accommodates butterflies, which fly but are not birds, and penguins, which are birds but do not fly. In the case of parameter measurements, the histogram of values gives a direct way to measure the conditional probabilities.

Fuzzy logic has been applied to expert systems and neural networks (both discussed below as engines for assigning classifications based on multiple rules). Typically, the result is to slow the convergence process because it is necessary to evaluate all paths and find the most likely, not simply to find one successful path through the rules. In a formal sense, fuzzy logic is equivalent to Bayesian logic with multileveled classic sets. For comprehensive information on fuzzy logic, refer to the literature (Negoita and Ralescu 1975, 1987; Sanchez and Zadeh 1987; Zadeh 1965; Zimmerman 1987).

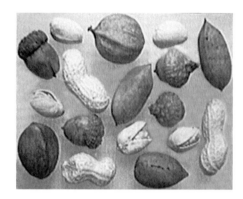

Figure 11.21 A few of the nuts used in the learning example discussed in the text.

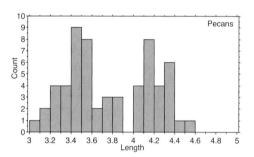

Figure 11.22 A bimodal length distribution for two species of pecans.

As an illustration of a learning system that uses histograms to establish decision points and works in multiparameter space using linear-discriminant- or context-line methods, populations of nine kinds of natural nuts were used (**Figure 11.21**). This is a much more difficult combination of nut types than the previous example (**Figure 11.14**) and requires more measurement parameters. Some of the nuts used represented more than one species (e.g., one class included both white and red oak acorns, both with and without their caps, and another included several kinds of pecans), so that histograms were generally not Gaussian and sometimes were multimodal (**Figure 11.22**). Images from an initial training population of about 20 of each variety of nut were captured with a monochrome video camera (this work was done in the 1980s, so much of the hardware was primitive by current standards), and the features measured to obtain a total of 40 parameters for each feature.

Some parameters such as location and orientation were discarded based on human judgment that they were not meaningful. Others were discarded by subsequent statistical analysis, leaving a net of 17 that were actually used, so discrimination was performed in a 17-dimensional space. However, not all of the dimensions are truly independent (orthogonal) because many of the shape parameters are based on size measures used in various combinations. Linear-discriminant lines were constructed in this space between each pair of nut classes, using stepwise regression (Draper and Smith 1981). Parameters were added to or removed from the equation of the context line based on the F-value (an arbitrary cutoff value of 4.0 was used), eliminating variables that did not improve the ability to distinguish particular population groups.

This elimination helps toward the goal of using independent parameters, as well as simplifying the total problem and reducing the number of training examples required. Many of the shape parameters, for example, use some of the same size information. For example, the convexity and formfactor defined in **Chapter 10** both use the perimeter. If one of them shows a high correlation with category discrimination, there is a good chance that others that incorporate perimeter will also show a correlation. Stepwise regression will select the one that has the highest correlation and predictive power, and discard the others.

The resulting context lines used as few as two or as many as eight terms. Some parameters were used in several cases (e.g., average brightness), while others appeared in only one or two equations but were then often the most important single parameter (e.g., convex area was highly important in distinguishing pistachios from almonds). On the average, each of the 17 parameters was used 11 times in the total of 55 pairwise context lines, and each context-line equation included an average of five parameters. **Figure 11.23** shows several examples. The

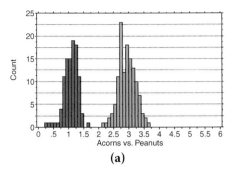

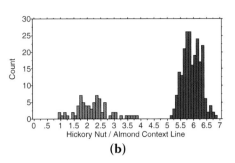

(a)   (b)

Figure 11.23 *Context lines and frequency distributions for hickory nuts-almonds and acorns-peanuts, examples of entirely separated classes. The regression equations are:*
(a) *Acorns (type 1) vs. Peanuts (type 3) =*
3.928 + 0.773·Aspect Ratio − 5.007·Fractal Dimension + 0.068·Brightness;
(b) *Hickory Nuts (type 2) vs. Almonds (type 6) =*
−2.266 − 2.372·Breadth + 2.184·Width + 0.226·Brightness + 0.318·Contrast + 2.374·Texture

coefficients in the equations for the linear-discriminant or context lines are derived by regression and represent the angles between the line and each of the parameter axes in *N*-space.

Discrimination of hickory nuts from almonds, and acorns from peanuts, is easy because the distributions are entirely separate, even though the distributions are somewhat irregular in shape. The acorn-pecan distribution (**Figure 11.24**) shows a slight overlap, which was the case in about 16% of the pairwise discriminant plots. Using the logic shown earlier in **Figure 11.12**, the decision point was located to make the probability of misclassification errors equal for both classes. In the acorn-pecan case, this amounted to about 1% and rose when a large acorn was viewed from the side without its end cap, as shown in **Figure 11.25**. The most likely error was confusion of an acorn with a filbert.

Once the discriminant functions (the equations of the context lines) have been established and distributions of derived parameter values along those lines set up, the system can go to work identifying nuts. The decision points along each context line position the planes (perpendicular to the lines and which form polyhedra around each class) in the high-dimensionality space. The problem is that with a training population of only 20 nuts from each class, the positions of those decision points are imperfect.

As the system examines more images (eventually a total of about 1000 nuts), the derived parameter values (positions along each context line) are calculated and the histograms are updated. This does not require any additional computer memory, since the histogram bins have already been established. Identification of nut types proceeds on the basis of the stored decision points. But whenever a value is added to the end of a histogram (within the last 5%

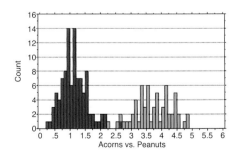

Figure 11.24 *Context line and frequency distribution for acorns-pecans, showing overlap. The regression equation is Acorns (type 1) vs. Pecans (type 4) = 1.457 + 6.141·Formfactor − 2.153·Convex Perimeter + 1.768·Convex Area + 2.926·Length − 1.575·Breadth − 1.131·Extent*

of its area), the program asks the operator to confirm the identification and then reestablishes the decision threshold using the then-current histogram. In this way the system learns from the additional specimens to which it has been exposed, which gradually increases the number of observations near the important limits of each distribution.

Figure 11.26 shows a table with the final results. Some 3.7% of the nuts were misidentified, but most of these errors occurred very early in the learning process; there was only one error in the last 200 nuts. The system started out with an approximate idea of the limits of each class and refined these limits with more information. It should be noted that many of the parameters used for each identification were not familiar to the human operators, and almost certainly did not represent the logic they used to identify the nuts. But the system quickly became as proficient as the humans.

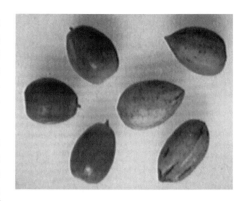

Figure 11.25 View of several large acorns without their end caps and pecans, showing a situation in which confusion between the two classes may arise.

In other examples, an automated system based on this same logic has surpassed the humans who trained it (Russ and Rovner 1987). In the study of archaeological sites in the American southwest and much of Central America, a subject of considerable interest is the process of domestication of corn, *Zea mays*. It is widely believed, although not proven, that corn is a domesticated offshoot of the wild grass teosinte, of which there are many varieties. Little remains of corn in an archaeological context that can be dated, but it happens that corn, like all grasses (and many other plants) produces small silica bodies called opal phytoliths in and between the cells on the stalk, leaves, and other parts of the plant. They are generally a few micrometers in size and act to stiffen the plant tissue. They are also selectively produced at any site of injury (including cropping by animals).

From an anthropological point of view, phytoliths are of interest for two reasons. First, they survive in the soil for long periods of time and can be recovered from layers that are datable and show other signs of human habitation. Second, they have shapes that are distinctive. Research over several decades has shown that phytoliths can be used taxonomically to identify species of grasses, including corn and its precursors (Pearsall 1978; Piperno 1984; Rovner 1971; Twiss et al. 1969). Most of this identification has been carried out by humans, who have accumulated photographs (mostly using the scanning electron microscope [SEM], since the particles are only a few micrometers in size and have significant three-dimensional structure so that they cannot be studied satisfactorily with the light microscope) and built catalogs from which matching com-

Initial Nut Identification

Actual Nut Type	Acorns	Hickory Nuts	Peanuts	Pecans	Pistachios	Almonds	Brazil Nuts	Filberts	Walnuts
Acorns	91			1					10
Hickory Nuts		70		1			1		
Peanuts			126			1			
Pecans	2	1		54			3		
Pistachios					126				
Almonds						224			
Brazil Nuts		3		6			115		
Filberts	8							67	
Walnuts									107

Figure 11.26 *"Confusion matrix" showing successes (green) and errors (red) in initial nut identification, as described in the text.*

parison to unknowns can be performed. The success rate for skilled observers in blind tests is generally better than 95%. However, this has been at the cost of a very substantial amount of effort, and the knowledge and experience is not readily transferred to other researchers. The human eye does not deal well with the need to characterize variation, and the individual phytoliths vary widely in shape. Such a situation is ripe for the use of computer image analysis methods.

Slides were prepared with phytoliths extracted from a training suite of five known species of maize and teosinte, and SEM images were analyzed to determine several size and shape parameters, which were used as described above to establish discriminant classes. On the original set of objects, this produced a better than 99% correct identification. After applying the results to a total of 300 objects from five additional species of plants (three maize and two teosinte), the results had improved to better than 99.6% accuracy in distinguishing the two classes. Furthermore, the system can examine hundreds of phytoliths (enough to produce statistically significant results) from more species of corn or other grasses in 1 month than have been done by hand and eye in the last 20 years. The same system has recently been used for classification of squash seeds (I. Rovner, personal communication).

kNN and cluster analysis

There are other methods used to establish limits for classes in parameter space. The two most widely used, k-nearest-neighbor (kNN) and cluster analysis, share the drawback that, unlike the histogram and linear-discriminant method described above, it is necessary to save the actual coordinates (measurement values for multiple parameters) for each identified feature, which means that storage requirements grow continually if the system is to continue learning. The other difficulty with these methods is that the time required to make an identification rises with the number of stored values, even with efficient algorithms to sort or prune the data set, and they work with only a reasonable number of candidate points. On the other hand, these methods do not presuppose any particular shape for the class regions, such as the rectangular prism, ellipsoid, or polyhedral methods described above. It is even possible to handle such situations as shown in **Figure 11.27**, in which one class is nonconvex, disjoint, or is largely or completely surrounded by another.

The kNN classification works by searching the database of previously identified features for those that are "most like" the current measurement, as shown in **Figure 11.28**. This amounts to finding the distance between the coordinates of the current feature's parameters and those for other features. The distance is generally calculated in a simple Pythagorean sense (square root of the sum of squares of differences), but this overlooks the important fact that the different axes in parameter space have different units and metrics. Often the distance along each axis is simply expressed as a fraction of the total range of values for that parameter, but there is no real justification for such an assumption. It is better to use a normalizing scale such as the standard deviation of values

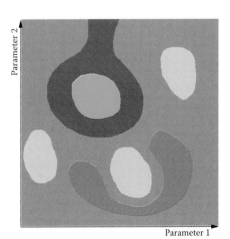

Figure 11.27 *Examples of nonconvex, disjoint, or surrounded classes (indicated by different colors) that are difficult to represent by simple geometric shapes.*

within each class, if this is available (the same logic with Mahalanobis distance, as used previously for the ellipsoid class limits).

In the simplest form of k-neighbor comparison, k is equal to 1, and the search is simply for the one single prior measurement that is most similar, which is then assumed to identify the class of the new feature. For features near the boundary between classes, single-nearest-neighbor matching proves to be quite noisy and produces irregular boundaries that do not promote robust identification, as shown in **Figure 11.29**. Using the identification of the majority of five, nine, or even more nearest neighbors produces a smoother boundary between classes, but it is still highly sensitive to the relative size of the populations. If one population has many more members than the other, it effectively shrinks the class limits for the minor group by making it more likely that the majority of matches will be with members of the more numerous population.

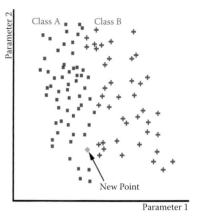

Figure 11.28 *A k-nearest-neighbor classification: three of the five nearest neighbors to the new point lie in Class B, so it is assigned to that class.*

The methods described so far presume that some training population, in which the features belong to known classes, can be used to construct the class limits. As noted before, this is known as "supervised learning," in which the operator identifies the actual class or population to which each feature belongs (based on whatever criteria or prior knowledge is available), and the software uses that information along with whatever measurement parameters are available to determine an identification strategy (which is generally quite different from the strategy used by the human). There are some situations in which it is not known *a priori* what the classes are, or perhaps even how many of them are present. In these cases, it is still useful to plot each feature's measured parameters as values in a parameter space, and then look for clusters of points. Cluster analysis with nonsupervised training is a rich topic that extends beyond the scope of this text. (See, for instance, Bow 1992; Fukunaga 1990; James 1988; Pentland 1986.)

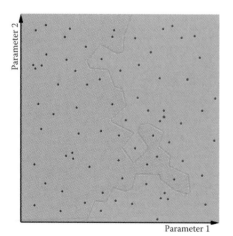

Figure 11.29 *The irregular boundary that forms between two classes (whose individual members have parameter values indicated by the colored points) using single-nearest-neighbor classification.*

One typical way that cluster analysis proceeds uses the distance between points to identify the members of a cluster. For example, start with the two points closest together. Assume that these represent a class and then add to the class other nearby points until the distance from the nearest point already assigned to the cluster exceeds some (arbitrary) limit, which can be calculated from the size of the growing class region. The method can obviously be generalized to use more than a single nearest neighbor. Once a given class has stopped growing, begin again with the remaining points and continue until all have been assigned. There are many refinements of this approach that allow for assigned class regions to be merged or split.

A somewhat complementary method for finding clusters uses all of the points simultaneously. It starts by constructing a minimal spanning tree for all of the points present (an intensive amount of computation for large data sets). The links in this tree can be weighted either by their Euclidean or Mahalanobis length, or by the number of matches present in a table of *k*-nearest neighbors for each point. In other words, if the same points are each listed in each other's nearest-neighbor lists, they are probably in the same cluster. The spanning tree is then pruned by cutting the links with the greatest length or the smallest number of matches, thus leaving the identified clusters. **Figure 11.30** shows an example of a sparse cluster of points, the minimal spanning tree, and the clusters that result from pruning (after Bow 1992).

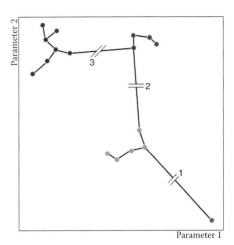

Figure 11.30 *Parameter values plotted as points and the minimal spanning tree connecting them. Cutting the branches with the greatest length separates the clusters (indicated by different colors).*

Another, somewhat different approach to find clusters in data, particularly when there is only one significant measured variable, is the dendrogram. **Figure 11.31** shows an example. The features are ranked into order based on the value of the measured variable, such as formfactor. Then the features that have the smallest value differences are connected (numbers 7 and 21 in the example, followed by 4 and 23, 27 and 14, 13 and 16, etc.) by horizontal lines positioned according to the difference value. Groups of features are usually linked based on the smallest difference between any two members of the group, although it is also possible to use the difference between the mean or median values in each group. Eventually all of the features and groups are connected into a single tree.

If multiple independent measurement parameters (e.g., shape, size, and color) are used, the difference between features is calculated as the distance between the vector representation of the multiple values in *N*-dimensional space. This typically presents a problem because the units of the various parameters are quite different and the lengths of the various axes are not compatible, so there is no natural way to scale them in proportion. This can sometimes be handled by normalizing each measured parameter based on (for example) the total range or standard deviation of the measured parameters, but such a method is inherently arbitrary. Without a full characterization of the statistical distributions of each parameter, it is not possible to calculate a true Mahalanobis distance for the parameter space.

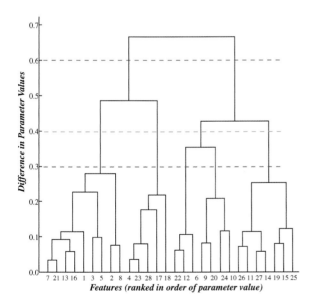

Figure 11.31 *Example dendrogram, as discussed in the text. The red, green, and blue lines indicate the effect of selecting different threshold values for the difference between feature measurements on the number of classes.*

Once the dendrogram has been constructed, it can be used to determine any number of clusters by selecting a different threshold value for the difference. For example, in **Figure 11.31** a value of 0.6 would yield two clusters, while a value of 0.4 would yield four clusters and a value of 0.3 would yield five clusters. Since, by definition, we do not know *a priori* how many classes are present in the unsupervised clustering situation, the decision requires human judgment.

Expert systems

After clusters have been identified by one of these methods, the class limits must still be constructed by one of the methods shown above. This could be a geometric shape (rectangular prism, ellipsoid, polyhedron) or a *k*NN boundary. Now we will consider how to apply these class boundaries as a set of rules for the identification of subsequent features.

The simplest and most common method is the traditional expert system. A set of rules (such as the limits — either hard or fuzzy — for the class boundaries) is created and applied to each new set of feature measurements. Returning to the example of the letters A through E, **Figure 11.32** shows a very simple expert system with four rules, requiring measurement of only three parameters. In the most efficient implementation, only those parameters required would be measured, so for the letter B (which is identified by the number of holes in the shape) the roundness and aspect-ratio parameters, which are not needed, would not be determined at all. When they are used, the cutoff values of the parameters for each letter type are determined experimentally by measuring characters from a few different fonts. In situations like this, it becomes important to design the system so that the least "expensive" parameters are determined first, as this reduces the time and effort needed for the overall identification. Counting holes requires less computation than measuring dimensions needed for the shape factors. Also notice that, unlike the template-matching and cross-correlation examples shown

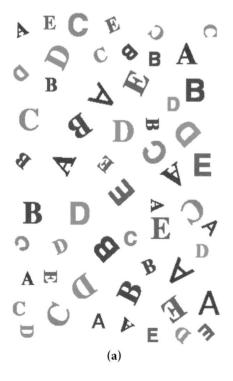

(a)

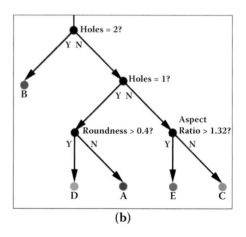

(b)

Figure 11.32 Expert system to classify the letters A through E. The colors shown in image **a** were assigned using the logic in image **b**. Note that the shape factors used as parameters do not depend on size, orientation, or position, and that several different fonts (with and without serifs) are present.

earlier, this method is insensitive to position, size, or orientation of the letters, and tolerates several different fonts.

Simple classification systems like this are sometimes called decision trees or production rules, consisting of an ordered set of IF/THEN relationships. Classic expert systems separate the database (rules) from the inference engine used to find a solution (Black 1986; Rolston 1988; Slatter 1987; Walters 1988; Winstanley 1987). One of the drawbacks to such systems is that the addition of another class (e.g., the letter F) does not simply graft on another step, but may completely reshuffle the order in which the rules should be applied, or even eliminate some rules altogether and replace them with others. The optimum decision tree is not necessarily the one with the fewest branches. "Knowledge shaping" procedures such as including the cost of obtaining each input value can greatly improve overall efficiency and determine an optimum search-and-solution tree (Cockett 1987).

Most real expert systems have far more rules than this one, and the order in which they are to be applied is not necessarily obvious. The complexity of decision paths increases rapidly with a large number of rules. General-purpose expert systems try to find a path between the various input values and a conclusion in one of two ways. If, as shown in **Figure 11.33**, the number of observations is less than the number of possible conclusions, forward chaining that starts at the left and explores pathways through various rules toward a conclusion would be used. In other cases, backward chaining that works from conclusions back toward observations may be more efficient. In the schematic diagram shown in the figure, there are 6 initial observations (measurements), 21 rules, and 12 possible conclusions; real systems are several orders of magnitude more complex. Some of the rules shown have more than two possible outcomes; in some systems, each possible outcome would represent a separate rule.

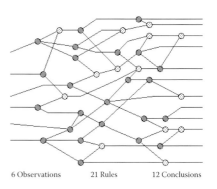

6 Observations   21 Rules   12 Conclusions

Figure 11.33 *Schematic diagram for an expert system.*

Normal forward searching for a successful path through this network would start at some point on the left, follow a path to a rule, and follow the outcome until a contradiction was met (a rule could not be satisfied). The system would then backtrack to the preceding node and try a different path until a conclusion was reached. This approach does not test all possible paths from observations to conclusions. Heuristics to control the order in which possible paths are tested are very important. In cases of realistic complexity, it is not possible to test all consequences of applying one rule, and so simplifications such as depth-first or breadth-first strategies are employed. Pruning, or rejecting a path before working through it to exhaustion, is also used. (As a rough analogy, you can use the search for a move in a chess program. Some initial moves are rejected immediately, while others are searched to various depths to evaluate the various possible responses and the outcomes.) Reverse searching works in the same way, starting from possible conclusions and searching for paths that lead to observations. Some search "engines" combine both forward and reverse searching methods.

When fuzzy logic is used, the various rules contain probabilities. In that case, it is ideally necessary to construct a total probability by combining the values for nodes along each path to select the most likely path and hence the most probable result. The heuristics that control search order are less important, but the total computation load can be much greater.

Neural networks

Searching the multiple pathways through an expert system, especially one utilizing fuzzy logic probabilities, is an inherently parallel problem. An attractive way to solve it uses neural networks, an implementation of a simplified and idealized model of the functioning of biological processes. Each element in a neural network is a threshold logic unit, illustrated in **Figure 11.34** (which was introduced in **Chapter 2**). It is analogous to a simplified model of a functioning neuron, as shown in the classic McCulloch-Pitts model (Grossberg 1988; Lettvin et al. 1959; McCulloch and Pitts 1943; Minsky and Papert 1969; Rosenblatt 1958). Multiple inputs (which in the image-analysis case could be either measured parameter values or pixel intensities) are weighted and summed, and the total compared with a threshold value. If the threshold is exceeded, the neuron "fires." In a biological system it sends a train of pulses as inputs to other neurons; in a neural network it transmits a calculated output value (a probability) to another threshold logic unit.

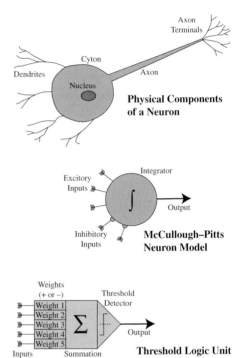

Figure 11.34 *Schematic diagram for an expert system.*

To understand the functioning of these simple units, it is worthwhile to consider again a classical description of a theoretical construct called the "grandmother cell." Imagine a cell that has been trained to recognize your grandmother, patiently examining every image that is transmitted from your eyes searching for clues. Earlier logic units, some of them in the eye and some in the visual cortex, find low-level structures. So the presence of white hair, blue eyes, and the spacing of eyes, nose, mouth, cheekbones, etc., are all inputs to the grandmother cell. It has been shown that human vision is very efficient at locating facial features (even babies do it, immediately after birth) and that, as illustrated previously, it is the ratios of spacings between these features that are important clues to recognition of individuals.

As described in **Chapter 2**, other clues might include the presence of a familiar dress, jewelry, or glasses. Some of these are more important than others (have larger weighting), and some factors may simply be missing (e.g., if your view of the person prevents seeing the color of her eyes). There may also be some factors with large negative weights, such as the presence of a bushy red mustache or a height over six feet tall. When all of the inputs are summed, if the total is large enough (exceeds a threshold value), the cell alerts your conscious brain that grandmother is present. Such a system accounts for the occurrence of false positives (thinking that you see someone familiar, who on close examination turns out not to be the expected person). The result will not always be correct (we may miss grandma in some situations, or mistake someone else for her occasionally), but it is very efficient and works quickly and well enough.

Connecting a network of these simple devices (perceptrons) in multiple layers, with some low-level decisions passing information to higher levels, produces a system capable of making decisions based on diverse types of inputs. The classic topology of a neural network is shown in **Figure 11.35**. Each artificial neuron calculates like the perceptron, producing an output that is a weighted combination (not necessarily linear) of its input values. These outputs are routed through at least one hidden layer before reaching the output layer. The output layer produces outputs that are discrete, selecting one (or at most a few) values. Training the neural network adjusts the weights in the neurons to produce the desired output patterns for the various training patterns (Hebb 1949). This is typically accomplished by training the system with examples. When a correct conclusion is reached, the weights of the inputs from the neurons that contributed to the decision are increased, and vice versa. This feedback system eventually results in pathways that correspond to descriptions of the objects being recognized. Various methods for adjusting the weights are in use, some working forward and some backward through the network (Rumelhart et al. 1986).

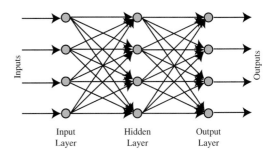

Figure 11.35 *Schematic diagram of a minimal neural network with one hidden layer.*

In principle, the weights in the various units describe the shape of each class space in a high-dimensional space (corresponding to the number of inputs). In practice, it is very difficult if not impossible to interpret the weights, particularly in the inner layers of the system. Dealing with overlapping classes (the possibility that the same set of inputs may lead to more than one output) is exactly analogous to the situation shown earlier in **Figure 11.11**. Many systems cannot explain the reasons for the answers they deliver; indeed, it is difficult to find just where the "knowledge" resides in the system (like in our own brains, it seems to be distributed widely throughout the network). It is difficult to assign probabilities or confidence limits to the result, but neural-network systems usually fail gracefully. Unlike classic expert systems, the solution time for a neural system decreases as more information is made available. Their principal shortcoming is the need for unusual computer architectures for efficient realization. Although the neural network is in theory a parallel device, many actual implementations use traditional serial computers to perform all of the calculations, simulating a parallel structure, and in this case the speed advantage is lost.

The weights in a neural network typically take a long time to stabilize, which is another way to say that it takes a lot of training to produce a network that gives correct answers most of the time. The same requirements for finding representative training populations exist as for the statistical classification methods discussed previously. The quality of the training is usually more important than how the solution is implemented. The only real difference between a neural network and one of the previously described statistical methods is the intricacy with which parameter space can be dissected into the various class regions. Neural networks can fit very complex functions to describe surfaces separating regions, and these may perform better in some cases than simple rectangular prisms, ellipsoids, or polyhedra, without encountering the problems of storage, sensitivity to outliers, and slow speed inherent in kNN methods.

This description tacitly assumes that the input values to the neural network are a set of measurements on the image or on the features within the image, each of which is obtained using the conventional procedures outlined in previous chapters. It is also possible to use the entire image itself as the input, namely the individual pixel values (Bollmann et al. 2004; Egmont-Petersen et al. 2002; France et al. 2004). In that case, the early layers of the net are also responsible for determining what in the image should be measured and how to measure it. This approach hides the details from the user, which may seem convenient but in practice makes the training process longer and the resulting decisions harder to decipher, explain, and debug. Applications involving global color and texture are generally more appropriate for this than applications involving discrete features.

Syntactical models

There is another approach to feature recognition that is quite different from the previously described parameter-space methods (Fu 1974, 1982; Pavlidis 1977; Schalkoff 1991; Tou and Gonzalez 1981). Syntactical models deal primarily with shape information, usually derived from the feature outline or skeleton. This is broken down into the important pieces, and their relative positions recorded. This recording can be likened to a set of characters that spell a word, and compared with other words on the basis of the number of missing, substituted, or rearranged characters.

To give an example, **Figure 11.36** shows the key elements of the letter *A*. The two branch points at the sides and the corner or apex at the top identify this letter visually, and no other letter in the alphabet has the same key points nor the same arrangement of them. The "springs" in the figure indicate that the key points can move around quite a bit without changing their usefulness for identification, as long as their relative positions remain in the same topological order. Extracting these key points and their arrangement provides a very robust identifier of the letter, which is quite insensitive to size and font. Some OCR (optical character recognition) programs that convert printed text to computer-readable files use similar methods.

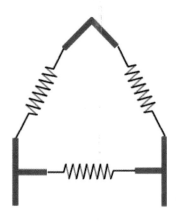

Figure 11.36 The important branch and corner points that identify the letter A. The springs that connect them indicate that shifting their positions, as long as their relative order remains the same, does not interfere with the identification.

Key points such as branches and ends can be obtained directly from the skeleton, as shown in **Chapter 8**. Corners can be isolated in several ways. **Figure 11.37** shows one in which convolution with a simple 3 × 3 kernel can select a corner in any specified orientation. A more general corner-finding method traverses the skeleton or outline of the feature using chain code, introduced in **Chapter 8**. A sequence of links in the chain that gives a net 90° (or more) change in direction within a certain (arbitrary) distance along the chain is interpreted as a corner. Fitting functions — polynomials or splines — to the edge points can also be used to locate corners.

Figure 11.38 shows another example of letters A through E, in several fonts, with the key identifying points of each (ends, branches, and corners). There is actually more information than needed to uniquely identify each character; some of the points can be missing (e.g., due to extreme alterations in letter shape in handwritten characters) without compromising readability. Similar schemes

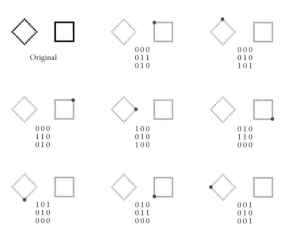

Figure 11.37 Extracting corner points from a skeleton or outline by using a 3 × 3 convolution kernel. Each kernel finds the points in the square and diamond shape that are marked in red. In general, any pattern can be found by applying a kernel that has the same shape as the desired pattern.

are used in some of the efforts to develop computer programs that read handwriting. Syntactical characterization of the shape and density patterns in human chromosomes is routinely used in karyotyping.

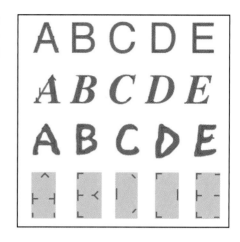

Figure 11.38 *The letters A through E with their key branch, corner, and endpoints.*

12

Tomographic Imaging

Volume imaging vs. sections

The study of three-dimensional structures of solid objects can utilize two-dimensional (2-D) or three-dimensional (3-D) imaging. Many of the 2-D images used in the preceding chapters have been sections through 3-D structures. This is especially true in the various types of microscopy, where either polished flat planes or cut thin sections are needed to form the images in the first place. But the specimens thus sampled are three-dimensional, and the goal of the microscopist is to understand the 3-D structure.

There are quantitative tools of great power and utility that can interpret measurements on 2-D images in ways that characterize 3-D structures. As summarized in **Chapter 9**, these enable the measurement of volume fraction of structures, surface area of interfaces, mean thickness of membranes, and even the size distribution of particles seen only in a random section. But there are many aspects of structure, both quantitative and qualitative, that are not accessible from a 2-D section image. Topological properties comprise a major category of such information, including such "simple" properties as the number of separate objects in a volume. Features visible in a single 2-D section do not reveal the actual 3-D structure present, as shown in **Figure 12.1**. In **Chapter 9**, a method was shown for unfolding the distribution of circles to determine the size distribution and total number of spheres in a sample. However, this procedure requires making a critical assumption that the objects are all spheres. If the shape of features is unknown, is variable, or is a function of size, then this method fails.

Furthermore, as valuable as numerical measurement data may be, they cannot provide the typical viewer with a real sense of the structure. As pointed out in **Chapter 2**, we are overwhelmingly visual creatures — we need to *see* the 3-D structure. Our world is 3-D, and we are accustomed to looking at external surfaces, or occasionally through transparent media, not at thin sections or polished cut surfaces. Try to imagine (again the need to resort to a word with its connotation of vision) standing by a busy street in which an imaginary plane exists transverse to traffic flow, and that you can see that plane but nothing else. What do people, cars and bicycles look like as they pass through that plane?

If you have a well-developed geometric sense, or experience as a radiologist or draftsman, you may be able to accurately visualize the appearance of that plane as portions of torsos, engine blocks, and even simple shapes like tires are cut by the plane. Most people will have difficulty

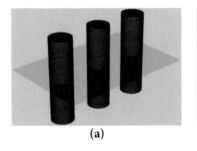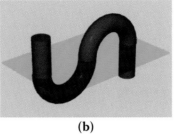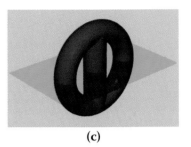

(a)   (b)   (c)

*Figure 12.1 Examples of sections through three different structures that produce the same 2-D section image: **(a)** three discrete objects; **(b)** one object with simple connectivity; **(c)** one object with multiple connectivity.*

imagining such collections of sections, and when asked to sketch the sections of even simple shapes will produce wildly inaccurate results.

If you doubt this, give yourself a simple test. Get some Cheerios®, or rotini noodles, or some other simple food object that has a well-defined shape (**Figure 12.2**). Then mix up an opaque matrix (fudge is good) and stir in the objects. While it is hardening, try to draw what various representative random slices through the structure might look like. After it has hardened, cut slices through the sample and compare the actual results to your sketches. My experience in conducting this experiment with students is that they have a strong tendency to imagine sections through the object that are parallel or perpendicular to principal axes, and ones that pass through the geometrical center of the objects. For the Cheerios (little tori), few actual sections consist of two side-by-side circles or one annulus, and are not necessarily even convex (**Figure 12.3**). For the rotini, most people do not realize that sections through the curved surfaces actually produce straight lines.

As difficult as this particular visualization task may be, even fewer people can make the transition in the opposite direction: given a collection of section data, to reconstruct in the mind a correct representation of the 3-D structure. This is true even of those who feel quite comfortable with the 2-D images themselves. Within the world of the 2-D images, recognition and understanding can be learned as a separate knowledge base that need not relate to the 3-D world. Observing the characteristic appearance of dendrites in polished metal samples, or that

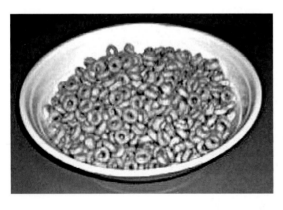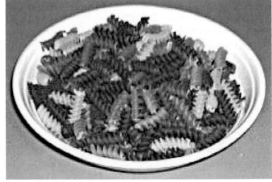

Figure 12.2 Food objects (Cheerios and rotini noodles) that are useful for experimenting with the relationship between 3-D shapes and 2-D section images. These are simpler and much more consistent than many natural structures we would like to understand.

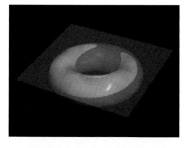 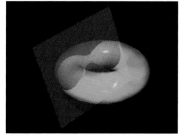 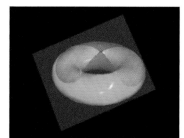

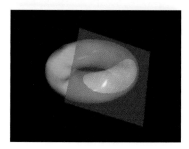

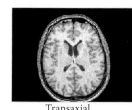

Figure 12.3 A few sections through a torus, producing one or two intersections that can be either convex or concave.

of mitochondria in thin electron microscope sections of cells, or internal organs in medical images (especially since these latter images are almost always oriented in transaxial, coronal, or sagittal views, as shown in **Figure 12.4**) does not necessarily mean that the complex 3-D shapes of these objects become familiar. In fact, there are numerous instances of erroneous 3-D interpretations that have persistently been made from 2-D section images.

Because of this difficulty in using 2-D images to study 3-D structure, there is interest in performing 3-D imaging. It can be performed directly, as discussed in this chapter, by actually collecting a 3-D set of information all at once, or indirectly by gathering a sequence of 2-D (slice) images and then combining them, as discussed in **Chapter 13**. Sometimes these slices must be obtained by physically sectioning the sample, and sometimes (as in the confocal light microscope) they can be nondestructive. There are a variety of ways to acquire 2-D images to assemble the data needed for 3-D imaging, and also a great variety of ways to present the information to the user. Several of each are discussed in **Chapter 13**. The large number of approaches suggests that no one way is best, either for most viewers or for most applications.

Any method that reconstructs internal structural information within an object by mathematically reconstructing it from a series of projections is generally referred to as tomography. It can be used to obtain true 3-D arrays of voxels (the 3-D analog of the pixel in a 2-D image) or to obtain a 2-D image from a series of one-dimensional line projections. The latter method is used in most medical imaging, which is by far the most common application of CT (computed tomography) at the present time. However, the same basic techniques are used for 3-D imaging and for a variety of imaging signals.

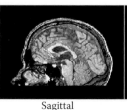 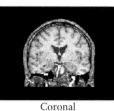

Transaxial   Sagittal   Coronal

Figure 12.4 Standard orientations (transaxial, sagittal, and coronal) for viewing medical slice images.

Medical tomography primarily uses X-ray absorption, magnetic resonance (MRI), emission of photons (single-photon emission spectroscopy, SPECT) or positrons (positron-emission tomography, PET), and sound waves (ultrasound). Comparisons of the various methods and the information they provide can be found in recent textbooks (Jan 2005; Rangayyan 2005). Other fields of application and research use many different frequencies of electromagnetic radiation, from X and gamma rays (nanometer wavelengths) through visible light and even microwave radiation (wavelengths from centimeters up). Besides using photons, tomography is regularly performed using electrons and neutrons. In addition to absorption of the particles or radiation, tomography can be based on the scattering or emission of radiation as well. Tomography of mixing fluids can sometimes be performed by measuring the electrical resistance or impedance between multiple points around the containment vessel (Mann et al. 2001; York 2001).

Sound waves produced by small intentional explosions or by "ground thumpers" are used to image underground strata for prospecting, while naturally occurring noise sources such as earthquakes are used to perform seismic tomography, imaging underground faults, rock density beneath volcanoes, and locating discontinuities between Earth's mantle and core. There are also devices listening for Moon- and Mars-quakes that will reveal their internal structure, and studies of the seismic structure of the Sun have been performed.

Basics of reconstruction

X-ray absorption tomography is one of the oldest, most widely used methods and will be used here to illustrate the various parameters, artifacts, and performance possibilities. Images produced by computer-assisted tomography (CAT or CT scans) and similar methods using magnetic resonance, sound waves, isotope emission, X-ray scattering, or electron beams deserve special attention. They are formed by computer processing of information from many individual pieces of projection information obtained nondestructively through the body of an object, which must be unfolded to see the internal structure. The mathematical description of the process presented here is that of X-ray absorption tomography, as it is used both in medical applications and in industrial testing (Herman 1980; Hsieh 2003; Kak and Slaney 1988, 2001; Natterer 2001; Natterer and Wubbeling 2001). Similar sets of equations and methods of solution apply to the other signal modalities.

Absorption tomography is based on physical processes that reduce intensity as radiation or particles pass through the sample in straight lines. In some other kinds of tomography, the paths are not straight and the reconstruction takes place along curved lines (e.g., magnetic resonance imaging and X-ray scattering tomography) or even along many lines at once (seismic tomography). This makes the equations and graphics slightly more confusing, but does not affect the basic principles involved.

X-rays pass through material but are absorbed along the way according to the composition and density that they encounter. The intensity (number of photons per second) is reduced according to a linear attenuation coefficient μ, which for an interesting specimen is not uniform but has some spatial variation so that we can write $\mu(x,y,z)$ or, for a 2-D plane through the object, $\mu(x,y)$. The linear attenuation coefficient is the product of the density and the mass-absorption coefficient, which depends on the local elemental composition. In medical tomography, the composition varies only slightly, and density variations are primarily responsible for producing images. For industrial applications, significant variations in composition are also usually present. The measured intensity along a straight-line path through this distribution is given by

$$\int \mu(x,y)\,dS = \log_e \frac{I_o}{I_d}$$

(12.1)

where I_0 is the incident intensity (from an X-ray tube or radioisotope) that is known and generally held constant, and I_d is the detected intensity. This is called the ray-integral equation and describes the result along one line projection through the object.

If a series of parallel lines are measured, either one at a time by scanning the source and detector or all at once using many detectors, a profile of intensity is obtained, which is called a view. As shown schematically in **Figure 12.5**, this function is usually plotted as the inverse of the intensity or the summation of absorption along each of the lines. The function is written as $P(\varphi,t)$ to indicate that it varies with position along the direction t as rays sample different portions of the object, and also with angle φ as the mechanism is rotated around the object to view it from different directions (or, equivalently, as the object is rotated).

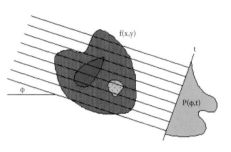

Figure 12.5 *Illustration of a set of projections through an object at a viewing angle φ forming the function P.*

Each of the views is a one-dimensional profile of measured attenuation as a function of position, corresponding to a particular angle. The collection of many such views can be presented as a 2-D plot or image in which one axis is position t and the other is angle φ. This image is called a sinogram or the Radon transform of the 2-D slice. **Figure 12.6** and **Figure 12.7** show a simple example. The construction of a planar figure, as shown in **Figure 12.6a**, is called a phantom, which is used to evaluate the important variables and different methods for reconstructing the object slice from the projection information. Such phantoms typically mimic the important structures of real interest as an aid to evaluating reconstruction algorithms. Compare it with **Figure 12.6b** showing an actual MRI image of a brain tumor.

The individual projection profiles shown in **Figure 12.7a** show some variation as the angle is changed, but this presentation is difficult to interpret. The sinogram in **Figure 12.7b** organizes the data so that it can be examined more readily. The name "sinogram" comes from the sinusoidal variation of position of projections through the various structures within the phantom as a function of rotation, which is evident in the example. The name "Radon transform" acknowledges the fact that the principles of this method of imaging were published in 1917 by Radon (1917). However, the equations he presented did not provide a practical way to imple-

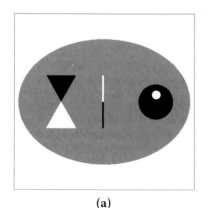

(a)

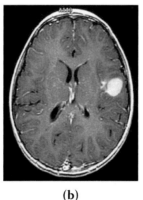

(b)

Figure 12.6
  (a) *A phantom or test object with geometrical shapes of known density, and*
  (b) *a real magnetic resonance image of a tumor (bright area) in a section through a head.*

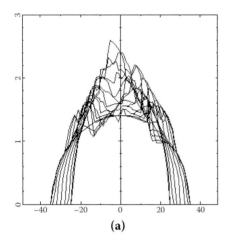

(a)

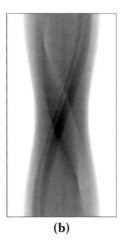

(b)

Figure 12.7 Sixteen attenuation profiles **(a)** for the phantom in *Figure 12.6a* and the sinogram or Radon transform; **(b)** produced by plotting 180 such profiles (each as one horizontal line).

ment a reconstruction, since they required a continuous array of projections, and it was not until Hounsfield and Cormack developed a practical reconstruction algorithm and hardware that CAT scans became a routine medical possibility. A. M. Cormack (1963, 1964) developed a mathematically manageable reconstruction method at Tufts University in 1963–64, and G. N. Hounsfield designed a working instrument at EMI Ltd. in England in 1972. They shared the Nobel Prize in physiology or medicine in 1979.

The Fourier transform of the set of projection data in one view direction can be written as

$$S(\phi,\varpi)= \int P(\phi,t)e^{-j2\pi\varpi}dt$$

(12.2)

Radon showed that this could also be written as

$$S(\phi,\varpi)= \int\int f(x,y)e^{-j2\pi\varpi(x\cos\phi+y\sin\phi)}dxdy$$

(12.3)

which is simply the 2-D Fourier transform $F(u,v)$ for the function $f(x,y)$ with the constraints that $u = \omega \cos \varphi$ and $v = \omega \sin \varphi$. This is consequently the equation of the line for the projection.

What this relationship means is that starting with the original image of the phantom, forming its 2-D Fourier transform as discussed in **Chapter 6**, and then looking at the information in that image along a radial direction from the origin normal to the direction φ would give the function S, which is just the one-dimensional Fourier transform of the projection data in direction φ in real space. The way this can be used in practice is to measure the projections P in many directions, calculate the one-dimensional transforms S, plot the complex coefficients of S into a 2-D transform image in the corresponding direction, and after enough directions have been measured, perform an inverse 2-D Fourier transform to recover the spatial-domain image for the slice. This permits a reconstruction of the slice image from the projection data so that a nondestructive internal image can be obtained. It is the principle behind tomographic imaging.

Figure 12.8 shows an example. Eight views or sets of projections are taken at equal-angle steps, and the Fourier transform of each is calculated and plotted into a 2-D complex image, which is then reconstructed. The image quality is only fair, because of the limited number of views. When 180 views at 1° intervals are used, the result is quite good. The artifacts that are still present arise because of the gaps in the frequency-space image. This missing information is especially evident at high frequencies (far from the center), where the lines from the individual views become more widely spaced. All tomographic reconstruction procedures are sensitive to the number of views, as we will see.

By collecting enough views and performing this Fourier space reconstruction, it is possible to perform tomographic imaging. In practice, few systems actually work this way. An exactly equivalent procedure that requires less computation and is more suitable for "real time" implementation is also available, known as filtered back-projection. This is the method used in most medical scanners and some industrial applications.

The principle behind back-projection is simple to demonstrate. The attenuation plotted in each projection in a view is due to the structure of the sample along the individual lines, or ray integrals. It is not possible to know from one projection just where along the line the attenuation occurs, but it is possible to evenly distribute the measured attenuation along the line. If this is done for only a single view, the result is not very interesting. But if it is done along projections from several views, the superposition of the density or attenuation values should correspond to the features present in the structure.

Figure 12.9 illustrates this result for the same phantom. It is possible to see the dense (dark) cylinder with its hollow (light) core in the projections. Data from several views overlap to delineate the cylinder in the reconstructed image. There is a problem with this result, however. The attenuation or density of uniform regions in the original phantom is not constant, but increases toward the center of the section. Also, edges are blurred.

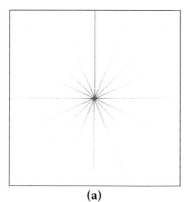
(a)

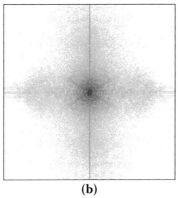
(b)

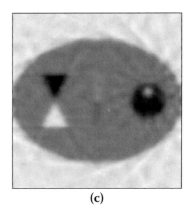
(c)

Figure 12.8 Reconstruction in frequency space using the projection data in Figure 12.7. The (complex) one-dimensional Fourier transforms of projection sets or views at different angles are plotted into a 2-D frequency domain image, which is then reconstructed:
(a) 8 views in frequency space;
(b) 180 views in frequency space;
(c) reconstruction from image a;
(d) reconstruction from image b.

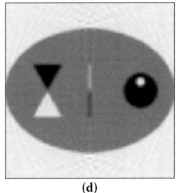
(d)

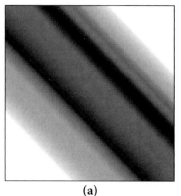

(a)

Figure 12.9 *Back-projection in the spatial domain. The attenuation values in each view are projected back through the object space along each projection line. Adding together the data from many view directions does show the major features, but the image is blurred:*
(a) *1 view;*
(b) *6 views;*
(c) *30 views;*
(d) *180 views.*

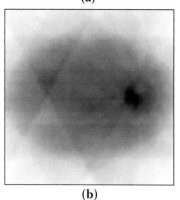

(b)

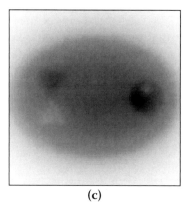

(c)

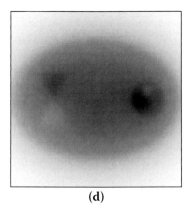

(d)

The cause of this problem can be described in several different but equivalent ways. The projections from all of the views contribute too much to the center of the image, where all projections overlap. The effect is the same as if the image were viewed through an out-of-focus optical system whose blur or point-spread function is proportional to $1/r$, where r is the frequency, or the distance from the center, of the frequency transform.

Chapter 6 showed how to remove a known blur from an image: apply an inverse function to the frequency-space transform that corrects for the blur, in this case by attenuating low frequencies before retransforming. Based on the Fourier approach, and writing the reverse transformation in terms of polar coordinates, this gives

$$f(x,y)=\int_{0^-}^{\varsigma}\int S(\phi,\varpi)|\varpi|e^{-j2\pi\omega}d\varpi d\phi$$

(12.4)

or, in terms of x and y,

$$f(x,y)=\int_0^\pi Q_\phi(x\cos\phi+y\sin\phi)d\phi$$

(12.5)

where

$$Q_\phi = \int_-^+ S(\phi, \varpi) |\varpi| e^{-j2\pi \varpi t} d\varpi \qquad (12.6)$$

This is just the convolution of S, the Fourier transform of the projection, by $|\omega|$, the absolute value of frequency. In frequency space, this is an ideal inverse filter that is shaped as shown in **Figure 12.10**. But, as was pointed out in **Chapter 6**, convolutions can also be applied in the spatial domain. The inverse transform of this ideal filter is also shown in **Figure 12.10**. Note its similarity to the shape of a Laplacian (LoG) or difference of Gaussians (DoG), as discussed in **Chapter 5**.

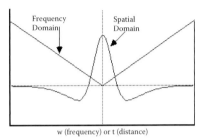

w (frequency) or t (distance)

Figure 12.10 An ideal inverse filter, which selectively removes low frequencies, and its spatial-domain-equivalent kernel.

As a one-dimensional kernel or set of weights, this function can be multiplied by the projection P, just as kernels were applied to 2-D images in **Chapters 4** and **5**. The weights are multiplied by the values, and the sum is saved as one point in the filtered projection. This is repeated for each line in the projection set or view. **Figure 12.11** shows the result for the projection data, presented in the form of a sinogram. Edges (high frequencies) are strongly enhanced, and low-frequency information is suppressed.

The filtered data are then projected back, and the blurring is corrected, as shown in **Figure 12.12**. Filtered back-projection using an ideal or inverse filter produces results identical to the previously described inverse Fourier transform method. The practical implementation of filtered back-projection is easier because the projection data from each view can be filtered by convolution (a one-dimensional operation) and the data spread back across the image as it is acquired, with no need to store the complex (i.e., real and imaginary values) frequency-space image needed for the Fourier method or to retransform it afterward.

Notice in **Figure 12.12** that the quality of the image, and the effect of the number of views on the artifacts, is identical to that shown for the frequency-space method in **Figure 12.8**. In the absence of noise in the data and other effects that will be discussed below, these two methods are exactly equivalent. Filtered back-projection is the method actually used in the majority of CT instruments in current use.

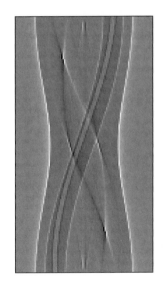

Figure 12.11 The filtered projection data from Figure 12.7, shown as a sinogram.

Algebraic reconstruction methods

The problem of solving for the density (actually, for the linear attenuation coefficient) of each location in the image can also be viewed as a set of simultaneous equations. Each ray integral (or summation, in the finite case we are dealing with here) provides one equation. The sum of the attenuation coefficients for the pixels (or voxels) along the ray, each multiplied by a weighting factor that takes into account the actual path length of that ray through the pixel, is

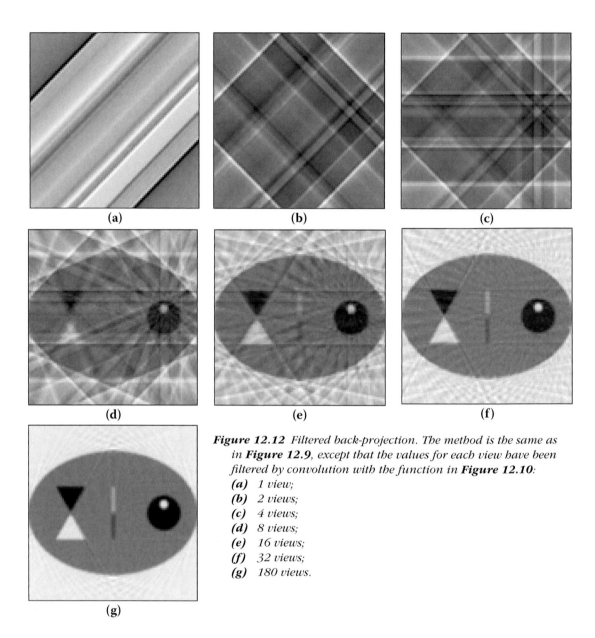

(a)

(b)

(c)

(d)

(e)

(f)

(g)

Figure 12.12 Filtered back-projection. The method is the same as in *Figure 12.9*, except that the values for each view have been filtered by convolution with the function in *Figure 12.10*:
(a) 1 view;
(b) 2 views;
(c) 4 views;
(d) 8 views;
(e) 16 views;
(f) 32 views;
(g) 180 views.

equal to the measured absorption. **Figure 12.13** illustrates the relationship between the pixels and the ray-integral equations.

The number of unknowns in this set of equations is the number of pixels in the image of the slice through the specimen. The number of equations is the number of ray integrals, which is generally the number of detectors used along each projection profile times the number of view angles. This is a very large number of equations, but many of the weights are zero (most pixels are not involved in any one particular ray-integral equation). Furthermore, the number of equations rarely equals the number of unknowns. But fortunately there are a number of practical and well-tested computer methods for solving such sets of sparse equations when they are under- or overdetermined.

It is not our purpose here to compare the various solution methods. A suitable understanding of the method can be attained using the simplest of the methods, known as the algebraic reconstruction technique or ART (Gordon 1974). In this approach, the equations are solved iteratively. The set of equations can be written as

$$\mathbf{A}^{mn}\,\mathbf{x}^n = \mathbf{b}^m \qquad (12.7)$$

where n is the number of voxels, m is the number of projections, and $\mathbf{A}$ is the matrix of weights that correspond to the contribution of each voxel to each ray path (which can be precalculated for any particular instrument and geometry). The voxel values are the $\mathbf{x}$ values and the projection measurements are the $\mathbf{b}$ values. The classic ART method calculates each iterative set of $\mathbf{x}$ values from the preceding ones as

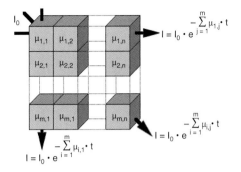

Figure 12.13 *Schematic drawing of pixels (or voxels, since they have depth) in a plane section of the specimen, and the ray-integral equations that sum up the attenuation along a few paths through the array.*

$$\mathbf{x}^{k+1} = \mathbf{x}^k + \mathrm{A}_i(b_i \pm \mathrm{A}_i^{\lambda}\mathbf{x}^k)\,\|\,\mathrm{A}_i\,\|^2 \qquad (12.8)$$

The value of λ, the relaxation coefficient, generally lies between 0 and 2, and controls the speed of convergence. When λ is very small, this becomes equivalent to a conventional least-squares solution. Practical considerations, including the order in which the various equations are applied, are dealt with in detail in the literature (Censor 1983, 1984).

Figure 12.14 shows a simple example of this approach. The 16 × 16 array of voxels has been given density values from 0 to 20 as shown in **Figure 12.14b**, and three projection sets at view angles of 0, 90, and 180° were calculated for the fan-beam geometry shown in **Figure 12.14a**. For an array of 25 detectors, this gives a total of 75 equations in 256 unknowns. Starting with an initial guess of uniform voxels (with density 10), the results after 1, 5, and 50 iterations are shown. The void areas and internal square appear rather quickly, and the definition of boundaries gradually improves. The errors — particularly in the corners of the image, where fewer ray equations contain any information, and at the corners of the internal dense square, where the attenuation value changes abruptly — are evident. Still, considering the extent to which the system is underdetermined, the results are rather good.

Kacmarz's method for this type of solution is illustrated in **Figure 12.15** for the very modest case of three equations and two unknowns, with $\lambda = 1$. Beginning at some initial guess, for instance that all of the pixels have the same attenuation value, one of the equations is applied. This is equivalent to moving perpendicular to the line representing the equation. This new point is then used as a starting point to apply the next equation, and so on. In the real case, the equations do not all meet in a perfect point because of finite precision in the various measurements, counting statistics, machine variation, etc.; thus there is no single point that represents a stable answer. Instead, the solution converges toward a region that is mostly within the region between the various lines and then oscillates there. However, in a high-dimensionality space with some noisy equations, it is possible for the solution to leave this region and wander away after many iterations.

In real cases with many dimensions, the convergence may not be very fast. The greatest difficulty in using the iterative algebraic technique is deciding when to stop. Logically, we would like to continue until the answer is as good as it can get, but without knowing the "truth," it

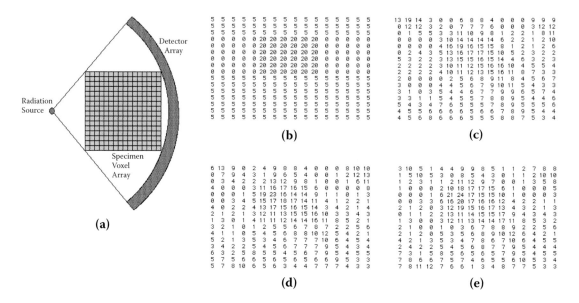

Figure 12.14 *Example of the application of an iterative solution. Three projection sets were calculated for an array of 25 detectors, (a) with view directions of 0, 90, and 180°. (b) The simulated specimen contains a 16 × 16 array of voxels. The calculation results after: (c) 1 iteration; (d) 5 iterations; (e) 50 iterations.*

is not possible to determine this stopping point exactly. Some methods examine the change in the calculated image after each iteration and attempt to judge from that when to stop (for instance, when the normalized total variation in pixel values falls below some arbitrary limit, or when it begins to increase from the previous iteration). This method is prone to serious errors in a few cases, but is used nonetheless. It should be noted that the penalty for continuing the iteration is not simply the computational cost, but also the possibility that, for some sets of data, the answer may start to diverge (leave the bounded region near the crossover point). This condition is, of course, highly undesirable.

Given the drawbacks to the algebraic approach and the relative simplicity and straightforward approach of the filtered back-projection method, why would we use this method? There are several potential advantages of algebraic methods such as ART. First, the filtered back-projection method, and the Fourier transform method that it embodies, require that the number of views be rather large and that they be equally spaced so that the frequency space is well filled with data. Missing angles, or entire sets of angles that may be unattainable due to physical limitations, present problems for filtered back-projection and introduce significant artifacts. ART methods can still produce an acceptable reconstruction. There may be a lack of detail in portions of the reconstructed image that are undersampled by the projections, but the artifacts do not spread throughout the entire image. In fact, acceptable reconstructions are often obtained with only a very few views (examples are shown below).

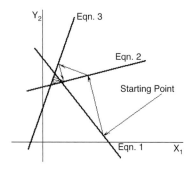

Figure 12.15 *Schematic diagram of Kacmarz's method for iteratively solving a set of equations, shown here for the case of two unknowns.*

Another advantage to ART is the ability to apply constraints. For instance, it is possible, in a filtered back-projection or Fourier transform method, to calculate negative values of density (attenuation) for some voxels because of the finite measurement precision. However, such values have no physical meaning. In the iterative algebraic method, any such values can be restricted to zero. In the schematic diagram of **Figure 12.15**, this amounts to restricting the solution to the quadrant of the graph with positive values.

In fact, any other prior knowledge can also be applied. If it is known that the only possible values of density and attenuation in the specimen correspond to specific materials, then the values can be easily constrained to correspond. Any geometric information, such as the outside dimensions of the object, can also be included (in this case, by forcing the voxels outside the object boundaries to zero density).

It is even possible to set up a grid of voxels that are not all of the same size and spacing. This setup might allow, for instance, the use of a fine voxel spacing in the interior of an object, where great detail is desired, but a much coarser grid outside (or vice versa). This would still allow the calculation of the contribution of the outside material to the ray integrals, but it would reduce the number of unknowns to produce a better solution for any given number of views and projections. Sets of nonsquare pixels or noncubic voxels can also be used when these are needed to conform to specific object shapes and symmetries.

The flexibility of the algebraic method and its particular abilities to use *a priori* information, often available in an industrial tomography setting, compensates for its slowness and requirements for large amounts of computation. The calculation of voxel weights (the **A** matrix) can be tedious, especially for fan-beam or other complex geometries, but no more so than back-projection in such cases, and it is a one-time calculation whose results can be stored and used for many reconstructions using the same geometry. The use of solution methods other than the simple iterative approach described here can provide improved stability and convergence.

Maximum entropy

There are other ways to solve these huge sets of sparse equations. One is the so-called maximum entropy approach. Maximum entropy was mentioned in **Chapter 4** as an image processing tool to remove noise from a 2-D image. Bayes's theorem is the cornerstone for the maximum entropy approach, given that we have relevant prior information that can be used as constraints. In the case where no prior information is available but noise is a dominant factor, Bayes's theorem leads to the classical or "least squares" approximation method. It is the use of prior information that permits a different approach.

The philosophical justification for the maximum entropy approach comes from Bayesian statistics and information theory. It has also been derived from Gibbs's concept of statistical thermodynamics (Jaynes 1985). For the nonspecialist, it can be described as follows: find the result (distribution of brightnesses in pixels of image, distribution of density values in a voxel array, or practically anything else) that is feasible (consistent with the known constraints, such as the total number of photons, the nonnegativity of brightness or density at any point, the physics involved in the detector or measurement process, etc.) and has the configuration of values that is most probable.

This most probable result is defined as the one that can be obtained in the greatest number of ways. For an image formed by photons, all photons are considered indistinguishable, and the order in which they arrive is unimportant, so the distribution of photons to the various pixels can be carried out in many ways. For some brightness patterns (images), the number of ways to form the pattern is much greater than that for other patterns. We say that these images with greater multiplicity have a higher entropy. Nature can form them in more ways, so they are more likely to occur. The entropy is defined as $S = -\Sigma\, p_i \log p_i$, where p_i is the fraction of pixels with brightness value i.

The most likely image (from a simple statistical point of view) is for all of the pixels to get the same average number of photons, producing a uniform gray scene. However, this result may not be permitted by our constraints, one of which is the measured brightness pattern actually recorded. The difference between the calculated scene and the measured one can only be allowed to have a set upper limit, usually based on the estimated noise characteristics of the detector, the number of photons, etc. Finding the feasible scene that has the highest multiplicity is the goal of the maximum entropy method.

For instance, in solving for the tomographic reconstruction of an object from the set of ray-integral equations obtained from various view angles, we have a large set of simultaneous equations in many unknowns. Instead of formally solving the set of simultaneous equations, for instance by a traditional Gauss-Jordan elimination scheme, which would take far too many steps to be practical, the maximum entropy approach recasts the problem. Start with any initial guess (in most "well-behaved" cases, the quality of that guess matters little to the end result), and then iteratively, starting at that point, find another solution (within the class of feasible solutions as defined by the constraints) that has a higher entropy. Deciding which way to move in the space defined by the parameters (the values of all the voxels) is usually done with La-Grange multipliers by taking partial derivatives and trying always to move "uphill," where the objective function used to evaluate each set of values is the entropy.

It is usually found that the solution having the maximum feasible entropy (i.e., permitted by the constraints) is hard against the boundary formed by those constraints, and if they were relaxed the solution would move higher (toward a more uniform image). Knowing or assuming that the solution lies along the constraint boundaries allows use of more efficient schemes for finding the best solution. For the noise removal problem discussed in **Chapter 4**, the constraint is commonly the chi-squared value of the smoothed image as compared with the measured one. This is generally assumed to be due to classical noise, and so should have an upper limit and a known distribution.

For tomographic reconstruction, the constraints are based on satisfying the ray-integral equations. These are not all consistent, so a weighting scheme must be imposed on the error; linear weighting is the simplest and most often used. It turns out that in most cases, the cluster of solutions with high entropies, all permitted by the constraints, are virtually indistinguishable. In other words, the maximum entropy method does lead to a useful and robust solution. While the solution is still iterative, the method is quite efficient as compared with other solution techniques.

Defects in reconstructed images

The reconstructed example shown in **Figure 12.8** and **Figure 12.12** was calculated using projection data simulated by computation, with no noise or any other defects. In real tomography, a variety of defects may be present in the projection sets that propagate errors back into the reconstructed image. Using the same phantom, several of the more common defects can be demonstrated.

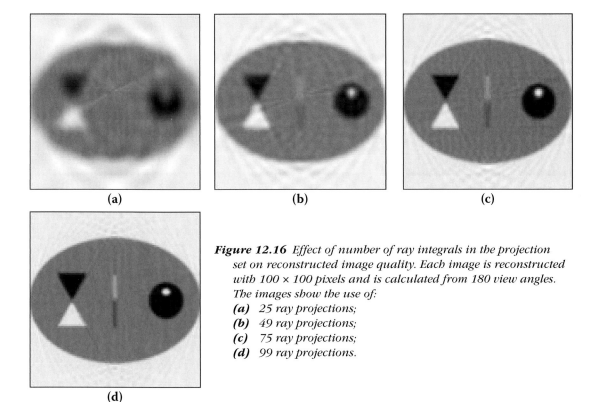

(a)   **(b)**   **(c)**

Figure 12.16 Effect of number of ray integrals in the projection set on reconstructed image quality. Each image is reconstructed with 100 × 100 pixels and is calculated from 180 view angles. The images show the use of:
(a) 25 ray projections;
(b) 49 ray projections;
(c) 75 ray projections;
(d) 99 ray projections.

(d)

Ideally, a large number of view angles and enough detector positions along each projection set will be used to provide enough information for the reconstruction. In the event that fewer projections in a set or fewer views are used, the image has more reconstruction artifacts and poorer resolution, definition of boundaries, and precision and uniformity of voxel values. **Figure 12.16** shows the effect of fewer projections in each set but still uses 180 view angles. The reconstructed images are displayed with 100 × 100 pixels. This ideally requires a number of ray integrals in each projection set equal to at least $\sqrt{2}$ times the width, or 141 equations for each view. With fewer, the resolution of the reconstruction degrades.

If fewer view angles are used (but the angular spacing is still uniform), the artifacts in the reconstruction increase, as was shown in **Figure 12.12**. If the view angles are not uniformly spaced, the results are much worse, as shown in **Figure 12.17**.

In real images, the number of X-ray photons detected at each point in the projection set is subject to fluctuations due to counting statistics. In many cases, both in medical and industrial tomography, the number of photons is limited. In medical applications, it is important to limit the total exposure to the subject. In industrial applications, the limitation is due to the finite source strength of either the X-ray tube or radioisotope source, and the need to acquire as many views as possible within a reasonable time. In either case, the variation in the number of detected X-rays varies in an approximately Gaussian or normal distribution whose standard deviation is the square root of the number counted. Counting an average of 100 X-rays produces a variation whose standard deviation is 10% ($\sqrt{100} = 10$), while an average of 10,000 X-rays is needed to reduce the variation to 1% ($\sqrt{10^4} = 10^2$).

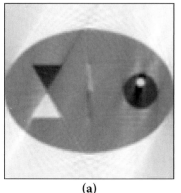

(a)

Figure 12.17 *Effect of using a set of view angles that do not uniformly fill the angular range:*
(a) *150° coverage;*
(b) *120° coverage;*
(c) *90° coverage;*
(d) *a different 90° range.*

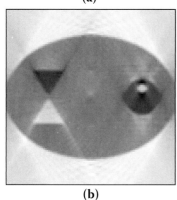

(b)

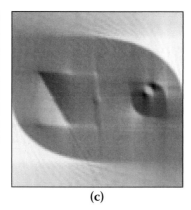

(c)

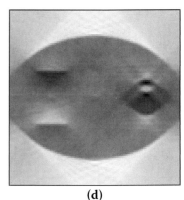

(d)

The process of reconstruction amplifies the effect of noise in the projections. This is the same effect of noise seen in **Chapter 6** for removing blur by deconvolution, and arises from the same mathematical causes. The filtering process suppresses the low frequencies and keeps the high frequencies, and the counting fluctuations vary randomly from point to point and so are represented in the highest frequency data. **Figure 12.18** shows the result. Adding a statistical or counting fluctuation of a few percent to the simulated projection data produces a much greater noise in the reconstructed image. Although the density differences in the three regions of the phantom vary by 100%, some of the regions disappear altogether when 10 or 20% noise is added to the projection data.

Suppression of the high-frequency noise in the projection data by the filtering process can reduce the effect of the noise somewhat, as shown in **Figure 12.19**. Notice that the noise variations in the reconstructed images are reduced, but that the high-frequency data needed to produce sharp edges and reveal the smaller structures are gone as well.

Several different filter shapes are used for this purpose. **Figure 12.20** shows representative examples in comparison with the shape of the ideal inverse filter that was discussed previously. The plots are in terms of frequency. All of the filters reduce the low-frequency values, which is required to prevent blurring, and all of the noise-reduction filters also attenuate the high frequencies to suppress the noise.

Another important source of errors in the reconstruction of images is imprecise knowledge of the location of the center of rotation, or variation in that center due to imperfect mechanical mechanisms (Barnes et al. 1990). As shown in **Figure 12.21**, this variation also produces an effect in the reconstructed image that is magnified. The characteristic U-shaped arcs result

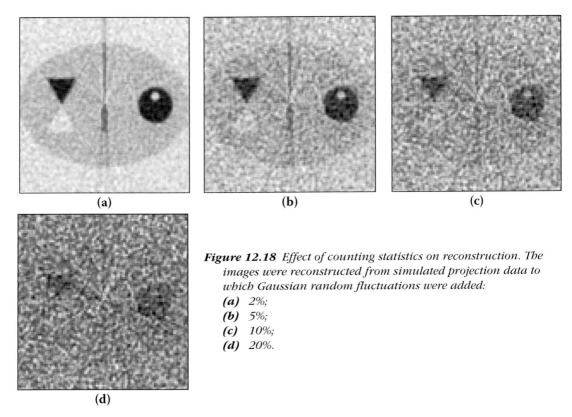

(a)   **(b)**   **(c)**

(d)

Figure 12.18 *Effect of counting statistics on reconstruction. The images were reconstructed from simulated projection data to which Gaussian random fluctuations were added:*
(a)   *2%;*
(b)   *5%;*
(c)   *10%;*
(d)   *20%.*

Figure 12.19 *Reconstructions from the same projection data with superimposed counting statistics variations as in* ***Figure 12.16****, but using a Hann filter instead of an ideal inverse filter to reduce the high-frequency noise.*

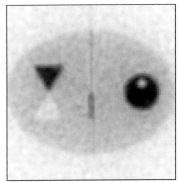

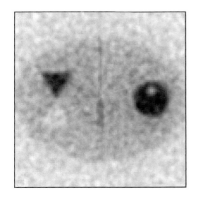 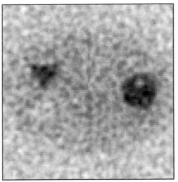 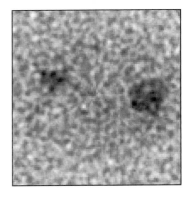

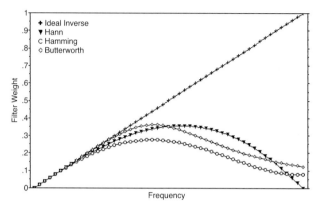

Figure 12.20 *Filter profiles for noise reduction in filtered back-projection: Ideal inverse: Weight = |f|; Hann: Weight = |f| ([0.5 + 0.5 cos [(π/2) (f/fm)]]; Hamming: Weight = |f| ([0.54 + 0.46 cos (π f/fm)]; Butterworth (n = 3): Weight = |f| (1/[1 + (f/2fm)2n].*

from an off-center rotation because view angles in a range of 180° were used. If 360° rotation is used, a complete circular arc is present (**Figure 12.22**) that also distorts the reconstruction but is more difficult to recognize. Note that it is not common to collect data over a complete 360° set of angles because, in the absence of off-center rotation or beam hardening (discussed below), the second half of the data would be redundant. The effect of a variable center is equal in magnitude with 360° rotation, but harder to recognize. In general, it is required that the location of the center of rotation and its constancy should be less than about one-tenth of the expected spatial resolution or voxel size in the reconstructed images.

Similarly, the motion of the object should be restricted during the collection of the multiple views. In medical imaging, where the most common imaging geometry is to place the subject inside a circular track on which the source or detectors rotate, this means that the patient must not breathe during the scanning process. If the images are expected to show the heart, the entire collection of views must be obtained in a time much shorter than the single beat, or else some stroboscopic triggering scheme must be used to collect images at the same relative timing over many beats. Both methods are used.

Beam hardening

Beam hardening is the name used to describe the effect in which the lower-energy or "softer" X-rays from a polychromatic source such as a conventional X-ray tube are preferentially absorbed in a sample. The consequence is that the effective attenuation coefficient of a voxel is different depending on whether it is on the side of the specimen near the source or farther away. This variation along the path is indicated schematically in **Figure 12.23**. Beam hardening is not a major problem in medical tomography because the variation in composition of the various parts of the human body is only slight. Everything is mostly water with some addition of carbon, a trace of other elements, and for bones, some calcium. The density is variable, and this is in fact what the reconstructed image shows, but the range of variation is small. This uniformity makes X-ray tubes an acceptable source and simple filtered back-projection a suitable reconstruction method.

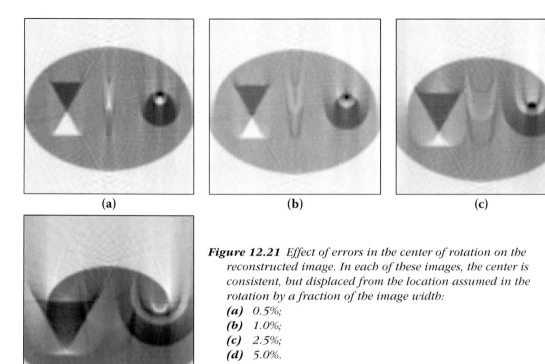

(a) (b) (c)

Figure 12.21 *Effect of errors in the center of rotation on the reconstructed image. In each of these images, the center is consistent, but displaced from the location assumed in the rotation by a fraction of the image width:*
(a) *0.5%;*
(b) *1.0%;*
(c) *2.5%;*
(d) *5.0%.*

(d)

Figure 12.22 *Repeating the reconstructions of* **Figure 12.21** *using the same number of views (180) but spread over 360° instead of 180°, with the center of rotation displaced from the assumed location by a fraction of the image width:*
(a) *0.5%;*
(b) *1.0%;*
(c) *2.5%;*
(d) *5.0%.*

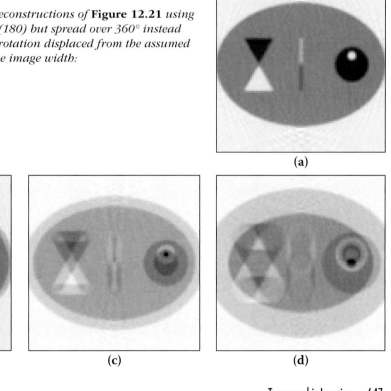

(a)

(b) (c) (d)

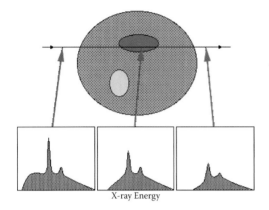

X-ray Energy

Figure 12.23 Schematic diagram of beam hardening. The energy spectrum of X-rays from an X-ray tube is shown at the beginning, middle, and end of the path through the specimen. As the lower-energy X-rays are absorbed, the attenuation coefficient of the sample changes independent of any actual change in composition or density.

Industrial applications commonly encounter samples with a much greater variation in composition, ranging across the entire periodic table and with physical densities that vary from zero (voids) to more than ten times the density of biological tissue. This large range of variation makes beam hardening an important problem. One solution is to use a monochromatic source such as a radioisotope or a filtered X-ray tube. Another is to use two different energies (Schneberk et al. 1991) or a combination of absorption and X-ray scattering data (Prettyman et al. 1991) and to use the two projection sets to correct for the change in composition in the reconstruction process. However, this method increases the complexity significantly and requires an algebraic solution method rather than back-projection or Fourier techniques.

Figure 12.24 shows a representative example of the beam-hardening effect in the same phantom used above. In this case, the sample composition is specified as void (the lightest region and the surroundings), titanium (the medium gray region of the elliptical object), and iron (the dark region). The total width is 1 cm, and the X-ray tube is assumed to be operating at 100 kV. This is in fact a very modest amount of beam hardening. A larger specimen, a lower tube voltage, higher atomic number elements, or a greater variation in atomic number of density, would produce a much greater effect.

Figure 12.25 shows reconstructions of the image using view angles that cover 180° and 360°. In most tomography, 180° is adequate, since the projections are expected to be the same regardless of direction along a ray path. This assumption is not true in the case of beam hardening (as it also was not for the case of off-center rotation), and so better results are obtained with a full 360° of data. Notice, however, that artifacts are still present. This is particularly true of the central feature, in which the narrow void is hardly visible. **Figure 12.26** shows the same phantom with no beam hardening, produced with a monochromatic X-ray source.

When X-rays pass through material, the attenuation coefficient that reduces the transmitted intensity consists of two principal parts: the absorption of the X-rays by the excitation of a bound electron, and the scattering of the X-rays either coherently or incoherently into a different direction. In either case, the photons are lost from the direct ray path, and the measured intensity decreases. However, in the case of scattering, the X-rays may be redirected to another location in the detector array. (See the subsequent discussion of the geometries of various generations of instrument designs.)

When this scattering takes place, the measured projection profiles contain additional background on which the attenuation data are superimposed. The presence of the background also produces artifacts in the reconstruction, as shown in **Figure 12.27**. The effect is visually similar to that produced by beam hardening.

Figure 12.24 Example of beam-
hardening effect on
(a) the sinogram or Radon
transform
(b) and the inverse-filtered
data.
Notice that the contrast
of each feature changes
according to where it lies
within the rotated object.

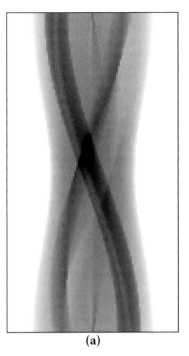
(a)

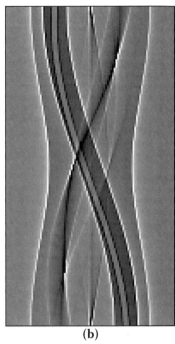
(b)

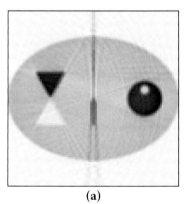
(a)

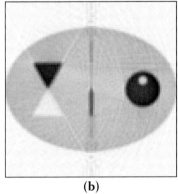
(b)

Figure 12.25 Reconstruction
of the beam-hardened data
from *Figure 12.24*:
(a) 180 views covering
180°;
(b) 180 views covering
360°.

Figure 12.26 Reconstruction of the same
phantom as *Figure 12.25*, but using
a monochromatic 50-kV X-ray source.
Notice particularly the void in the center
of the object, which is not visible in
Figure 12.25.

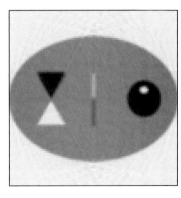

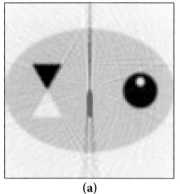

(a)

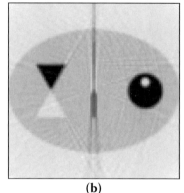

(b)

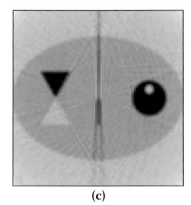

(c)

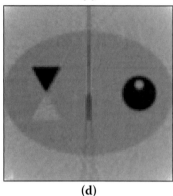

(d)

*Figure 12.27 Reconstruction of the phantom in **Figure 12.26**
when the measured projection sets include scattered background
radiation of:*
(a) 5%,
(b) 10%,
(c) 20%, and
(d) 40% of the average intensity.
*The effect on the image is similar to beam hardening. Small
features are obscured by artifacts, and the overall contrast
changes.*

In addition, the uniform regions in the object are reconstructed with a variable density due to the background. **Figure 12.28** shows this reconstruction for a simple annular object (a simplified model for bone cross section), and **Figure 12.29** shows plots across the center of the reconstructions. The deviation from a uniform density in the reconstruction is called cupping. Note that this example uses materials similar to those in the human body. However, medical tomography is not usually required to produce a quantitatively accurate measure of density, but only to show the location of internal structures and boundaries. In some applications, this may not be true; for example radiography and computed tomography are used to measure bone density loss due to osteoporosis. Industrial tomography is often called upon to measure densities accurately so as to quantify gradients in parts due to processing (e.g., pressing powders to make sintered ceramic parts), and this source of error is therefore of concern. **Figure 12.30**

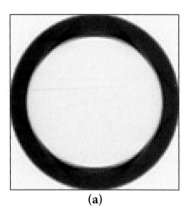

(a)

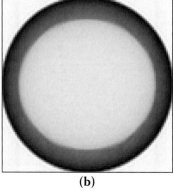

(b)

*Figure 12.28 Reconstruction
of a simple annulus with
outer composition of
calcium carbonate (an
approximation to bone) and
an inner composition of
water (an approximation to
tissue):*
*(a) no scattered
background;*
*(b) 10% scattered
background in
projection data.*

shows an interesting application (Sirr and Waddle 1999) in which precise measurement of both density and dimensions is important.

Although medical applications rarely need to measure densities exactly, they do require the ability to show small variations in density. A test phantom often used to demonstrate and evaluate performance in this category is the Shepp and Logan (1974) head phantom. Composed of ellipses with densities close to 1.0, it mimics in simplified form the human head, surrounded by a much denser skull, and containing regions very slightly lower or higher in density that model the brain structure and the presence of tumors. The ability to image these areas is critical to the detection of anomalies in real head scans.

Figure 12.31 shows a reconstruction of this phantom. Using the full dynamic range of the display (values from 0 to 255) linearly to represent the image does not reveal the internal detail within the phantom. Applying histogram equalization (as discussed in **Chapter 5**) expands the contrast in the center of the histogram so that the different regions become visible. The figure shows the cumulative histograms of display brightness for the original and histogram-equalized images. A profile plot across the center of the structure shows the different regions with nominally uniform density values (**Figure 12.32**).

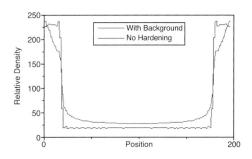

Figure 12.29 Line profiles of the density in the images in *Figure 12.28*.

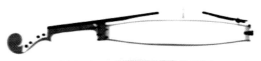

Figure 12.30 CT scan of a Stradivarius violin called the "Harrison." This violin was constructed in Cremona, Italy, in the 17th century and is thought to be nearly completely original (without patches or "modern" additions). (Courtesy of Dr. S. Sirr, Abbott Northwestern Hospital, Minneapolis, MN. With permission.)

As noted above, tomography can be performed using other modalities than X-ray absorption. One is emission tomography, in which a radioactive isotope is placed inside the object and then reveals its location by emitting gamma ray photons. Collimated detectors around the object can specify the lines along which the source of the photons lie, producing data functionally equivalent to the attenuation profiles of the conventional case.

Figure 12.33 shows an example of emission tomography using real data in which another artifact is evident. The bright areas in the reconstruction are cavities within a machined part that contain a radioactive isotope. The same technique is used to measure the internal contents of 55-gallon drums used to store radioactive waste materials. The sinogram shows the detected emission profiles as a function of view angle. Notice that the width of the regions varies with angle. This variation is due to the finite width of the collimators on the detectors, which cover a wider dimension on the far side of the object, as indicated schematically in **Figure 12.34**. This effect is also present in X-ray absorption tomography, due to the finite size of apertures on the source and the detectors. Using narrow collimators that further restrict the angle of acceptance also reduces the measured signal. If the angle of the collimators is known, this effect can be included in the reconstruction, either by progressively spreading the data as the filtered profile is spread back across the voxel array, or by adjusting the voxel weights in the algebraic reconstruction technique.

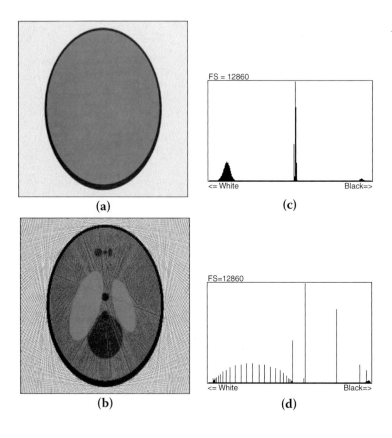

Figure 12.31 Shepp and Logan phantom, intended to represent the difficulty of visualizing a tumor inside the human head. The regions of varying density inside the "brain" have a range of relative densities from 1.0 to 1.04, while the "skull" has a density of 2.0. They are not visible in the reconstructed image

(a) unless some contrast expansion is applied.
(b) Here, histogram equalization is used to spread the gray scale nonlinearly to show the various ellipses and their overlaps (and also to increase the visibility of artifacts in the reconstruction).
(c, d) The brightness histograms show the effect of the equalization.

Figure 12.32 *Brightness profiles across the images in* **Figure 12.31,** *showing the uniformity and sharpness of transitions for the regions and the effect of histogram equalization, which increases the noise but also the magnitude of steps between regions.*

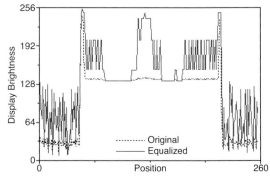

Imaging geometries

First-generation tomographic systems collected projection sets at a variety of view angles by moving a source and detector, as shown in **Figure 12.5. Figure 12.35** shows the procedure used to collect a complete set of projection data. This is called a pencil-beam or parallel-beam geometry, in which each ray integral is parallel and the projection set can be directly backprojected. It is not very efficient, since only a small solid angle of the generated X-rays can be used, and only a single detector is in use, but it is still used in a few industrial imaging situations where time of data acquisition is not a major concern.

Second-generation instruments added a set of detectors so that a fan beam of X-rays could be detected and attenuation measured along several lines at the same time, as shown in **Figure 12.36.**

Figure 12.33 *Emission tomography.*
The sample is a block of aluminum
containing several cylindrical cavities
containing radioactive cobalt. The
detector collects a series of intensity
profiles as a function of rotation,

(a) *shown in the form of a sinogram.*
Note that the width of the trace for
each cylinder varies as the sample
is rotated, due to the finite angle
of the entrance collimator to the
detector.

(b) *The reconstruction of the cross*
section.

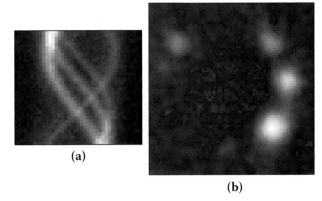

(a)

(b)

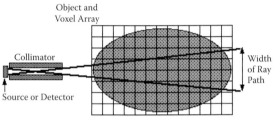

Figure 12.34 *Schematic diagram showing the effect*
of a finite collimator angle on the dimensions and
voxels covered in different parts of the object.

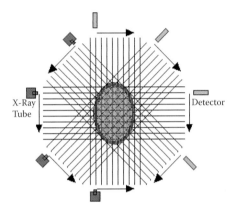

This procedure requires fewer view angles to collect the same amount of data, but the attenuation measurements from each detector are actually for different angles, and there is some rearrangement of the data needed before it can be used.

Figure 12.35 *First-generation geometry.*
The detector and source move together
to collect each projection set, rotating
to many view angles to collect all of
the required data.

The so-called fan-beam geometry is appealing in its efficiency, and the next logical step, in so-called third-generation instruments used for medical imaging, was to use a larger array of detectors (and to arrange them on an arc so that each covered the same solid angle and had normal X-ray incidence) with a single X-ray tube. The detectors and tube rotate together about the object as the X-ray tube is pulsed to produce the series of views (**Figure 12.37**). In fourth-generation systems, a complete ring of detectors is installed, and only the source rotates (**Figure 12.38**). Notice that the X-rays are no longer normally incident on the detectors in this case. There is a fifth-generation design in which even less hardware motion is required: the X-rays are generated by magnetically deflecting an electron beam against a fixed target ring, rotating the source of X-rays to produce the same effective geometry as in fourth-generation systems, but with even shorter exposure times and without moving mechanical parts.

These latter types of geometry are less used in industrial tomography, since they are primarily intended to speed image acquisition, minimize exposure, and acquire all of the projections before anything can move in the person being imaged. First- or second-generation (pencil or fan beam) methods, in which a series of discrete views are collected, provide greater flexibility in dealing with industrial problems. However, all of the methods are equivalent if the various

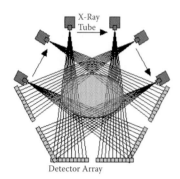

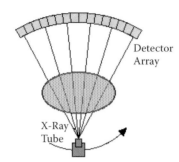

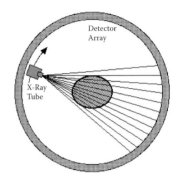

Figure 12.36 *Second-generation geometry. The detector array simultaneously measures attenuations in a fan beam, requiring fewer view angles than first-generation systems to collect the data.*

Figure 12.37 *Third-generation geometry. The X-ray tube and detector array rotate together around the object being imaged as the tube is rapidly pulsed to produce each view.*

Figure 12.38 *Fourth-generation geometry. The detector array forms a complete ring and is fixed. The X-ray tube rotates around the object and is pulsed. Data from the detectors is sorted out to produce the projection sets.*

ray integrals using individual detectors in the fan-beam geometry are sorted out according to angle and either back-projected, used in a Fourier transform method, or used to calculate an algebraic reconstruction with appropriate weights.

Some imaging technologies use different geometries and reconstructions. For instance, ultrasound images, most familiarly used for examining a fetus *in utero* or imaging blood flow to monitor heart problems, are obtained as fan-beam sections (**Figure 12.39**), but these can also be reconstructed to visualize surfaces (as shown in **Chapter 13**). Positron-emission tomography (PET), single-photon emission spectroscopy (SPECT), and magnetic resonance imaging (MRI) are somewhat different in geometry than CT scans and record different information about internal structure.

PET and SPECT localize specific atomic isotopes by their decay. In PET, the positron produced by the atomic nucleus gives rise to a pair of 511-keV photons that travel in exactly opposite directions. Detecting them with a ring of detectors locates the original isotope tag somewhere on the line between the two points, which becomes the line integral used in the reconstruction. PET scans are used most often to detect cancer and to examine the effects of cancer therapy by characterizing biochemical changes in the cancer. It is also used in research to localize brain activity, to study decreased metabolism associated with Alzheimer's, and to detect damaged portions of heart muscle after heart attacks. Radionuclides used in PET scanning are typically isotopes with short half-lives, such as car-

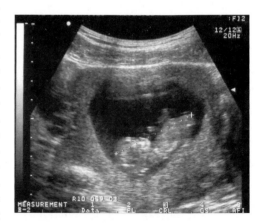

Figure 12.39 *Ultrasound image of an 11-week-old fetus. (Courtesy of J. Russ.)*

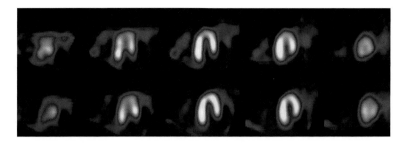

Figure 12.40 SPECT images showing blood flow to the heart. The series of images are parallel sections, with color and brightness representing the isotope concentration.

bon-11, nitrogen-13, oxygen-15, and fluorine-18 (half-lives of 20, 10, 2, and 110 min, respectively).

SPECT detects gamma rays from isotope decay with collimated detectors. The most commonly used isotopes are technetium-99 (6-h half-life) and iodine-123 (13-h half-life). An array of detectors collects information from a parallel set of projections and is scanned across and around the subject to collect multiple projections. The most common use of SPECT is to visualize the blood flow reaching the heart muscle (**Figure 12.40**), to detect areas of insufficiency and coronary artery disease, often as part of a stress test in which images are taken before and after exercise. Both PET and SPECT have poor resolution when compared with MRI or CT methods, but are adequate for their diagnostic and research purposes, particularly when combined with other higher-resolution imaging modalities. PET and MRI data can be very complementary to the density information from X-ray tomography, and in many cases scans using the different modalities are combined by overlaying the section images in registration (**Figure 12.41**). Registration of these images, which typically have quite different resolutions and voxel dimensions, as well as showing contrast for different structures, can be challenging (Hajnal et al. 2001).

When protons are placed in a magnetic field, they oscillate (resonate, hence "magnetic resonance imaging" or MRI, considered to be a more socially acceptable name than NMR or "nuclear magnetic resonance," which is the underlying technology) at a frequency that depends on the field strength, and absorb energy at the oscillation frequency. This energy is reradiated as the protons return to their ground state. The reradiation involves processes (relaxation of the magnetization components parallel and perpendicular to the field) with different time

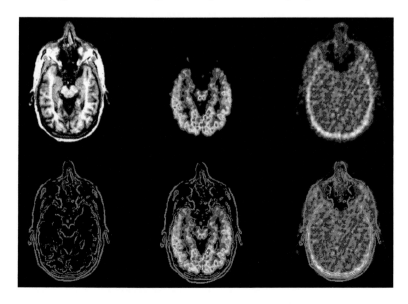

Figure 12.41 Coregistration of PET and MRI scans. (Courtesy of K. A. Paller, Northwestern University, Evanston, IL.)

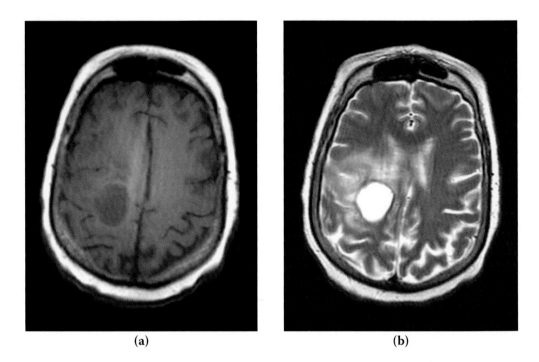

(a) (b)

Figure 12.42 *MRI slices with **(a)** T1 and **(b)** T2 weighting.*

constants T1 and T2. MRI signal strength depends on the proton concentration (essentially the water concentration in the tissue for medical imaging), but the contrast depends on T1 and T2 (as shown in **Figure 12.42**), which are strongly influenced by the fluid viscosity or tissue rigidity. Weighting the combination of the two signals provides control over the observed image. Reconstruction of MRI images is geometrically more complex than CT, but the principles are similar. MRI is used to image virtually all of the soft tissues in the body, which generally do not produce good contrast in CT (although ingestion or injection of contrast agents can be used in specific situations). **Figure 12.43** shows typical CT views of a human abdomen.

Three-dimensional tomography

While the most common application of tomography is still to form images of planar sections through objects without physical sectioning, the method can be directly extended to generate complete 3-D images. **Chapter 13** shows several examples of 3-D displays of volume data. Most of these, including many of the tomographic images, are actually serial-section images. Whether formed by physical sectioning, optical sectioning (for instance, using the confocal light microscope), or conventional tomographic reconstruction, these methods are not ideal 3-D data sets.

The distinction is that the pixels in each image plane are square, but as they are extended into the third dimension as voxels, they do not necessarily become cubes. The distance between the planes, or the depth resolution, is not inherently the same as the pixel size or resolution within the plane. In fact, few of these methods have depth resolution that is even close to the lateral resolution. Some techniques such as physical or optical sectioning have poorer depth resolution. Others such as the secondary ion mass spectrometer (SIMS) have depth resolution

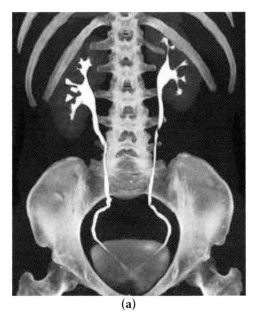

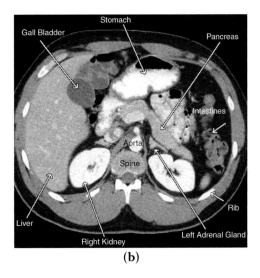

(b)

(a)

*Figure 12.43 Reconstructed views of the abdomen: **(a)** coronal view of the kidneys and ureters connecting to the bladder, with part of the ribs, spine, and pelvis visible; **(b)** transaxial slice showing several labeled organs.*

that is far better than the lateral resolution of images. This has profound effects for 3-D image presentation, for image processing, and especially for 3-D structural measurement.

True 3-D imaging is possible with tomographic reconstruction. The object is represented by a 3-D array of cubic voxels, and the individual projection sets become 2-D arrays (projection images). Each projection is from a point and is referred to as a cone-beam geometry (Shih et al. 2001) by analogy to the fan-beam method used for single-slice projections. The set of view directions must include orientations that move out of the plane and into three dimensions, described by two polar angles. This does not necessarily require rotating the object with two different polar angles, since using a cone-beam imaging geometry provides different angles for the projection lines, just as a fan-beam geometry does in two dimensions. However, the best reconstructions are obtained with a series of view angles that cover the 3-D orientations as uniformly as possible.

Several geometries are possible. One of the simplest is to rotate the sample about a single axis, as shown in **Figure 12.44**. This method offers the advantage of precise rotation, since as seen before, the quality of the reconstruction depends on the consistency of the center of rotation. On the other hand, artifacts in the reconstructed voxels can be significant, especially in the direction parallel to the axis and near the top and bottom of the sample. The single-axis rotation method is most often used with X-ray, neutron, or gamma-ray tomography, because the samples may be rather large and are relatively equiaxial, so that the distance that the radiation must pass through the sample is the same in each direction. Improved resolution in the axial direction can be obtained using a helical scan (Wang et al. 1991) in which the specimen rotates while moving in the axial direction (**Figure 12.45**). This has become the preferred geometry, particularly for small industrial objects.

For electron tomography, most samples are thin sections, and few transmission electron microscope (TEM) stages permit complete movement of the sample about its axis. For a sample that

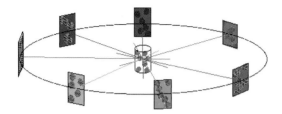

Figure 12.44 *Geometry for volume imaging using radial cone-beam projections obtained by rotating the sample about a single axis.*

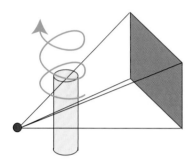

Figure 12.45 *In helical scanning, the specimen is raised as it rotates so that multiple cone-beam projections measure absorption along different angles through the voxels.*

Figure 12.46 *Tilting the sample in a conical pattern produces a series of parallel-beam projections used for reconstruction in transmission electron microscopy. The spacing along the cone trace is not necessarily uniform.*

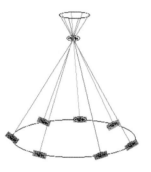

is essentially slablike, the geometry that is usually adopted is a series of tilt angles that project along the limbs of a cone, as shown in **Figure 12.46**. Collecting these projections by controlling the tilt and rotation of the sample in its holder with enough precision to allow good reconstructions is very difficult. Some TEM samples consist of many repeating structures (macromolecules, virus particles, etc.), so that a single image of the sample can collect enough different projected views to be used for reconstruction. Because of the use of many different individual (but presumably identical) objects with various orientations, this method is described as random projections, in contrast to the use of equal angular increments. The very small aperture angle of the beam in the TEM produces essentially parallel rather than cone-beam projections, which does simplify the reconstruction and makes back-projection straightforward. But the use of a limited set of views arranged in a cone produces artifacts because little information is available in the axial direction (sometimes referred to as the missing cone of information). Frank (1992) and Kubel et al. (2005) present thorough reviews of the current state of the art in electron microscope tomography.

From a theoretical viewpoint, the best reconstruction for any given number of projections is obtained when they are uniformly distributed in 3-D space (**Figure 12.47**). However, constructing a mechanism to achieve accurate rotations about two precisely centered axes is difficult, and this technique is rarely used.

Three-dimensional reconstruction can be performed with any of the methods used in two dimensions. For Fourier inversion, the frequency space is also a 3-D array, and the 2-D images produced by each projection are transformed and the complex values plotted on planes in the array. As for the 2-D case, filling the space as completely and uniformly as possible is desirable. The Fourier inversion is performed in three dimensions, but this is a direct extension of methods in lower dimensions, and in practice, the inversion can be performed in one dimension at a time (successively along rows in the u, v, and w directions).

Back-projection can also be used for 3-D reconstruction, and as in the 2-D case is simply an implementation of the Fourier-transform mathematics. The filtering of the 2-D images must be performed with a 2-D convolution, which can be carried out either by kernel operation in the spatial domain or by multiplication in the Fourier domain. The principal difficulty with the back-projection method is that calculation of the matrix of weights can be tricky for cone-beam geometry, especially when combined with helical scanning. These values represent the attenuation path length along each of the ray integrals through each of the voxels. The use of back-projection requires a large number of views to avoid artifacts and is most commonly used with single-axis rotation or with helical scans about a single rotational axis, with either cone-beam or parallel-beam projections (Feldkamp et al. 1984; Shih et al. 2001; B. Smith 1990). It is difficult to apply to a full 3-D set of cone beams because they are spaced at relatively large angles.

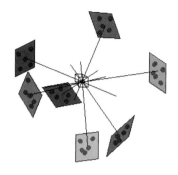

Figure 12.47 *Optimum 3-D reconstruction is possible, when a series of 3-D projections is used, by rotating the sample about two axes.*

Algebraic reconstruction (ART) methods are also applicable to voxel arrays. The difficulty in obtaining a uniform set of view angles, which is particularly the case for electron microscopy, can make ART methods more attractive than the inverse Fourier approach. In fact, when using an iterative technique such as ART, good results are often obtained with a surprisingly small number of views. **Figure 12.48** and **Figure 12.49** show an example. The specimen (about 2 cm on a side) consists of three different metal cylinders in a plastic block. Chromium, manganese, and iron are consecutive elements in the periodic table, with similar densities. Tomographic reconstruction from only 12 views with 3-D rotations, using a low-power industrial X-ray source, shows the inserts quite well (Ham 1993).

Of course, more views should produce a better reconstruction. But in most tomography situations, the total dose is a fixed constraint. In some cases, this can be because of concerns about radiation damage to the sample. Dosage to the sample is a concern for medical X-ray tomography, of course. But it also creates problems for electron tomography. The amount of energy deposited in each cubic nanometer of the sample from a focused electron beam is great enough to cook biological tissue, disrupt molecules, and change the structure we want to image.

But even for industrial tomography, the total flux of radiation that can be generated and the time spent acquiring the images usually is limited. There is a necessary trade-off between the number of projections and the time spent acquiring each one. More time on each projection improves the statistical quality of the view image, so acquiring more projections makes each one noisier, and vice versa. In some experiments with a limited total photon budget, the best quality reconstructions with full 3-D rotation were obtained with a very small number of projections (Ham 1993). This approach requires an iterative method rather than back-projection.

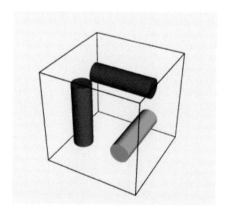

Figure 12.48 *Geometry of a test sample. Three cylindrical inserts of different metals (Cr, Mn, and Fe) are placed in a plastic block (2 cm on a side).*

The limited number of photons becomes particularly critical when low-intensity sources are used. Synchrotrons (Helfen et al. 2003) are excellent sources of X-rays with high brightness and the ability to select a specific

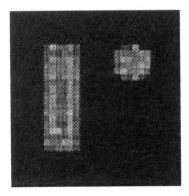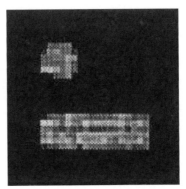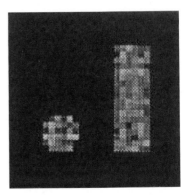

Figure 12.49 Tomographic reconstruction of three planes in the xy, yz, and zx orientations passing through the metal inserts in the plastic block shown in Figure 12.48, reconstructed using just 12 cone-beam projections with rotations in three dimensions.

monochromatic energy, but these are not usually conveniently available for tomographic work. Radioactive sources of gamma rays present handling difficulties and have low intensities as well. X-ray tubes are a convenient source for tomography, with adjustable voltage and a variety of target materials that emit different X-ray spectra. Such a source is not monochromatic, which can cause significant beam-hardening effects for many specimens, as discussed previously.

Absorption filters can be used to select just a single band of energies from a polychromatic source. For each view angle, two projection images are collected using filters whose absorption edge energies are different. The ratio of the two images yields the attenuation information for the elements whose absorption edges lie between the two filter energies, as indicated in **Figure 12.50**. A series of such image pairs can provide separate information on the spatial distribution of many elements. **Figure 12.51** shows an example in which the use of filters has selected two of the three metal inserts in the sample from **Figure 12.49**. The use of the filters reduces the already low intensity from the X-ray tube, and the use of the ratio of the two images presents a further limitation on the statistical quality of the projections. It is therefore important to use a small number of views to obtain the best possible projection images. In this example, 12 projections with full 3-D rotation of axes were obtained. **Figure 12.52** shows the artifacts present in the reconstruction when the same number of views is obtained with single-axis rotation.

The electron microscope produces images in which contrast is due to attenuation, and a series of views at different angles can be reconstructed to show 3-D structure. The use of an arbitrary series of angles is quite difficult to achieve for specimens of crystalline materials

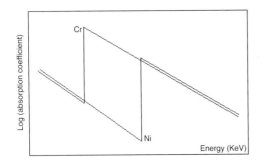

Figure 12.50 Diagram of the use of balanced absorption edge filters to isolate a single energy band. The plots show the absorption coefficient as a function of energy for two different filters containing the elements chromium and nickel. Elements in the sample with absorption edges between these two energies, such as manganese, iron, and cobalt, will be imaged in the ratio of the two intensities.

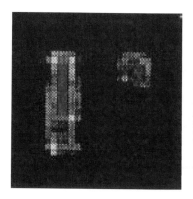 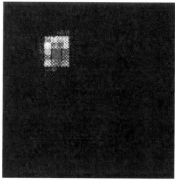 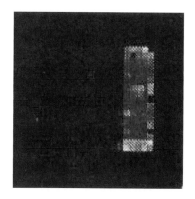

Figure 12.51 *Reconstruction of the same three planes as shown in **Figure 12.49**, but using images obtained as a difference between two projections through different filters (Cr and Fe metal foils), which form a band-pass filter to select a narrow band of X-ray energies. Note that one of the inserts (Cr) is excluded but the Mn and Fe inserts are visible. Reconstructed using 12 cone-beam projections with rotations in three dimensions.*

because of diffraction of the electrons from planes of atoms in the crystal structure. This source of contrast is not easily modeled by the usual attenuation calculation, since one voxel can have quite different values in different directions. However, for noncrystalline materials such as biological specimens, the reconstruction is straightforward (Engel and Massalski 1984; Hegerl 1989).

Even more efficient than collecting a series of different views using multiple orientations of a single specimen is using images of many different but identical specimens that happen to have different orientations, as mentioned previously. **Figure 12.53** shows an example. The 2-D image is an electron micrograph of a single virus particle. The specimen is an adenovirus that causes respiratory ailments.

The low dose of electrons required to prevent damage to the specimen makes the image very noisy. However, in a typical specimen there are many such particles, each in a different, essentially random orientation. Collecting the various images, indexing the orientation of each image by referring to

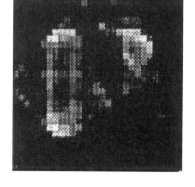

Figure 12.52 *Reconstruction of the same plane as shown in **Figure 12.51** left, reconstructed in the same way using two filters, but using 12 radial projections (rotating the sample about one axis only). Note the artifacts between and within the inserts.*

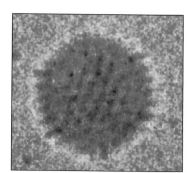

Figure 12.53 *TEM image of single adenovirus particle.*

the location of the triangular facets on the virus surface, and performing a reconstruction produces a 3-D reconstruction of the particle in which each voxel value is the electron density. Modeling the surface of the outer protein coat of the virus produces the surface-rendered image shown in **Figure 12.54** (Stewart and Burnett 1991).

At a very different scale, tomography has also been performed on the Earth itself using seismography. Seismic waves are created by earthquakes or large explosions such as nuclear weapons tests. Such large-magnitude events generate two types of waves that propagate through the Earth to receivers (seismographs) at many different locations. P-waves (pressure waves) are compressional pulses that can penetrate through every part of Earth's interior, while S-waves (shear waves) are transverse deformations that cannot propagate through the liquid core. In fact, the presence of a liquid core was deduced in 1906 by the British seismologist R. D. Oldham from the shadow cast by the core in seismic S-wave patterns.

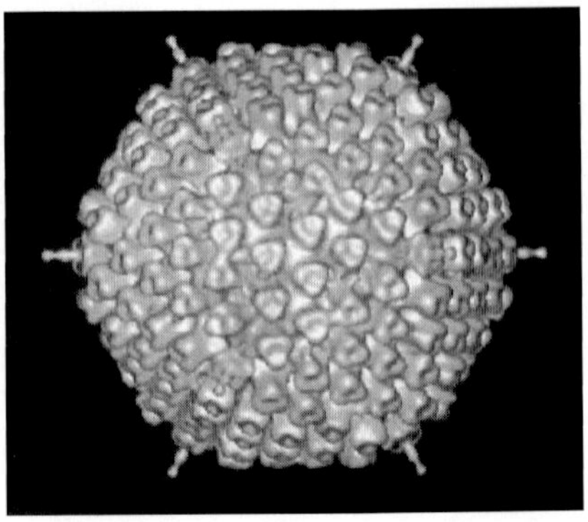

The paths of seismic waves are not straight (**Figure 12.55**); rather, they bend because of the variations in temperature, pressure, and composition within the Earth, which affect the speed of transmission just as the index of refraction of glass affects light and causes it to bend in a lens system. Similar to the behavior of light,

Figure 12.54 Reconstruction of the adenovirus particle from many randomly oriented transmission images.

the seismic waves can reflect at interfaces where the speed of propagation varies abruptly. This happens at the core–mantle boundary and the surface of the inner core. The propagation velocities of the P- and S-waves are different, and they respond differently to composition.

Collecting many seismograms from different events creates a set of ray paths that do not uniformly cover the Earth, but rather depend on the chance and highly nonuniform distribution of earthquakes and the distribution of seismographs. Nevertheless, analysis of the travel times of waves that have taken different paths through the Earth permits forming a tomographic reconstruction. The density of the material (shown by shading in **Figure 12.56**) indicates the temperature and the direction of motion (cool, dense material is sinking through the mantle toward the core, while hot, light material is rising). Convection in the mantle is the driving force behind volcanism and continental drift.

Also of great utility are waves that have reflected (one or more times) from the various surfaces. For instance, the difference in travel times of S-waves that arrive directly vs. those that have reflected from the core–mantle boundary permits mapping the elevation of that boundary with a resolution better than 1 kilometer, thus revealing that the boundary is not a smooth spherical surface. Since the relatively viscous mantle is floating on a low-velocity liquid core, and it is the relatively fast motion of the latter that produces Earth's magnetic field, the study of this interface is important in understanding Earth's dynamics.

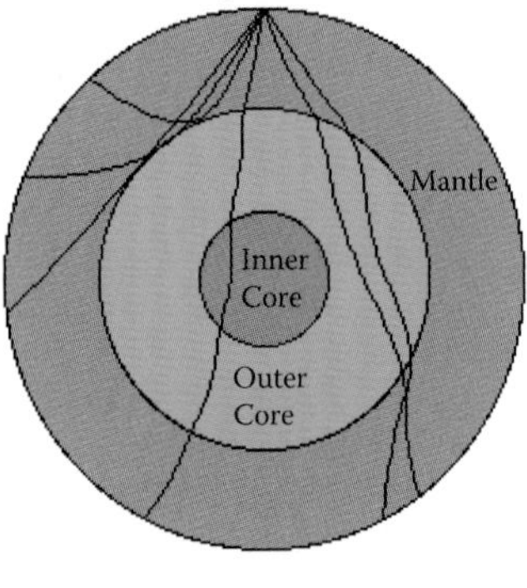

Figure 12.55 Diagram of paths taken by pressure and shear waves from earthquakes, which reveals information about the density along the paths through the core and mantle, and the location of discontinuities.

Global tomographic reconstruction is generally insensitive to the small details of structure such as faults, but another ongoing program to perform high-resolution tomography under the state of California (where there are many faults of more than casual interest to the surface-dwelling humans) employs an array of high-sensitivity seismographs and uses the very frequent minor earthquakes there to map out the faults through the reflections that they produce.

High-resolution tomography

Medical tomography has a typical resolution of about 1 mm, which is adequate for its purpose, and radiologists generally feel comfortable with a series of planar section images in standardized orientations in which they have been trained to recognize normal and abnormal features. But there is considerable interest in applying true 3-D tomographic imaging to study the microstructure of various materials including metals, ceramics, composites, and polymers, as well as larger industrial components. Some of the structural features cannot be determined from conventional 2-D microscopy of cross-section surfaces. This includes determining the number of particles of arbitrary or variable shape in a volume and the topology of networks or pore structures that control the permeability of materials to fluids (including, for instance, the flow of oil through porous rock strata).

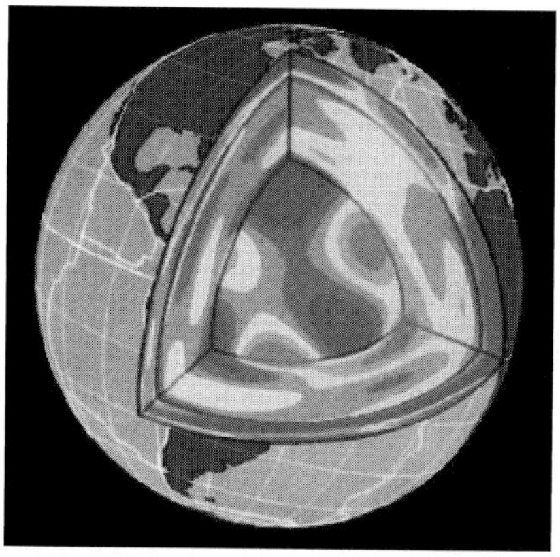

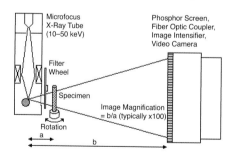

Figure 12.56 Computed tomogram of the mantle, showing rock densities (light shades indicate hot, light rocks that are rising, and conversely).

This information can only be determined by having a 3-D data set, with adequate resolution, and ideally with cubic voxels. Resolution of better than 1 μm has been demonstrated using a synchrotron as a very bright point source of X-rays. Similar resolution is possible using more readily available sources such as microfocus X-ray tubes. Filtering such sources to produce element-specific imaging is also possible, as illustrated previously.

Cone-beam geometry is well suited to this type of microstructural imaging, since it provides magnification of the structure (Deckman 1989; Johnson et al. 1986; Kinney et al. 1989, 1990; Russ 1988). **Figure 12.57** shows this schematically. The magnification is strictly geometric, since X-rays are not refracted by lenses, but can amount to as much as 100:1. The projected images can be collected using conventional video technology after conversion to visible light by a phosphor or channel plate and suitable intensification. Since the intensity of conventional small-spot X-ray sources is very low, the use of high-brightness sources such as are available at a synchrotron is particularly desirable for high-resolution imaging. So is image averaging, which can be done using the same cooled CCD (charge-coupled device) cameras used for astronomical imaging.

As discussed in **Chapter 13**, 3-D imaging requires many voxels, and the reconstruction process is computer-intensive. The time required to perform the reconstruction is, however, still shorter than that required to collect the various projection images. These images are generally photon-limited, with considerable noise affecting the reconstruction, as indicated previously. To collect reasonable-quality projections from a finite intensity source, the number of view angles must be limited. The views should be ideally arranged to cover the polar angles optimally in 3-D space. This arrangement of course places demands on the quality of the mechanism used to perform the rotations and tilts, because the center of rotation must

Figure 12.57 Diagram of a cone-beam imaging system. The projection image magnification is the ratio of b:a. The attainable resolution is limited by the spot size of the X-ray source and possibly by the spatial resolution of the detector.

be constant and located within a few micrometers to preserve the image quality, as discussed previously. Helical scanning is usually easier to accomplish and is more commonly used.

The presentation of 3-D information requires extensive use of computer graphics methods, as shown in **Chapter 13**. **Figure 12.58** shows a simple series of planes of voxels from a 3-D tomo-

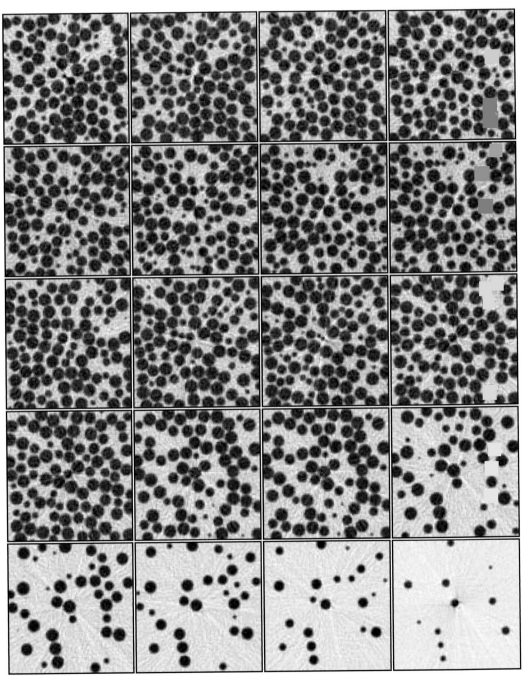

Figure 12.58 *Twenty individual planes of reconstructed voxels showing a sintered alumina ceramic consisting of 100-µm-diameter spheres.*

graphic reconstruction of a porous alumina ceramic. The individual particles are approximately 100-μm-diameter spheres that fill about 60% of the volume of the sample. The voxels are 10-μm cubes. **Figure 12.59** shows one of the projection sets through this specimen, a 2-D image in which the spherical particles overlap along the lines of sight and are partially transparent. A 3-D presentation of these data is shown in **Figure 12.60**.

The first edition of this book (1990) showed these examples from our own experimental setup. Since then, technology has progressed, and several commercial implementations of such instruments have become available (Chappard et al. 2005; Wang and Vannier 2001). **Figure 12.61** shows an image of wood in which the resolution of the cells and growth rings is comparable with a light-microscope image. A wide range of applications has been opened up by the availability of this technology, including microelectronic devices, materials, and more, creating a 3-D microscope with submicron resolution. Reconstructions of 1000 slices of 1000 × 1000 voxels that in 1990 required a Cray supercomputer are now routinely performed on a desktop workstation. **Figure 12.62** shows a few additional examples.

The overwhelming majority of applications for the various tomographic imaging methods produce visualizations, either as a set of 2-D slices or 3-D renderings (as shown in **Chapter 13**), for human examination and interpretation. Some quantitative measurement procedures are carried out (Hanke 2003; Rangayyan 2005), but in general the stereological methods described in **Chapter 9** are more efficient for obtaining numeric values that characterize the metric properties of 3-D structures.

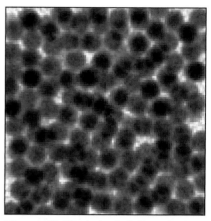

Figure 12.59 A single 2-D projection set through the structure shown in *Figure 12.58*.

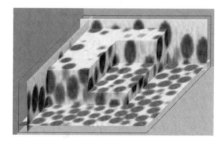

Figure 12.60 Three-dimensional presentation of the data from *Figure 12.58*, artificially stretched in the vertical direction.

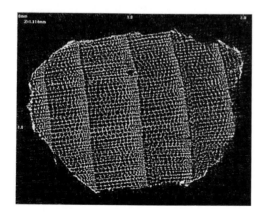

Figure 12.61 Microtomographic image of a section through a piece of wood, showing cells and annual growth rings. (Courtesy of Skyscan, Aartselaar, Belgium.)

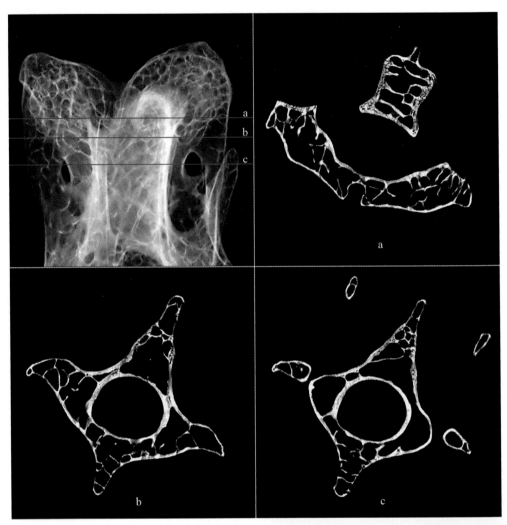

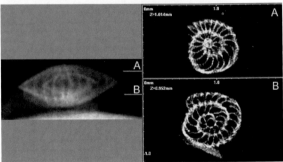

Figure 12.62 *Examples of microtomographic sections:*
(a) *projected image of bone with reconstructed transverse slices at the positions marked;*
(b) *projected image of a foraminifer with reconstructed transverse slices at the positions marked.*
(Courtesy of Skyscan, Aartselaar, Belgium.)

13

3-D Image Visualization

Sources of 3-D data

Three-dimensional (3-D) imaging is becoming more accessible with the continued development of instrumentation for generating 3-D image data (tomographic equipment of various kinds, confocal microscopes, etc.) and the availability of versatile software for increasingly powerful computers. Just as the pixel is the unit of brightness measurement for a two-dimensional image, the voxel (volume element, the three-dimensional analog of the pixel or picture element) is the unit for three-dimensional imaging. And just as processing and analysis is much simpler if the pixels are square, so the use of cubic voxels is preferred for three dimensions, although it is not as often achieved.

There are several basic approaches to volume imaging. **Chapter 12** described 3-D imaging by tomographic reconstruction. This is the best method for measuring the density and, in some cases, the composition of solid specimens. It can produce a set of cubic voxels, although that is not the only or even the most common way that tomography is presently used. Most medical and industrial applications produce a series of two-dimensional section planes that are spaced farther apart than the lateral resolution within the plane (Baba et al. 1984, 1989; Briarty and Jenkins 1984; Johnson and Capowski 1985; Kriete 1992).

As described in **Chapter 12**, tomography can be performed using a variety of different signals, including seismic waves, ultrasound, magnetic resonance, conventional X-rays, gamma rays, neutron beams, electron microscopy, as well as other less familiar methods. The resolution can vary from kilometers (seismic tomography) to centimeters (most conventional medical scans), millimeters (typical industrial applications), micrometers (microfocus X-ray or synchrotron sources), and even nanometers (electron-microscope reconstructions of viruses and atomic lattices). The same basic presentation tools are available for visualizing the resulting data regardless of the imaging modality or the dimensional scale.

An important distinction in tomographic imaging, as for all of the other 3-D methods discussed here, is whether the data set is planes of pixels or an array of true voxels. As discussed in **Chapter 12**, it is possible to set up an array of cubic voxels, collect projection data from a series of views in three dimensions, and solve (either algebraically or by filtered back-projection) for the density of each voxel. However, the most common way to perform tomography is to define one plane at a time as an array of square pixels, collect a series of linear views, solve for the two-dimensional array of densities in that plane, and then proceed to the next plane. When used in this way, tomography shares many similarities (and problems) with other essentially two-dimensional imaging methods that we will collectively define as serial imaging or serial-section techniques.

A radiologist viewing an array of such images is expected to combine them in his or her mind to "see" the three-dimensional structures present. (This process is aided enormously by the fact that the radiologist already knows what the structure is, and is generally looking for things that differ from the familiar, particularly in a few characteristic ways that identify disease or injury.) Only a few current-generation medical systems use the techniques discussed in this chapter to present three-dimensional views directly. In industrial tomography, the greater diversity of structure (and the correspondingly lesser ability to predict what is expected) and the greater amount of time available for study and interpretation has encouraged the use of computer graphics. However, such displays are still the exception rather than the rule, and an array of two-dimensional planar images is commonly used for volume imaging. This chapter emphasizes methods that use a series of parallel, uniformly spaced two-dimensional images that are presented in combination to show three-dimensional structure.

Rendered visualizations of 3-D structure can be quite dramatic in their appearance, and these are often used to communicate the important details of the structure. Animations in which the presentations rotate (**Figure 13.1**) or dynamically change transparency, etc., are even more powerful tools for this purpose, although they cannot be well represented in printed communications. Most software and computer systems that generate these images are not fast enough to generate such images in real time, although some high-end workstations do offer interactive rotational capability. Typically, the final graphics or animations are produced after the human operator has detected the important structural information and decided how it can be effectively presented. So the graphics become primarily a means to communicate the results of research rather than a research or diagnostic tool.

In the most common approach to 3-D imaging, a series of images is obtained by dissecting the sample into a series of planar sections, which are then piled up as a stack of voxels. Sometimes the sectioning is physical. Blocks of embedded biological materials, textiles, and even some metals can be sliced with a microtome, and each slice imaged (just as individual slices are normally viewed). Collecting and aligning the images produces a three-dimensional data set in which the voxels are typically very elongated in the z direction because the slices are much thicker or more widely spaced than the lateral resolution within each slice.

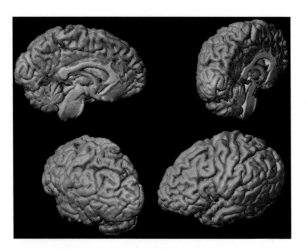

Figure 13.1 *Selected still frames from an animation in which a reconstructed view of one-half of a brain is continuously rotated. (Courtesy of M. Dow, University of Oregon, Eugene.)*

At the other extreme, the secondary ion mass spectrometer (SIMS) uses an incident ion beam to remove one layer of atoms at a time from the sample surface. These pass through a mass spectrometer to select atoms from a single element, the results of which are then amplified and imaged on a fluorescent screen or recorded by a camera. Collecting a series of images from many elements can produce a complete three-dimensional map of the sample. One difference from the imaging of slices is that there is no alignment problem, because the sample block is held in place as the surface layers are removed. On the other hand, the erosion rate through different structures can vary so that the surface does not remain planar, and this roughening or differential erosion is very difficult to account for. In this type of instrument, the voxel height can be very small (essentially atomic dimensions) while the lateral dimension is many times larger.

Serial sections

Most physical sectioning approaches are similar to one or the other of these examples. They are known collectively as serial-section methods. Although it applies equally well to many different situations, including for example the sequential removal of material from an archaeological site, the name serial section comes from the use of light microscopy imaging of biological tissue, in which blocks of tissue embedded in resin are cut using a microtome into a series of individual slices. Collecting these slices (or at least some of them) for viewing in the microscope enables researchers to assemble a set of photographs that can then be used to reconstruct the 3-D structure. A variety of commercial and free (Fiala 2005) software tools to assemble the images and generate the graphics are available.

The serial-section technique illustrates most of the problems that can be encountered with any 3-D imaging method based on a series of individual slices. If the surface revealed by removing each slice is imaged, there is minimal distortion or difficulty in aligning the sequential images. However, if the slice is collected and imaged, the individual images must first be aligned. The microtomed slices are collected on slides or grids and viewed in arbitrary orientations. So, even if the same structures can be located in the different sections (not always an easy task, given that some variation in structure with depth must be present or there would be no incentive to do this kind of work), the pictures do not line up.

Using the details of structure visible in each section provides only a coarse guide to alignment. The automatic methods generally seek to minimize the mismatch between sections either by aligning the centroids of features in the planes so that the sum of squares of distances is minimized, or by overlaying binary images from the two sections and shifting or rotating to minimize the area resulting from combining them with an Ex-OR (exclusive OR) operation, discussed in **Chapter 8**. This procedure is illustrated in **Figure 13.2**. When gray-scale values are present in the image, cross-correlation can be used, as discussed in **Chapter 6**. Unfortunately, neither of these methods is easy to implement in the general case when sections can be shifted in the x and y directions, stretched or compressed (causing local distortion), or rotated by large and arbitrary angles. Solving for the "best alignment" is difficult and must usually proceed iteratively and hence slowly.

Furthermore, there is no reason to expect the optimum point reached by these algorithms to really represent the true alignment. As shown in **Figure 13.3** and **Figure 13.4**, shifting or rotating each image to visually align the structures in one section with the next can completely alter the reconstructed 3-D structure. It is generally assumed that given enough detail present in the images, some kind of average alignment will avoid these major errors. However, it is far

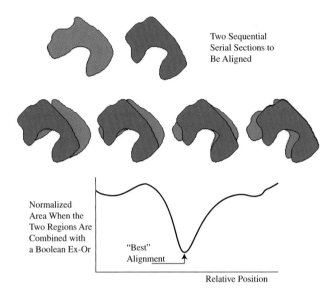

Two Sequential
Serial Sections to
Be Aligned

Figure 13.2 *Alignment of serial*
sections by the "best fit" of features
seeks to minimize mismatched area,
measured by Ex-OR function, as a
function of translation and rotation.

Normalized
Area When the
Two Regions Are
Combined with
a Boolean Ex-Or

"Best"
Alignment

Relative Position

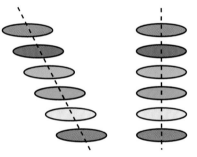

Figure 13.3 *Alignment of serial*
sections with translation:
sections through an inclined
circular cylinder may be
misconstrued as a vertical
elliptical cylinder.

from certain that a best visual alignment is the correct one, nor that automated methods that overlap sequential images produce the proper alignment.

One approach that improves on the use of internal image detail for alignment is to incorporate fiducial marks in the block before sectioning. These could take the form of holes drilled by a laser, threads or fibers placed in the resin before it hardens, or grooves machined down the edges of the block, for example. For some opaque materials that are processed by imaging a surface and then polishing down to reveal another surface, hardness indentations or scratches can be used for alignment. With several fiducial marks that can reasonably be expected to maintain their shape from section to section and continue in some known direction through the stack of images, improved alignment is possible. However, placing and finding fiducial marks in the close vicinity of the structures of interest is often difficult. In practice, if the sections are not contiguous there may still be difficulties, and alignment errors may propagate through the stack of images. Distortions in the sections, such as those produced by cutting, create additional difficulties, particularly if they are not uniform but vary from location to location.

Most fiducial marks are large enough to cover several pixels in each image. As discussed in **Chapter 9**, this size allows locating the centroid to a fraction of one pixel accuracy, although not all systems take advantage of this capability. Once the alignment points are identified (either from fiducial marks or internal image detail), the rotation and translation of one image to line up with the next is performed as discussed in **Chapter 4**. Resampling of the pixel array and interpolation to prevent aliasing produces a new image. This process takes some computational time, but this is a minor problem in comparison with the difficulty of obtaining the images in the first place.

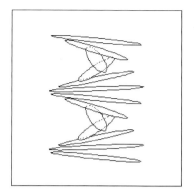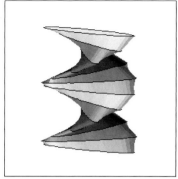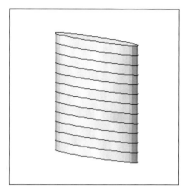

Figure 13.4 *Alignment of serial sections with translation: sections through an inclined circular cylinder may be misconstrued as a vertical elliptical cylinder.*

Unfortunately, for classic serial sectioning the result of this rotation and translation is not a true representation of the original 3-D structure. The act of sectioning using a microtome generally produces some distortion in the block. This 5 to 20% compression in one direction is usually assumed to be nearly the same for all sections (since they are cut in the same direction and generally have only small differences in structure that would alter their mechanical properties). If the fiducial marks have known absolute coordinates, then stretching of the images to correct for the distortion is possible. It is usually assumed that the entire section is compressed uniformly, although for some samples this may not be true.

If the only purpose of the 3-D reconstruction is to view, rather than measure, the structure, the distortion may not be considered important. And in some situations it may be possible to use internal information to estimate the distortion. For example, if there is no reason to expect cells or cell nuclei to be elongated in any preferred direction in the tissue, then measurement of the dimensions of many cells or nuclei can be used to determine an average amount of compression. Obviously, this approach includes some assumptions and can only be used in particular circumstances.

Another difficulty with serial sections is calibration of dimension in the depth direction. The thickness of the individual sections is known only approximately (for example, by judging the color of the light produced by interference from the top and bottom surfaces, or based on the mechanical feed rate of the microtome while typically ignoring any compliance in the material being cut). It can vary from section to section, and even from place to place within the section, depending on the local hardness of the material being cut. Constructing an accurate depth scale is quite difficult, and dimensions in the depth direction may be much less accurate than those measured within one section plane.

If only some sections are used, such as every second or fifth (to reduce the amount of work required to image them and then align the images), then this error increases. It also becomes difficult to follow structures from one image to the next with confidence. However, before computer reconstruction methods became common, this kind of skipping was often necessary simply to reduce the amount of data that the human observer had to juggle and interpret.

Using only a fraction of the sections is particularly common when ultrathin sections are cut for viewing in an electron microscope instead of the light microscope. As the sections become thinner, they increase in number and are more prone to distortion. Some may be lost (for instance due to folding) or intentionally skipped. Portions of each section are obscured by the support grid, which also prevents some from being used. One consequence is that the spacing of the images that are actually acquired may not be uniform. At higher magnification, the fiducial marks become larger, less precisely defined, and above all more widely spaced, so that they may not be in close proximity to the structure of interest.

Figure 13.5 shows a portion of a series of transmission electron microscope (TEM) images of tissue in which the 3-D configuration of the membranes (dark stained lines) is of interest. The details of the edges of cells and organelles have been used to approximately align pairs of sections through the stack, but different details must be used for different pairs, as there is no continuity of detail through the entire stack. The membranes can be isolated in these images by thresholding (**Figure 13.6**), but the sections are too far apart to link the lines together to reconstruct the 3-D shape of the surface. This problem is common with conventional serial-section images.

Metallographic imaging typically uses reflected rather than transmitted light. As discussed below, serial sectioning in this context is accomplished by removing layers of materials sequentially by physical polishing. The need to locate the same sample position after polishing, and to monitor the depth of polishing, can be met by placing hardness indentations on the sample, or by laser ablation of pits. These serve as fiduciary marks for alignment, and the change in size of the mark allows calculating the depth. In archaeological excavation, the fiduciary marks may be a network of strings and a transit, and the removal tool may be a shovel. In some mining and quarrying examples it may be a bulldozer, but the principles remain the same regardless of scale.

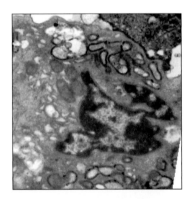

*Figure 13.5 Four serial-section images from a stack, which have already been rotated for alignment. The membranes at the upper left corner of the images are thresholded and displayed for the entire stack of images in **Figure 13.6**. (Courtesy of Dr. C. D. Bucana, University of Texas and M. D. Anderson Cancer Center, Houston.)*

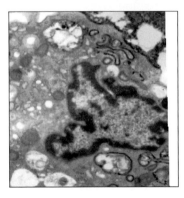
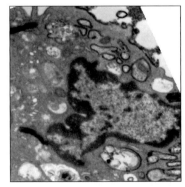
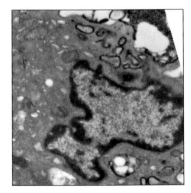

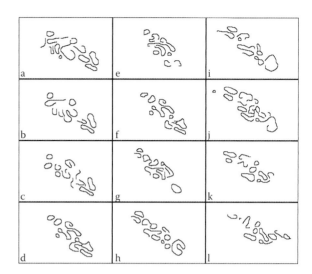

Figure 13.6 *Membranes from the sequential images illustrated in* **Figure 13.5**, *showing the changes from section to section. Because of the separation distance between the planes, these variations are too great to model the shape of the surfaces in 3-D.*

In most of these surface-imaging methods, the sequential 2-D images represent the sample along planes that are separated in the z direction. The intervening material that has been removed must be inferred or interpolated from the planes. In these cases, the voxel value is not really an average over its extent, as most pixel values are. Nor is the voxel truly a discrete point value in space, since it does represent an average in the section plane. Interpolation between sections that are too far apart (in terms of the scale of the structure) can lead to some serious errors and misinterpretation.

For the serial-sectioning method in which slices are viewed in transmission, the voxel value is a volume average, which is easier to interpret. In most cases, the voxel value is a measure of density of the material. Depending on what the radiation is (visible light, X-rays, electrons, neutrons, sound, and so forth), the value may represent the local concentration of some element or compound, including those introduced as tracers or markers. In some cases, emitted radiation from voxels also gives concentration information (examples include fluorescence light microscopy and positron-emission tomography).

Optical sectioning

Physical sectioning on any scale is a difficult technique that destroys the sample. Controlling and measuring the section thickness and aligning the sections or at least locating the same position on the sample can become a major source of error. In some cases, it is possible to image sections through a sample without performing physical sectioning. The confocal scanning light microscope (CSLM) offers one way to accomplish this (tomographic slice images, described in **Chapter 12**, are another). Depth information can also be obtained in some cases by interpreting the phase shift introduced by objects viewed in light microscopy, as well as by neutron or X-ray transmission imaging (Barty et al. 2000).

The normal operation of the transmission light microscope does not lend itself to optical sectioning. The depth of field of high numerical aperture optics is small (just a few times the lateral resolution), so that only a small "slice" of the image will be sharply focused. However, light from locations above and below the plane of focus is also transmitted to the image, out of focus, and this both blurs the image and includes information from an extended distance in the z direction. In some cases, deconvolution of the point-spread function can be accomplished (as discussed in **Chapter 6**), but in many cases this is of limited value, since the blurring varies from one location to another. An example shown below (**Figure 13.38**) illustrates the processing of images to remove some of the artifacts that result from the passage of light through the sample above and below the plane of focus.

The confocal scanning microscope eliminates this extraneous light, and so produces useful optical section images without the need for processing. This is possible because the sample is imaged one point at a time (hence the presence of "scanning" in the name). The principle of the confocal microscope, introduced in **Chapter 5**, is that light from a point source (often a laser) is focused on a single point in the specimen and collected by an identical set of optics, reaching a pinhole detector. Any portion of the specimen away from the focal point, and particularly out of the focal plane, cannot return light to the pinhole to interfere with the formation of the image. Scanning the beam with respect to the specimen (by moving the light source, the specimen, or using scanning elements in the optical path) builds up a complete image of the focal plane.

If the numerical aperture of the lenses is high, the depth of field of this microscope is very small, although still greater than the lateral resolution within individual image planes. Much more important, the portion of the specimen that is away from the focal plane contributes very little to the image. This makes it possible to image a plane within a bulk specimen, even one that would ordinarily be considered translucent because of light scattering. This method of isolating a single plane within a bulk sample, called optical sectioning, works because the confocal light microscope has a very shallow depth of field and a high rejection of stray light. Translating the specimen in the z direction and collecting a series of images makes it possible to build up a 3-D data set for viewing.

Several imaging modalities are possible with the confocal light microscope. The most common are (a) reflected light, in which the light reflected from the sample returns through the same objective lens as used to focus the incident light and is then diverted by a mirror to a detector, and (b) fluorescence, in which light is emitted from points within the specimen and is recorded using the same geometry. It is less common to use the microscope to view transmitted light images. This mode permits acquiring transmitted light images for focal-plane sectioning of bulk translucent or transparent materials. **Figure 13.7** shows an example of a transmitted light focal-plane section.

Both transmitted- and reflected-light images of focal-plane sections can be used in 3-D imaging for different types of specimens. The characteristic of reflected-light confocal images is that the intensity of light reflected to the detector drops off very rapidly as points are shifted above or below the focal plane. Therefore, for structures in a transparent medium, only the surfaces will reflect light. For any single image plane, only the portion of the field of view where some structure passes through the plane will appear bright, and the rest of the image will be dark. This characteristic permits straightforward reconstruction algorithms.

A widely used imaging method for the confocal microscope is emission or fluorescence, in which the wavelength of the incident light is able to cause excitation of a dye or other fluorescing probe introduced to the specimen. The lower-energy (longer wavelength) light emitted by this probe is separated from the incident light, for instance by a dichroic mirror, and used to form an image in which the location of the probe or dye appears bright. Building up a series of images in depth allows the structure labeled by the probe to be reconstructed.

The principal advantages of optical sectioning are speed and ease of use, avoiding physical distortion of the specimen due to cutting, and preserving alignment of images from the various imaging planes. The depth resolution, while inferior to the lateral resolution in each plane by

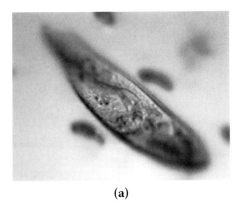

(a)

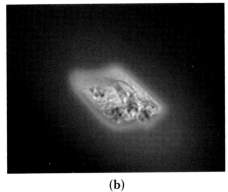

(b)

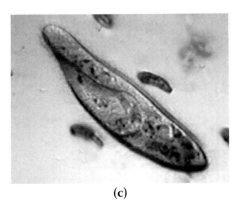

(c)

Figure 13.7 *Images of a paramecium swimming in a droplet of water:*
(a) conventional transmission light microscope;
(b) transmission confocal microscope (only the portion in the focal plane is seen);
(c) extended-focus image produced by merging all of the planes from the confocal series.

about a factor of two to three times, is still useful for many applications. However, this difference in resolution does raise some difficulties for 3-D image processing, even if the distance between planes is made smaller than the resolution so that the stored voxels are cubic.

By measuring or modeling the 3-D shape of the microscope's point-spread function, it is possible by deconvolution to improve the resolution of the confocal light microscope. The method is identical to that shown in **Chapter 6** for 2-D images, but carried out with a 3-D Fourier transform. (The Fourier transform is separable, meaning that it can be performed individually and sequentially along rows and columns of pixels or voxels, and so it is directly extended from two to three dimensions.)

Sequential removal

Many materials are opaque and therefore cannot be imaged by any transmission method, preventing optical sectioning. Indeed, metals, composites, and ceramics are usually examined in the reflected light microscope. However, it is still possible to collect a series of depth images for 3-D reconstruction by sequential polishing of such materials, as mentioned previously.

The means of removal of material from the surface depends strongly on the hardness of the material. For some soft metals, polymers, and textiles, the microtome can be used just as for a block of biological material, except that instead of examining the slice of material removed, the surface left behind is imaged. This approach avoids most problems of alignment and distortion, especially if the cutting can be done *in situ* without removing the specimen from the viewing position in the microscope. It is still difficult to determine precisely the thickness of material removed in each cut and to assure its uniformity, but it is generally estimated from the mechanical settings on the device (ignoring any permanent or temporary distortion in the material).

For harder materials, the grinding or polishing operations used to produce conventional sections for 2-D images can be used. Such operations generally require removing and replacing the specimen, so fiducial marks are needed to locate the same region. Probably the most common approach to this marking is the use of hardness indentations. Several pyramid-shaped impressions are made in the surface of the specimen so that after additional abrasion or polishing, the deepest parts of the indentations are still visible. These can be accurately aligned with the marks in the original image. In addition, the reduction in size of the impression, whose shape is known, gives a measure of the depth of polish and hence of the spacing between the two images. With several such indentations, the overall uniformity of polish can also be judged, although local variations due to the hardness of particular phases may be present.

For harder materials or ones in which conventional polishing might cause surface damage, other methods can be used. Electrolytic or chemical etching is generally difficult to control and is thus rarely used. Ion beam erosion is slow, but is already in use in many laboratories for the cutting and thinning of transmission electron microscope specimens, and may be utilized for this purpose. Controlling the erosion to obtain uniformity and avoid surface roughening presents challenges for many specimens.

In situ ion beam erosion is used in the scanning electron microscope (SEM) and scanning Auger microscope, for instance to allow the removal of surface contamination. Focused ion beams (FIB) are also used to cut slices in the z direction to examine microstructures. This capability can be used to produce a series of images in depth in these microscopes, which generally have resolution far better than the light microscope. The time involved in performing the erosion or slicing may be quite long (and hence costly), and the uniformity of eroding through complex structures (the most interesting kind for imaging) may be poor.

FIB machining has been used primarily for cutting through microelectronic devices to measure critical thicknesses and dimensions with the SEM. In those cases, the geometry of the cut is controlled according to the known geometry of the specimen, often producing a vertical cut through a structure on which the important dimensions are directly revealed. Of course, it is also possible to use FIB machining to produce sections on which stereological measurements can be made, or to use a series of sections as a serial-sectioning device to directly reveal 3-D structure. This has been done to a limited degree for measurements of metal and ceramic microstructures (Holzer et al. 2004). FIB has also been used for sectioning of some tissue specimens. However, the primary use of these images has been for visual presentation rather than measurement.

One kind of microscope erodes the specimen surface automatically as part of its imaging process. The ion microscope (secondary ion mass spectrometer, SIMS) uses a beam of heavy ions to erode a layer of atoms from the specimen surface. The secondary ions are then separated according to element in a mass spectrometer and recorded, for example using a channel plate multiplier and more-or-less conventional video or digital camera, to form an image of one plane in the specimen for one element at a time. The depth of erosion is usually calibrated for these instruments by measuring the signal profile of a known standard, such as may be produced by the same methods used to produce modern microelectronics.

The rate of surface removal is highly controllable (if somewhat slow) and capable of essentially atomic resolution in depth. The lateral resolution, by contrast, is of about the same level as in the conventional light microscope, so in this case instead of having voxels that are high in resolution in the plane but poorer in the depth direction, the situation is reversed. As always, the noncubic voxels create problems for processing and measurement.

Furthermore, the erosion rate for ion beam bombardment in the ion microscope or SIMS may vary from place to place in the specimen as a function of composition, structure, or even crystallographic orientation. This variation does not necessarily show up in the reconstruction, since each set of data is assumed to represent a plane, but it can cause significant distortion in the final interpretation. In principle, stretching of the data in 3-D can be performed just as images can be corrected for deformation in 2-D. However, without fiducial marks or accurate quantitative data on local erosion rates, it is hard to accomplish this with real data.

The ability to image many different elements with the SIMS creates a rich data set for 3-D display. A color 2-D image has three channels (whether it is saved as RGB [red, green, blue] or HSI [hue, saturation, intensity], as discussed in **Chapter 1**), but the SIMS data can have practically any number. The ability of the instrument to detect trace levels (typically parts per million or better) of every element or even isotope in the periodic table, plus molecular fragments, means that even for relatively simple specimens the multiband data present a challenge to store, display, and interpret.

Another type of microscope that removes layers of atoms as it images them is the atom probe ion microscope. In this instrument, a strong electrical field between a sharply curved sample tip and a display screen causes atoms to be desorbed from the surface and accelerated toward the screen, where they are imaged. The screen can include an electron channel plate to amplify the signal so that individual atoms can be seen, or it can be used as a time-of-flight mass spectrometer with pulsed application of the high voltage so that the different atom species can be distinguished. With any of the instrument variations, the result is a highly magnified image of atoms from the sample, showing atom arrangements in 3-D as layer after layer is removed. Examples of images from all these types of instruments are shown in **Chapter 1**.

Stereo measurement

There is another way to see 3-D structures, the same way that humans can perceive depth in some real-world situations. Having two eyes that face forward so that their fields of view overlap permits us to use stereoscopic vision to judge the relative distance to objects. In humans, this is done point by point, by moving our eyes in their sockets to bring each subject to the fovea, the portion of the retina with the densest packing of cones, as discussed in **Chapter 2**. The muscles in turn tell the brain what motion was needed to achieve convergence, and so we know whether one object is closer or farther than another. Stereo vision is used below as a means to transmit 3-D data to the human viewer.

It would be wrong to think that all human depth perception relies on stereoscopy. In fact, much of our judgment about the 3-D world around us comes from other cues such as shading, relative size, precedence, atmospheric effects (e.g., fog or haze), and motion flow (nearer objects move more in our visual field when we move our head) that work just fine with one eye and are used in some computer-based measurement methods (Carlsen 1985; Horn 1970, 1975; Pentland 1986; Roberts 1965; Woodham 1978). But stereo images can be used to determine depth information to put information into a 3-D computer database.

The light microscope has a rather shallow depth of field, which is made even less in the confocal scanning light microscope discussed previously. Consequently, looking at a specimen with deep relief is not very satisfactory except at relatively low magnifications. However, the electron microscope has lenses with very small aperture angles, and hence has very great depth of field. Stereoscopy is most commonly used with the scanning electron microscope (SEM) to produce in-focus images of rough surfaces. Tilting the specimen, or equivalently deflecting the scanning beam, can produce a pair of images from different points of view that form a stereo pair. Looking at one picture with each eye fools the brain into seeing the original rough surface.

Measuring the relief of surfaces from such images is the same in principle and in practice as using stereo-pair images taken from aircraft or satellites to measure the elevation of topographic features on Earth or another planet. The rich detail in the satellite photos makes it easier to find matching points practically anywhere in the images, but by the same token requires more matching points to define the surface than the simpler geometry of typical specimens observed in the SEM. The mathematical relationship between the measured parallax (the displacement of points in the left- and right-eye image) and the relative elevation of the points on the surface is presented in **Chapter 1**.

Automatic matching of points from stereo pairs is a difficult task for computer-based image analysis (Grimson 1981; Kayaalp and Jain 1987; Marr and Poggio 1976; Medioni and Nevatia 1985; Smith and Elstrom 2001). It is usually performed by using the pattern of brightness values in one image, for instance the left one, as a template to perform a cross-correlation search for the most nearly identical pattern in the right image. The area of search is restricted to a horizontal band in the second image covering the possible displacement, which depends on the angle between the two views and the maximum roughness of the surface. Some points will not be matched by this process because they may not be visible in both images (or are lost off the edges of one or the other image). Other points will match poorly because the local pattern of brightness values in the pixels includes some noise, and several parts of the image may have similar noise levels. Specular reflections, which can move on the surface as the point of view changes, also interfere with matching of locations.

Matching many points produces a new image in which each pixel can be given a value, based on the parallax, that represents the elevation of the surface. This range image will contain many false matches, but operations such as a median filter usually do a good job of removing the outlier points to produce an overall range image of the surface. In the example of **Figure 13.8**, cross-correlation matching of every point in the left-eye view with points in the right-eye view produces a disparity map (the horizontal distance between the location of the matched points) that contains false matches, which are filled in by a median filter as shown. The resulting elevation data can be used for measurement of points or line profiles, or used to reconstruct surface images, as illustrated. This use of surface range data is discussed further in **Chapter 14**.

A second approach to matching stereo pairs is based on the realization that many of the points in each image will not match well because they are just part of the overall surface or structure and not the "interesting" points where surfaces meet or other discontinuities are present. This approach is presumably related to human vision, which usually spends most of its time concentrating on only the few points in each scene where discontinuities are found. Locating these interesting points, based on some local property such as the variance, entropy, or result of a high-pass filter, produces a comparatively short list of points to be matched between the two images (Moravec 1977; Quam and Hannah 1974). A typical case may have only thousands of points instead of the million or so pixels in the original images.

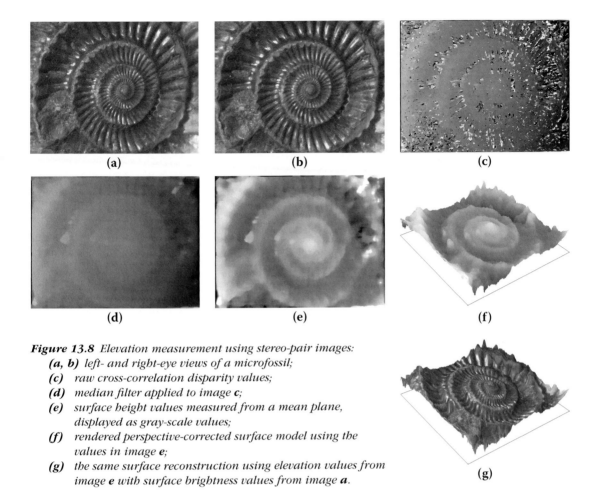

Figure 13.8 *Elevation measurement using stereo-pair images:*
(a, b) *left- and right-eye views of a microfossil;*
(c) *raw cross-correlation disparity values;*
(d) *median filter applied to image **c**;*
(e) *surface height values measured from a mean plane,*
displayed as gray-scale values;
(f) *rendered perspective-corrected surface model using the*
*values in image **e**;*
(g) *the same surface reconstruction using elevation values from*
*image **e** with surface brightness values from image **a**.*

Somewhat better selection of points is obtained by fitting a cubic polynomial to the pixel brightness values in each neighborhood. Then, if the polynomial is written as

$$f(i, j) = c_1 + c_2 x + c_3 y + c_4 x^2 + c_5 xy + c_6 y^2 +$$

$$+ c_7 x^3 + c_8 x^2 y + c_9 xy^2 + c_{10} y^3 \tag{13.1}$$

the Zuniga-Haralick operator (Haralick and Shapiro 1992; Zuniga and Haralick 1983) used to detect corner points is

$$\frac{-2 \cdot (c_2^2 c_6 - c_2 c_3 c_5 - c_3^2 c_4)}{(c_2^2 + c_3^2)^{3/2}} \tag{13.2}$$

The points on the resulting short list are then matched in the same way as above, by correlation of their neighborhood brightness patterns. Additionally, for most surfaces (i.e., simply connected ones that do not have loops or bridges), the order of points from top to bottom and left to right is preserved. This, and the limits on possible parallax for a given pair of images, reduces the typical candidate list for matching to a small number (typically ten or less), and the result produces a list of surface points and their elevations. It is then assumed that the

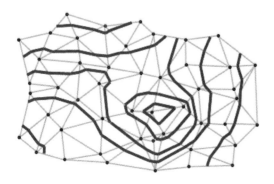

Figure 13.9 *Diagram showing contour lines (isoelevation lines) on the triangular facets joining an arbitrary arrangement of points whose elevations have been determined by stereoscopy.*

surface between these points is well behaved and can be treated as consisting of planar facets or simple spline patches, which are constructed by linking the points in a Delaunay tessellation. If the facets are small enough, it is possible to generate a contour map of the surface, as shown in **Figure 13.9**, by interpolating straight-line segments or spline curves between points along the edges of each planar facet. A complete display of elevation, called a range image, can be produced by interpolation, as shown in **Figure 13.10**.

The transmission electron microscope (TEM) also has a very large depth of field. In most cases, the specimens observed in the TEM are very thin (to permit electron penetration), and the optical depth of field is unimportant. However, with recent generations of high-voltage microscopes, comparatively thick samples (on the order of micrometers) can be imaged. This thickness is enough to contain a considerable amount of 3-D structure at the resolution of the TEM (on the order of a few nanometers). Hence, using the same approach of tilting the specimen to acquire stereo-pair images, it is possible to obtain information about the depth of points and the 3-D structure.

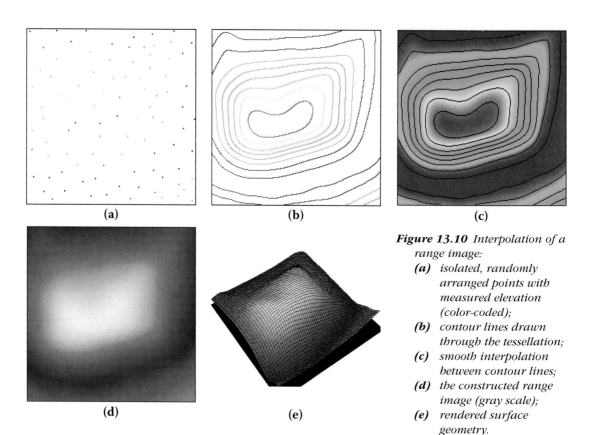

(a)

(b)

(c)

(d)

(e)

Figure 13.10 *Interpolation of a range image:*
(a) isolated, randomly arranged points with measured elevation (color-coded);
(b) contour lines drawn through the tessellation;
(c) smooth interpolation between contour lines;
(d) the constructed range image (gray scale);
(e) rendered surface geometry.

Presenting the images of scenes with discrete objects distributed in distance to a human viewer's eyes so that two pictures acquired from different viewpoints can be fused in the mind and examined in depth is not difficult (although it does not work for a significant fraction of viewers). Stereo imagery has been accomplished for years photographically. The technique seems to undergo a resurgence of interest every decade or so, either for still images or movies. Similar displays are now often generated using computers to display — or even generate — the images. The methods discussed below for using stereo-pair displays to communicate 3-D information from generated images are equally applicable here.

However, it is far more difficult to have the computer determine the depth of features in the structure from the images and construct a 3-D database of points and their relationship to each other. Part of the problem is that there is so much background detail from the (mostly) transparent medium surrounding the features of interest that it may dominate the local pixel brightnesses and make matching impossible. Another part of the problem is that it is no longer possible to assume that points maintain their order from left to right. In a 3-D structure, points may change their order as they pass in front or in back of each other.

The consequence of these limitations has been that only in a very few, highly idealized cases has automatic fusion of stereo-pair images from the TEM been attempted successfully. Simplification of the problem using very-high-contrast markers, such as small gold particles bound to selected surfaces using antibodies, or some other highly selective stain, helps. In this case only the markers are considered. There are only a few dozens or at most hundreds of these, and like the interesting points mentioned above for mapping surfaces, they are easily detected (being usually far darker than anything else in the image), and only a few could possibly match.

Even with these markers, a human may still be needed to identify or edit the matches. Given the matching points in the two images, the computer can construct a series of lines that describe the surface that the markers define, but this surface may only be a small part of the total structure. **Figure 13.11** shows an example of this method in which human matching was performed. Similar methods can be applied to stained networks (Huang et al. 1994) or to the distribution of precipitate particles in materials, for example.

In most matching procedures, the points in left- and right-eye images are defined in terms of pixel addresses. The error in the vertical (height) dimension determined by stereoscopy is typically an order of magnitude greater than the precision of measurement of the parallax, because the vertical height is proportional to the lateral parallax times the cosecant of the small angle between the views. Improving the measurement of parallax between features to subpixel

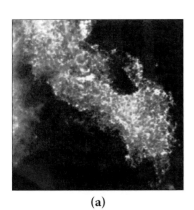

(a)

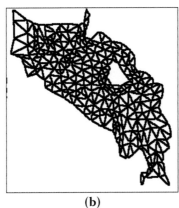

(b)

Figure 13.11

(a) Example of decorating a surface with metal particles (Golgi stain) shown in transmission electron micrographs

(b) whose elevations are measured stereoscopically to form a network describing the surface. (From Peachey, L. D. and Heath, J. P., J. Microsc. 153: 193, 1989. With permission.)

accuracy is therefore of considerable interest. Such improvement is possible in some cases, particularly when information from many pixels can be combined. As described in **Chapter 10**, the centroids of features or the location of lines can be specified to accuracy of 1/10th pixel or better.

3-D data sets

In the case of matching of points between two stereo-pair images, the database is a list of a few hundreds or thousands of coordinates that usually define either a surface or perhaps nodes in a network structure. If these points are to be used for measurement, the coordinates (and perhaps some information on which points are connected to which) are all that is required. If image reconstruction is intended, it will be necessary to interpolate additional points between them to complete a display. This is somewhat analogous to the use of boundary representation in two dimensions. It may offer a very compact record of the essential (or at least of the selected) information in the image, but it requires expansion to be visually useful to the human observer.

The most common way to store 3-D data sets is as a series of 2-D images. Each single image, which we have previously described as an array of pixels, is now seen to have depth. This depth is present either because the plane is truly an average over some depth of the sample (as in looking through a thin section) or because it is based on the spacing between that plane and the next (as for instance a series of polished planes observed by reflected light). Because of the depth associated with the planes, we refer to the individual elements as voxels (volume elements) rather than pixels (pixel elements).

For viewing, processing and measurement, the voxels will ideally be regular and uniformly spaced. This goal is best accomplished with a cubic array of voxels, which is easiest to address in computer memory, is compatible with processing and measurement operations, and corresponds to the way that some image-acquisition devices function (e.g., the confocal scanning light microscope). Other arrangements of voxels in space offer some theoretical advantages. In a simple cubic arrangement, the neighboring voxels are at different distances from the central voxel, depending on whether they share a face, edge, or corner. Deciding whether voxels touch and are part of the same feature requires a decision to include 6-, 18-, or 26-neighbor connectedness, even more complicated than the 4- or 8-connectedness of square pixels in a two-dimensional image, discussed in **Chapter 7**.

More-symmetrical arrangements are possible. The arrangements of atoms in metal crystals typically occupy sites in one of three lattice configurations: body-centered cubic (BCC), face-centered cubic (FCC), or hexagonal close packed (HCP). The first of these surrounds each atom (or voxel) with 8 touching neighbors at the same distance, and the other two have 12 equidistant neighbors.

The advantages of these voxel-stacking arrangements are that processing of images can treat each of the neighbors identically, and that measurements are less biased as a function of direction. A more symmetrical neighborhood with neighbors at uniform distances also simplifies processing, including the application of filters and morphological operations. Of course, to fill the space, the shapes of the voxels in these cases are not simple. Storing and addressing the voxel array is difficult, as is acquiring images or displaying them. Usually the acquired image must be resampled by interpolation to obtain voxels in one of these patterns, and a reverse interpolation is needed for display. For most purposes, these disadvantages outweigh the theoretical advantages, just as the use of a hexagonal pixel array is rarely used for 2-D images. Cubic arrays are the most common 3-D arrangement of voxels, just as square arrays of pixels are used for most 2-D images instead of a theoretically more attractive hexagonal pattern.

If the voxels are not cubic because the spacing between planes is different from the resolution within each plane, it may be possible to adjust things so that they are. In the discussion that follows, we will assume that the depth spacing is greater than the spacing within the plane, but an analogous situation could be described for the reverse case. The adjustment might be done by interpolating additional planes of voxels between those that have been measured. Unfortunately, doing this will not help much with image processing operations, since the assumption is that all of the neighbors are equal in importance, and with interpolation they become redundant.

The alternative approach is to reduce the resolution within the plane by sampling every nth pixel, or perhaps by averaging pixels together in blocks, so that a new image is formed with cubic voxels. This resolution reduction also reduces the amount of storage that will be required, since many fewer voxels remain. Although it seems unnatural to give up resolution, this is done in a few cases where cubic voxels are required for analysis.

A variety of different formats are available for storing 3-D data sets, either as a stack of individual images or effectively as an array of voxel values with x,y,z indices. Such arrays become very large, very fast. A 1024 × 1024-pixel 2-D monochrome 8-bit image occupies 1 MB of storage, using 1 byte per pixel (256 gray values). This is easily handled in the memory of a desktop computer. Even with modern digital cameras, a typical color image occupies only a few megabytes. But a 1024 × 1024 × 1024 3-D image would occupy 1 GB of memory, about the upper limit for practical processing on a desktop machine. Larger files present difficulties just in storing or transmitting from place to place, let alone processing. Many of the data sets used in this chapter are smaller arrays cut from or sampled from larger ones. The same operations can be used for larger data sets, given time, computer power (speed and memory), or both.

It is instructive to compare this situation with that of computer-aided drafting (CAD). For human-made objects with comparatively simple geometric surfaces, only a tiny number of point coordinates are required to define the entire 3-D structure. This kind of boundary representation is very compact, but it often takes some time (or specialized display hardware) to render a drawing with realistic surfaces from such a data set. For a voxel image, the storage requirements are great, but information is immediately available without computation for each location, and the various display images shown in this chapter can usually be produced very quickly (sometimes even at interactive speeds) by modest computers, provided that the data are held in memory.

For instance, given a series of surfaces defined by boundary representation or a few coordinates, the generation of a display can proceed by first constructing all of the points for one plane, calculating the local angles of the plane with respect to the viewer and light source, using those to determine a brightness value, and then plotting that value on the screen. At the same time, another image memory is used to store the actual depth (z-value) of the surface at that point. After one plane is complete, the next one is similarly drawn, except that the depth value is compared point by point with the values in the z-buffer to determine whether the plane is in front of or behind the previous values. Of course, each point is only drawn if it lies in front. This procedure permits multiple intersecting planes to be drawn on the screen correctly. (For more information on graphic presentation of three-dimensional CAD data, see Foley and Van Dam [1984] or Hearn and Baker [1986].)

Additional logic is needed to clip the edges of the planes to the stored boundaries, to change the reflectivity rules used to calculate brightness depending on the surface characteristics, and so forth. Standard texts on computer graphics describe algorithms for accomplishing these tasks and devote considerable space to the relative efficiency of various methods because the time involved can be significant. By comparison, looking up the value in a large array, or even running through a column in the array to add densities or find the maximum value, is very fast. This is particularly true if the array can be held in memory rather than requiring disk access.

The difficulties of aligning sequential slices to produce a 3-D data set were discussed above. In many cases, there may be several 3-D data sets obtained by different imaging techniques (e.g., MRI, X-ray, PET images of the head) that must be aligned to each other. They also commonly have different resolutions and voxel sizes, so that interpolation is needed to adjust them to match one another. The situation is similar to the 2-D problems encountered in geographical information systems (GIS), in which surface maps, images in different wavelengths from different satellites, aerial photographs, and other information must be aligned and combined.

The general problem is usually described as one of registering the multiple data sets. The two principal techniques, which are complementary, are to use cross-correlation methods on the entire pixel or voxel array, as discussed in **Chapter 6**, or to isolate specific features in the multiple images and use them as fiducial marks to perform warping (Besl 1992; Brown 1992; van den Elsen et al. 1993, 1994, 1995; Frederik et al. 1997; Goshtasby 2005; Hajnal et al. 2001; Modersitzki 2004; Reddy and Chatterji 1996; Rehm et al. 1994; West et al. 1997).

Slicing the data set

Since most 3-D image data sets are actually stored as a series of 2-D images, it is usually easy to access any of the individual image planes, commonly called slices. Playing the series of slices back to create an animation or "movie" is perhaps the most common tool available to let the user view the data. It is often quite effective in letting the viewer perform the 3-D integration, and as it recapitulates the way the images may have been acquired (but with a much-compressed time base), most viewers can understand images presented in this way. A simple user interface need only allow the viewer to vary the speed of the animation, change direction, or stop at a chosen slice, for example. This is by far the most common way that 3-D data sets are actually examined.

One problem with presenting the original images as slices of the data is that the orientation of some features in the 3-D structure may not show up very well in the slices. It is useful to be able to change the orientation of the slices to look at any plane through the data, either in still or animated playback. This change in orientation is quite easy to do as long as the orientation of the slices is parallel to the x-, y-, or z-axes in the data set. If the depth direction is understood as the z-axis, then the x- and y-axes are the horizontal and vertical edges of the individual images. If the data are stored as discrete voxels, then accessing the data to form an image on planes parallel to these directions is just a matter of calculating the addresses of voxels using offsets to the start of each row and column in the array. This addressing can be done at real-time speeds if the data are held in memory, but is somewhat slower if the data are stored on a disk drive because the voxels that are adjacent along scan lines in the original slice images are stored contiguously on disk and can be read as a group in a single pass. However, when a different orientation is required, the voxels must be located at widely separated places in the file, and it takes time to move the disk head and wait for the disk to rotate.

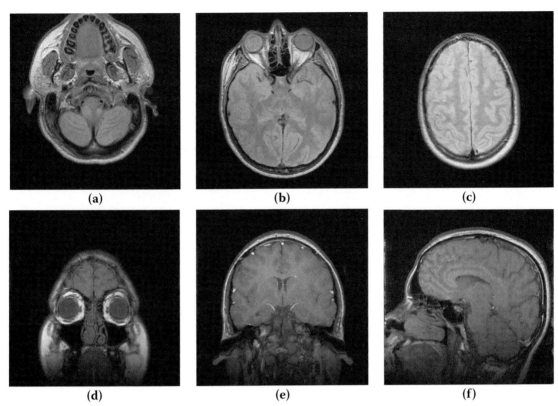

Figure 13.12 *A few slices from a complete set of MRI head-scan data. Images **a, b, c** show transaxial sections (3 from a set of 46); images **d** and **e** are coronal sections (2 from a set of 42); and image **f** is a sagittal section (1 from a set of 30).*

Displaying an image in planes parallel to the x-, y-, and z-axes was introduced in **Chapter 12**. **Figure 13.12** shows another example of orthogonal slices. The images are magnetic resonance images (MRIs) of a human head. The views are generally described as transaxial (perpendicular to the subject's spine), sagittal (parallel to the spine and to the major axis of symmetry), and coronal (parallel to the spine and perpendicular to the "straight ahead" line of sight). Several individual sections are shown representing each orientation.

This kind of resectioning with MRI data (or most other kinds of medical images) suffers in quality because the spacing of the planes is usually greater than the resolution within the plane, and the result is a visible loss of resolution in one direction in the resectioned slices due to interpolation in the z direction. The alternative to interpolation is to extend the voxels in space; in most cases, this is even more distracting to the eye, as shown in **Figure 13.13**. Interpolation between planes of pixels can be done linearly, or using higher-order fits to more than two planes, or more than just the two pixels immediately above and below. But while interpolation produces a visually acceptable image, it can ignore real structure or create apparent structure. **Figure 13.14** shows an example of interpolation that creates an impression of structure that is not actually present (and hides the real structure).

When data can be obtained with cubic voxels, this interpolation is not a problem. In several of the figures later in this chapter, much greater loss of resolution in the z direction will be evident when plane images are reconstructed by sampling and interpolation of the original data. In the case of **Figure 13.12**, the MRI images were actually obtained with uniform

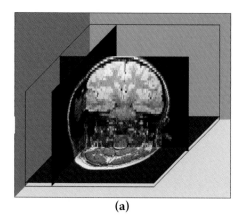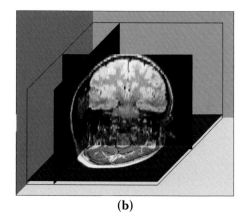

(a)   (b)

Figure 13.13 Comparison of two vertical slices through the 3-D MRI data set from Figure 13.12: (a) slices extended vertically; (b) linear interpolation between slices.

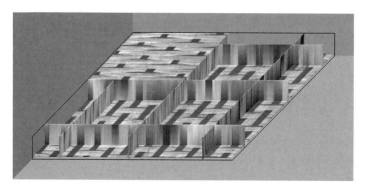

Figure 13.14 Interpolation in a 3-D array. In this example, only two images of the top and bottom of a woven fabric are used. The points between the two surfaces are linearly interpolated and bear no relationship to the actual 3-D structure of the textile.

resolution in each of the three directions. Many current diagnostic procedures acquire multiple sets of scans in different orientations to provide high-quality viewing of sections in any of these primary directions.

Combining several views at once using orthogonal planes adds to the feeling of three-dimensionality of the data. **Figure 13.15** shows several examples of this using the same MRI head-scan data based on plane images obtained in the transaxial direction. The poorer resolution in the z direction is evident, but still the overall impression of 3-D structure is quite good. These views can also be animated by moving one (or several) of the planes through the data set while keeping the other orthogonal planes fixed to act as a visual reference.

Unfortunately, there is no good way to demonstrate this time-based animation in a print medium. Once upon a time, children's cartoon books used a "flip" mode with animation printed on a series of pages that the viewer could literally flip or riffle through at a fast enough rate to cause flicker-fusion in the eye and create the visual impression of continuous motion. That form of animation takes a lot of pages and is really only good for very simple images such as cartoons. It is unlikely to appeal to the publishers of books and technical journals. All that can really be done here is to show a few of the still images from such a sequence and appeal to the reader's imagination to supply a necessarily weak impression of the effect of a live animation. There are many online Web sites that show such animations as QuickTime® movies.

Chapter 2, **Figure 2.32** showed a series of images that can be used to show "moving pictures" of this kind (the Muybridge "running horse" sequence). There is current interest in the use of

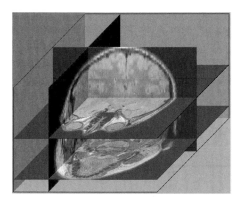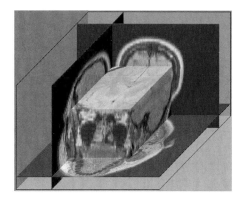

Figure 13.15 *Several views of the MRI head-scan data from* **Figure 13.12** *along section planes normal to the axes of the voxel array. The voxels were taken from the transaxial slices, and so the resolution is poorer in the direction normal to the planes than in the planes.*

online delivery and compact discs for the distribution of technical papers, which will perhaps offer a medium that can use time as a third axis to substitute for a spatial axis and show 3-D structure through motion. The possibilities will be mentioned again in connection with rotation and other time-based display methods.

Motion, or sequences of images, is used to show multidimensional data in many cases. Rapidly accessing a series of planes provides a crude method of showing data sets that occupy three spatial dimensions. Another effective animation shows a view of an entire 3-D data set while varying the opacity of the voxels. Even for a data set that occupies two spatial dimensions, transitions between many kinds of information can be used effectively. **Figure 13.16** illustrates this multiplicity with weather data, showing temperature, wind velocity, and other parameters displayed on a map of the United States. In general, displays that utilize a two-dimensional map as an organizing basis for multidimensional data such as road networks, geological formations, and so on — called geographic information systems (GIS) — have many types of data and can only display a small fraction of it at any one time.

Of course, time itself is also a valid third dimension, and the acquisition of a series of images in rapid succession to study changes in structure or composition with time can employ many

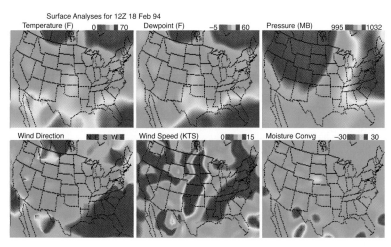

Figure 13.16 *Weather data for the United States is a richly multidimensional data set tied to a geographic base.*

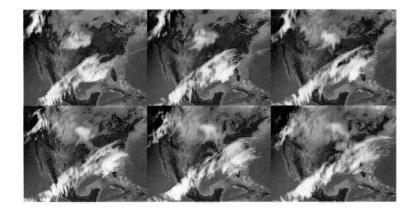

Figure 13.17 A series of
satellite images taken at
3-hour intervals showing
the motion of cloud
patterns over the United
States.

Figure 13.18 A series of
images of adult rat atrial
myocytes loaded with
the calcium indicator
fluo-3. The images were
recorded at video rate
(30 frames per second)
from a confocal light
microscope. (Courtesy of
Dr. W. T. Mason and Dr. J.
Hoyland, Department of
Neurobiology, Babraham
Institute, Cambridge,
U.K.)

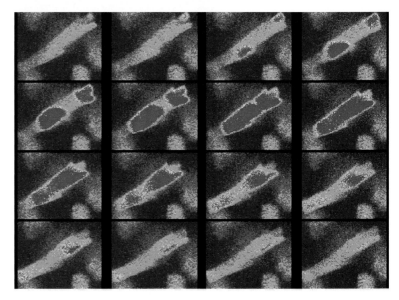

of the same analytical and visualization tools as images covering three spatial dimensions. We
see this routinely on TV as satellite images of weather patterns are shown that compress hours
or days into a few seconds to show cloud motion (**Figure 13.17**). The same approach is useful in other fields. **Figure 13.18** shows a series of images recorded at video rate (30 frames
per second) from a confocal light microscope. Such data sets can be assembled into a cube in
which the *z* direction is time, and changes can be studied by sectioning this volume in planes
along the *z* direction, or they can be viewed volumetrically or as a time sequence.

Arbitrary section planes

Restricting the section planes to those perpendicular to the *x*-, *y*-, or *z*-axes is obviously limiting for
the viewer. It is done for convenience in accessing the voxels in storage and creating the display. If
some arbitrary planar orientation is selected, the voxels must be found that lie closest to the plane.
As for the case of image warping, stretching, and rotating discussed in **Chapter 4**, these voxels
will not generally lie exactly in the plane, nor will they have a regular gridlike spacing that lends

itself to forming an image. **Figure 13.19** shows a detailed example of a plane section through an array of cubic voxels, in which portions of various size and shape are revealed. These variations complicate displaying the voxel contents on the plane.

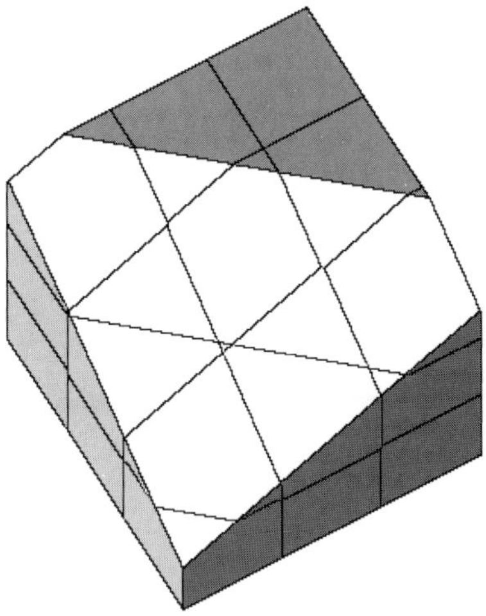

The available solutions are either to use the voxels that are closest to the section plane, plot them where they land, and spread them out to fill any gaps that develop, or to establish a grid of points in the section plane and then interpolate values from the nearest voxels, which can be up to eight in number. As for the case of rotation and stretching, these two solutions have different shortcomings. Using the nearest voxel preserves brightness values (for whatever the voxel value represents) but may distort boundaries and produce stair-stepping or aliasing. Interpolation makes the boundaries appear straight and smooth, but also smoothes the brightness values by averaging so that steps are blurred. It is also slower, because more voxels must be located in the array and the interpolation performed.

Figure 13.19 Intersection of a plane with an array of cubic voxels. The plane is viewed perpendicularly, showing the different areas and shapes of the intersection regions.

Producing an animation by continuously moving a section plane at an arbitrary orientation requires a significant amount of computation and access to the data (which may not all be in active memory), even if it is simple calculation of addresses and linear interpolation of values. Instead of doing this calculation in real time, many systems instead create new images of each of the plane positions, store them, and then create the animation by playing them back. This procedure is fine for demonstrating something that the user has already found, but because of the time delay, it is not a particularly good tool for exploring the 3-D data set to discover the unexpected.

The ultimate use of planar resectioning would be to change the location and orientation of the section plane dynamically in real time, allowing instant response to the scene. **Chapter 2** pointed out that humans study things by turning them over, either in the hand or in the mind. This act of turning over is a natural way to study objects, but it requires a fairly large computer memory (to hold all of the voxel data), a fairly speedy processor and display, and a user interface that provides the required number of degrees of freedom. Modern desktop computers are approaching this

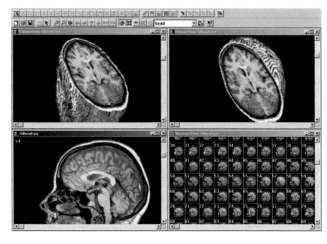

Figure 13.20 Presentation of serial sections, 3-D reconstruction, and arbitrary plane slice on a desktop computer. (Courtesy of Able Software, Lexington, MA.)

level of performance; **Figure 13.20** shows a typical display in which arbitrary sections can be accessed in real time.

Positioning an arbitrary plane can be done in two different ways, both of which produce the same results but feel quite different to the user. One is to move the plane with respect to a fixed 3-D voxel array. This can be done, for example, by dragging the corners of the plane along the x-, y-, z-axes, or by positioning a center point and then tilting the plane around two axes through that point. A different method is to keep the section plane fixed perpendicular to the direction of view while allowing the data set to be rotated in space. Combined with the ability to shift the section plane toward or away from the viewer (or equivalently to shift the data set), this method allows exactly the same information to be obtained.

The principal difference between these approaches is that, in the latter case, the image is seen without perspective or foreshortening, so that size comparisons or measurements can be made. Obtaining such data can be important in some applications. On the other hand, keeping the data set fixed and moving the section plane seems to aid the user in maintaining orientation within the structure. There are as many different modes of human interaction with 3-D data sets as there are programs, and as yet no general consensus on which are most useful has emerged. The control mechanisms for such interactions are also primitive. Using a mouse to scroll multiple sliders for angles or positions is clumsy, but few 3-D tools are available. Using an instrumented glove to "turn over" a data set while viewing it on a large screen or personal head-mounted display is an entertaining possibility, but is not within reach for many potential viewers.

Figure 13.21 shows the voxels revealed by an arbitrary section plane through the 3-D data set from the MRI head-scan image series (see **Figure 13.12**). The appearance of the voxels as a series of steps is rather distracting, so it is more common to show the value of the voxels nearest to the plane, or to interpolate among the voxels to obtain brightness values for each point on the plane, as shown in **Figure 13.22**.

Also useful is the ability to make some of the pixels in section planes transparent, allowing the viewing of other planes behind the first, and making the 3-D structure of the data more apparent. **Figure 13.23** shows an example of this for the spherical particle data shown in **Chapter 12**. The series of parallel slices are not contiguous planes of voxels, and the separation of the planes has been increased by a factor of two in the z direction. The voxels whose density falls below a threshold that roughly corresponds to that of the particles have been

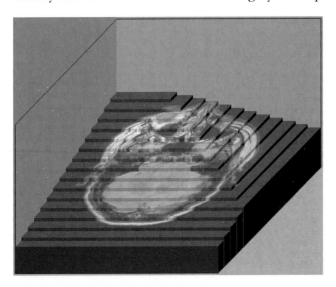

Figure 13.21 Sampling voxels along inclined planes in the 3-D array from the MRI head-scan data from Figure 13.12. Showing each entire voxel is visually distracting and does not produce a smooth image.

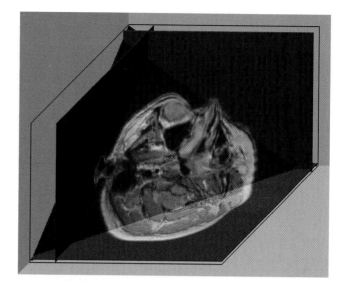

Figure 13.22 *Smooth interpolation of image pixels on arbitrary planes positioned in a voxel array.*

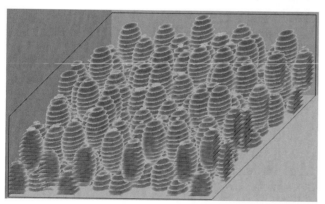

Figure 13.23 *"Exploded" view of voxel layers in the tomographic reconstruction of spherical particles (see* **Figure 12.59***). The low-density region surrounding the particles is shown as transparent.*

made transparent. This allows seeing voxels that are part of particles in other section planes behind the first.

Figure 13.24 shows a similar treatment for the MRI data set of the human head (see **Figure 13.12**). The threshold for choosing which voxels to make transparent is more arbitrary than that for the spheres, since there are void and low-density regions inside as well as outside the head. However, the overall impression of 3-D structure is clearly enhanced by this treatment.

The use of color

Assignment of pseudocolors to gray-scale 2-D images was discussed in earlier chapters. It sometimes permits distinguishing subtle variations that are imperceptible in brightness in the original. But, as noted previously, it more often breaks up the overall continuity and gestalt of the image so that the image is more difficult to interpret. Of course, the same display tricks can be used with three-dimensional sets of images, with the same consequences.

A subtle use of color or shading is to apply slightly different shading to different planar orientations shown in **Figure 13.15** and **Figure 13.22** to increase the impression of three-

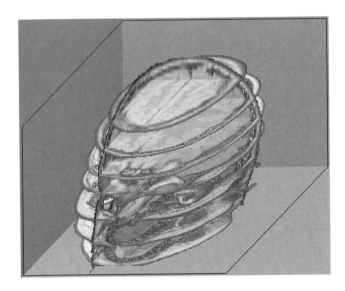

Figure 13.24 View of several orthogonal slices of the MRI head-scan data from *Figure 13.12*, with transparency for the low-density regions in the planes.

dimensionality. In this example, a gray-scale difference between the x,y,z orientations is evident. Light tints of color can be used for this as well.

It is more useful to employ color scales to distinguish different structures, as was also demonstrated for 2-D images. It requires separate processing or measurement operations to distinguish the different structures, or postprocessing to apply colors to various regions of a reconstruction, as shown in **Figure 13.25**. When applied to 3-D data sets, the colored scales assist in seeing the continuity from one image to another, while providing ranges of brightness values for each object (Parker et al. 2005).

One of the most common ways that multiple colors can be used to advantage in 3-D image data is to code multiband data, such as the elemental concentrations measured from the SIMS. This use of pseudocolor is analogous to similar coding in 2-D images, frequently used for X-ray maps from the SEM and for remotely sensed satellite images, in which the colors can either be "true" or be used to represent colors beyond the range of human vision, particularly infrared. Of course, the other tools for working with multiband images in 2-D, such as calculating ratios, can also be applied in 3-D.

Figure 13.25 Volume-rendered image of vasculature in the lung, with color tinting. (Courtesy of TeraRecon, Inc., San Mateo, CA.)

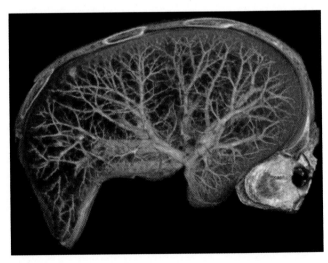

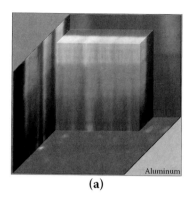 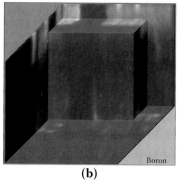 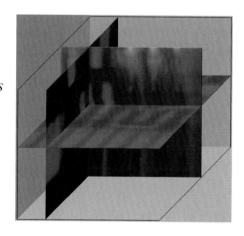

(a)   (b)   (c)

Figure 13.26   *Views of plane sections for the elements aluminum **(a)**, boron **(b)**, and oxygen **(c)** in a silicon wafer, imaged by SIMS. **Figure 13.27** shows a color image of all three elements on another orthogonal set of planes.*

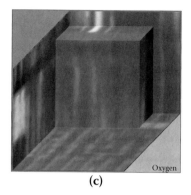

Figure 13.27   *Color coding of elemental intensity from SIMS images in **Figure 13.26**. The multiband 3-D data set is sectioned on x, y, and z planes, and the 256-level (8 bit) brightness scale for the elements aluminum, boron, and oxygen are assigned to red, green, and blue, respectively.*

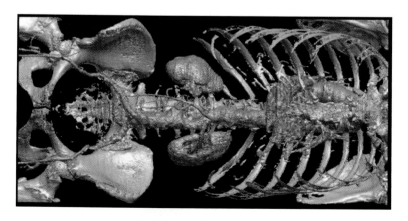

Figure 13.28   *Volume-rendered image with multimode fusion and color tinting. (Courtesy of A. Quon, Stanford University, Stanford, CA.)*

Figure 13.26 shows example images for the SIMS depth imaging of elements implanted in a silicon wafer. Comparing the spatial location of the different elements is made easier by superimposing the separate images and using colors to distinguish the elements. This is done by assigning red, green, and blue to each of three elements and then combining the image planes, with the result shown in **Figure 13.27**.

The use of distinct colors to label different structures can be very useful for visualizations. In **Figure 13.28**, the merging of reconstructions of CT and MRI data has been done using tints of different colors to show bone structures and blood vessels. Merging multiple data sets adds important complementary information to presentations (Ruiz-Alzola et al. 2005; Spetsieris 1995). The use of surface rendering (described below) for each data set, and their registration in 3-D, makes this an extremely realistic and powerful visualization.

Volumetric display

Sectioning the data set, even if some regions are made transparent, obscures much of the voxel array. Only the selected planes are seen, and much of the information in the data set is not used. It has been pointed out before that the topological properties of 3-D structures are not revealed on section planes. However, the volumetric display method shows all of the 3-D voxel information. For simple structures, displaying everything can be an advantage, while for complex structures the overlapping features and boundaries can become confusing.

A volumetric display is produced by ray tracing. In the simplest model used, a uniform, extended light source is placed behind the voxel array. For each parallel straight-line ray from the light source to a point on the display screen, the density value of each voxel that lies along the path is used to calculate a reduction in the light intensity following the usual absorption rule:

$$\frac{I}{I_0} = e^{-\sum \rho}$$

(13.3)

Performing this calculation for rays reaching each point on the display generates an image. The total contrast range can be adjusted to the range of the display by introducing an arbitrary scaling constant. This scaling can be important because the calculated intensities may be quite small for large voxel arrays.

Notice that this model assumes that the voxel values actually correspond to density or to some other property that can be adequately modeled by the absorption of light. The image shown in **Figure 12.59** in **Chapter 12** corresponds to this model, since it shows the projected view through a specimen using X-rays, although the geometry is cone beam rather than parallel projection. In fact, X-ray tomographic reconstruction, discussed in **Chapter 12**, proceeds from such views to a calculation of the voxel array. Having the array of voxel values then permits generating many kinds of displays to examine the data. It seems counterproductive to calculate the projection view again, and indeed in such a view as shown in those figures, the ability to distinguish the individual features and see their relationship is poor.

One of the advantages of this mode is that the direction of view can be changed rather easily. For each, it is necessary to calculate the addresses of voxels that lie along each ray. When the view direction is not parallel to one of the axes, this addressing can be done efficiently using sine/cosine values or a generalization of the Bresenham line-drawing algorithm (see, for instance, Foley and Van Dam 1984). Also, in this case, an improved display quality is obtained

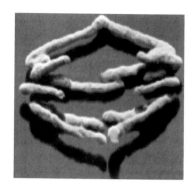

Figure 13.29 Reconstruction of chromosomes in a dividing cell from CSLM 3-D data. The chromosomes are opaque and the matrix around them transparent, and shadows have been ray cast on the rear plane to enhance the 3-D appearance.

by calculating the length of the line segment along each ray through each pixel. The absorption rule then must include those distances t in the summation:

$$\frac{I}{I_0} = e^{-\sum \rho t}$$

(13.4)

This method is far short of a complete ray tracing, although it is sometimes described as one. In a true ray-traced image, refraction and reflection of the light is included along with the absorption. **Figure 13.29** shows an example in which the inclusion of shadows greatly increases the 3-D impression. More complex shading, in which features cast shadows on themselves and each other, requires calculations that are generally too time-consuming for routine use in this application. With the simple absorption-only method, it is possible to achieve display speeds capable of rotating the array (changing the view direction) interactively with desktop computers.

Of course, it is always possible to generate and save a series of projection images that can then be played back as an animation or movie. But as with the other animation techniques discussed here, these are primarily useful for communicating some information that is already known to a new viewer, while interactive displays may assist in discovering the structural relationships in the first place.

These types of volumetric displays are often isometric rather than perspective-corrected. In other words, the dimension of a voxel or feature does not change with distance. This is equivalent to looking at the scene through a long-focal-length lens, and given the inherent strangeness of data in most 3-D image sets, it does not generally cause significant additional discomfort to viewers. True perspective correction requires that x,y dimensions on the screen be adjusted for depth. Particularly for rotated views, perspective adds a significant amount of computation, and this is incorporated in many modern general-purpose graphics packages such as OpenGL.

Figure 13.30 shows such a view through a joint in the leg of a head louse. The original series of images were obtained with a transmission confocal light microscope, with nearly cubic voxels (the spacing between sequential focal planes was 0.2 μm in depth). The individual muscle fibers are visible but overlapped. Shifting the stack to approximate rotation as described below gives the viewer the ability to distinguish the various muscle groups. Again, a time sequence (hard to show in print media) can be used as a third dimension to display 3-D data as the planes are shifted, and since no complex arithmetic is needed to run this sequence, it is practical to create such animations in a small computer.

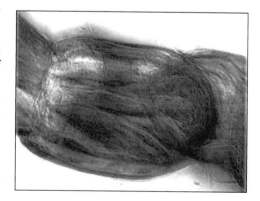

Figure 13.30 Volumetric projection image through a stack of 60 CSLM images of a joint in the leg of a head louse. Each plane is displaced by one voxel dimension to produce a view at 45°.

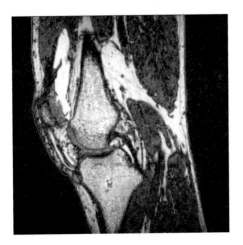

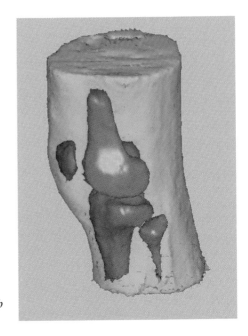

Figure 13.31 *Viewing the surface reconstruction from serial sections through a knee joint, with the surrounding tissue shown as a transparent volume with no internal detail.*

A much more limited approach to volumetric presentation is to show one portion of the image as a surface-rendered model, as discussed below, but to show the surrounding tissue as a transparent volume. Usually no detail is preserved in this volume, and it is included only to provide a point of reference for the structure of interest, as shown in **Figure 13.31**.

Very rapid generation of projection images is possible if the addressing can be simplified and the variation in distance through different voxels can be ignored. **Figure 13.32** shows an approximation that facilitates these changes. Each plane of voxels is shifted laterally by a small amount, which can be an integer number of voxel spaces (thus making the address calculation particularly simple), but in any case requires no more than simple 2-D interpolation. The planes remain normal to the view direction, so that all distances through pixels are the same. This kind of shifting can give the impression of rotation for small angles. Beyond about 30°, the distortion of the 3-D structure due to stretching may become visually objectionable. However, this method provides a fast way to cause some relative displacement of features as a function of depth to better understand the structure.

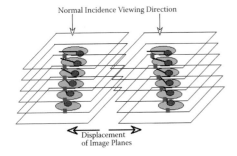

Figure 13.32 *Schematic diagram of shifting image planes laterally to create illusion of rotation or to produce stereo-pair images for viewing.*

Stereo viewing

In many of the images in this chapter, two adjacent images in a rotation or pseudorotation sequence can be viewed as a stereo pair. For some readers, looking at them will require an inexpensive viewer that allows one to focus on the separate images while keeping the eyes looking straight ahead (which the brain expects to correspond to objects at a great distance). Other readers may have mastered the trick of fusing such printed stereo views without assistance. Some, unfortunately, will not be able to see them at all. A significant portion of the population seems not to actually use stereo vision, due for instance to uncorrected amblyopia ("lazy eye") in childhood.

Stereo views are so useful to a reasonable fraction of people that it may be useful to display them directly on the viewing screen. Of course, with a large screen, it is possible to draw the two views side by side. **Figure 13.33** and **Figure 13.34** show examples of stereo-pair presentation of 3-D images, using both the volumetric display method discussed above and the surface-rendered method discussed below, for the same specimen (derived from confocal light-microscope images of a sea urchin embryo). **Figure 13.35** shows another stereo-pair presentation of skeletonized data obtained from neurons imaged in the confocal light microscope.

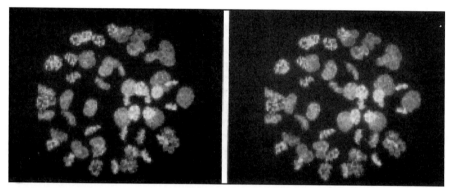

Figure 13.33 *Stereo-pair presentation of Feulgen-stained DNA in a sea urchin embryo. The cells form a hollow sphere, evident in the stereo images, with some cells in the act of cell division. This image shows a volumetric image that is "ray cast" or "ray traced," using an emission model, with different offsets for the individual optical sections to produce a stereo effect. See also **Figure 13.34** for a surface image of the same data. (From Summers, R. G. et al.,* J. Electron Microscope Tech. *18: 24, 1991. With permission.)*

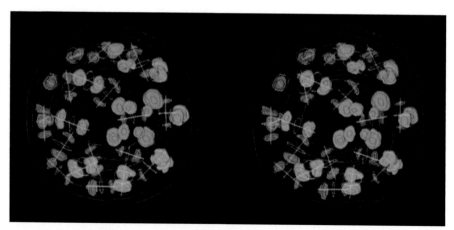

Figure 13.34 *Stereo view of the data set from **Figure 13.33**, but surface rendered and color-coded. The surface image shows contours within each section that render the surfaces of the chromosomal masses but obscure any internal detail or structures to the rear. Contour lines for the embryo are also shown.*

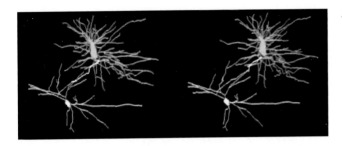

Figure 13.35 Stereo images of skeletonized lines (manually entered from serial-section data) from two neurons in hippocampus of 10-day-old rat, showing branching and 3-D relationships. (From Turner, J. N. et al., J. Electron Microscope Tech. 8: 11, 1991. With permission.)

A more direct stereo display method uses color planes in the display for the left- and right-eye views. For instance, **Figure 13.36** shows a stereo pair of blood vessels in the skin of a hamster, imaged live using a confocal light microscope in fluorescence mode. The 3-D reconstruction method used pseudorotation by shifting of the focal-section planes combined with the emission rules discussed below. Merging these images using red and green to display two views of the same 3-D data set is shown in **Figure 13.37**. The images are overlapped, and a viewer equipped with glasses having appropriate red and cyan filters can easily see the depth information in the combined images. Of course, this method cannot be used for color images, as discussed below.

These stereo views were constructed from multiple sections by projecting or ray tracing through a stack of images, as shown previously. The individual sections were obtained by confocal microscopy, which because of its very shallow depth of field can be used to obtain a continuous set of voxel planes. Other techniques that produce continuous arrays of thin sections can also be used, of course. But it is even possible to perform this type of reconstruction using a conventional optical microscope, despite the blurring of the images due to the large depth of field and the effect of light passing through the specimen above and below the image planes.

Removing artifacts such as blur from images by processing in frequency space was discussed in **Chapter 6**. For three dimensions, the procedure is identical except that the point-spread

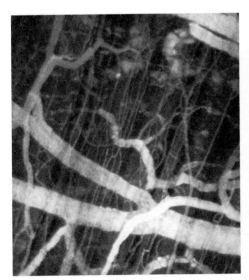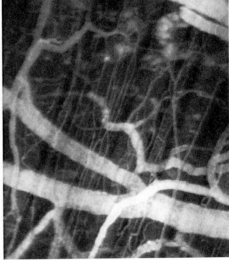

Figure 13.36 Stereo view of multiple focal-plane images from a confocal light microscope showing light emitted from fluorescent dye injected into the vasculature of a hamster and viewed live in the skin. This image is also shown in *Figure 13.37*. (Courtesy of C. Russ, University of Texas, Austin, TX.)

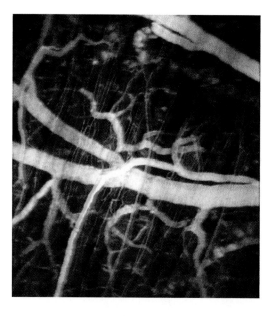

Figure 13.37 Stereo pair of the same image pair shown in *Figure 13.36*, using red and cyan for the different eye views. This allows viewing the image with normal eye vergence, using glasses (red lens on left eye, green or blue on right).

function and the Fourier transform are three-dimensional. **Figure 13.38** shows an example of using Wiener inverse filtering to accomplish this deblurring in the creation of a stereo pair. The images were reconstructed from 90 optical sections spaced through a 50-μm-thick section, which is much closer than the depth of field of the optics. The use of the inverse filter removes most of the artifacts from the images and produces a clear stereo-pair image (Lin et al. 1994). Another approach to the same kind of sharpening is to apply an iterative procedure that uses neighboring images to estimate the artifacts in each plane. This Van Cittert filter requires using neighbor planes on each side out to about twice the dimension of the point-spread function, which in this case is the depth of optical focus (Jain 1989). Because it uses only a few planes at a time, this method may be faster than full 3-D deconvolution in cases where computer memory is insufficient to hold the full data set.

For projection of stereo-pair images, it is possible to use two slide projectors or digital computer projectors equipped with polarizing filters that orient the light polarization at right angles (usually 45° to the right and left of vertical) and superimpose the two images. Viewers wearing polarized glasses can then see the stereo effect, and color can still be used. This display method requires special specular projection screens that reflect the light without

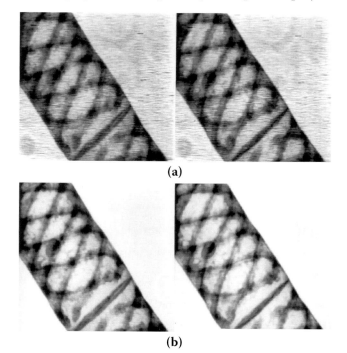

(a)

(b)

Figure 13.38 Sharpening of 3-D images by Wiener filtering. The stereo-pair images are produced by ray tracing two projections at angles of about ±2.4° through 90 serial optical sections in a 50-μm-thick section. The sample is spirogyra:
(a) original images;
(b) Wiener inverse filtered.
(From Lin, W. et al., J. Computer Assisted Microsc. 6: 113, 1994. With permission.)

losing the polarization, and it works best for viewers in line with the center of the screen. It has become a rather popular method of displaying 3-D data. Of course, it is not as practical for interactive exploration of a data set if photographic slides must be made first. Polarization can also be used with displays on a single computer monitor, as discussed below.

The difference in viewing angle for the two images can be adjusted somewhat arbitrarily to control the visual impression of depth. The angle can be made to correspond to the typical vergence angle of human vision for normal viewing. Using a typical interocular distance of 7.5 cm, and a viewing distance of 1 m, the actual vergence angle is 4.3°. For closer viewing, larger angles are appropriate. The judgment of depth thus depends on our brain's interpretation of the viewing distance, which is based on the focus distance to the image in combination with the vergence angle of the eyes in their sockets. If the angle is varied, the impression of depth can be adjusted to expand or compress the z dimension, as shown in **Figure 13.39**.

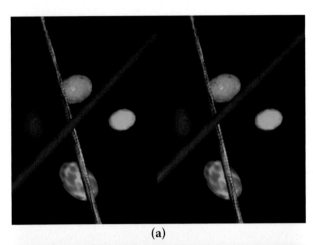

(a)

Special display hardware

Specialized display hardware for 3-D image analysis can be useful in some cases. Holography offers the promise of realistic three-dimensional display that can be viewed from different directions (Blackie et al. 1987). Attempts to generate such displays by calculating the holograms have been experimentally successful, although they are still too slow for interactive use (and far from the "stand-alone"

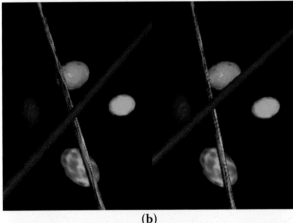

(b)

Figure 13.39 Stereo-pair images of a generated structure with varying angles to control the apparent depth of the structure in the z direction:
(a) ±1°;
(b) ±3°;
(c) ±5°.
Visual fusion of the images becomes increasingly difficult with the larger angles.

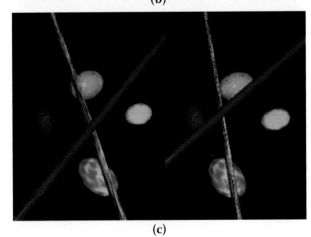

(c)

three-dimensional presentation of Princess Leia generated by R2-D2 in *Star Wars!*). At present, the best holograms are displayed using coherent light from a laser and high-resolution film. To produce live displays from a computer, multiple screens such as the LCDs used for flat-screen displays can be used in place of the film. However, the resolution and control of the light modulation (relative intensity) is not really adequate.

Another custom approach is called a varifocal mirror (Fuchs et al. 1982). Each plane of voxels in the 3-D array is drawn one at a time on the display CRT. The screen is not viewed directly by the user, but is reflected from a mirror. The mirror is mounted on a speaker voice coil so that it can be moved. As each different plane of voxels is drawn, the mirror is displaced slightly, as shown schematically in **Figure 13.40**. This movement changes the distance from the viewer's eye to the screen and gives the impression of depth. To achieve high drawing speeds (so that the entire set of planes can be redrawn at least 30 times per second), this technique is usually restricted to simple outline drawings rather than the entire voxel data set. The successive outlines are perceived as surfaces in three-dimensions.

Another, more recent development for real-time viewing of 3-D computer graphics displays uses stereo images. The computer calculates two display images for slightly different orientations of the data set or viewing positions. These are displayed alternately using high-speed display hardware, which typically shows 120 images per second. Special hardware is then used to allow each eye to see only the correct images at a rate of 60 times per second, fast enough to eliminate flicker. (The minimum rate for flicker fusion, above which we see continuous images rather than discrete ones, is usually at least 20 frames per second; commercial moving pictures typically use 24 frames, and television uses 25 in European and 30 in U.S. systems.)

The visual switching can be done by installing a liquid-crystal device on the display monitor that rapidly switches the polarization direction of the transmitted light, thus allowing viewers to watch through glasses containing polarizing film. A second approach is to wear special glasses containing active liquid-crystal devices that can rapidly turn clear or opaque. Synchronizing pulses from the computer cause the glasses to switch as the images are displayed, so that each eye sees the proper view.

Such devices have been used primarily for graphics design, in which substantial computer resources are used to model three-dimensional objects, generate rendered surface views, and allow the user to freely rotate and zoom. With the number of disciplines interested in using 3-D computer graphics, it seems assured that new hardware (and the required corresponding software) will continue to evolve for this purpose. The economic breakthrough that would impact scientific uses will probably come when game-console manufacturers decide to deliver 3-D displays.

These various display tools can be adapted to the display of 3-D image data and used at scales ranging from nanometers (electron and ion microscopy) to kilometers (seismic exploration). It is possible to imagine using other senses than visual to deal with multiband data (e.g., sound that changes pitch and volume to reveal density and composition as you move a cursor over

Figure 13.40 *Diagram of the operation of a varifocal mirror to show depth in images. The speaker voice coil rapidly varies the position of the mirror, which changes the distance from the viewer's eye to the cathode ray tube display as it draws information from different depths in the data set.*

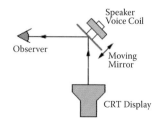

the display of a voxel array), but as emphasized in **Chapter 2**, we are overwhelmingly visual creatures who expect to get information through images.

There is no consensus on the best input and control devices for complex computer graphics displays. Rotating or shifting the viewpoint in response to horizontal or vertical motion of the now-ubiquitous mouse gives a rather crude control. For moving points, lines, and planes in 3-D, some more-flexible device will be required. Simply locating a specific voxel location in the array can be done in several different ways. One is to use an x,y input device (mouse, trackball, etc.) for two axes and periodically shift to a different control, typically a scroll bar on the screen, to adjust the distance along the third axis. Another is to move two cursors, one on an x–y projection and one on an x–z projection, for example. Such approaches usually feel rather clumsy because of the need to move back and forth between two areas of the screen and two modalities of interaction. Appropriate color coding of the cursor to report depth can help. Three-axis joysticks and sonic digitizers that allow the user to point in space (multiple sensors triangulate the position) exist, but these are hardly standard.

Immersive virtual reality (VR) was first suggested by Sutherland (1965). Practical working systems have now been used for more than a decade and have been written about extensively (Rheingold 1991). One approach to VR is that of the head-mounted display (HMD) coupled with head tracking. The user is presented with a stereo binocular view of the virtual world. By tracking the orientation of the viewer's head, the content and perspective of the virtual images are drawn consistent with what one would experience in the physical worlds. More elaborate "cave"-based VR systems cover some or all of the walls of a room with rear-projection stereo displays. The user wears glasses to permit viewing the stereo images, and there is a head-tracking mechanism to control what is projected (i.e., the view), depending on where the viewer moves and looks.

In addition, for either system, there is usually some mechanism for interacting with what is seen, such as a "dataglove" (Zimmerman et al. 1987) or some other high-degree-of-freedom input to support manipulation of the displayed virtual world. The dataglove has been used, for example, to move molecules around each other to study enzyme action. Supplemented by force feedback, this method gives the researcher rich information about the ways that molecules can best fit together. VR, while expensive and still relatively new, is a powerful technology. It is being applied in a range of contexts ranging from entertainment to automotive design. Few of these systems can accommodate more than a single viewer at a time; there is still a long way to go before the *Star Trek* "holodeck" arrives.

At the other extreme, it is important to remember the history of 3-D visualization (Cookson 1994), which began with physical models constructed of wood, plastic, or plaster. Building such a model from a series of section planes was very difficult and time consuming, and still could not reveal all of the internal detail. Computer modeling has progressed from simple outlines to hidden line removal, surface construction, shading and rendering, and full volumetric or ray-traced methods. Clearly there are rich future possibilities.

Ray tracing

The previous example of volumetric display performed a simplified ray tracing to sum the density values of voxels and calculate a brightness based on light being absorbed as it propagated from back to front through the 3-D data set. While this model does correspond to some imaging situations such as the transmission light or electron microscope and tomography, there are many other situations in which different rules are appropriate.

In the process of traversing a voxel array while following a particular line of sight that will end in one pixel of a ray-traced image, the available variables include:

1. The brightness and perhaps color of the original light source placed behind the array, and whether it is an extended source (producing parallel rays of light) or a point source (producing a cone beam of light). This illumination source will control the contribution that transmission makes to the final image.
2. The location of the first or last voxels with a density above some arbitrary threshold taken to represent transparency. These voxels will define surfaces that can be rendered using reflected light. Additional rules for surface reflectivity as well as the location, brightness, and color of the light sources, and so forth, must be added.
3. The location of the maximum or minimum values or large gradients, which can define the location of some internal surface for rendering.
4. The rule for combining voxel values along a path. This can be multiplication of fractional values, which models simple absorption according to Beer's law for photons, provided that the voxel values are linear absorption values. In some cases, density is proportional to attenuation, so this rule can produce interpretable images. There are other convolution rules available as well, including linear summation and retention of maximum or minimum values. While these may also correspond to some physical situations, their greatest value is that they produce images that can delineate internal structure.
5. The relationship between the voxel values and the intensity (and perhaps color) of light originating in each voxel, which represents fluorescence or other emission processes.

The combining rules mentioned briefly in no. 4 of the above list correspond to the various image processing tools described in **Chapter 4** and **Chapter 5** for combining pixels from two or more images. They include arithmetic (multiplication, addition), rank ordering (minimum or maximum value), and Boolean logic. It is also possible to include lateral scattering, so that point sources of light spread or blur as they pass through the voxel array, or even to combine several modes. This approach to realism through computation is rarely justified, since the measured voxel values are not generally physically related to light transmission or scattering.

A software package for 3-D visualization can make any or all of these parameters accessible to the user, along with others. For example, control of the surface reflectivity and roughness, and the location of the incident light source(s), affects the appearance of rendered surfaces. In performing a convolution of transmitted light along ray paths from a light source behind the voxel array, the relationship between the voxel values and the absorption of the light is another parameter that offers control. By varying the relationship between voxel value and opacity (linear attenuation coefficient), or selectively introducing color, it is possible to make some structures appear or to remove them, allowing others to be seen.

Figure 13.41 shows an example of this presentation. The data set is the same MRI head-scan data used in **Figure 13.12**; the voxel values come from the MRI measurement technique and approximately correspond to the amount of water present. There is not enough information to fully describe the structures actually present in a human head, so there is no "correct" relationship between voxel value and light absorption for the volumetric rendering. Using different, arbitrary curves, it is possible to selectively view the outer skin, bone structure, or brain.

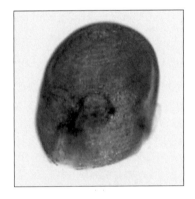

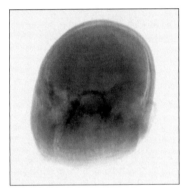

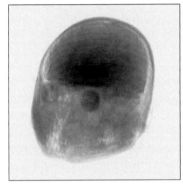

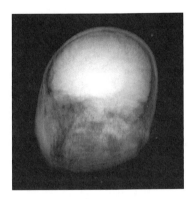

Figure 13.41 Volumetric imaging of the MRI head-scan data from Figure 13.12. Varying the relationship between voxel values and the opacity used to absorb light transmitted along each ray through the structure allows selection of which structures are revealed.

Using color permits even more distinctions to be made. **Figure 13.42** shows images of a hog heart reconstructed using different relationships for opacity vs. voxel value that emphasize the heart muscle or the blood vessels. In this example, each voxel is assumed both to absorb the light from the source placed behind the voxel array and to contribute its own light along the ray in proportion to its value, with color taken from an arbitrary table. The result allows structures with different measured values to appear in different colors.

Of course, with only a single value for each voxel, it is not possible to model absorption and emission separately. Such techniques become possible by performing dual-energy tomography, in which the average atomic number and average density are both determined; by performing multienergy tomography, in which the concentration of various elements in each voxel is measured; or by using the T1-, T2-relaxation time signals from MRI. These techniques represent

Figure 13.42 Volumetric rendering of MRI data for a hog heart specimen. Changing the arbitrary relationship between voxel value and display opacity for the voxels allows selectively showing the heart muscle or blood vessels. (Data courtesy of B. Knosp, R. Frank, M. Marcus, and R. Weiss, University of Iowa, Image Analysis Facility and Dept. of Internal Medicine.)

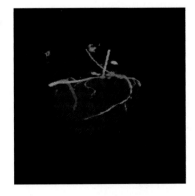

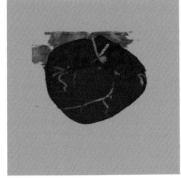

straightforward implementation of several of the multiband and color-imaging methods discussed in earlier chapters, but they are not yet common, as neither the imaging instrumentation nor the computer routines are yet widely available. It is consequently usually necessary to adopt some arbitrary relationship between the single measured set of voxel values and the displayed rendering that corresponds to the major voxel property measured by the original imaging process.

For example, in fluorescence light microscopy, or X-ray images from the SEM, or ion microscopy, the voxel value is a measure of emitted brightness that is approximately proportional to elemental or chemical concentration. These 3-D data sets can also be shown volumetrically by a simplified ray tracing. Instead of absorbing light from an external light source, the rule is to sum the voxel values as brightnesses along each path.

Figure 13.36 showed an application using the fluorescence confocal light microscope. A dye was injected into the blood vessel of a hamster, which was excited by the incident light from the microscope. The emitted light was collected to form a series of 2-D images at different focal depths, and these were then arranged in a stack to produce a 3-D data set. In this case, the spacing between the planes is much greater than the resolution within each image plane. Sliding the image stack laterally, as discussed previously, produces an approximation of rotation and an impression of depth. The brightness values for each voxel are then summed along vertical columns to produce each image.

This emission model is very easy to calculate, but it does not account for any possible absorption of the emitted light intensity by other voxels along the ray path. Generally, simple 3-D data sets have only one piece of data per voxel, and there is no separate information on density and emission brightness, so it is not possible to make corrections. Sometimes a simple reduction in intensity in proportion to the total number of voxels traversed (known as a "distance fade") can be used to approximate this absorption effect. However, it is usually assumed that the emission intensity is sufficiently high and that the structure is sufficiently transparent. Under these assumptions, no correction would be needed, since it would not change the interpretation of the structure, which is in any case qualitative rather than quantitative.

When multiband data are available, as for instance in the SIMS data set used in **Figure 13.26** and **Figure 13.27**, emission rules can be used with the assignment of different colors (up to three) to different signals. **Figure 13.43** and **Figure 13.44** show a volumetric view of these data using emission rules, presented as a stereo pair. The monochrome figure shows a single element (boron), while multiple elements are combined in the color image. The use of color in the images forces the use of two side-by-side images for viewing, and the density of information in the images that results from overlaying the 8-bit (256 gray level) values from each element at every point makes it quite difficult to fuse these images for satisfactory stereo viewing.

Using the same data set, it is possible to use the location of the frontmost voxel along each line of sight (whose value is above an arbitrary threshold) to define the location of an internal

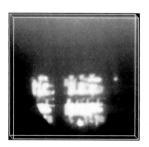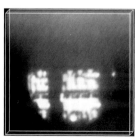

Figure 13.43 Stereo-pair display of emission-rule volumetric images of boron concentration in a silicon wafer, imaged by a SIMS (see Figure 13.26).

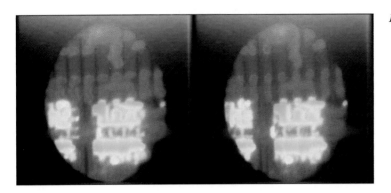

Figure 13.44 *Stereo pair of volumetric images from the SIMS data set. Colors assigned to the different elements are red = aluminum, green = boron, and blue = oxygen, with 256 brightness levels of each. The use of color for elemental information precludes color coding of views for stereo viewing. The density of information in this display is so great that fusing the images to see the depth is quite difficult.*

boundary. If this resulting surface is then rendered as a solid surface with incident reflected light, another representation of the data is obtained, as shown in **Figure 13.45**.

There are several different ways that an internal surface can be displayed. **Figure 13.46** shows several views of the spiral cochlear structure from the ear of a bat (Keating 1993). Slices through the 3-D voxel array do not show that the structure is connected. Thresholding to show all of the voxels within the structure reveals the topology of the spiral. A series of section images can be shown as either wire-frame outlines or as an image with a rendered surface. The outlines are more convenient for rotating to view the structure from different directions.

When color coding of structures, volumetric rendering, and selective transparency are combined with the display of internal surfaces (with shading as discussed below), the results can be quite striking. **Figure 13.47** shows an example, the brain of a fruit fly (*Drosophila melanogaster*), using data recorded with a confocal laser scanning microscope. The 3-D reconstruction shows surfaces rendered as partially transparent in a transparent medium, which reveals the surfaces of other structures behind them. While effective at communicating specific information to the viewer, these displays require prior decisions and selection, and thus are not so useful for exploring unknown data sets, as noted previously.

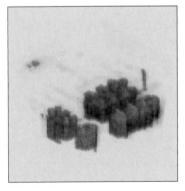

Figure 13.45 *Surface-rendered display of the same data as in* *Figure 13.43.* *The internal surface of the boron-rich region is determined by thresholding and then rendered using an arbitrarily placed light source.*

Reflection

Reflection from surfaces is an important imaging modality. The conventional CSLM, seismic reflection mapping, acoustic microscopy, ultrasound imaging, and so forth, acquire a 3-D image set whose voxel values record the reflection of the signal from internal locations. **Figure 13.48** shows the use of ultrasound to show the surface of a fetus *in utero*. In most of these technologies, a voxel array is generated and used to locate boundaries where strong reflections occur within a matrix that might otherwise be opaque. In the CSLM the matrix is transparent (either air or liquid), and the strongest reflection at each x,y point is where the specimen surface is in focus. This means that recording a set of images as a 3-D data array makes it possible to locate the surface in three dimensions. Most systems use the processing methods discussed in **Chapter 5** to find the brightest value at each pixel and thus construct the surface range image.

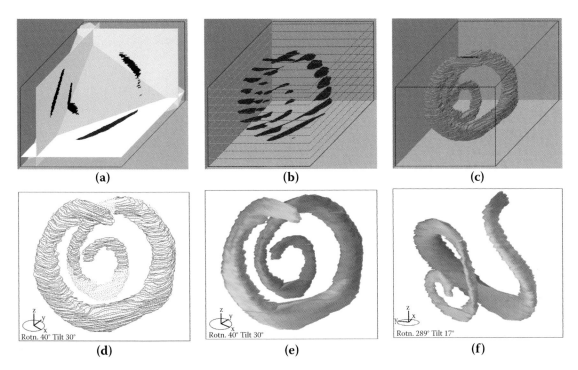

(a)   (b)   (c)

Rotn. 40° Tilt 30°

Rotn. 40° Tilt 30°

Rotn. 289° Tilt 17°

(d)   (e)   (f)

Figure 13.46 Cochlear structure from the ear of a bat: (a) arbitrary planar slices through the voxel array; (b) array of parallel slices through the array; (c) surface revealed by thresholding the voxels; (d) outlines delineating the structure in all voxel planes; (e) surface reconstructed from the outlines in image d; (f) the same structure as shown in image e, rotated to a different point of view. (Courtesy of A. Keating, Duke University, Durham, NC.)

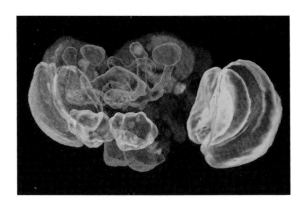

Figure 13.47 Reconstruction of a fruit-fly brain with transparent surfaces. (Data courtesy of K. Rein, University of Wuerzburg, Dept. of Genetics; visualization by M. Zoeckler, ZIB, using the Amira software, www.amiravis. com.)

One way to generate such a display is to go down columns of the data array (just as in volumetric ray tracing) looking for the maximum voxel value, or the first value to exceed some threshold, or a location of maximum change or gradient in value. Keeping only that value or location produces an image of the entire surface in focus, as was shown in **Chapter 5**. Since the same methods for rotating or shifting the data array to alter the viewing direction can be used, it is also possible to find the maxima or surface points along any viewing direction and display the surface as an animation sequence or to construct a stereo pair. In principle, fitting a curve based on the known depth-of-field characteristics of the optics to the brightness values along a vertical column of voxels can locate the surface with subvoxel

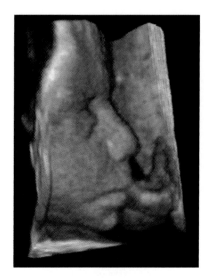

Figure 13.48 The face of a 26-week-old fetus, imaged by ultrasound.

accuracy. **Figure 13.49** shows an alumina fracture surface (from **Chapter 5**, **Figure 5.70**) both as an extended-focus image and as a range image (in which pixel brightness is proportional to elevation). Several presentation modes for range images are available to assist in visualizing the three-dimensional shape of the surface. One, shown in the figure, is simply to plot the brightness profile along any line across the image, which gives the elevation profile directly.

Figure 13.50 shows several of the presentation modes for range images of surfaces (**Chapter 14** goes into more detail). The specimen is a microelectronics chip imaged by reflection CSLM, so both an extended-focus image and a range image can be obtained from the series of focal-plane sections. From the range-image data, plotting contour maps, grid or mesh plots, or rendered displays is a straightforward exercise in computer graphics.

One of the classic ways to show surface elevation is a contour map (**Figure 13.51**), in which isoelevation lines are drawn, usually at uniform increments of altitude. These lines are of course continuous and closed. This is the way topographic maps are drawn, and the same methods are useful at any scale. Since the contour map reduces the pixel data from the original range image to boundary representation, the method for forming the boundaries is the same as discussed in **Chapter 7** for segmentation. The lines can be labeled or color-coded to assist in distinguishing elevations.

Presenting the data as a color-coded shaded isometric view is closely related to a contour map. **Figure 13.52** shows the elevation data for the alumina fracture surface of **Figure 13.49**. In this image, a 3-D representation (without perspective) is used to draw a vertical line for each pixel in the range image to a height proportional to the value. The image is also shaded so that each point has its gray-scale value. Replacing the gray-scale values with a pseudocolor table

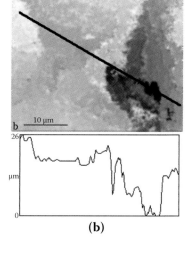

(a)   (b)

Figure 13.49 Depth measurement using the CSLM:

(a) extended-focus image of an alumina fracture surface obtained by keeping the brightest value from many focal planes at each pixel location;

(b) range image obtained by assigning a gray-scale value to each pixel according to the focal-plane image in which the brightest (in focus) reflectance is measured, with the elevation profile along the traverse line shown.

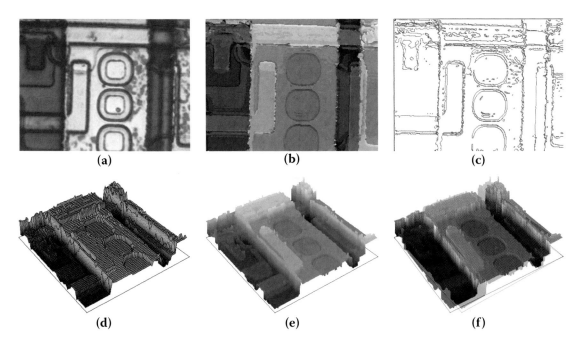

Figure 13.50 *Presentation modes for surface information from the CSLM (specimen is a microelectronics chip):* **(a)** *the in-focus image of the surface reflectance obtained by keeping the brightest value at each pixel address from all of the multiple focal-plane images;* **(b)** *the elevation or range image produced by gray-scale encoding the depth at which the brightest pixel was measured for each pixel address;* **(c)** *contour map of the surface elevation with color coding for the height values;* **(d)** *perspective-corrected rendering of the surface with grid lines and pseudocolor;* **(e)** *the same image as image* **d**, *with realistic shading;* **(f)** *the rendering from image* **e** *from two points of view, combined as a stereo pair.*

Figure 13.51 *Fragment of a conventional topographic map (Phantom Ranch in the Grand Canyon) showing isoelevation contour lines.*

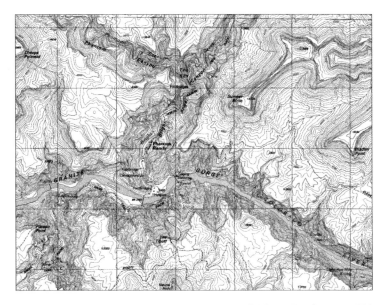

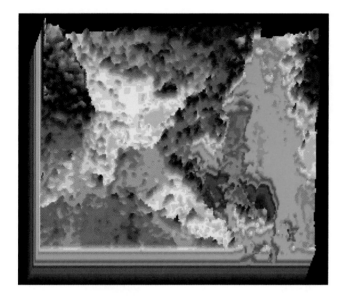

Figure 13.52 Isometric view of elevation data for the alumina fracture surface shown in *Figure 13.49*. A rapidly varying color palette is used to reveal small changes.

allows communication of the elevations in essentially the same way as contour lines, and many topographic maps use similar methods to show elevations.

Constructing a contour map can be either simple or complex. The simplest method merely locates those pixels that have neighbors that are above and below the threshold level. But, as shown in **Figure 13.53**, this produces a coarse approximation. Interpolating between pixel addresses produces a smoother map, as shown in the figure.

Figure 13.54 shows an example that looks broadly similar to the preceding case, but represents data at a very different scale. This is a three-dimensional view of Ishtar Terra on Venus. The data come from the spacecraft *Magellan*'s side-looking mapping radar. This synthetic-aperture radar bounces 12.5-cm-wavelength radar waves off the surface, using the echo time delay for range and the Doppler shift to collect signals from points ahead of and behind the direct line of sight. The two-dimensional images obtained by processing the signals are similar in appearance to aerial photographs.

Rendering of a surface defined by a range image produces a realistic image of surface appearance, as compared with grid or isometric contour map displays that are more abstract and more difficult for visual interpretation, as shown in **Figure 13.55**. The quantitative interpretation of the surface data is also more readily accessible in the range image. However, it is difficult to select realistic surface colors and textures to be applied. It is possible to apply brightness values to an isometric display of range data that come from another image of the same area, such as the original reflectivity or texture information. When multiband images are recorded, this combination is particularly effective.

The surfaces discussed in the preceding section are external physical surfaces of the specimen. Internal surfaces can be defined as boundaries between distinct regions, but there are other, more subtle definitions. For instance, **Figure 13.56** shows the data from the SIMS example used previously in this chapter, in which the depth of the voxel having the maximum concentration of silicon at any location is shown. This surface isolation provides a visualization of the shape of the implanted region. The image is shown as a shaded isometric display, as discussed previously.

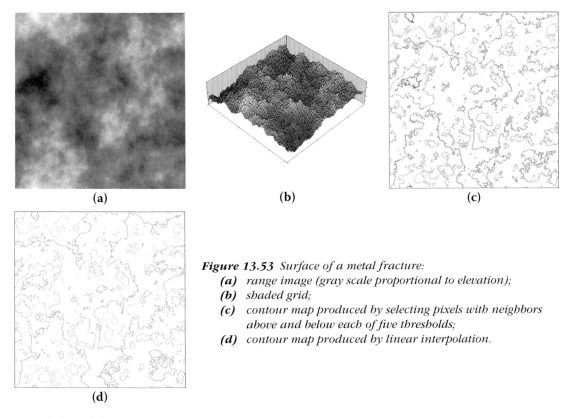

(a)   **(b)**   **(c)**

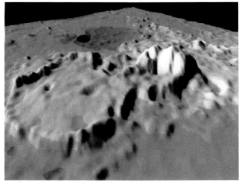

(d)

Figure 13.53 Surface of a metal fracture:
- **(a)** range image (gray scale proportional to elevation);
- **(b)** shaded grid;
- **(c)** contour map produced by selecting pixels with neighbors above and below each of five thresholds;
- **(d)** contour map produced by linear interpolation.

Figure 13.54 Reconstructed surface image of Ishtar Terra on Venus, looking northeast across Lakshmi Panum toward Maxwell Montes with an exaggerated vertical scale. (From Saunders, S., Eng. Sci. *Spring*, 15, 1991. With permission.)

Surfaces

Surfaces to be examined can be either physical surfaces revealed directly by reflection of light, electrons, or sound waves, or they can be surfaces internal to the sample and revealed only indirectly after the entire 3-D data set has been acquired. The use of computer graphics to display them is closely related to other graphics display modes used in computer-assisted design (CAD), for example. However, the typical CAD object has only a few numbers to describe it, such as the coordinates of vertices. Generating the interpolated surfaces and calculating the local orientation, and hence the brightness of the image at many points, requires a significant amount of computing.

In contrast, the image data discussed typically comprise a complete 3-D data set, or at least a complete 2-D range image derived from the 3-D set. Consequently, there is elevation data

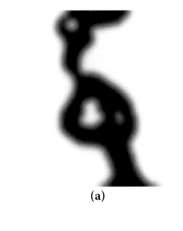

(a)

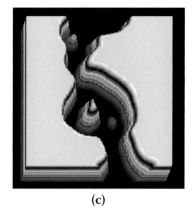

(c)

Figure 13.55 *Display modes for surface information:*
(a) range image;
(b) grid mesh;
(c) isometric view;
(d) rendered terrain.

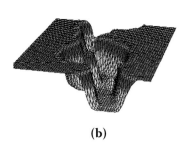

(b)

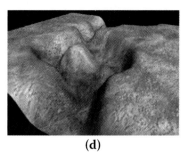

(d)

at every pixel location in the display image, which allows for an extremely rapid image generation. Rendering the surface images shown here is essentially instantaneous on a desktop computer. Doing the same for a typical CAD object would take longer or require dedicated processing in the display hardware.

Some instruments produce range images directly. Large-scale examples include radar mapping, elevation measurement from stereo-pair calculations, and sonar depth ranging. At a finer scale, a standard tool for measuring precision machined surfaces is interferometry, which produces images such as those shown in **Figure 13.57**. The brightness is a direct measure of elevation, and the image can be comprehended more easily with appropriate rendering. Notice that the lens artifact (the faint ring structure at the left side of the image) is not true elevation data and, when presented as such, looks quite strange.

Figure 13.56 *Isometric display of elevation data within a volume: the height of the surface having the maximum concentration on Si in the SIMS voxel array.*

Displays of surface images (more formally of range images, since real surfaces can be complex and multivalued, but range images are well behaved and single valued) can use any of the techniques described above. These include wire-mesh or line-profile displays, contour maps, and shaded isometric displays, all described in more detail in **Chapter 14**. These all involve a certain level of abstraction.

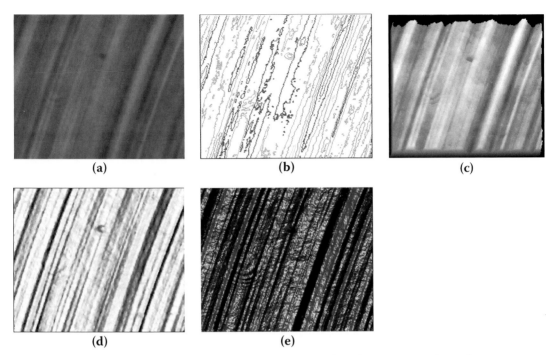

(a) (b) (c)

(d) (e)

Figure 13.57 *Presentation modes for the surface elevation data from an optical interferometer (specimen is a machined surface of nickel): **(a)** original image, in which the gray-scale brightness encodes height; **(b)** a contour map with gray-scale shading to indicate the height of lines; **(c)** isometric view with superimposed gray-scale values from image **a**; **(d)** the surface data rendered as it would appear with a diffuse material; **(e)** the surface data rendered as it would appear with a specular material.*

A simple set of line profiles gives an impression of surface elevation and requires no computation, although the need to space the lines apart loses some detail. Consequently, it is sometimes used as a direct display mode on instruments such as the SEM or STM (scanning tunneling microscope). Unfortunately, the signal that is displayed in this way may not actually be the elevation, and in this case the SEM pseudotopographic display can be quite misleading. Adding grid or mesh lines in both directions requires additional computation, but also increases the effective spacing and decreases the lateral resolution of the display.

Generating an image of a surface that approximates the appearance of a real, physical surface is known generically as rendering and requires more computational effort. The physical rules that govern the way real surfaces look are simple and are summarized in **Figure 13.58**. The important variables are the intensity and location of the light source and the location of the viewer. Both are usually given in terms of the angles between the normal vector of the surface and the vectors to the source and viewer. The absolute reflectivity of the surface (or albedo) must be known; if this varies with wavelength, we say that the surface is colored because some colors will be reflected more than others.

Finally, the local roughness of the surface controls the degree of variation in the angle of reflection. A very narrow angle for this spread corresponds to a smooth surface that reflects specularly. A broader angle corresponds to a more diffuse reflection. One of the very common tricks in graphic arts, routinely seen in television advertising, is the addition of bright specular reflections to objects to make them appear metallic and hopefully more interesting.

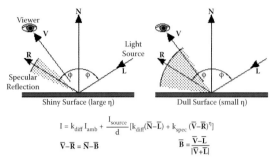

$$I = k_{diff} I_{amb} + \frac{I_{source}}{d} [k_{diff}(\overline{N}-\overline{L}) + k_{spec}(\overline{V}-\overline{R})^{\eta}]$$

$$\overline{V}-\overline{R} = \overline{N}-\overline{B} \qquad \overline{B} = \frac{\overline{V}-\overline{L}}{|\overline{V}+\overline{L}|}$$

Figure 13.58 Lambertian rules for light scattering from surfaces with different specularity. The vectors are N (surface normal), L (light source), R (reflection), and V (viewing direction). The k factors are the diffuse and specular reflection coefficients. The I values are the intensities of the principal and ambient light sources, and h is a constant describing the breadth of the specular reflection, which depends on the fine-scale surface roughness.

For a typical surface defined by a few points, as in CAD drawings, the surface is broken into facets, often triangular, and the orientation of each facet is calculated with respect to the viewer and light source. The reflected light intensity is then calculated, and the result plotted on the display screen or other output device to build the image. This would seem to be a rather fast process with only a small number of facets, but the problem is that such images do not look natural. The large flat facets and the abrupt angles between them do not correspond to the continuous surfaces we encounter in most real objects.

Shading the brightness values between facets (Gouraud shading) can eliminate these abrupt edges and improve the appearance of the image, but this requires interpolation. Better smoothing can be achieved (particularly when there are specular reflections present) by interpolating the angles between the centers of the facets rather than simply the mean brightness values. The interpolated angles are used to generate local brightness values, which vary nonlinearly with angle and hence position. This Phong shading is even more computer-intensive.

For continuous pixel images, each set of three pixels can be considered to define a triangular facet, as shown schematically in **Figure 13.59**. The difference in value (elevation) of the neighboring pixels gives the angles of the local surface normal directly. A precalculated lookup table (LUT) of the image brightness values for a given light-source location and surface characteristics completes the solution with minimum calculations. Since this is done at the pixel or voxel level in the display, no interpolation of shading is needed.

When the surface rendering is accomplished in this way using section planes that are relatively widely spaced, it often produces artifacts in the reconstruction that appear to be grooves parallel to the section direction (**Figure 13.60**). The use of relatively large voxels can produce rendered results that have an artificial blocky appearance (**Figure 13.61**). Applying image processing operations beforehand to range-image data is often used to improve the resulting surface image. Smoothing with kernels that calculate a weighted average can produce Gouraud shading. Applying a median filter removes noise that would show up as local spikes or holes in the surface. The names of filters such as the rolling-ball operator discussed in **Chapter 4** come directly from their use on range images. This particular operator tests the difference between the minimum value in two neighborhood regions of different sizes and eliminates points that are

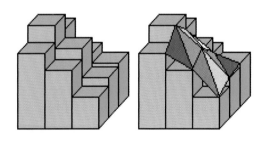

Figure 13.59 Diagram showing the construction of a triangular tessellation on a surface formed by discrete height values for an array of pixels.

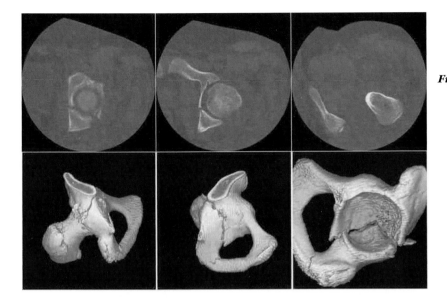

Figure 13.60 *Rendered surface of a fractured pelvis created from sequential tomographic section images. Note the appearance of grooves and other surface artifacts due to the section-plane spacing.*

too low. The analogy is that depressions that a ball of defined radius cannot touch as it rolls across the surface are filled in.

Surface rendering of structures isolated within a voxel array can be enhanced by adding stereo views (**Figure 13.62**) and shadows (**Figure 13.63**). Rendered surface images have the appearance of real physical objects and so communicate easily to the viewer. However, they obscure much of the information present in the original 3-D image data set from which they have been extracted. More complex displays, which require real ray tracing, can make surfaces that are partially reflecting and partially transmitting, so that the surface can be combined with volumetric information in the display. This presentation has somewhat the appearance of embedding the solid surface in a partially transparent medium, like fruit in JELL-O®. Such displays can be dramatic in appearance and useful for communicating complex three-dimensional information, but they are too slow to generate and have too many variable parameters to be used for most interactive explorations of complex data sets.

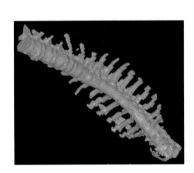

Figure 13.61 *Rendered surface of a spine in which the coarse voxel size produces a blocky appearance.*

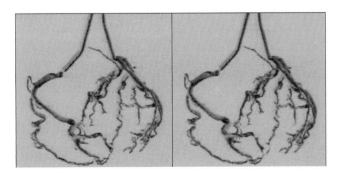

Figure 13.62 *CT slices of arteries in a human heart, combined and surface rendered, shown as a stereo pair. (Courtesy of General Electric Co.)*

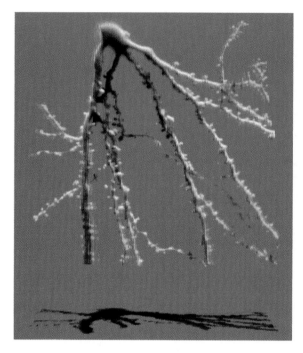

Figure 13.63 Stereo view of rendered dendrites, with shadows.

Because surface images are what human vision encounters in everyday life, they are easily interpreted. This makes the use of surface rendering very useful for presenting volumetric data. Surfaces are defined as a location where some voxel property changes significantly, very much the same criterion that was used in **Chapter 7** for contouring 2-D images. Many systems that acquire 3-D data now have sufficient computational power to generate rendered surface images in real time. Ultrasound scans, like the one in **Figure 13.48**, are very well accepted and used in routine practice despite the noise inherent in the technique.

Multi-ply connected surfaces

Rendering techniques are most needed for complex, multi-ply connected surfaces, since the topology of such structures cannot be studied in 2-D images. Rendering these more complex surfaces is also possible, but takes a little longer. **Figure 13.64** shows a series of 2-D planes in a 3-D data set from an ion microscope. The sample, a two-phase metal alloy, shows many regions in each image. It is only in the full 3-D data set that the connection between all of the regions is evident. In fact, each of the two phase regions in this specimen is a single, continuous network intimately intertwined with the other. This cannot be seen by using resectioning in various directions (**Figure 13.65**).

Volumetric displays of this data set can show some of the intricacy, especially when the live animation can be viewed as the rotation is carried out. **Figure 13.66** shows a few orientations of the data set using ray tracing to produce a volumetric display; viewed rapidly in sequence, these produce the visual effect of rotation. However, the complexity of this structure and the precedence in which features lie in front and in back of others limits the usefulness of this approach. Isolating the boundary between the two phases allows a rendered surface to be constructed, as shown in **Figure 13.67**. With the faceting shown, this display can be drawn quickly enough to support interactive viewing as an analysis tool. A complete smoothed rendering (**Figure 13.68**) takes somewhat longer.

When cubic voxel images are obtained from 3-D tomography, rendering of internal surfaces produces a high-quality result, as shown in **Figure 13.69**. In this case, the pore structure in the sandstone has been rendered as a solid, while the matrix has been made transparent. Such reversals of contrast can be extremely useful for visualizing complex structures.

The rendering of a surface follows the determination of the various surface facets. The simplest kind of facet is a triangle. In the example shown in **Figure 13.67**, a series of narrow rectangles or trapezoids are used to connect points along each section outline. For features in which the sections are similar in shape and size, this faceting is fairly straightforward. When the shapes

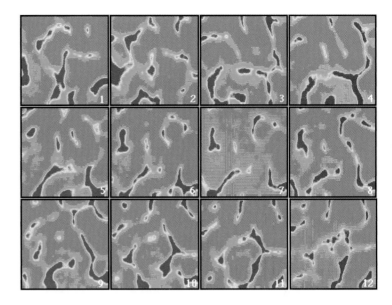

Figure 13.64 *Sequential images from an ion microscope, showing two-phase structure in an Fe-45% Cr alloy aged 192 h at 540°C. (Courtesy of M. K. Miller, Oak Ridge National Laboratories, Oak Ridge, TN.)*

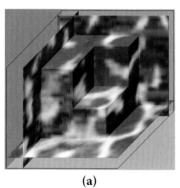

(a)

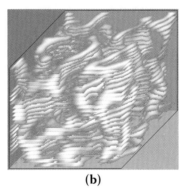

(b)

Figure 13.65 *Section views of the 3-D voxel array formed from the images in* **Figure 13.64***:*

(a) *stored brightness values along several arbitrary orthogonal planes;*

(b) *stored values on a series of parallel planes, with dark voxels made transparent.*

Figure 13.66 *Volumetric displays using ray tracing and absorption rules as the planes from* **Figure 13.64b** *are shifted to produce the effect of rotation. Viewing these images in rapid succession produces a movie that shows the 3-D structure.*

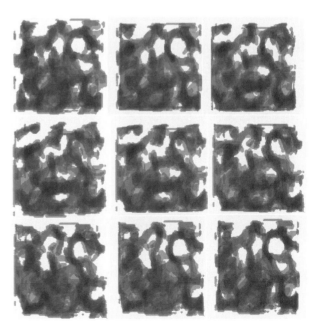

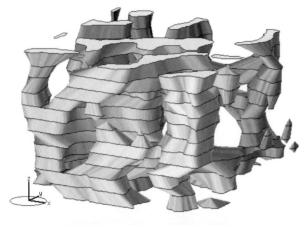

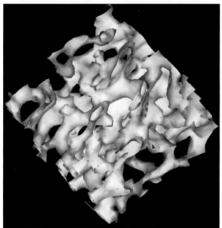
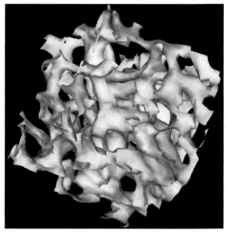

Figure 13.67 Simple rendering of the boundary surface between the two phases in the specimen from *Figure 13.64* by interpolating planar facets between the planes.

Figure 13.68 Two high-resolution rendered views of the boundary surface between the two phases in the specimen from *Figure 13.64*.

change considerably from section to section, the resulting facets offer a less realistic view of the surface shape.

The greatest difficulty is dealing with splits and merges in the structure. This means that the number of outlines in one section is greater than in the next, and so the surface must somehow divide. **Figure 13.70** shows two ways to do this. In one, the junction lies in one of the planes. It can either be located manually or by various algorithms, such as dividing the feature normal to its moment axis at a point that gives area ratios equal to those of the two features in the next section. The rendered result is fairly easy to draw, since no surface facets intersect.

The second method constructs surface facets from sets of points along the feature boundaries from the single feature in one section to both of the features in the next section plane. This technique moves the junction into the space between planes and produces a fairly realistic picture, but it requires more calculation. The intersecting planes must be drawn with a *z*-buffer, a computer graphics technique that records the depth (in the viewing direction) of each image point and only draws points on one surface where they lie in front of the other.

The major drawback to this kind of surface rendering from serial-section outlines is that the surfaces hide what is behind them, and even with rotation it may not be possible to see all parts of a complex structure. Combining surface rendering with transparency (so that selective features are shown as opaque and others as partially or fully transparent, thus letting other structures behind become visible) offers a partial solution. **Figure 13.71a** shows an example in which one kind of feature (the white spheres) has been made opaque, the matrix is entirely transparent, and the remainder of the structure is volumetrically rendered with transparency. The example in **Figure 13.71b** shows internal surfaces in a microelectronics device, rendered with the matrix entirely transparent to show the geometry of the embedded structure. The combination of colors to identify particular structures, selective transparency, and surface rendering produces very effective visualization, especially when combined with the ability to rotate the data set.

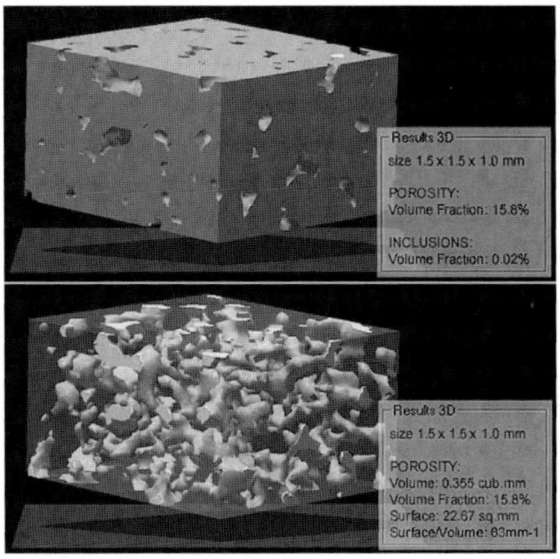

In the example shown in **Figure 13.67**, the boundary was determined by thresholding in each of the 2-D image planes, since the plane spacing was not the same as the in-plane resolution. A certain amount of interpolation between the planes is required, which makes the curvature and roughness of surfaces different in the depth or z direction. For data sets with true cubic voxels, as for example those in **Chapter 12**, the resolution is the same in all directions, and greater fidelity can be achieved in the surface rendering.

Figure 13.69 Rendered surface image from micro-CT data set. The porosity in the sandstone has been rendered as a solid object and the solid matrix made transparent to show the connectivity and complexity of the pore structure. (Courtesy of Skyscan, Aartselaar, Belgium.)

Multiple colors are useful to distinguish the many features that can be present in a complex structure. **Figure 13.72** shows the approximately 200 roughly spherical particles from the data in **Figure 13.23** individually color labeled. This use of pseudocolor can be particularly important to identify the continuity of multi-ply connected surfaces.

Serial-section reconstruction for 3-D displays is certainly not restricted to microscopy and medical applications. The study of woven textiles and fibers used in composite materials uses the same methods (Gowayed and Russ 1991). **Figure 13.73** uses color coding to identify the muscles and bones in a common everyday example of serial sectioning. The images were acquired by visiting the local supermarket and photographing each roast sliced from a side

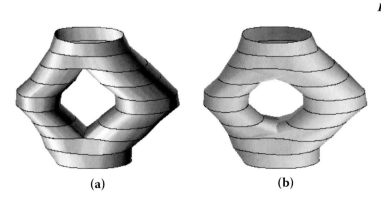

(a)   (b)

Figure 13.70 Two ways to render a surface from serial-section outlines where splits or merges occur:
- *(a) dividing one plane into arbitrary regions that correspond to each branch;*
- *(b) continuous surfaces from each branch to the entire next outline, forming an intersection between the planes.*

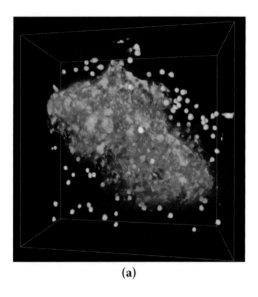

(a)

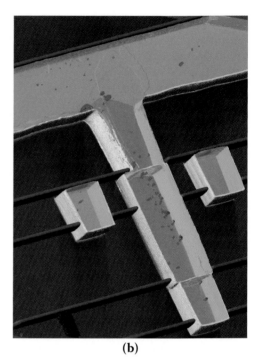

(b)

Figure 13.71 *Combining surface rendering with full or partial transparency to show internal structures, as described in the text:* **(a)** *white gold marker particles and a high-density region in hydrogen storage medium, imaged by TEM tomography;* **(b)** *green-shaded copper interconnect lines containing red voids, with blue etch-stop layers, imaged by high-angle annular dark-field scanning transmission electron microscope (STEM) tomography. (From Kubel, C.,* Microsc. Microanal. *11: 378, 2005. With permission.)*

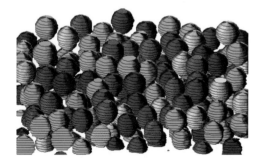

Figure 13.72 *Rendered surface image of spherical particles from reconstruction created by interpolating surface tiles between the slices shown in* **Figure 13.23** *and then assigning arbitrary colors to each feature.*

of beef. After aligning the images and thresholding them to delineate the various structures, the stack of slices can be rendered to reveal the three-dimensional structure of the muscles and bones. However, the volume, surface area, and length of these structures can be determined much more efficiently by using stereological procedures to draw grids and count points on the individual slices, as discussed in **Chapter 9**.

Image processing in 3-D

The emphasis so far has been on the display of 3-D image data, with little mention of processing. Most of the same processing tools that were described in the preceding chapters for 2-D images can be applied more or less directly to 3-D images for the same purposes (Nikolaidis and Pitas 2001). Arithmetic operations such as ratios in multiband data are used, for instance, in exactly the same way.

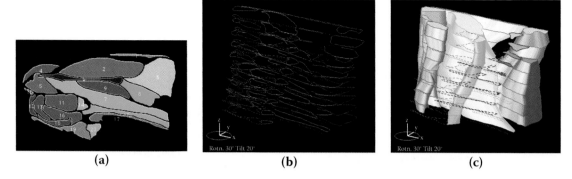

(a)   **(b)**   **(c)**

Figure 13.73 *Serial sections through a side of beef: **(a)** one section with features numbered; **(b)** stack of slices; **(c)** rendered result, showing selected muscles with solid surfaces and several bones with dashed outlines.*

Each voxel value is combined with the value of the voxel at the same location in the second image. This kind of operation does not depend on the images having cubic voxels.

However, many processing operations that use neighborhoods, e.g., for kernel multiplication, template matching, rank operations, and so forth, do expect cubic voxel arrays. In a few instances, a kernel can be adapted to noncubic voxels by adjusting the weight values so that the different distance to the neighbors in the z direction is taken into account. This adjustment only works when the difference in z distance is small as compared with the x,y directions, for instance a factor of 2 or 3 as can be achieved in the confocal light microscope. It will not work well if the image planes are separated by ten (or more) times the magnitude of the in-plane resolution. And any departure from cubic voxel shape causes serious problems for ranking or template-matching operations.

In these cases, it is more common to perform the processing on the individual planes and then form a new 3-D image set from the results. **Figure 13.74** shows a series of pseudorotation views of the MRI head images used previously. Each slice image has been processed using a Frei and Chen operator (see **Chapter 5**) to extract edges. These edges show the internal structure as well as the surface wrinkles in the brain. Image processing was also used to form a mask to delineate the brain (defined as the central bright feature in each slice) and isolate it from other portions of the image. The result is a series of slice images that show only the brain, processed to show the internal edges.

Another display trick has been used here. It is not clear just what volumetric display mode is appropriate for such processed images. Instead of the conventional absorption mode, in which transmitted light is passed through the data array, these images use the emission mode, in which each voxel emits light in proportion to its value. That value is the "edgeness" of the voxel as defined by the Frei and Chen operator. In other words, we see the edges glowing in space. In a live animation, or for those readers who can use pairs of the images to view the 3-D data set stereoscopically, this image creates a fairly strong impression of the 3-D structure of the brain. The same type of display of lines in space can be used to display contours within a 3-D data set.

This illustration can serve as an indication of the flexibility with which display rules for 3-D images can be bent. Nontraditional display modes, particularly for processed images, are often quite effective for showing structural relationships. There are no guidelines here, except for

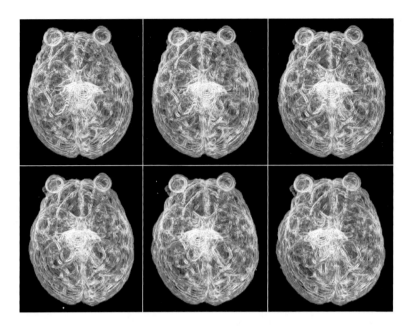

Figure 13.74 *Several views of the brain from the MRI data set in* **Figure 13.12**. *The skull has been eliminated, individual image planes have been processed with an edge operator, and the resulting values have been used with emission rules to create a volumetric display. Lateral shifting of the planes produces pseudorotation. Each pair of images can be viewed in stereo, or the entire sequence used as an animation. Structures are visible from the folds in the top of the brain to the spinal column at the bottom.*

the need to simplify the image by eliminating extraneous detail to reveal the structure that is important. An experimental approach is encouraged.

The use of two-dimensional processing of image planes in a 3-D data set should be used with some care. It is only justified if the planes have no preferred orientation and are random with respect to the structure, or conversely if the planes have a very definite but known orientation that matches that of the structure. The latter condition applies to some situations involving coatings. When possible, 3-D processing is preferred, even though it imposes a rather significant computing load. The size of neighborhoods increases as the cube of dimension. A kernel of modest size, say 7×7, may be fast enough for practical use in 2-D, requiring 49 multiplications and additions for every pixel. In 3-D, the same $7 \times 7 \times 7$ kernel requires 343 multiplications and additions per voxel, and of course the number of total voxels has also increased dramatically so that processing takes much more time.

For complex neighborhood operations such as gradient or edge finding in which more than one kernel is used, the problem is increased further because the number of kernels must increase to deal with the higher dimensionality of the data. For instance, the 3-D version of the Sobel gradient operator would use the square root of the sum of squares of derivatives in three directions. And since it takes two angles to define a direction in three dimensions, an image of gradient orientation would require two arrays, and it is not clear how it would be used or displayed.

The Frei and Chen operator (Frei and Chen 1977), a very useful edge detector in 2-D images introduced in **Chapter 5**, can be extended to three dimensions by adding to the size and number of the basis functions. For instance, the first basis function (which measures the gradient in one direction and corresponds to the presence of a boundary) in a 2-D image is

$$
\begin{array}{ccc}
-1 & 0 & +1 \\
-\sqrt{2} & 0 & +\sqrt{2} \\
-1 & 0 & +1
\end{array}
$$

In three dimensions this becomes

$$
\begin{array}{ccccccccc}
-\sqrt{3}/3 & -\sqrt{2}/2 & -\sqrt{3}/3 & & & & & & \\
-\sqrt{2}/2 & -1 & -\sqrt{2}/2 & 0 & 0 & 0 & & & \\
-\sqrt{3}/3 & -\sqrt{2}/2 & -\sqrt{3}/3 & 0 & 0 & 0 & +\sqrt{3}/3 & +\sqrt{2}/2 & +\sqrt{3}/3 \\
& & & 0 & 0 & 0 & +\sqrt{2}/2 & +1 & +\sqrt{2}/2 \\
& & & & & & +\sqrt{3}/3 & +\sqrt{2}/2 & +\sqrt{3}/3
\end{array}
$$

Similar extensions are made for the other kernels from two dimensions to three dimensions. In three dimensions, it is also possible to construct a set of basis functions to search for lines as well as surfaces. It remains to find good ways to display the boundaries that these operators find.

Three-dimensional processing can be used in many ways to enhance the visibility of structures. In **Figure 13.43**, the boron concentration was shown volumetrically using emission rules. However, the overlap between front and rear portions of the structure makes it difficult to see all of the details. The surface rendering in **Figure 13.45** also suffers in this regard. **Figure 13.75** shows the same structures after 3-D processing. Each voxel in the new image has a value that is proportional to the variance of voxels in a $3 \times 3 \times 3$ neighborhood in the original image set. These values are displayed volumetrically as a transmission image. In other words, the absorption of light coming through the 3-D array is a measure of the presence of edges; uniform regions appear transparent. The visibility of internal surfaces in this "cellophane" display is much better than in the original, and the surfaces do not obscure information behind them, as they would with rendering.

The time requirements for neighborhood operations are much worse for ranking operations. The time required to rank a list of values in order increases not in proportion to the number of entries, as in the kernel multiplication case, but as $N \cdot \log (N)$. This assumes a maximally efficient sorting algorithm and means that ranking operations in really large neighborhoods take quite a long time.

For template-matching operations such as those used in implementing erosion, dilation, skeletonization, and so forth, the situation is worse still. The very efficient methods possible in 2-D by using a lookup or fate table based on the pattern of neighbors will no longer work. In 2-D, there are eight neighbors, so a table with $2^8 = 256$ entries can cover all possibilities. In 3-D there are 26 adjacent neighbors and $2^{26} = 67$ million patterns. Consequently, either fewer neighboring voxels can be considered in determining the result (e.g., just the six face-touching

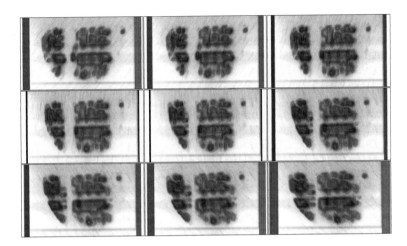

Figure 13.75 Volumetric display of boron concentration from SIMS image data set in *Figure 13.26*. The series of images shows pseudorotation by shifting of planes, using the local 3-D variance in pixel values to locate edges. The magnitude of the variance is used as an effective density value to absorb light along rays through the voxel array.

neighbors), or a different algorithm must be used, for instance one that takes advantage of all of the symmetries in neighbor patterns.

All of the morphological operations (erosion, dilation, etc.) have direct generalizations in three dimensions (Gratin and Meyer 1992). When cubic voxels are used, consideration must be given to the difference between face-, edge-, and corner-touching neighbors. Just as in two dimensions it is necessary to distinguish between 4-connectedness (touching pixels share an edge) and 8-connectedness (touching pixels share a corner), so in three dimensions there are 6-, 18-, and 26-connectedness possibilities for voxels (sharing a face, edge, or corner, respectively). For practical reasons, many methods use 6-connectedness as the simplest definition.

This has particular impact on thresholding and feature enumeration. In many 3-D data arrays, thresholding based on voxel value is a simple and effective method. But in complex structures, methods based on region growing are widely used, in which the user identifies a seed pixel and then all connected voxels having values within some tolerance band are selected. Another approach to segmentation of features uses a 3-D extension ("balloons") of the active contours ("snakes") used in two dimensions (Cohen 1991; Kaes et al. 1987).

The 3-D analog of a Euclidean distance map can be constructed by a direct extension of the 2-D method, and has the same advantages both for improving isotropy and for distance measurement from surfaces or boundaries (Borgefors 1996). However, watershed segmentation in three dimensions has only rarely proved useful.

Skeletonization in three dimensions analogous to that in two dimensions would remove voxels from a binary image if they touched a background or OFF voxel, unless the touching ON voxels did not all touch each other (Borgefors et al. 1999; Halford and Preston 1984; Lobregt et al. 1980). If touching is considered to include the corner-to-corner diagonal neighbors as well as edge-to-edge touching and face-to-face touching, then a minimum skeleton can be constructed. However, if a table for the 26 possible touching neighbors cannot be used, then it is necessary to actually count the touching voxels for each neighbor, which is much slower.

It should be noted that skeletonization in 3-D is entirely different than performing a series of skeletonizations in the 2-D image planes and combining or connecting them. In 3-D, the skeleton becomes a series of linear links and branches that correctly depict the topology of the structure. If the operation is performed in 2-D image planes, the skeletons in each plane form a series of sheetlike surfaces that twist through the 3-D object and have a different topological relationship to the structure. A skeleton of linear links and branches in three dimensions can be formed by connecting the ultimate eroded points (UEPs) in each section, and a different skeleton can be constructed by joining the branch points in the 2-D sections.

Measurements on 3-D images

As discussed in **Chapters 9** and **10**, one of the reasons to collect and process images is to obtain quantitative data from them. This is true for 3-D imaging as well as 2-D, although most of the use of 3-D images to date has been for visualization rather than measurement. Some additional comments about the kinds of measurements that can be performed, their practicality, and the accuracy of the results seem appropriate.

Measurements are broadly classified into two categories: feature-specific and global or scene-based. The best-known global measurement is the volume fraction of a selected phase or region. Assuming that the phase can be selected by thresholding (perhaps with processing, as discussed in earlier chapters), then the volume fraction could be estimated simply by counting the voxels in the phase and dividing by the total number of voxels in the array or in some other separately defined reference volume. The result is independent of whether the voxels are cubic. In fact, the same result can be obtained by counting pixels on image planes and does not depend in any way on the arrangement of the planes into a 3-D array.

A second global parameter is the surface area per unit volume of a selected boundary. There are stereological rules for determining this value from measurements on 2-D images, as presented in **Chapter 9**. One method counts the number of crossings that random lines (for a random structure, the scan lines can be used) make with the boundary. Another method measures the length of the boundary in the 2-D image. Each of these values can be used to calculate the 3-D surface area.

It might seem that directly measuring the area in the 3-D data set would be a superior method that does not require so many assumptions. In practice, it is not clear that this is so. First, the resolution of the boundary, particularly if it is irregular and rough, depends critically on the size of pixels or voxels. The practical limitation on the number of voxels that can be dealt with in 3-D arrays can force the individual voxels to be larger than desired. It was pointed out before that a 1024 × 1024 image in 2-D requires 1 MB of storage, while the same storage space can hold only a 128 × 128 × 64 3-D array.

The use of smaller pixels to better define the boundary is not the only advantage of performing measurements in 2-D. The summation of boundary area in a 3-D array must add up the areas of triangles defined by each set of three voxels along the boundary. The summation process must be assured of finding all of the parts of the boundary, but there is no unique path that can be followed along a convoluted or multi-ply connected surface that guarantees finding all of the parts. For other global properties such as the length of linear features or the curvature of boundaries, similar considerations apply. The power of unbiased 2-D stereological tools for measuring global metric parameters is such that the efficiency and precision of measurement make them preferred in most cases.

Feature-specific measurements include measures of size, shape, position, and density. Examples of size measures are volume, surface area, length (maximum dimension), and so forth. In three dimensions, these parameters can be determined by direct counting. The same difficulties for following a boundary in 3-D mentioned above still apply. But in 2-D images, the measurements of features must be converted to 3-D sizes using relationships from geometric probability. These calculations are based on shape assumptions and are mathematically ill-conditioned. This means that a small error in measurements or assumptions is magnified in the calculated size distribution.

Simple shapes such as spheres produce reasonable results. **Figure 13.76** shows the result for the tomographic image of spherical particles shown in **Figure 13.72**. The measurement on 2-D plane slices gives circle areas that must be unfolded to get a distribution of spheres, as discussed in **Chapter 9**. The result shows some small errors in the distribution, including negative counts for some sizes, which are physically impossible. But the total number and mean size are in good agreement with the results from direct 3-D measurement and require much less effort. When feature shapes are more complicated or variable, 2-D methods simply do not work. If information on the distribution of shapes and sizes is needed, then measurement in 3-D, even with the problem of limited resolution, is the only available technique.

The position of features in 3-D is not difficult to determine. Counting pixels and summing moments in three directions provides the location of the centroid and the orientation of the moment axes. Likewise, feature density can be calculated by straightforward summation. These properties can be determined accurately even if the voxels are not cubic and are affected only slightly by a reduction in voxel resolution.

Shape is a difficult concept even in two dimensions. The most common shape parameters are formally dimensionless ratios of size, such as (volume)$^{1/3}$/(surface area)$^{1/2}$ or length/breadth. (Length is easy to define as the longest dimension, but just as for the 2-D case, the proper definition and measurement procedure and even the definition for breadth is not so obvious.) The selection of a parameter that has meaning in any particular situation is very *ad hoc*, either based on the researcher's intuition or on trial and error and statistical analysis. In 3-D, the values may be less precise because of the poorer voxel resolution, but the accuracy may be better because the size parameters used are less biased. And it may be important to the user's intuition to consider 3-D shape factors, which are less unfamiliar than 2-D ones.

The other approaches to shape in 2-D are harmonic analysis (which unrolls the feature boundary and performs a Fourier analysis on the resulting plot) and fractal-dimension determination; both were discussed in **Chapter 10**. These parameters can be determined rather efficiently in two dimensions, but only with greater difficulty in three dimensions. Since the 2-D results are related stereologically to 3-D structure, it is usually preferable to perform these measurements on the individual 2-D image planes.

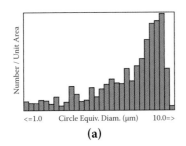
(a)

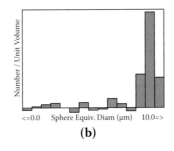
(b)

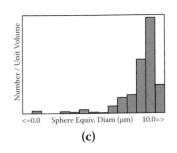
(c)

Figure 13.76 *Comparison of 2-D and 3-D measurement of size of spherical particles in structure shown in **Figure 13.72**: **(a)** size distribution of circles in 2-D plane sections; **(b)** estimated size distribution of spheres by unfolding the circle data in image a (note negative values); **(c)** directly measured size distribution of spheres from 3-D voxel array.*

Closely related to shape is the idea of topology. This is a nonmetric description of the basic geometrical properties of the object or structure. Topological properties include the numbers of loops, nodes, and branches (Aigeltinger et al. 1972). The connectivity per unit volume of a network structure is a topological property that is directly related to such physical properties as permeability. It is not possible to determine topological properties of 3-D structures from single 2-D images (although minimal 3-D probes such as the Disector can provide unbiased estimates). These can be measured directly on the 3-D data set, perhaps after skeletonization to simplify the structure (Russ and Russ 1989b). An example, a 3-D reconstruction showing the topology of an overhand knot, was shown in **Chapter 9**, **Figure 9.24**.

There is little doubt that 3-D imaging will continue to increase in capability and popularity. It offers direct visualization and measurement of complex structures and 3-D relationships, which cannot be as satisfactorily studied using 2-D imaging. Most of the kinds of imaging modalities that produce 3-D images, especially tomographic reconstruction and optical sectioning, are well understood, although the hardware will benefit from further development (as will the computers and software).

Current display methods are barely adequate to the task of communicating the richness of 3-D image data sets to the user. New display algorithms and interface control devices will surely emerge, driven not only by the field of image processing but also by other related fields such as visualization of supercomputer data and interactive computer games. The ability of humans to interpret (usually correctly) realistic surface renderings of complex structures makes these displays very important for many applications. The continued increase in computer power and memory is certain. The quality of surface renderings, in particular, will continue to improve as developments flow from corporate and university research facilities to routine use in hospitals and industry. Watching and using these developments offers an exciting prospect for the future.

14

Imaging Surfaces

In many disciplines, surfaces are more important than bulk structures. Mechanical interaction between parts involves friction and wear between surfaces; many chemical interactions take place on surfaces (including catalysis); and most modern electronic devices consist of thin layers of materials laid down in intricate patterns on the surface of substrates. Similarly, the appearance of an object is dominated by its surface characteristics, texture, and coating. In these and many other cases, scientists and engineers need to characterize surfaces and the ways in which they are modified through fabrication and use. Imaging plays an important role in obtaining information as well as presenting it for human visualization and analysis. As pointed out in Chapter 2, human vision is well adapted to interpreting images of surfaces, and presentation of various types of data rendered as a surface is a common data-visualization tool.

Producing surfaces

Surfaces are produced in a wide variety of processes, some tightly controlled and some quite chaotic. One of the oldest techniques by which mankind has produced intentional surfaces is by removal of material, for instance creating a statue or a stone tool by removing chips from a larger block of stone. Modern fabrication of parts typically involves machining, grinding, and polishing to remove material and to create a surface with specific macroscopic dimensions and microscopic roughness.

Machining is a process in which a cutting tool removes chips from the material as it is moved relative to the workpiece. The shape of the tool's cutting tip or edge, its speed, and the depth of cut control the dynamics of chip formation, which can be either ductile (long continuous chips) or brittle (short broken ones). The surface typically displays long grooves in one direction whose shape is determined in large part by the shape of the tool. Grinding is a process in which many small cutting points, typically facets of hard particles cemented together into a wheel, simultaneously remove material from a surface. A third mode of surface modification, polishing, results when many loose hard particles slide and roll between two surfaces, removing material as the surfaces move relative to one another. Impact erosion (such as sandblasting) uses particles to produce small craters on the surface. Each of these processes involve both plastic deformation and fracture, and they have many variables such as applied forces, the presence of liquids, etc., that dramatically modify the appearance and performance of the resulting surface (as well as the tools or particles doing the work). There are a wide variety of other methods — ranging from fracture to electrical spark discharges; plastic deformation of surfaces by rolling, forging, or extrusion; chemical etching; and so on — that modern technology employs to produce surfaces of parts by the removal or rearrangement of material. **Figure 14.1** shows a few different surfaces.

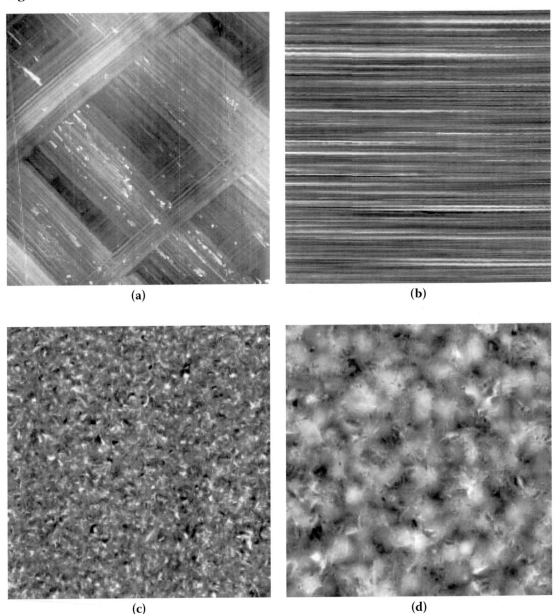

(a) (b)

(c) (d)

Figure 14.1 *Range images of metal surfaces (images obtained with a scanning-probe instrument with 5-μm-radius diamond stylus; each shows 1 mm² with gray scale proportional to elevation):* **(a)** *machined (flycut) surface of aluminum;* **(b)** *ground surface of stainless steel;* **(c)** *vapor-polished surface of aluminum;* **(d)** *shot-blasted surface of brass. (Courtesy of Rank Taylor Hobson, Ltd. Leicester, U.K.)*

There are also methods that build up surfaces by deposition. Again, this may be physical or chemical. Liquids solidify to leave solid coatings, sometimes accompanied by polymerization or formation of crystalline structures. Liquids can solidify in a mold, which controls some of the surface morphology, while in some cases other forces such as viscosity and surface tension are more important than the actual mold surface. Freezing of liquids or gases onto a substrate can produce either very smooth or extremely rough surfaces, depending on how the particles and molecules can move on the surface (**Figure 14.2**). Electroplating typically produces quite smooth surfaces by deposition of atoms from chemical solution, while ballistic deposition and aggregation of particles can generate ones with porous fractal surfaces. Some deposited layers are then subjected to selective removal, either by chemical or physical processes. This is the process by which complex multilayer electronic chips and micromechanical devices are fabricated.

Another concern about surfaces is their cleanliness. The presence of molecules or particulates, either lying loosely on the surface or attached by electrostatic or chemical forces, can disrupt the deposition of the carefully controlled layers used in microelectronics, so elaborate clean rooms and handling methods are required. Surface defects such as pits and scratches are also of concern. Chemical modification of surfaces is called contamination, oxidation, or corrosion, depending on the circumstances. This is strongly controlled by the environment. Sometimes such processes are carried out intentionally to protect the original surface from other environmental effects (for instance, aluminum is anodized to produce a thin oxide layer that provides a chemically inert, mechanically hard surface resistant to further contamination in use). Electrical and optical properties of surfaces can be modified greatly by extremely thin contamination layers.

In all these cases, there is a great need to characterize the surfaces so that the topography of the surface, and perhaps other properties such as chemical composition or electrical parameters, can be determined. Some of the surface characterization data are obtained directly by imaging methods. Even when the data are obtained in other ways, visualizing the surfaces is an imaging technique, relying on the human interpretation of the images to detect important

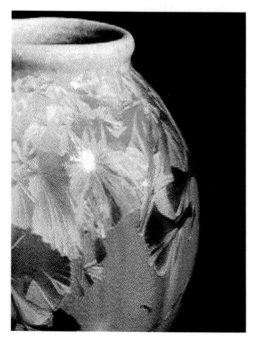

Figure 14.2 *Photograph of a glaze covering a ceramic pot. The glaze flows down the surface in a molten state and solidifies to an amorphous glass under the forces of surface tension. Subsequently, the atoms rearrange themselves to form crystals that nucleate and grow in the glaze, producing visually interesting patterns and also modifying the surface geometry.*

information about the surfaces. Measurement often follows visualization, to reduce the image data to a few selected numbers that can be used for process control, and to correlate the structure of the surfaces with their fabrication history on the one hand and with their performance and behavior on the other.

Devices that image surfaces by physical contact

Most of the measurement methods used to characterize surfaces are based on either some kind of microscope that provides magnified images of the surface, or scattering of radiation or particles from the surface. The methods can provide measurement of either composition or geometry, including the thickness of thin layers. Many different kinds of microscopes (and some tools that may not be conventionally thought of or named as microscopes) are used to study surfaces (Castle and Zhdan 1997; Castle et al. 1998; Russell and Batchelor 2001; Van Helleputte et al. 1995). Many of these require no surface preparation, or at most minimal cleaning; a few such as the scanning electron microscope (SEM) may require the application of conductive coatings to electrical insulators. The common methods use visible light, electrons, ions, physical contact, electron tunneling, sound waves, and other signals to produce images that sometimes can be directly related to the surface geometry and in other cases are primarily influenced by the surface slope, composition, coating thickness, or microstructure. The most immediately useful and interpretable imaging methods are those whose output consists of "range" values in which the elevation of the surface is directly represented in the values often shown as either profile traces or gray-scale images. Although most of the examples shown here will be ones in which the gray scale directly encodes elevation, it should be understood that a similar display of chemical information or elemental concentration can be dealt with using the identical measurement and visualization tools.

One method that covers some of the newest devices, such as the atomic force microscope (AFM), and quite old and well-established methods used in industrial manufacturing, such as profilometers, is the use of a mechanical stylus that is dragged across the surface. Motion of the stylus is amplified to record the elevation of the surface point by point. If a full raster scan is used, this produces an array of elevation data that can be displayed as an image, as shown by the examples in **Figure 14.1**. If the mass of the moving parts of the stylus assembly is kept as low as possible, forces of milligrams or less can keep the stylus in contact with the surface (at least for surfaces that have slopes up to about 45°) at quite high scanning rates. The images in **Figure 14.1** were obtained in about 50 sec each, as an array of 500 × 500 points covering a 1-mm^2 area.

Stylus instruments used in industry typically use diamond-tipped styli with a tip radius of about 1 micrometer, which defines the lateral resolution that the instruments can provide. Vertical motion can be sensed using inductive, capacitance, or interference gauges, all of which are capable of subnanometer sensitivity. With suitable calibration, which is typically provided by scanning over known artifacts, these methods are routinely used to quantitatively measure surface elevations in many industrial settings to measure surface finish, the thickness of layers, etc. These instruments have primarily been used with metal and ceramic parts, but are also capable of measuring a wide variety of softer and more fragile materials, as shown in **Figure 14.3**.

The AFM also uses a stylus, but a much smaller one (Binnig et al. 1986; Quate 1994; Wickramasinghe 1991). The scanning tunneling microscope (STM) stimulated a range of new microscopy techniques that use essentially the same scanning and similar feedback principles to obtain

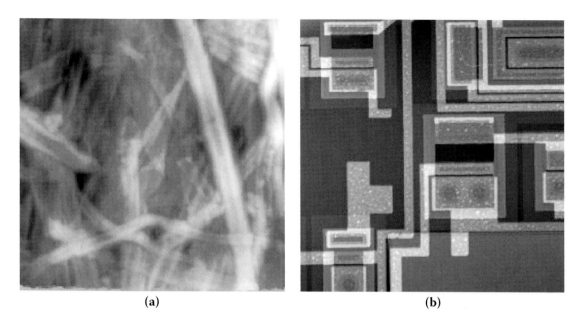

Figure 14.3 *Range images obtained with a scanned stylus instrument:* **(a)** *paper;* **(b)** *microelectronic chip.*

images with nanometer lateral as well as height resolution. The atomic force microscope was introduced in 1986 as a new instrument for examining the surface of insulating crystals. There was a clear implication from the first that it would be capable of resolving single atoms, although unambiguous evidence for atomic resolution did not appear until 1993. The AFM has evolved into a flexible instrument that provides new insights in the fields of surface science, electrochemistry, biology, and physics, and new adaptations of the technology continue.

By etching silicon or silicon nitride to a sharp point, by depositing carbon in such a way that it grows into a long thin spike, or by utilizing carbon nanotubes ("buckytubes"), a stylus can be fabricated with a tip radius of a few nanometers (**Figure 14.4**). This allows much greater lateral resolution than profilometer styli. But such tips are extremely fragile and easily deformed, so a variety of techniques have been devised to utilize them to probe a surface. Classically, the tip is used as a reference point and the surface is translated in the z (elevation) direction to contact it. The tip is attached to or a part of a cantilever arm whose deflection is monitored by deflection of a light beam on the rear face or sometimes by interference measurement, and vertical sensitivity below 1 nm is easily obtained. Either the sample or the stylus can be translated in an x,y raster pattern to cover the entire surface to create a complete image. The translation is typically accomplished with piezoelectric devices, which limits the total range of motion.

The traditional and still most common mode of operation places the tip in sliding contact with the surface. To reduce the lateral and shear forces on the stylus and the surface, the stylus may be rapidly raised and lowered ("tapping mode"), or the lateral forces may be measured by the twisting of the stylus to determine either the elastic modulus of the surface material or the friction between the stylus and surface. Additional modes can be used in which physical contact is not actually required. For example, the stylus can track the surface without touching it with somewhat lower resolution by using attractive Van der Waals forces. In addition, some systems use strategies such as heating the tip and measuring the heat loss when it is close to the surface, vibrating it and measuring a change in characteristic frequency when it is close to

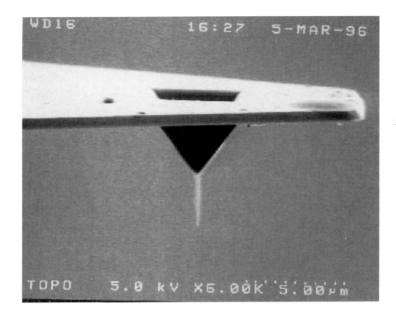

Figure 14.4 SEM image of an ultrafine tip used for high-resolution atomic force microscopy. (Courtesy of Topometrix Corp., Santa Clara, CA.)

the surface, or using it as a guide for light photons that interact with the surface and detect its presence without contact. The electric or magnetic force gradient and distribution above the sample surface can be measured using amplitude, phase, or frequency shifts, while scanning capacitance microscopy measures carrier (dopant) concentration profiles on semiconductor surfaces. The original operational mode, whose development won a Nobel Prize, was scanning tunneling microscopy (STM), which measures the surface electronic states in semiconducting materials. The variety of operational modes of the scanned probe microscope seems nearly unlimited as manufacturers and users experiment with them, but many of these techniques are applicable only to a particular set of materials and surface types. The same technology has been used to modify surfaces, either by pushing individual atoms around or by writing patterns into masks used for lithographic manufacture of microelectronic and micromechanical devices.

One of the problems faced by AFMs is the difficulty in making quantitative dimensional measurements. The original designs used open-loop piezoelectric ceramic devices for scanning, which suffer from hysteresis and nonlinearity. Software correction, no matter how elegant, can only go so far in correcting the resulting image distortions and measurement errors due to its inability to adapt to the topography of each individual sample. This particularly affects the use of the AFM in the metrology-intensive semiconductor industry. Some more recent designs use a more expensive approach that employs a separate measurement device in each axis to provide a closed-loop measurement of the piezoelectric scanner's movement. Using either interference or capacitance gauges, these permit accurate measurements to be made on small structures such as microelectronic and micromechanical devices, magnetic storage devices, and structures such as the compact disc stamper shown in **Figure 14.5**.

The AFM is limited in the area that it can scan and the speed with which it can do so, in the relief of the specimen that can be present without interfering with the cantilever arm, and the steepness of slopes (or undercuts) that can be accessed by the tip. Special designs that attempt to alleviate one or more of these limitations are required for specific applications, as is true for all surface-measurement approaches. But it is useful to have an overview of the general range of capabilities of the different techniques. **Figure 14.6** shows of graph (a Stedman diagram, named after Margaret Stedman of the British National Physical Laboratories) that plots the

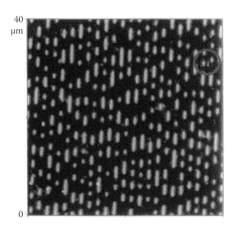

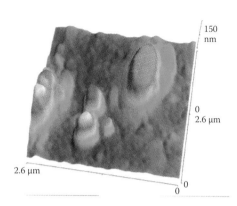

Figure 14.5 *AFM images of a defect on a CD stamper. (Courtesy of Topometrix Corp., Santa Clara, CA.)*

range of lateral and vertical distances that can be accommodated by various surface-measurement techniques. Notice that the minimum vertical dimensions detected by the AFM and traditional stylus instruments is about the same, but the AFM has much better lateral resolution, while the stylus instruments have a much larger range. Some of the other techniques plotted on the diagram will be discussed later in this chapter, but none of them offers a perfect combination of range and resolution in both vertical and lateral directions along with quantitative accuracy and an ability to deal with most kinds of surfaces.

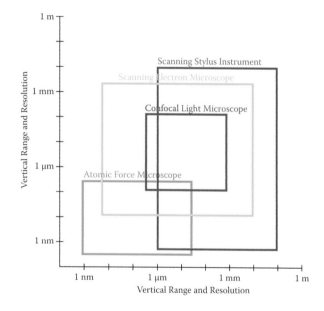

Figure 14.6 *Comparison of the typical range and resolution of several surface imaging technologies (Stedman diagram).*

Noncontacting measurements

All stylus instruments, indeed all techniques that examine one point at a time, are limited in speed by the need to move a probe with finite mass across the specimen one line at a time. Most stylus methods also touch the surface, which raises concerns about specimen damage. Indeed, AFMs have been used to create surface topography as well as to image it, and industrial stylus instruments are often accused of leaving surface markings where they have been used on soft metal surfaces. For some surfaces, the best solution is to make a replica that can be scanned. Plastic replicas can preserve fine detail, as shown in **Figure 14.7**, and alleviate concern about damage to the original specimen.

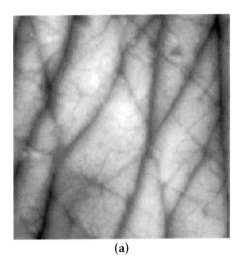

(a)

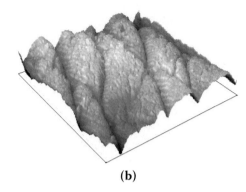

(b)

Figure 14.7 Scanned stylus image of a plastic replica of human skin:
(a) gray-scale representation of the elevation data;
(b) photorealistic visualization of the surface.

It would seem that using light as a probe should make it possible to overcome concerns about speed or damage. Unfortunately, it also raises others. The principal drawback is that the light does not interact with the same surface that the tip feels, so that the measured elevation does not agree with that from the stylus methods (which are accepted according to various international standards for surface measurement). In many materials the light waves penetrate to a small distance beneath the surface as they are reflected, and this surface impedance depends upon the dielectric properties of the material (which can be modified near the surface by contamination or oxidation layers). Very-fine-scale structure can also produce speckle and interference effects that alter the returned light in ways that mimic quite different surface structures and give incorrect results. Also, the presence of contaminant or oxidation films or local surface tilt angles of more than a few degrees can reduce the amount of light scattered back to the detector so that some points on the surface are not measured at all.

There are a variety of ways that light can be used to probe surfaces. One choice is to use a beam of light focused to a point that is then scanned over the sample in the same way that a stylus would be, while other instruments image light from the entire area of interest at once. Point probes can use confocal optics to detect the distance to the specimen (also called focus detection), which also requires vertical scanning of either the sample or the optics. This can be done for each point, which is slow because of the need to move a finite mass, or the scan can be performed over the entire area for each z setting, as in most confocal light microscopes. In this method, the light intensity at each location is stored for each z setting, and then the peak intensity value (which can be interpolated between settings) is used to determine the surface elevation at that location. It is also possible to construct an optical point probe that uses a lens with large chromatic aberrations, and to detect the wavelength of light that is most strongly reflected. Because the lens brings each wavelength to focus at a different working distance, this provides a measure of the surface elevation. Other optical techniques such as triangulation are very sensitive to the local surface slope and have relatively poor lateral resolution.

The method that provides the greatest resolution over the greatest range is interference, and this can be done with either a point probe or for the entire surface, and with either monochromatic (usually laser) light or with white light. The classic Michelson-Morley interferometer uses mirrors to send light along two pathways, and then recombines them to produce interference patterns that show fringes corresponding to differences in dimensions that can be much smaller than the wavelength of the light. When one leg of the interferometer reflects light from the sample surface, these fringes can be used to directly measure surface elevations. The lateral resolution is only as good as the light microscope used to collect the reflected light, or about 1 μm, but the depth resolution can be 1 nm or better. However, for samples that do not reflect light well or that have steep cliffs or deep pits, there may not be enough light reflected, or the spacing of the fringes may be too close together, to provide results.

When monochromatic light is used it is possible to interpolate the elevation of a point to about 1 nm, about 1/1000th the wavelength of light. However, the fringes must be far enough apart (the surface elevation must vary gradually) that it is possible to keep track of the changes in elevation, because the interference pattern repeats with every multiple of the light wavelength. Many modern systems use more than one wavelength of light or white light instead. This produces constructive interference only at one focal depth, where the path lengths are equal and all of the wavelengths are in phase. When a surface is being imaged, this means that only points along one isoelevation contour are bright. Varying the distance between the specimen and the optics allows scanning in z to determine the elevation of points over the entire image. This takes longer than a simple monochromatic interference pattern and is limited in precision of elevation values to the performance of the scanning hardware, but it can handle surfaces with much more relief and steeper slopes.

Indirect interference techniques such as projection of grids to produce moiré patterns, also produce two-dimensional arrays of elevation data. Imagine light streaming through Venetian blinds onto the floor of a room. If the floor is flat, the strips of light will be straight when viewed from above. If there are irregularities, they show up directly as deviations in the lines of light and shadow. Scaled down to the dimensions of a few micrometers, which is the resolution of the light optics used to view the stripes, this same structured light method is easily used to measure surface geometry. Image processing can be used to detect the edges of the shadows, interpolating along each scan line to accuracies much better than the pixel spacing. Depending on the geometry, this can produce vertical measurement accuracy similar to the lateral resolution of the optics, typically about 1 μm (Sciammarella et al. 2005), but of course for only a few locations across the sample surface unless the line pattern is scanned. Toolmakers' microscopes and quality control examination of planed surfaces of lumber (among other applications) use the same basic method. One unusual modification (Ghita et al. 2005) of a structured light measurement measures the defocus (spreading) of the projected pattern to determine depth.

In modern implementations of the technique (Masi 2005), mirrors or prisms are used to deflect a beam of laser light in patterns across the workpiece to produce the same type of image. This has the advantage of being able to measure in various orientations and directions. Closely related to the idea of structured light is shadowing of surfaces with evaporated or deposited metal or carbon coatings, followed by measurement of the shadows cast by features and irregularities on the surface. If the image of the grid pattern in the incident light passes through another similar grid, it produces a moiré pattern, whose dark lines can be used to reveal the shape of the object. This technique is particularly useful for revealing local strains and deviations of surfaces from ideal geometric forms. Because it is fast and noncontacting, this method is often used in medical applications, ranging from orthopedic work on curvature of the spine to measuring the curvature of the lens of the eye before and after corrective surgery.

Microscopy of surfaces

Most forms of microscopy produce images in which intensity is related to the reflection of light (or some other signal) from the surface. This is only indirectly related to the surface geometry, and includes other information such as composition. Despite the difficulties in interpretation, this is still the most widespread procedure for surface examination because of its speed and convenience.

The standard light microscope at moderately high magnification has a comparatively shallow depth of field. This creates many problems for examining surfaces. If the surface is not extremely flat and perpendicular to the optical axis (for example, a metallographically polished specimen), it cannot all be focused at the same time. Only low-magnification light microscopes can be used to examine rough surfaces (e.g., for fractography), and these do not give much information about surface geometry. The pattern of light scattered by rough surfaces under diffuse lighting can be used to determine the roughness. It has been shown (Pentland 1983; Russ 1994) that a surface with fractal geometry will scatter diffuse light to produce a fractal pattern, and that there is a relationship between the fractal dimension of the surface and that of the image. This has also been reported for SEM images of such surfaces. But measuring the overall roughness dimension of the surface is not the same thing as determining the actual coordinates of points on the surface.

On the other hand, the depth of field of the conventional light microscope is too great to measure the important dimensions in the vertical direction on rough surfaces. Paradoxically, the confocal light microscope (CLM) has a much shallower depth of field (and, more importantly, rejects stray light from locations away from the plane and point of focus), which allows it to produce true range images from irregular surfaces. In the confocal microscope, the image is built up one point at a time (usually in a raster pattern). Each image corresponds only to points at a particular focal depth, but repeating this operation at many focal depths produces both an extended-focus image in which the entire surface is imaged and a range image in which the elevation at each point is recorded. The resolution in both vertical and lateral directions is much worse than the scanned-probe microscopes or interferometers, but this technique is quite useful for many surface measurement applications, including metrology of some microelectronic devices. For dielectric materials, capturing multiple images with different orientations of polarized light can be used to compute the surface geometry (Miché et al. 2005).

Because of its very large depth of field, coupled with excellent resolution (typically <10 nm, much better than the light microscope), the SEM is often a tool of choice for the examination of rough surfaces. Furthermore, the appearance of the secondary electron image that is most often recorded from this instrument looks reasonably "familiar" to most observers, who therefore believe they can interpret the image to obtain geometric information. Unfortunately, this is not at all simple. **Figure 14.8** shows an SEM image of a surface consisting of sintered tungsten carbide particles. This is a relatively simple surface composed of particles of uniform composition with relatively flat facets. But there is no unique or simple relationship between elevation or slope and the local pixel brightness. For relatively smooth surfaces without sharp edges, "shape from shading" methods can convert changes in intensity to changes in slope and thus extract the geometry. The influence of fine-scale roughness, edges, surface contamination, compositional variation, etc., prevents shape-from-shading from being a general-purpose approach. Backscattered electron imaging is less sensitive to many of these effects and is used for some metrology applications, but this only gives "real" geometric dimensions when standards are available for comparison or when extensive modeling of the interactions between electron and sample is performed.

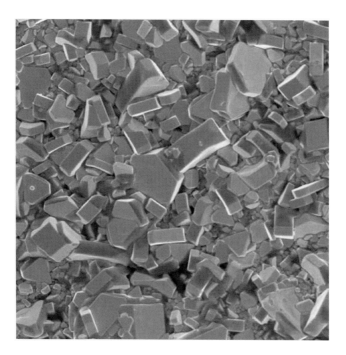

Figure 14.8 *SEM image of the surface of sintered tungsten carbide.*

The great frustration in using the SEM to examine surfaces is that while the images look quite natural to human viewers, and seem to represent surface geometry in a familiar way, determining actual dimension values from them is nearly impossible except in very constrained cases. Metrology of integrated circuits is used to determine lateral dimensions, but even in these cases the definition of just what the relationship is between the physical contour of an edge and the voltage profile of the signal is far from certain (and highly dependent upon the voltage used, the material being imaged, the detector type and location, etc.). Metrology is used for quality control in which consistency rather than absolute accuracy is important, and there is no attempt to extract measurements in the z direction from such images. (Indeed, even the visibility of points near the bottoms of grooves or contact holes is a problem.)

Stereoscopic imaging in which two (or more) different views of the surface are combined to measure elevation is the same in principle as the generation of topographic contour maps from aerial photographs (Wang 1990; Wong 1980). However, this is not an easy technique to automate (Abbasi-Dezfouli and Freeman 1994; Barnard and Thompson 1980; Heipke 1992; Park et al. 2005; Raspanti et al. 2005; Tang et al. 2005; Wrobel 1991; Zhou and Dorrer 1994), and even with careful control of imaging conditions and measurement of angles, the vertical resolution is typically much worse than the lateral resolution of the individual images. This is because the tilt angle δ between the two views must usually be small (7 to 10° is typical) to prevent points being hidden in one of the two views, and the angle enters the calculation as $1/\sin(\delta)$. The precision of lateral dimensions is magnified by any uncertainty in angle and limits the precision of the final result.

Measurement of the elevation difference between individual points is in principle quite straightforward when a human can locate the same points in the two images. The parallax or offset of the points gives the elevation by straightforward trigonometry (**Chapter 1**). However, to generate an elevation map for an entire surface involves matching a great many points and requires automation to be practical. The two methods used for this are area-based or feature-based matching. Area-based matching uses cross-correlation (either in the spatial domain or the frequency domain) to find the location of an area in the second image that most closely matches each area in the first. However, changes in the visibility or contrast of the area between the two images, the presence of specular reflections, or repetitive structures that produce multiple matches can produce problems for this approach.

Feature matching detects locations in each image that have some characteristic such as a maximum local value of variance or entropy, or a high local brightness gradient. These points are then matched against the similar list of points in the other image. This is generally more successful, but may match only a few thousand locations in the two images out of perhaps a million pixels, so that the intervening locations can only be interpolated. In all cases, constraints such as preserving the order of points from left to right and knowing the direction of tilt so that searching for matches need only occur in a small fraction of the total image area are important aids to the practical implementation of the methods.

Figure 13.8 in **Chapter 13** shows a typical result in which two stereo images have been matched by cross-correlation, testing each point in the left-eye view with possible points in the right-eye view to find the best match. The horizontal displacement (disparity or parallax) where the match was found measures the elevation of the point. Mismatched or unmatched points are typically present and are filled in using a median filter. The calculated elevation values can then be used for measurement or visualization. Highly specialized software for the purpose of fusing stereo-pair images, usually from the SEM, has been developed (www.alicona.com; Ponz et al. 2006) to produce both visualizations and measurements of surfaces (**Figure 14.9**). Because of its great depth of field, the scanning electron microscope is very often used to obtain stereo-pair images of surfaces. The SEM is also used to generate X-ray maps of surface composition, discussed separately below. The Alicona programs include corrections for lens focal length (short working distances produce additional distortions in the images) and can accommodate more than two images for greater precision. The surface visualizations can be freely rotated on the display, and a variety of profile and area measurements can be carried out.

Instead of using electrons, light, or other radiation to form an image of the surface, quite a lot of information is available from the scattering or diffraction patterns that are produced. X-ray patterns contain data about the structure of either crystalline or amorphous layers. Electron scattering patterns contain information on the crystallographic arrangement and also on local strains in the material (which show up as the displacement or broadening of lines in the pattern). Visible-light scattering patterns contain information on the distribution of surface orientations (Zhu and Zhang 2005). Scattered patterns of electromagnetic radiation are in effect the Fourier transform of the elevation profiles of the surface, and their measurement is therefore a direct method to study the surface elevation in a way that separates the information on the form or figure (the intended large-scale geometry of the part), the waviness (medium-scale departures from the figure), and the texture or roughness (the fine-scale details on the surface). In many cases, the scattering of reflected light can also be directly related to the intended use of the surface, for instance a high-precision mirror. Images such as diffraction patterns can be processed and measured using many of the same techniques as more conventional images, but these are not discussed here in detail.

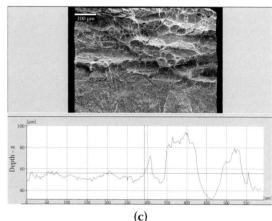

(a)

(c)

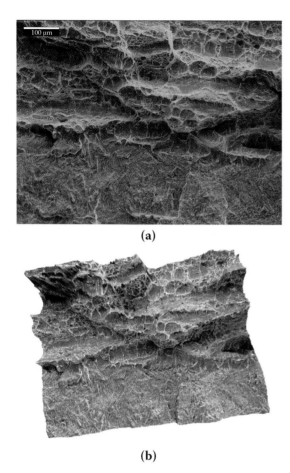

(b)

Figure 14.9 *Visualization and measurement of a surface computed from stereo-pair SEM images:*

(a) *anaglyph presentation of stereo-pair images of a metal fracture surface;*

(b) *rendered-surface representation of the fracture surface computed from the stereo-pair images by the Alicona software;*

(c) *measured elevation profile across the fracture surface.*

(Courtesy of Dr. S. Scherer, Alicona Imaging GmbH, Graz, Austria; www.alicona.com.)

Surface composition imaging

The variety of techniques for probing surface composition is astoundingly broad. Some of the more common ones are the SEM using an X-ray detector, the ion microscope or microprobe using secondary ion mass spectrometry (SIMS), and Fourier transform infrared (FTIR) spectroscopy. There are many other tools used as well, particularly for measuring the thickness and composition of coatings. These include the backscattering of particles, which samples the composition and density of the sample at depths up to several micrometers beneath the surface. Also of rather specialized interest is acoustic microscopy, which is sensitive to debonding between the coating layer and substrate. Gigahertz acoustic waves have a wavelength similar to visible light and can be used to image surface and near-surface structures that are difficult to detect with other signals. Surface waves are strongly reflected by cracks (even closed ones that cannot be seen otherwise), and bulk waves are similarly reflected by the surfaces of pores (although these subsurface waves only propagate at lower frequencies, with correspondingly poorer resolution). The speed of sound in the material can also be measured to determine the modulus of elasticity and other physical properties. Ellipsometry takes advantage of the fact that for many types of thin-layer dielectric coatings, the plane of polarized light is rotated as it passes through the coating. Measurement of that rotation can provide highly precise coating thickness measurements, and the use of different wavelengths of light (or a spectrometer to scan an entire range of wavelengths) can also reveal details about the internal structure of the coating. However, this method is primarily used to measure relatively large spots and not to produce images of the surface. Similarly, another spot-analysis analytical technique uses a laser beam directed at a selected point on the surface with a light microscope to vaporize material from a pit (typically several micrometers across and deep) blasted from the surface so that the atomic and molecular fragments can be weighed in a mass spectrometer.

There are several different types of ion microscopes. Many can produce elemental composition maps of the surface, or a series of such images at various depths in the material. An incident beam of ions knocks the uppermost layer of atoms loose from the specimen, either one point at a time (the ion microprobe) or over the entire surface at once. These atoms are ionized and are then accelerated into a mass spectrometer that separates them according to their mass/charge ratio, identifying specific elements and isotopes. A detector or detector array then produces an image. This typically represents the spatial distribution of one selected element at a time across the imaged area, with a lateral resolution of about 1 µm (depending on the diameter of the incident beam in the case of the ion microprobe and the resolution of the ion optics in the case of the ion microscope) but with a depth resolution of one atomic layer. Rapidly switching the spectrometer from one element to another as layers are removed produces complete data sets of the structure of the material.

Compositional mapping of surfaces is particularly important for examination of deposited coatings and the identification of contamination. The most common approach to this mapping uses a raster-scanned electron beam to generate characteristic X-rays from the atoms present, which are then detected. The unique energy or wavelength of the X-rays identify the elements, and calculations based on the physics of X-ray generation can be used to determine their amounts. The lateral and depth resolution is limited to the order of 1 µm by the range of the electrons. Several different types of X-ray spectrometers are used; the diffractive or wavelength-dispersive type measures X-rays from one element at a time, but with good trace-element sensitivity, while the more common energy-dispersive type can measure all of the elements present at the same time, but with poorer detectability. These typically produce "dot map" images for several elements at once, as shown in **Figure 1.31** of **Chapter 1**, which only approximately delineate the regions containing the elements and must be processed and combined, as discussed below. Other signals, such as Auger electrons, come from a smaller region near the point of entry of the focused electron beam and have better spatial and depth resolution, but because the signal-to-noise level is poor, these are not so good at detecting minor and trace elements.

Molecular identification of coatings and contamination can be made using infrared spectroscopy, in which various vibratory modes of the molecules are excited to produce characteristic spectral peaks. This method is most suitable to the analysis of organic materials and coatings, such as plastics. The spatial resolution of this approach is limited to several micrometers by the light optics used.

Compositional maps of surfaces are often displayed, processed, and analyzed by treating the signal strength (which is approximately proportional to concentration) as a range image, and interpreting it visually as a surface whose elevation represents concentrations. These images often contain many channels of information, representing different elements, and their display using colors is shown below. Principal-components analysis, discussed in **Chapter 5**, can also be used to delineate the various phases present.

Processing of range images

Elevation data from surfaces produced by the various methods discussed above are typically recorded as 8- or 16-bit gray-scale images, or more rarely as an array of real numbers. Each pixel has a value that represents the physical elevation or composition of the corresponding surface location. Since most of the techniques described look vertically down upon the surface, the data are single valued and represent only the uppermost point for surfaces in which undercuts and bridges can occur. The SEM is an exception to this, as shown in **Figure 14.10**, which shows a complex polymer surface with undercuts and bridges that a range image cannot reveal. Integer data stored for each pixel in a range image can be converted to an elevation value in appropriate units (nanometers, micrometers, etc.) using scale data that are usually stored in the file header. There is unfortunately no standard

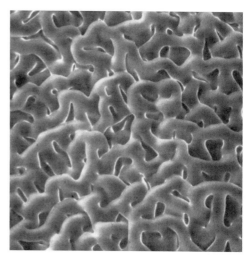

Figure 14.10 *SEM image of the complex surface of a polymer, with undercuts and bridges.*

format for these data, and not only does each manufacturer have its own (which is not always generally readable or well documented), but some have more than one corresponding to different instruments.

Reading in these different file formats and storing the data in some standardized format such as TIFF (tagged image file format) files may require custom programming. Some image processing and display programs do have the ability to read arrays of data (i.e., images) in a wide variety of data formats, provided that the user can specify (or deduce) the necessary format information. This typically includes at least the length of the header and perhaps where specific scaling or other information is stored within, the dimensions of the array and whether the data are stored in rows or columns, and the data format (byte, integer, long integer, real, etc., and whether the byte order is Intel or Motorola — low word first or high word first).

Once the data are available, the kinds of processing that are required for surface images depend strongly on what kind of instrument was used. Some examples will serve to illustrate the possibilities:

Interference microscopes often have dropout pixels where the local slope of the surface was too great to return enough light to the optics to permit measurement. These points can be detected by filling the array beforehand with an illegal or impossible value that is replaced by real measurement data. Any pixel that retains the illegal value is a dropout point and must be filled in, and the most common way to do this is with a median or smoothing filter. A simple median would suffice for single points, but in many cases, regions several pixels across or arranged as a line corresponding to some step or ridge on the surface may be missing. In this case, several approaches are possible. An iterated median, perhaps weighting the neighboring pixel values inversely by their distance, will fill in even large areas from their periphery. Linear or spline interpolation between pixels around the dropout produces smoothed results.

Reducing or removing noise in range images uses the same methods as other images: either a median filter or some type of averaging filter such as the Gaussian. But for surface images, these are best not applied in the same type of round neighborhood, as shown in **Chapter 4.** Instead, the neighborhood is restricted to pixels that lie on the same portion of the surface, excluding points at a different elevation or on a surface with a different slope. This was described as conditional smoothing in **Chapter 4** and is an example of an adaptive neighborhood filter, similar to the procedures used to smooth geographic data (also a range map) called "kriging." In the example shown in **Figure 14.11**, the neighborhood restriction provides superior noise reduction while preserving fine lines and corners.

Stylus instruments, whether macroscopic ones with diamond tips several micrometers in diameter or atomic force microscopes using Buckytubes to probe much smaller lateral dimensions, share some of the same image-analysis problems and require anisotropic filtering. The scan rate along each line (the *x* direction) is typically determined by the dynamics of the stylus itself — the mass of the moving tip and the applied force — which determines the maximum speed at which the tip can move across the surface while remaining in contact with it. Too high a force will result in damage to the surface or the tip, but too low a restoring force will allow the tip to skip over holes or fly from rising slopes. Depending on whether the stylus moves some sensing element (an interferometer or a capacitance or inductance gauge, for example, or perhaps just a beam of light) or the surface is moved to null the position of the stylus (the classical AFM mode of operation) and the signal to the piezoelectric drivers is recorded, the output signal for the surface elevation is usually an electrical voltage. This must be amplified and then digitized, and in the process suitable filtering can be applied with a time constant appropriate for the scanning speed. This reduces the noise along each scan line and eliminates the need for subsequent digital processing to reduce noise. Filtering can be used, as discussed below, to separate the low-frequency signals related to surface form and waviness from the high-frequency roughness value, but that is part of the process of measurement rather than image enhancement.

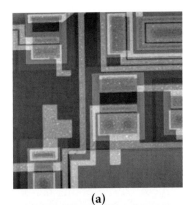
(a)

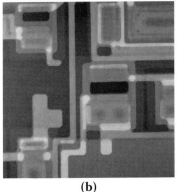
(b)

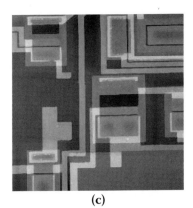
(c)

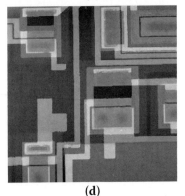
(d)

Figure 14.11 Noise reduction using a restricted neighborhood:
  (a) *original image showing noise;*
  (b) *conventional median filter (7-pixel diameter) applied;*
  (c) *mean filter in a 9-pixel diameter with a threshold to exclude values more than 40 gray levels different from the local surface;*
  (d) *median filter with the same neighborhood as image c.*

The situation is quite different in the y direction (from one line to the next). A significant amount of time passes between sequential lines in the raster scan, allowing for changes in the mechanical and electronic components. Most systems scan in one direction only (to minimize hysteresis problems) and have a retrace scan during which the stylus is raised and not in contact with the sample. Repositioning the stylus to the exact same value is very difficult when the resolution of these methods in the vertical direction is on the order of a nanometer, The result is that subsequent scan lines tend to be offset from each other either vertically or laterally. Since the eye is sensitive to abrupt changes in brightness that extend over large distances, this produces images in which a visible horizontal-stripe pattern can be seen. Some AFM manufacturers attempt to alleviate this problem by adjusting each line so that the average value is the same as that of the preceding line. This is rarely a good idea; it means for example that if there is a rising peak or depression somewhere in the image area, the background around the feature will be shifted, producing false data and even an incorrect visual impression of the surface, as shown in **Figure 14.12**.

There is a better solution than the mean or average value for this line-to-line adjustment, although it requires more computation. The ideal solution would be to align the mode values of sequential lines of data. Under the assumption that the surface consists primarily of a background level with some roughness superimposed on it, plus major features of interest that rise or fall with respect to that plane, the mode is by definition the most probable surface elevation value. For a relatively small collection of data points (most area scans have only a few hundred data points along each line), the mode is not robustly determined. But for any distribution the median is closer to the mode than is the mean. Just as the median value is preferred over the mean for filtering noise from an array of pixels, so the median offers a workable solution for adjusting the scan lines in a raster scan stylus image. **Figure 14.13** shows this method applied to a typical image of a rough surface.

Another artifact in AFM images that is best avoided by proper attention to the hardware, but which is correctable to some extent in software, is the deconvolution of tip shape from the images. As shown in **Chapter 6**, if the point-spread function of an image can be measured, dividing the Fourier transform of the image by the transform of the point-spread function can remove much of the smearing or loss of resolution, so that the inverse transform yields an improved image. Real AFM tips are far from perfect, exhibiting various departures from an ideal symmetrical point. Scanning the tip over a known artifact such as a circular disk (Jarausch et

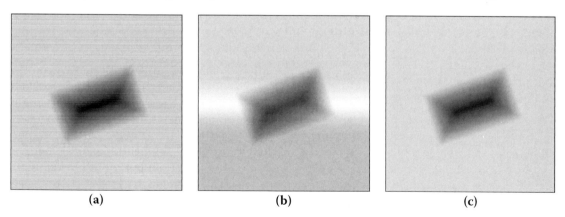

(a) (b) (c)

Figure 14.12 AFM scan of an etch pit in silicon, showing *(a)* the line offsets in the raw image, *(b)* the artifact resulting from correction by adjusting the mean value of each line, and *(c)* the improved result using the median value.

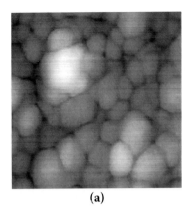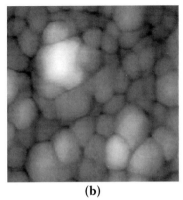

Figure 14.13 *AFM scan of a chemically deposited surface* **(a)** *before and* **(b)** *after the correction of line offsets.*

(a)   (b)

al. 1996; Keller 1991; Keller and Franke 1993; Markiewicz and Goh 1994, 1995; Villarrubia 1994, 1996, 1997) allows calculation of the tip shape, and permits this deconvolution. In practice the tips have a short life and no two are identical, so that frequent recalibration is required. However, tip deconvolution is only important at the highest magnification and finest resolution levels.

Processing of composition maps

Most surface composition maps that are obtained by ion mass spectroscopy, X-ray energy spectroscopy, or other methods suffer from low signal levels. As discussed in **Chapter 4**, this can in principle be rectified by collecting more data, but this is generally not desirable on economic grounds and sometimes is impossible because the analysis alters or consumes the surface. Hence noise-reduction methods such as weighted smoothing or median filtering are often applicable.

When multiple images are obtained of the same area showing the spatial distribution of different elements or other chemical data, it is very important to find ways to display them in combinations that will communicate the information to the observer, and to find ways to delineate and distinguish the various phases that are present. Combining multiple images as color planes offers one approach to this, as shown **Chapter 1**, **Figure 1.32**. However, because of the way that the display hardware (and human vision) works, this allows only three planes (red, green and blue, or RGB) to be assigned, and there may be many more individual images available than that. The situation is analogous to the situation for remote sensing of images; the *Landsat Thematic Mapper* satellite records seven wavelength bands from the visible into the infrared, and other satellites capture even more. There is no straightforward way to "see" all of this information at one time, and the choice of which planes to show and in which colors can be quite subjective and can reveal (or conceal) quite different aspects of the information.

If the individual elemental maps can be thresholded to correspond to the intensity levels from individual phases, then Boolean combinations of the planes using AND and NOT permit forming binary images of each phase, which can then be measured. This process corresponds to setting up threshold ranges in an N-dimensional intensity space corresponding to the number of elements present, in which the ranges are rectangular prisms in shape. This is often adequate to distinguish the phases present in real materials, but a more free-form shape that corresponded to the natural variations in intensity for each phase would be preferred.

There are statistical techniques that plot the intensity of each pixel in each of the image planes as a vector or point in N-space (nine dimensions for the example shown here), and then search for principal axes or clusters within that space. Principal-components analysis is shown in **Chapter 5**. Once clusters are identified and the boundaries around them are defined, the various phases present can be identified (Anderberg 1973; Hartigan 1975; MacQueen 1967). This is a direct extension of the classification methods discussed in **Chapter 11**. The pixels whose values lie within each cluster are then classified as belonging to the corresponding phase, and a new image can be generated with unique colors for each class so that the phases are delineated (Bright et al. 1988; DeMandolx and Davoust 1997; Mott 1995).

When there is *a priori* information about the composition of the various phases expected to be present, this method works quite well. However, cluster detection without such information suffers from several problems. First, the statistical techniques will always be better able (in a statistical sense) to segment the space by defining more clusters, so unless the number of phase clusters is known, the results are suspect. Second, clusters for minor phases representing only a few percent by volume of the structure will be represented by only a few percent of the points. Although these phases may be very important (e.g., for the properties of materials and the economics of mineral ores), they will be poorly defined in the n-space plot and very hard to detect. They are likely to be overlooked amid the background of points from pixels that straddle boundaries between major phases. Cluster detection methods, for example, are more likely to segment single-phase regions based on minor gradients in composition or statistical variations in intensity, rather than to identify the presence of important minor-phase regions.

Data presentation and visualization

Some types of surface-measurement instruments produce data arrays with very large range-to-resolution ratios. In other words, the number of bits that encode the elevation or other surface characterization data are very large. Most image processing and display programs cope adequately with 256 gray levels, but even this exceeds the ability of human vision to distinguish them on a computer screen. Resolution of 1 nm over a range of 1 mm, which is quite possible with a high-precision stylus or interferometric instrument, produces a million levels (20 bits). This far exceeds the capabilities of displays or of perception. Consequently, the display routines must either select one part of the entire range to display or compress the data to show the entire range. Processing can help, for instance by dealing with local slopes or derivatives rather than absolute values, but this also requires some user experience to interpret.

The large dynamic range of the data from surface measuring tools can only be displayed on the computer screen at the cost of making small but measurably different values appear with indistinguishably small differences in brightness. One particularly effective way of assisting in the visualization of such small changes, often associated with dirt or defects, is the adaptive neighborhood histogram equalization introduced in **Chapter 5**. **Figure 14.14** shows an example, a range image of the raised surface of a letter on a coin. Scratches on both the lower coin face and the raised letter can barely be detected in the original, but become visually quite evident after applying the equalization procedure, which makes small differences larger while suppressing large ones. Other processing techniques, discussed in preceding chapters, can also of course be employed on range images, but should be done while always recognizing that the actual numeric elevation values are altered and can no longer be used for measurement purposes.

Range images, in which the gray-scale value at each pixel represents the elevation (or some other surface parameter) at that point, contain all of the raw information in the data array. Even

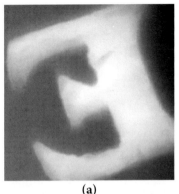

(a)

Figure 14.14 *Enhanced visibility for surface scratches by processing:*
(a) *original range image of letter on the surface of a coin;*
(b) *adaptive histogram equalization applied to image a;*
(c) *photorealistic surface rendering of image a;*
(d) *rendering of height information from image a with surface brightness values from image b.*

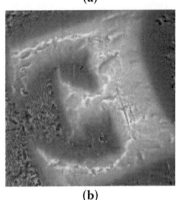

(b)

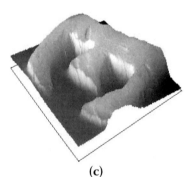

(c)

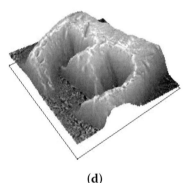

(d)

if the range can be accommodated by the display (for instance by dividing down the resolution with which the data were acquired, or using a local equalization technique or high-pass filter), the resulting image is an unfamiliar one to human observers and requires experience to interpret. Using false colors to increase the ability to visually discriminate small changes may make the resulting images even more unfamiliar.

Contour maps draw isoelevation lines, which are exactly the same as topographic maps of the Earth's surface. These are familiar to many people and can be more easily interpreted because they make it easy to follow the contour lines to identify the shape of protrusions and valleys, and to identify points at the same elevation. Of course, they also eliminate a great deal of information (the elevation data for all of the other pixels on the surface), but this is part of the simplification that makes interpretation easier. **Figure 14.15** shows the elevation of a coin displayed as a gray-scale range image, one that has been color-coded, and one reduced to a small number of contour lines (which have also been color-coded to make it easier to distinguish their elevation values).

Contour maps are less successful at communicating visual information when the lateral scale of detail is finer, or when the surface if very anisotropic, as shown in **Figure 14.16**. In these cases, the individual lines are close together and hard to distinguish, and the lines do not tie together different areas of the surface very well. Whenever contour lines become close together because of the presence of fine detail or steep slopes, it is helpful to reduce the number of contour lines or color code them to clarify the map.

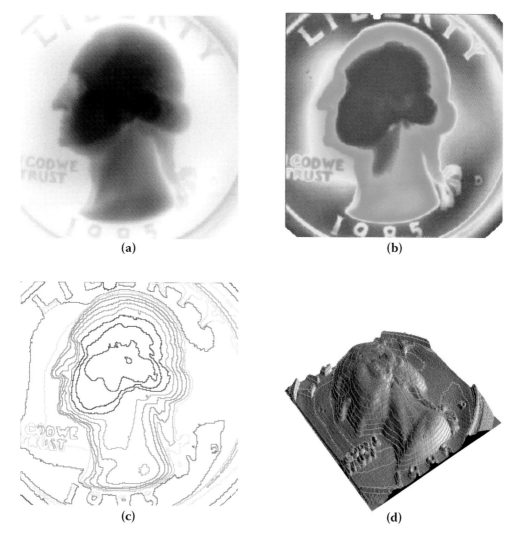

Figure 14.15 *Range image of a coin from a scanning stylus instrument, displayed as:*
- *(a)* *a gray-scale range image;*
- *(b)* *a color-coded range image;*
- *(c)* *a color-coded contour map with ten isoelevation lines;*
- *(d)* *a rendered isometric image with color-coded contour lines superimposed. (Courtesy of P. Scott, Rank Taylor Hobson, Ltd. Leicester, U.K.)*

The visual impression of surface relief can be improved by processing. A directional derivative creates an "embossed" appearance with light and dark contrast along edges and gradients. As discussed in **Chapter 5**, a convolution kernel of weights of the form

$$
\begin{array}{ccc}
+1 & +1 & 0 \\
+1 & 0 & -1 \\
0 & -1 & -1
\end{array}
$$

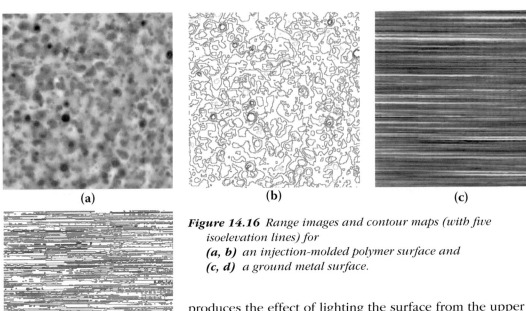

(a)   (b)   (c)

(d)

Figure 14.16 *Range images and contour maps (with five isoelevation lines) for*
(a, b) *an injection-molded polymer surface and*
(c, d) *a ground metal surface.*

produces the effect of lighting the surface from the upper left corner and produces the effect of shadows, which the eye interprets as relief. The direction should usually be from the top; if bright edges appear on the bottoms of edges, the human vision system (which is accustomed to lighting from above) inverts the interpretation of the data and perceives hills as pits, and vice versa.

The derivative image shows fine detail but hides the overall elevation changes in the data. This can be alleviated by combining the gray-scale range image with the derivative. This can be done by adding the two (simply change the central value in the kernel from 0 to 1), but results that correspond more closely to the way vision perceives texture on surfaces can be obtained by multiplying the two images together. This is shown in **Figure 14.17**. A particularly attractive version of this display can be constructed by using the information from a color-coded range image as well. In **Figure 14.17d**, a hue, saturation, intensity (HSI) model was used, with the elevation assigned to the hue for each pixel and the derivative assigned to the intensity (saturation is set to 50%). The shadows create an impression of relief, while the color informs the eye about overall elevation values.

These results compare quite favorably with the results of a true rendering of the surface using each triangle of neighboring pixels as a facet and calculating the reflection of light from a light source in a fixed position, as shown in **Figure 14.18**. In this type of calculation, the surface can be given various reflectivity characteristics, either more diffuse or more specular. In the examples shown, a full ray tracing and Phong shading was used. The latter method varies the shade across each facet according to the angle variation between neighboring facets, and produces a very smooth and realistic rendered surface as used in computer-assisted drafting (CAD) workstations. The rendered image can also be color-coded by using the gray-scale rendering of reflectivity as the intensity channel and the elevation as the hue channel, as discussed above. Example of this are shown in **Figure 14.19**.

Altering the displayed lighting and shading of surfaces can be an extremely powerful visualization tool for surface examination, taking advantage of the abilities to interpret surface images

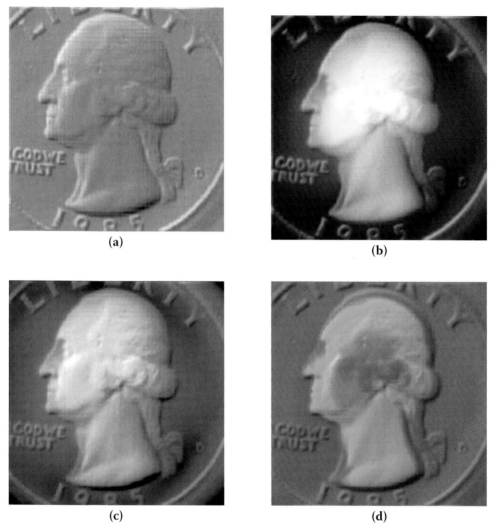

Figure 14.17 *Enhancement of the image of the coin from* **Figure 14.15**: *(a) directional derivative; (b) the derivative added to the original gray values; (c) the derivative multiplied by the original elevation values; (d) color image with the elevation in the hue plane and the derivative in the intensity image.*

that humans have evolved in response to real-world experiences. Specular enhancement of surface appearance has been demonstrated by Malzbender et al. (2001). This method, called surface relighting, uses multiple light sources (40 in the examples shown) to illuminate a specimen, which enables the local surface orientation at each location to be determined by shape-from-shading, also called photometric stereo. This data set is then represented mathematically as a polynomial map of orientation and texture, so that the appearance can be computed with altered surface reflectivity characteristics and any selected illumination direction. **Figure 14.20** shows the enhanced appearance of a clay tablet with synthetic specular shading computed from the local surface orientation.

With this data set, it is also possible to interactively alter the illumination direction by moving the mouse over the image. **Figure 14.21** shows four images from this procedure, in which fine details on the surface can be studied as the lighting is altered. For instance, one

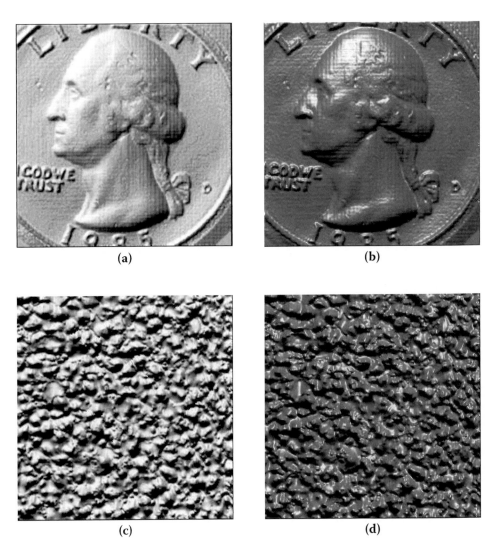

(a)　　　　　　　　　　　　　　　(b)

(c)　　　　　　　　　　　　　　　(d)

Figure 14.18 *Rendered surfaces of the coin (**a, b** from **Figure 14.15**) and the polymer (**c, d** from **Figure 14.16**), treating the surface as though it were a diffuse scatterer (**a, c**: plaster of Paris) or a specular one (**b, d**: shiny plastic or metal). The grid pattern visible in the coin image is an artifact of the scanner used to obtain the images and becomes more visually evident in this display mode.*

interesting note is the fingerprint left in the wet clay by the scribe who prepared this tablet 4000 years ago in Sumer, which can be discerned as a series of ridges near the upper left corner of the tablet. Such fine details are generally not observable without this enhancement technique.

Rendering and visualization

The views shown above look onto the surface from directly above. This normal view shows all of the data, but is not the most familiar to a human observer. The use of computer graphics to

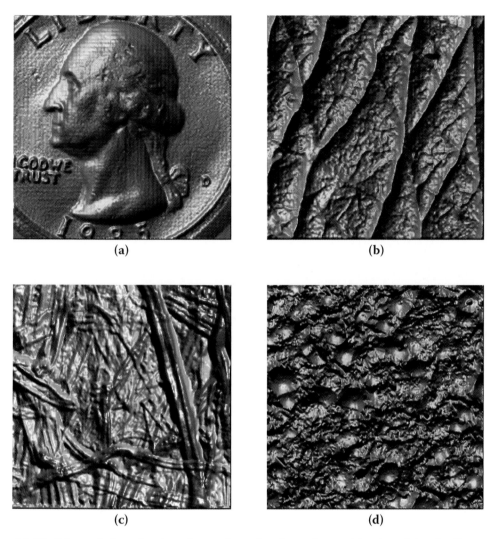

Figure 14.19 *Color-coded rendered surfaces using a hue/intensity combination:* **(a)** *coin (from* **Figure 14.15***);* **(b)** *skin (from* **Figure 14.7***);* **(c)** *paper (from* **Figure 14.3***);* **(d)** *shot-blasted metal (from* **Figure 14.1d***).*

render the surface from an oblique point of view (which many programs allow to be selected or even interactively rotated) produces an image that makes it easier to visualize the surface morphology, and perhaps to detect the features of interest. The oldest and simplest approach to this is to plot elevation profiles along some of the horizontal rows of pixels, displacing each line vertically and laterally to create the effect of a surface, and skipping some rows so that the lines are adequately spaced apart. **Figure 14.22** shows two examples of this. In the first, the coin image from **Figure 14.15**, the lines are well spaced and the surface slopes gradually enough so that there are only a few places where lines are hidden (and erased). The result is a fairly easy surface to interpret. In the second example, the polymer image from **Figure 14.16**, the presentation is harder to interpret because so many lines cross each other and the overall morphology is obscured. Also, in these displays the width of each line profile is the same, so that there is no perspective applied to the view. In this type of isometric presentation, the

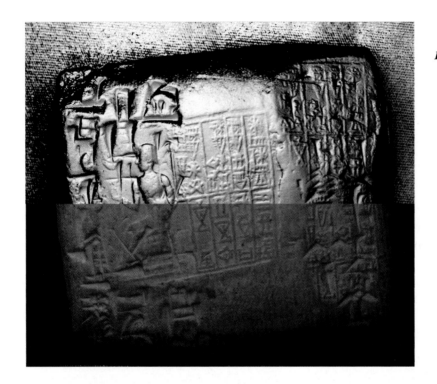

*Figure 14.20 Specular
enhancement of
the image of a clay
cuneiform tablet
by computing the
rendered reflection
from the surface
based on orientation
data calculated by
shape-from-shading
using multiple images
with different light-
source locations.
Bottom half of the
image shows the
original surface
appearance. (Courtesy
of T. Malzbender,
Hewlett Packard Labs,
Palo Alto, CA.)*

human familiarity with the rules of perspective causes this constant width of the data to be misinterpreted as giving the array a wider apparent dimension at the back than at the front.

With the continued advance in computer graphics capabilities, in the form of more process-ing power and displays with more gray levels and colors, much more realistic presentations can be generated. Adding perspective also makes the data seem more realistic, and adding cross lines that connect points on successive line profiles breaks the surface up into an array of square or rectangular tiles that improve the interpretability of the surface morphology by showing slopes in the second direction. Increasing the line density provides more informa-tion, but still must omit many lines and rows of pixels to avoid overwhelming the eye with too many disappearing lines. Coloring in the tiles according to the elevation of the points provides additional cues to depth. The results (shown in **Figure 14.23**) represented the state of the art only a few years ago, but are now easily performed on the typical desktop machine. Computer graphics packages such as OpenGL simplify the tasks of rendering realistic surface images for visualization.

The most visually realistic presentation uses actual surface rendering to control the brightness of each facet on the surface. Rather than square tiles that must be bent to fit the four corner points (which in general will not lie in a plane), triangular tiles are simpler to deal with. Three corner points define the triangle and the orientation of the facet with respect to the line of sight, and a light-source location permits calculation of the intensity to be assigned to the facet. This can be done with complete photorealism given the time and computing power, but there will in general be a very large number of facets to render, and faster methods are sought. We can perform this operation by shading each facet according to the product of its absolute height and its derivative to produce a very quick and visually realistic rendering.

Figure 14.24 illustrates this method. In **Figure 14.24a**, the edges of the individual triangular facets are drawn in for clarity. But with this method it is practical to create a facet for every

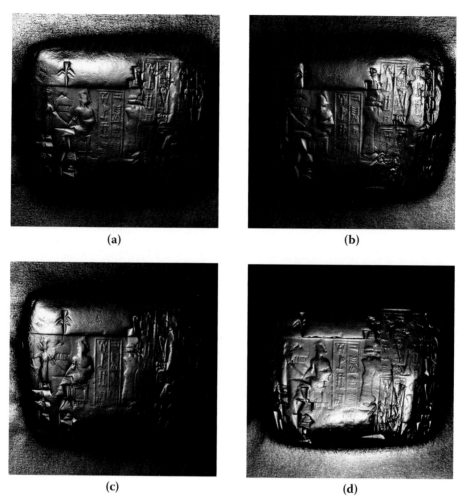

Figure 14.21 *Four images of the specularly enhanced surface of the same tablet shown in* **Figure 14.20** *as the location of the computed light source is interactively shifted. This happens in real time so that the observer can visually interpret the fine details. (Courtesy of T. Malzbender, Hewlett Packard Labs, Palo Alto, CA.)*

pixel and its immediate neighbors so that the full resolution of the data set can be displayed. The result is shown in **Figure 14.24b**. In computer graphics (as used in CAD programs, for example), it is common to apply shading to facets so that they blend in with their neighbors (Gourard or Phong shading) and to not reveal lines where they meet. But while that method is important for the small number of large facets encountered in CAD renderings, it is unnecessary for the tiny facets that correspond to each pixel, because the facets may cover only 1 or 2 pixels on the display. This also speeds up the process.

It is useful to compare this method against the slightly simpler display procedure of using the elevation to shade the facets, or of using false colors to indicate elevation. These methods produce much less realistic results for visualization, and require a more educated eye on the part of the user. It is important to understand that human vision is an important tool for examining surface images, since the presence of defects or other features of interest is usually far more readily discerned by an experienced observer than is possible with computer pattern-recognition programs.

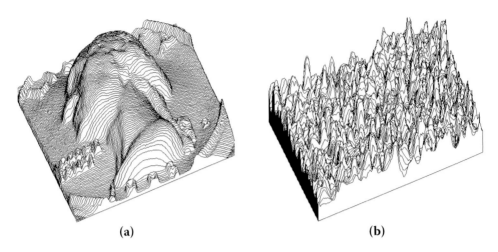

Figure 14.22 *Isometric line profile displays of the coin image from **Figure 14.15** and the polymer image from **Figure 14.16**.*

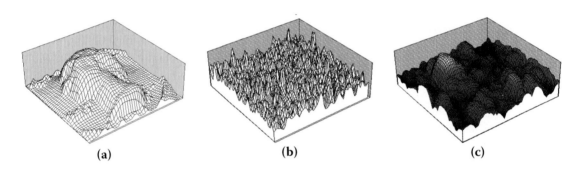

(a)   (b)   (c)

Figure 14.23 *Grid or mesh displays of the coin (**Figure 14.15**), polymer (**Figure 14.16**), and deposited surface (**Figure 14.13**).*

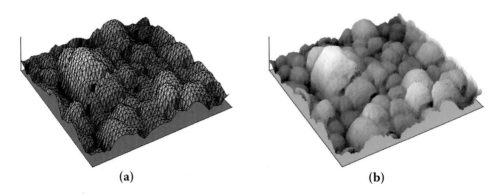

(a)   (b)

Figure 14.24 *Deposited surface rendered with triangular facets whose brightness is the product of the elevation and slope: **(a)** large facets that are 6 pixels wide; **(b)** facets connecting each pixel and its immediate neighbors.*

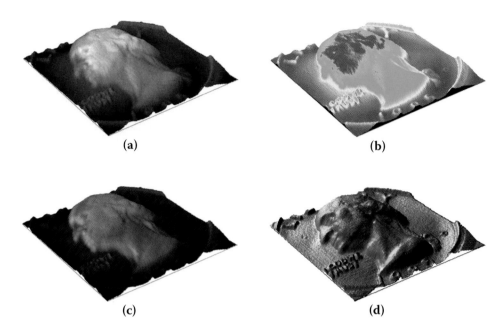

(a)   (b)

(c)   (d)

Figure 14.25 *Presentation of elevation data from the coin image: (a) each facet shaded according to the product of elevation and slope; (b) each facet assigned a color representing elevation; (c) using the hue to represent elevation and the intensity to represent slope; (d) using hue for elevation and the Phong-rendered surface values for intensity.*

It is also possible to introduce color to these displays using the same procedure as shown in **Figure 14.23**, applying the elevation as a color in the hue channel and the slope or Phong-rendered values in the intensity channel, while drawing each facet in its appropriate place on the screen to generate a perspective-corrected visual representation of the surface geometry. This is more readily visually interpreted than simply applying false color, as shown in **Figure 14.25**.

Using this type of presentation communicates a much more effective representation of the surface geometry to most users, even ones with some experience, than does the simple gray-scale range image. **Figure 14.26** shows this mode of presentation for the same surface images presented in **Figure 14.1** and **Figure 14.3**. Even though the range images contain all of the data, and the perspective-corrected visualizations actually obscure some of it, comparison suggests that the latter are more realistic in appearance and hence more useful for visual recognition of characteristics or defects, although not, of course, for surface measurements.

Modern computer graphics is also capable of rapidly redrawing surface views from different viewpoints. This can be used in several ways. Generating two realistic renderings of a surface from slightly different points of view allows using human stereo vision to interpret the depth of a surface. Creating a series of such images from different viewpoints can be used to display a "movie" showing a flyover across the surface, and with enough computer horsepower this can be done in real time as an operator manipulates a joystick to interactively control the flight path. Combining this with the stereo display (**Figure 14.27**) creates a virtual-reality world in which the surface can be viewed in detail. The figure illustrates this with an anaglyph image requiring red/green or red/blue glasses, but of course other computer display modes, including synchronized polarized glasses, can also be used.

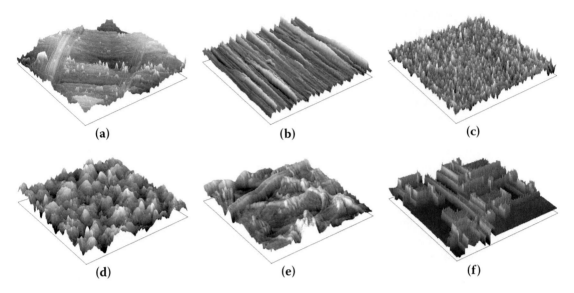

(a)   (b)   (c)

(d)   (e)   (f)

Figure 14.26 *The surface data from the four surfaces in **Figure 14.1** and the two surfaces in* **Figure 14.3** *rendered to show perspective-corrected visualizations with facets shaded according to the product of slope and elevation. The graphics have been expanded in the vertical (z) direction to increase the perception of roughness and relief in the data:* **(a)** *machined aluminum;* **(b)** *ground steel;* **(c)** *vapor-polished aluminum;* **(d)** *shot-blasted brass;* **(e)** *paper;* **(f)** *microelectronic device.*

Figure 14.27 *The surface rendering of **Figure 14.26f** performed from two slightly different viewpoints, which are combined to form a stereo pair.*

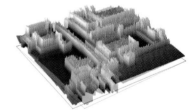

Analysis of surface data

There is no doubt that human visual examination of well-presented visualizations of the surface geometrical and compositional information offers a powerful tool for detecting and recognizing defects and other specific characteristics of the surface. But for many purposes there is a need for numerical measures of the surface that can be used for control purposes and to correlate the surface geometry or compositional variations with (a) the creation and processing history of the surface and (b) its performance behavior. For these purposes, analytical methods relying on computer processing of the data are needed, and it is far from clear just what should be measured to provide effective parameters for any given requirement.

The traditional measures of surfaces include the thickness of coatings and the geometric features of the surface geometry. Most of these values, while quite precise, are highly dependent on other factors such as the material composition (and spatial variations of composition), the particular measurement procedure used, and the size of the measured area. Most thickness-measuring procedures and some elevation-measuring instruments naturally average over a lateral distance that is at least several micrometers and often much more. This is much larger than the vertical resolution most techniques are capable of and may hide important details of the coating. Sampling strategies must be employed to determine spatial uniformity.

Dimensional measurement of surfaces is one application where coordinate measuring machines, stylus instruments, and optical interference techniques are all used. In many cases very exact dimensions are specified in the design of the part, and so the measurement does not require an area scan or an image, but simply the proper alignment of the measuring tool with the component. However, as dimensions become small, as in the case of microelectronic devices, it may be necessary to acquire an image to locate the point where measurement is to be performed. **Figure 14.28** shows an elevation profile taken from one scan line of an AFM, from which highly precise measurements can be taken on the width and height of the steps present. AFM data sets are generally presented as visualizations that represent surface relief, but quantitative measurements are gradually becoming more common (Shuman 2005).

Because the AFM is a relatively slow device that has difficulty handling large parts or scanning large areas, and because there is always concern about surface damage when a physical contact is made, many of the metrology measurements on these devices are presently made by SEM. (The light microscope was used with earlier generations of devices, but the dimensions are now too small for the wavelength of light to resolve.) **Figure 14.29** shows an SEM image

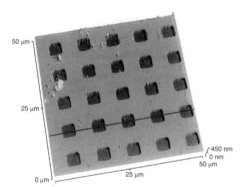

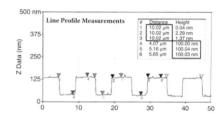

Figure 14.28 *AFM image of a lithographic test pattern used to select the location for a single line scan used for dimensional measurement. When used for this purpose, the AFM requires quantitative position sensing such as an interferometer, rather than relying on measuring the signals sent to the piezoelectric positioners.*

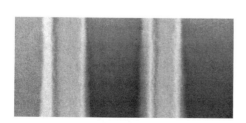

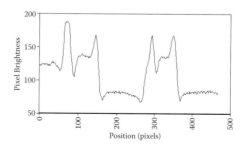

Figure 14.29 *Portion of an SEM image of two parallel lines of photoresist on a silicon wafer, and the signal profile across them. The relationship between the physical profile and the signal depends upon the slope and roughness of the sides of the lines, the composition of the material, the electron-accelerating voltage used, the electron detector used, and its placement relative to the specimen.*

of two lines of photoresist on a silicon wafer. Unfortunately, the SEM image is only indirectly related to the surface geometry. Consequently, the signal profile along a scan line (actually averaged over multiple scan lines to improve the signal-to-noise ratio) is difficult to interpret to determine the line width. The pitch or spacing of the lines can be determined with fair accuracy under the assumption that the lines have the same shape, and thus generate the same signal profile. Consequently selecting any reproducible characteristic of the signal — the peak, the maximum slope, etc. — can be used to measure the distance between the lines. But to measure the line width accurately there must be some absolute determination of where the edge lies (and even what that means, given the slightly irregular shape of typical lines).

Computer modeling of the process of generating the SEM image signal can be carried out for various specimen geometries (and as a function of composition, electron beam voltage, and detector characteristics and placement). This is a time-consuming process but is still easier than fabricating physical standards for comparison. Even so, little accurate metrology is done in reality. Most manufacturers that use SEM images for metrology select some arbitrary feature of the signal that can be easily and reproducibly measured, such as the point of maximum slope or halfway between the darkest and lightest signal levels, and use that to monitor changes in dimension but without trying to determine the actual dimension. This is the classic difference between accuracy and precision, and works adequately for production control but not for the development of new geometries and devices.

Profile measurements

Unlike the SEM, most instruments considered here do produce actual physical elevation profiles. Surface measurements have historically been assessed from these elevation profiles rather than using full two-dimensional images (because the instrumentation is simpler and less expensive, and the time required is much less, and hence because familiarity with the methods became established). By applying filters to the data (either digitally or in the amplifier electronics), different ranges of frequencies in the profiles can be separated that are traditionally described as the figure or form, waviness, and texture or roughness (**Figure 14.30**). Form is the overall gross geometrical shape, which is generally specified in engineering drawings, controlled by set dimensions, and described by conventional Euclidean geometry. The medium frequencies are called waviness and the high frequencies the texture or roughness. In machining processes, waviness is assumed to result from vibrations or deflections in the machine, while roughness results from more local interactions between the tool and the local microstructure in the material. These divisions are somewhat arbitrary and may differ according to the size of the part. It must also be remembered that the shape of the stylus itself is effectively a filter that removes the highest frequencies. The cutoff frequencies used to define the filters are typically set to wavelengths from about 0.25 mm up to several millimeters to separate waviness from roughness. International standards specify these as part of the measurement procedure for many mechanical engineering applications.

Filtering to separate roughness from waviness and form data was originally done using analog RC filters in the electronics. In modern systems, digital processing is used, with a least-squares line or arc fitted to remove the form and a spatial Gaussian filter to separate the waviness and

Figure 14.30 Deviations from intended shape are commonly divided into roughness (fine scale), waviness (intermediate scale), and form (large scale).

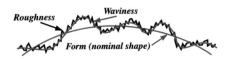

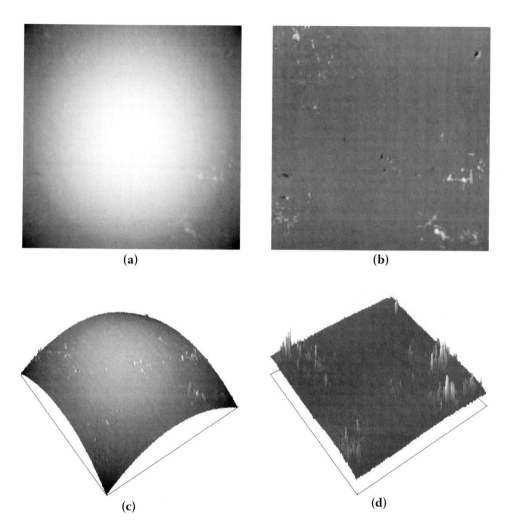

Figure 14.31 *Range images and surface visualizations of a ball-bearing surface showing the overall form* **(a, c)** *and the results of flattening the data by subtracting the spherical shape* **(b, d)**. *Gray-scale and vertical expansion of the data are facilitated after form removal.*

roughness. This generalizes directly to area scans that can also be filtered with an equivalent Gaussian filter, or the Fourier transform of the image can be filtered to select the desired range of frequencies. The form data are most often separated by least-squares fitting of a plane, or some other Euclidean shape such as a cylinder or sphere that corresponds to the known intended form, or a generalized polynomial. **Figure 14.31** shows a simple example of form removal, in which roughness on a ball bearing (spherical) surface is made more evident visually and also becomes easier to measure after the general curvature is subtracted. Deviations are then measured from the nominal form of the ball.

The roughness of surfaces is typically determined from the roughness profile after the low(er)-frequency components have been removed. A wide variety of measurement parameters are used, some of them codified in various ISO or other international standards, and some of them corresponding to specific industries or equipment manufacturers (Rosen and Crafoord 1997). A complete review of instrumentation and methods is in Whitehouse (1994), and up-to-date reviews of analysis procedures are covered in Thomas (1999) and Mainsah et al. (2001).

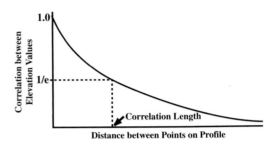

Figure 14.32 *The correlation plot shows the probability that points will have the same elevation value as a function of their lateral separation. The correlation length is defined as the point at which this plot drops to 1/e, or 36.79%.*

The most widely used procedures perform statistical analysis on the elevation data without regard to its spatial arrangement. Examples include the maximum peak-to-valley range of elevations along the profile, the average absolute value of the deviation from the mean (*Ra*), or the statistical standard deviation of the elevation data (*Rq*). Another measure of the magnitude of the roughness is the difference in elevation between the five highest peaks and five lowest valleys (*Rz*), but this requires defining a peak or a valley. This problem becomes more difficult when applied to area scans or images.

Information on the spatial distribution of the elevation data includes parameters such as the number of peaks along the profile and the correlation length. The latter can be defined as the average distance between successive peaks, or between points at some specific elevation such as the mean elevation line left after removing the form and waviness. A more general definition of the correlation length comes from a plot as shown in **Figure 14.32**; this is just the magnitude of the autocorrelation function, which can be determined from the Fourier transform of the profile. The autocorrelation function (ACF), described in **Chapter 6**, is also of interest because, for surfaces produced by a large number of independent events (shot blasting, grinding, ballistic deposition, etc.), it has the same shape as the ACF of the "average event" that produced the surface.

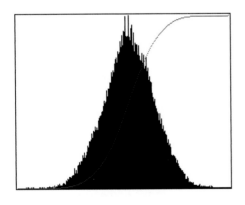

Figure 14.33 *The histogram (black) of the shot-blasted-surface range image (Figure 14.1d) and the same data shown as a cumulative histogram (red). The latter curve plots the fraction of points on the surface whose elevation is less than the value on the horizontal axes, and is called the Abbott-Firestone curve.*

Functional parameters are also used, which are presumed to correspond to particular usage of the surfaces. The Abbott-Firestone curve is simply the cumulative histogram of the elevation data (**Figure 14.33**); it gives the area of contact that would be obtained by removal of a portion of the surface, either by in-service wear or by an additional fabrication step such as plateau honing of automotive cylinder liners.

Another approach, called "Motif," originally introduced in the French automobile industry and now used throughout Europe (Dietzsch et al. 1997), simplifies the profile to just the peaks that would contact another surface based on the height of the peaks relative to the intervening valleys and the width of the valleys. **Figure 14.34** shows the principle. Peaks are characterized by their depth (the height above the valley) and their separation distance. Peak-and-valley patterns are then combined according to their separation distance and depth to eliminate the small peaks on the sides of larger ones, until a minimum representation is reached that contains just the most important peaks.

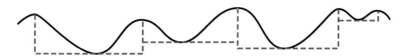

Figure 14.34 *The basics of motif combination: each peak-and-valley motif is measured by the depth (height of the smaller peak above the valley) and width. Motifs that have peaks smaller than the neighbor on either side, a width less than an arbitrary cutoff, and a depth less than 60% of the largest depth in the profile are combined with their neighbors to reduce the number of motifs present.*

All of these methods simplify the original data to extract a few key values, but they have serious limitations. They are highly dependent on the length of the profile scanned and the lateral resolution of the data points. They involve some very arbitrary definitions of what constitutes a peak or valley, ignore the fact that the profile path will not cross the highest or lowest points of most surface peaks and valleys, and do not correlate very well with the real subjects of interest, which are the processes by which surfaces are produced and their behavior for whatever service they are used. They are primarily suitable for specific quality control applications in which the real meaning of the parameters is hidden, but where the consistency of measurement results can be used to keep a working process in control. Furthermore, the line profile interpretations are very difficult to generalize to surface images produced by area scans of elevation (Balagurunathan and Dougherty 2003).

All profile methods suffer from the fact that most real surfaces are not isotropic but have some directionality that results either from the way the surface was generated, the characteristics of the material itself, or the use it has been subjected to. This so-called "lay" of the surface can be simple (e.g., the ground surface in **Figure 14.1b** is highly directional) or very complex and subtle. Measuring a profile perpendicular to the principal lay direction is the recommended approach, but for complicated surfaces this misses much of the actual character of the surface.

Because the history of profile measurements has generated (or accumulated) a rash of parameters, an effort is being made to rationalize the measurement of area scans. Supported by the ISO committee and spearheaded by researchers at the University of Birmingham (Stout et al. 1993), a set of statistical, spatial, and functional parameters has been proposed that will probably evolve to form the basis of future international standards. These still contain some of the same limitations as the profile measures, such as the need to define what constitutes a peak and a strong dependence upon the size of the scan area and the lateral resolution of the points. And they do not include some of the potentially important methods such as topographic analysis, envelope or motif analysis, and fractal geometry. But because they represent an important starting point for surface description, some consideration of them is appropriate.

The Birmingham measurement suite

Four classes of measurement parameters are proposed, ones that deal with the elevation values without regard to their location (called amplitude parameters), ones that deal with lateral distances on the surface (called spatial parameters), ones that combine these (called hybrid parameters), and ones that are believed to have some direct correlation with surface history and properties (called functional parameters). Within each group only a very few parameters, those that have the most direct relationship to the more widely accepted profile measurement parameters, are selected. The symbols proposed for these parameters use the same nomenclature as those for profiles, except that S (surface) is substituted for the R used in profile standards.

The amplitude parameters are simple extensions to area scans of the statistical measures that are used with profile plots. For instance, Sa is the analog to Ra, the arithmetic mean deviation. For an area scan, it is the arithmetic mean of the absolute values of the elevation values from the mean plane (fit as discussed previously). Sa is preserved only because Ra is widely used, and that is so, in turn, because it was comparatively easy in the precomputer days to design instruments to measure it. The root-mean-square deviation of the elevation points is a more robust measure, which is simply the standard deviation of the distribution of the elevation values, Sq. The variance (the square of the standard deviation) is the second moment of the distribution. The third and fourth moments are the skew and kurtosis, respectively, and these are also used as amplitude measurement parameters, called Ssk and Sku, respectively. For simple distributions that are not bimodal, these three parameters offer a reasonably compact statistical description of the surface heights.

The histogram of the surface elevation data (examples are shown in **Figure 14.35**) shows the overall range of surface elevation. The skew in the distribution distinguishes such cases as the narrow and deep grooves that may be important for distributing lubricant on plateau-honed cylinder liners in automobile engines (**Figure 14.35c**). In this case, most of the surface has a very narrow range of elevations, but the grooves, which cover only a small fraction of the area, reach down to much lower depths. A skew in the opposite direction would correspond to a surface with just a few high peaks or ridges rising up from a relatively smooth surface. But the histogram by itself contains no information on the spatial arrangement of the pits and valleys or the peaks and ridges. The same histogram would result from a surface with all of the high points collected together in one continuous ridge or distributed as thousands of tiny separate peaks. The properties of these two extreme surfaces would be quite different.

Just as for profiles, these statistical measures of amplitude are sensitive to the size of the sampled area. For most surfaces, the standard deviation increases with the number of points

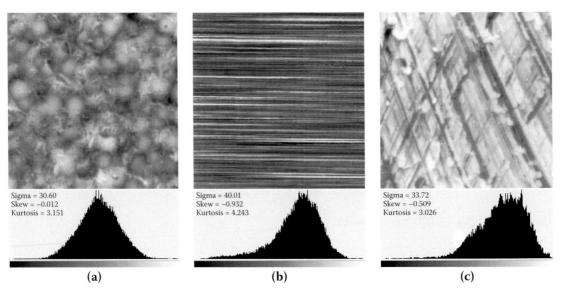

Sigma = 30.60
Skew = −0.012
Kurtosis = 3.151

Sigma = 40.01
Skew = −0.932
Kurtosis = 4.243

Sigma = 33.72
Skew = −0.509
Kurtosis = 3.026

(a) (b) (c)

Figure 14.35 *Histograms of elevation values for a few metal surfaces: (a) shot-blasted brass, which has a symmetrical distribution; (b) ground stainless steel, which has a slight negative skew due to the presence of a few deep but separated parallel grooves; (c) a plateau-honed cylinder liner with a negative skew resulting from the deep intersecting grooves that distribute lubricant.*

measured; in fact, for a fractal rough surface, the slope of a curve plotting the variance as a function of size on log-log axes is one of the ways used to measure the fractal dimension.

For profiles, the parameter Rz is the difference in elevation between the average of the five highest peaks and five lowest valleys. For an area scan of a surface, this is generalized to Sz, the difference between the ten highest peaks and ten lowest valleys. However, this is not purely an amplitude parameter because it depends critically on the definitions of a peak and a valley. They cannot be simply the highest and lowest points on the surface (or pixels in the surface image), since these could be (and often will be) adjacent to each other and would all represent a single peak and valley. For a profile, the presence of a low point separating two high points might be taken to indicate separate peaks. This is a flawed definition because infinitesimal irregularities should not be considered significant, and so some criterion for the depth and perhaps width of the valley between the peaks is required. But on an area scan of a surface, even more is needed because the peak (or valley) covers an area, and two or more local peaks may connect along intricate paths (a ridge) to be considered part of the same peak (and vice versa for valleys). In tracing this connectivity, it matters whether pixels are considered to touch all eight of their immediate neighbors or only the four that share edges with them.

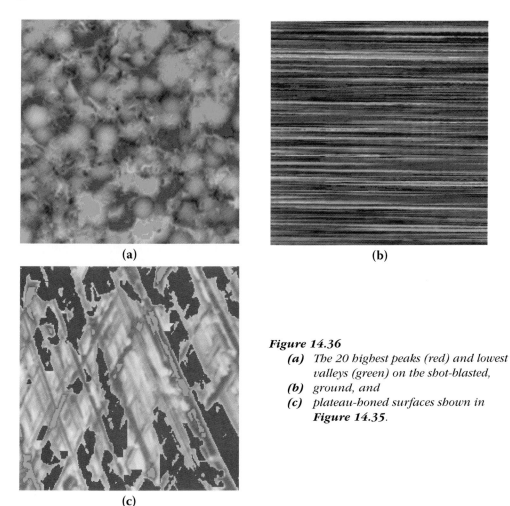

(a)

(b)

(c)

Figure 14.36
  (a) *The 20 highest peaks (red) and lowest valleys (green) on the shot-blasted,*
  (b) *ground, and*
  (c) *plateau-honed surfaces shown in Figure 14.35.*

There is much more information in the identification of peaks and valleys than just the Sz parameter that is the elevation difference between the average of the ten highest and ten lowest. Different surfaces give rise to very different shapes for peaks and valleys, and their sizes and shapes, orientation, and spacing can all contain important characterization information. In **Figure 14.36**, several examples are shown in which peaks are defined as eight-connected (pixels touch eight neighbors), and are required to be distinct down to 80% of the height of the peak. Valleys are defined in the same way. In this example, the 20 highest peaks and lowest valleys are found. The method is similar to the "flood fill" algorithm used in image processing, starting with the highest local maximum (and proceeding down) and including all touching pixels that extend down to the 80% limit, while checking to see if the peak merges into an existing labeled peak. Notice that, for the shot-blasted surface, the valleys are relatively smooth in outline, while the peaks are very irregular. Also, for the ground surface the peaks (ridges) tend to be broader than the valleys (crevices), and for the honed surface the peaks are very large, while the valleys are much smaller. All of these differences are consistent with our understanding of how such surfaces are produced, and they can give important insights into other surfaces and their functional performance (Sacerdotti et al. 2002).

Another parameter involving the peaks present on the surface is the number of them per unit area, called Sds. Again, this depends upon the definition of a peak as just discussed. It is likely that secondary information about the peaks will also be important in a variety of applications. For instance, the uniformity of spacing of the peaks can play a role in cases where the surfaces are involved in electrical or thermal contact, friction and wear, or to judge the visual and aesthetic appearance. As discussed under image measurement in **Chapter 10**, the mean nearest-neighbor distance can be used to determine the tendency toward uniform spacing or clustering by comparing the value with the mean distance that a Poisson random distribution of the same number of points per unit area would have. **Figure 14.37** shows the surface of an injection-molded polymer in which the peaks are relatively evenly spaced (a complex function of the surface finish of the die, the temperature, pressure and viscosity of the polymer, and its molecular weight). This uniformity, coupled with a spacing between peaks that is close to the spatial resolution limit of human vision, produces an aesthetically pleasing appearance for the product.

Note in the figure that the valleys have a very different shape and distribution than do the peaks. In some other applications, the same information about the density and uniformity of

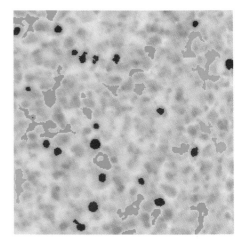

Figure 14.37 The highest 20 peaks and lowest 20 valleys in a 1-mm² area of the molded polymer surface from Figure 14.18. The peaks are color-coded from purple to red according to height and the valleys from green to cyan. Notice that one valley completely surrounds a small peak, and that the peaks are much more regular in shape than the valleys.

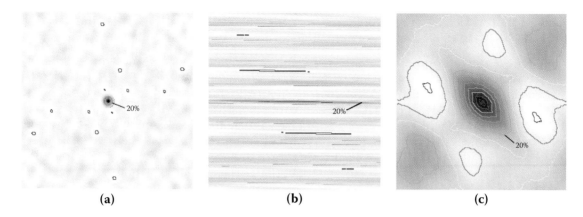

Figure 14.38 *Autocorrelation function calculated for: (a) the polymer surface from Figure 14.18; (b) the ground surface from Figure 14.1b; and (c) the flycut surface from Figure 14.1a, with superimposed contour lines indicating the shape of the function and the distance at which it drops to 20%.*

pits rather than peaks would be of interest. An example is the surfaces of plates used to retain ink for printing applications.

Surfaces with anisotropy or lay can be characterized by spatial parameters derived from the autocorrelation function. The autocorrelation function (ACF) is obtained by squaring the magnitude of the complex variables in the Fourier transform while setting the phase to zero, which removes all spatial location information. The inverse transform produces the two-dimensional spatial image of the ACF. The parameters defined from this function are the texture aspect ratio *Str*, the texture direction *Std*, and the autocorrelation length *Sal*. Understanding these may be helped by examining the ACF images in **Figure 14.38**. The autocorrelation length is defined in the Birmingham report as the shortest distance in which the magnitude of the ACF drops to 20%. For the examples shown, this is the minimum radius of the contour line drawn at the 20% intensity level. The texture aspect ratio is the ratio of the minimum radius to the maximum radius, and the texture direction is the orientation of the maximum radius.

For the examples in **Figure 14.38**, the ACF of the polymer surface (**Figure 14.18**) is quite isotropic (indicating that the surface is also isotropic), so the aspect ratio is unity and there is no pronounced direction. The ground surface (**Figure 14.1b**), on the other hand, has a strong preferred orientation that is evident in the ACF and can be measured there. For the flycut surface (**Figure 14.1a**), the texture is more complicated, as is indeed evident in the original image, which shows two predominant machining directions. The *Str*, *Std*, and *Sal* values as defined can, of course, be measured from the ACF, but it is not clear that they contain all of the information about the surface lay that would be desired for characterization.

The hybrid properties involve both the elevation and lateral data (as indeed do many of the preceding parameters). $S\Delta q$ is the root-mean-square slope of the surface, which can be calculated from the same triangular tiling procedure used to generate the visualizations shown earlier. Formally, it is defined as the square root of the mean value of the sum of squares of the derivatives of the image in the vertical and horizontal directions, which can be determined simply as the local difference of elevation values between adjacent pixels. The mean summit curvature *Ssc* is similarly related to the second derivatives of elevation, but calculated only for those pixels located at peaks. This depends, of course, on first arriving at a meaningful and accepted definition of which peaks are to be included. The third hybrid property is the ratio of the actual surface area to the projected area *Sdr*. This can be obtained by summing up the areas of the triangles making up the visualization.

None of these hybrid properties is very difficult to compute, but they all depend critically on the sampling interval or spacing of the pixels. Changing lateral resolution will alter the parameter values dramatically so that they are not really functions of the surface but of the measurement technique, and can be used only for comparisons in the most limited way. This is also the case for many of the profile-based measurements, but one of the goals in moving to area-based measurements was to overcome some of the limitations of the older methods. In fact, many engineering surfaces have been shown to have a fractal geometry whose actual surface area is undefined (it increases without limit as the lateral resolution of the measurements improves).

It is a more subtle point, but measurements like these also depend upon whether the elevation data at each pixel are samples of the surface or averages over the pixel area. The mathematics apply for the case of sampling, where the elevation at each pixel is measured at a precise mathematical point, and whatever happens between that pixel and the next is not taken into account. In fact, many measurement methods, such as those involving conventional stylus instruments and optical interferometers, perform some averaging of measurement over the entire area of the pixel, which can either report the maximum value in that area or a weighted average of the elevation values. The mathematics appropriate to these cases has not been worked out and would affect not just the hybrid parameters, but all of the parameters described here.

Functional parameters are intended to relate surface geometric data to specific aspects of surface performance, and these are generally related to mechanical engineering applications, since the greatest use of surface metrology has thus far been in that field. One typical example is the surface-bearing area ratio *Stp*, which is the fraction of the image area that would be in contact with a flat plane parallel to the base if a given height of all peaks was removed by wear (**Figure 14.39**). This value, of course, can be read directly from the histogram of the elevation data in the image.

Similarly, the amount of volume removed in the process (the material-volume ratio *Smr*) can be calculated by integrating the histogram or by using the cumulative histogram. The void-volume ratio *Svr* is the volume of empty space within the surface of the specimen that is available for retaining or distributing a lubricant. It is measured by integrating the spaces at each elevation level, but this can also be done efficiently using the cumulative histogram. **Figure 14.40** shows the same data from **Figure 14.39**, but here it is depicted as a surface visualization that reveals

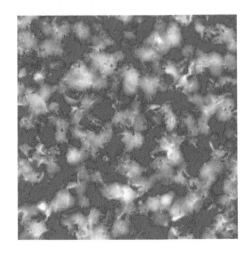

*Figure 14.39 Thresholding the range image (in this example the shot-blasted surface from **Figure 14.1d**) at any particular elevation (in this example 31% below the maximum value) shows the surface area that would be in contact with a plane after a corresponding amount of wear (in the absence of any elastic or plastic deformation).*

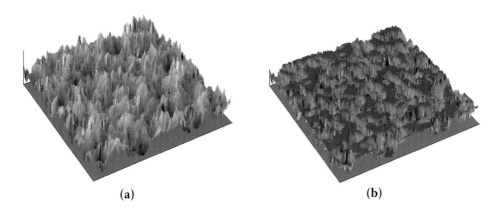

(a)   (b)

Figure 14.40 *Visualization of the data from **Figure 14.39**: (a) the original shot-blasted surface; (b) the same surface truncated 31% below the top of the highest peak, showing the contact areas and the void volume.*

the nature of the contact surface and the void volume after some of the peaks have been removed by wear (but assuming that there is no deformation of the remaining surface nor filling in of pits with debris).

There is really more information needed about the contact areas than these parameters provide. The size of the individual contacts is important for heating and deformation, and the void volume can either be completely connected, consist of isolated pockets, or be a mixture of the two, with very different consequences for lubrication. There are other functional parameters proposed to deal with these and other aspects of surface performance, but these become very specific to each application and will require considerable research to properly define or utilize. Many of them are handicapped to a significant degree because the surface elevation data in a range image are single-valued. The elevation recorded at each pixel is the maximum height at that point, as detected by a stylus or optical reflection, etc. Undercuts, caves, or pores within the surface that do not show up in the range image can become important if wear removes some of the surface overburden.

Image processing and analysis using the tools already developed in preceding chapters can be used to obtain many of the parameters of interest for surfaces from range images. For example, min and max ranking operators (gray-scale erosion and dilation) can be used to modify the image to form the envelope of the surface that a contact of known form would feel, creating a two-dimensional form of the previously mentioned motif logic for profiles. Cross-correlation with the image of a defect (crack, dust particle, etc.) can be used to locate such defects. Measurement of features obtained by thresholding can provide data on the contact areas and their distribution after wear has modified a surface. Skeletonization of the pore volume can be used to determine its connectivity as a pathway to distribute lubricants. Using these tools is straightforward once the significant parameters have been determined so that their relationships to surface behavior and history can be assessed.

Topographic analysis and fractal dimensions

The limitations and inadequacies of the traditional methods of analysis discussed above prevent them from fully describing real surfaces. They are primarily being used for process control

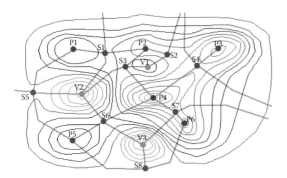

Figure 14.41 *A contour map representing a surface, with the peaks (red), valleys (green), and saddle points (purple) marked.*

applications in mechanical engineering, where comparison of measurements with prior history provides an indication of change, so long as the measurement technique and instrumentation remain unchanged. Newer methods have become available, but their full meaning and interpretation remain to be explored. It is hoped that these new approaches can provide more insight into the description and makeup of surfaces.

Human vision uses global topographic information to organize information on surfaces (Scott 1995). The arrangement of hills and dales, ridges, courses, and saddle points contains quite a bit of information for describing a surface. A landscape or surface can be divided into regions consisting of hills (points from which all uphill paths lead to one particular peak) and dales (points from which all downhill paths lead to a pit). Boundaries between hills are courses, and boundaries between dales are ridge lines (**Figure 14.41**).

A Pfalz graph (Pfalz 1976) or change tree (**Figure 14.42**) connecting the peaks and dales through the respective saddle points where ridge and course lines meet summarizes the topological structure. The change tree can represent directly the height difference and lateral distance between features, which makes decisions straightforward about eliminating features that have either small vertical or lateral extent. This is a direct extension to surfaces of the motif combination used for profiles. Scott (1997) has proposed methods for dealing with the finite extent of real images and the corrections necessary for dealing with the intersection of ridges and courses with the edges of the image area. It is not yet clear just how this information will

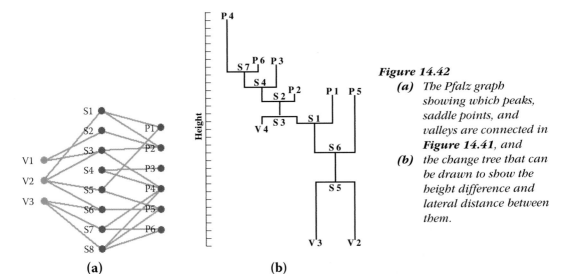

Figure 14.42
(a) *The Pfalz graph showing which peaks, saddle points, and valleys are connected in* **Figure 14.41**, *and*
(b) *the change tree that can be drawn to show the height difference and lateral distance between them.*

(a)

(b)

be used for surface measurement, but parameters such as the volume of connected valleys, the spatial distribution of valleys and peaks across the surface, and orientation of watercourses and ridges seem likely to be important for surface characterization.

At quite a different extreme of local roughness, many surfaces (but emphatically not all) are characterized by a self-similarity (or, more exactly, a self-affinity) that can be described by a fractal dimension. There are several ways to measure this (which do not exactly agree numerically), plus the need to provide an additional parameter that describes the magnitude of the roughness, and perhaps others to describe the directionality of the surface. The appeal of the fractal dimension is that it is not dependent on the measurement scale, and that it summarizes much of the "roughness" of surfaces in a way that seems to correspond to both the way nature works and the way humans perceive roughness. Given a series of surfaces, the "rougher" the surface as it appears to human interpretation (for a variety of basic reasons), the higher the fractal dimension. At the same time, it must be noted that the recognition of fractal geometry (even the name) is comparatively new, and there is a "bandwagon" tendency that probably causes it to be applied where it should not be, or to be used with more enthusiasm than critical thinking.

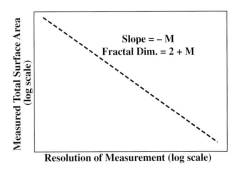

Figure 14.43 *Schematic diagram of fractal-dimension measurement: as the measurement resolution becomes smaller, the total measured area increases.*

The fractal dimension of a surface is a real number greater than 2 (the topological dimension of the surface) and less than 3 (the topological dimension of the space in which the surface exists). A perfectly smooth surface (dimension 2.0) corresponds to Euclidean geometry, and a plot of the actual area of the measured area as a function of measurement resolution would not change. But for real surfaces, an increase in the magnification or resolution with which it is examined will reveal more nooks and crannies, and the surface area will increase. For a surprising variety of natural and human-made surfaces, a plot of the area as a function of resolution is linear on a log-log graph, and the slope of this curve gives the dimension D, as shown in **Figure 14.43**.

This description comes directly from the earlier recognition that boundary lines around islands had a length that depended upon the measurement scale. A so-called Richardson plot of the length of the west coast of Britain (Mandelbrot 1967) as a function of the length of the measurement tool showed this log-log relationship and was one of the triggering ideas that led Mandelbrot to study the mathematics of self-similar structures (ones that appear equally irregular at all scales) and to coin the name "fractal" for the field. Many other subsequent publications have shown that an extremely broad variety of surfaces also exhibit this kind of geometry, have investigated a number of ways to measure the dimension, and have begun to study the relationships between the dimension and the history and performance characteristics of surfaces.

Measuring the surface area over a range of resolutions is in fact a rather difficult thing to do (one way is by adsorbing molecules of different sizes), and for basic reasons, measurement is not actually appropriate for many surfaces because they are not ideally self-similar. For most surfaces, the lateral directions and the normal direction are distinct in dimension and physical properties, which means that the scaling or self-similarity that exists in one direction may not be the same as in the others. At a sufficiently large scale, most surfaces approach an ideal Euclidean flat surface. For anisotropic surfaces, this situation is more severe, and even lateral directions are different. This means that the surfaces are mathematically self-affine rather than self-similar. The fact that elevation measurements are single-valued and cannot reveal undercuts means that the measured data would be self-affine even for a truly self-similar surface (for instance, one produced by diffusion-limited aggregation of particles on a substrate). For self-affine surfaces and data sets, there are still a variety of correct and practical measurement techniques. A few of the more practical ones are summarized here. (A more complete discussion is available in Russ [1994].)

In most cases, the most robust measure of the fractal dimension uses the same procedure that can characterize surfaces that are not ideally fractal or perfectly isotropic (Russ 2001b). The Fourier power spectrum can also be used to characterize the instrumental response function, to distinguish it from the surface information. Instead of the usual display mode for the power spectrum, a plot of log (magnitude) vs. log (frequency) reveals a fractal surface as a straight-line plot whose slope gives the dimension. The principal drawbacks to using the power-spectrum plot to measure the dimension are that it tends to overestimate the numerical value of the dimension for relatively smooth surfaces (dimensions between 2.0 and about 2.3), and that the numerical precision of the measured value is lower than some of the other methods can provide for images of a given size. **Figure 14.44** shows an example of the power-spectrum plot for a fractal surface, whose slope gives the fractal dimension.

Generating the two-dimensional Fourier transform of the surface range image reveals any fractal anisotropy (which can be either weak anisotropy in which the dimension is the same in all directions but the magnitude is not, or strong anisotropy in which the dimension also varies). Plotting the slope and intercept of the plot of log (magnitude) vs. log (frequency) as a function of orientation provides a quantitative tool to describe the fractal anisotropy. **Figure 14.45** shows an example. The separation of the low-frequency data that describes the figure and the high frequencies that often reveal instrument limitations from the intermediate frequencies can be used to isolate the surface fractal dimension.

By itself, the fractal dimension is only a partial description of surface roughness, even for ideally fractal surfaces. Stretching the surface vertically to increase the magnitude of the roughness does not change the slope of the power spectrum or the fractal dimension.

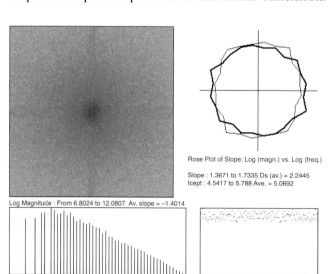

Rose Plot of Slope: Log (magn.) vs. Log (freq.)

Slope : 1.3671 to 1.7335 Ds (av.) = 2.2445
Icept : 4.5417 to 5.788 Ave. = 5.0692

Log Magnitude : From 6.8024 to 12.0807 Av. slope = −1.4014

0.4043   Log frequency ->   4.852   Phase (0.2π)

*Figure 14.44 The Fourier-transform power spectrum (upper left) of the shot-blasted metal image (**Figure 14.1d**), with its subsequent analysis. The plot of log magnitude vs. log frequency (lower left) averaged over all directions shows a linear relationship that confirms the fractal behavior, and whose slope gives the dimension (2.24). A rose plot of the slope of as a function of orientation (upper left, bold line) shows that the surface is isotropic and has the same dimension in all directions. The thin line on the same plot shows the intercept of the plot as a function of direction, which is a measure of the amplitude of the roughness and also shows isotropy for this surface. Finally, a plot of the distribution of phases of the terms in the Fourier transform shows them to be uniformly random, which is required for a fractal.*

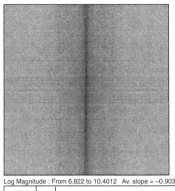

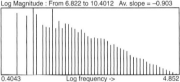

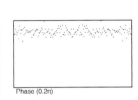

Rose Plot of Slope: Log (magn.) vs. Log (freq.)

Slope : 0.8218 to 1.1862 Ds (av.) = 2.509
Icept : 4.966 to 6.5227 Ave. = 5.5424

Log Magnitude : From 6.822 to 10.4012   Av. slope = –0.903

0.4043   Log frequency ->   4.852

Phase (0.2π)

*Figure 14.45 The same data presentation as in **Figure 14.44**, but for the anisotropic ground surface shown in **Figure 14.1b**. Both the slope and intercept of the power-spectrum plot are different in the vertical and horizontal directions. The surface is an anisotropic fractal.*

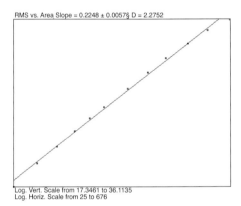

RMS vs. Area Slope = 0.2248 ± 0.0057§ D = 2.2752

Log. Vert. Scale from 17.3461 to 36.1135
Log. Horiz. Scale from 25 to 676

***Figure 14.46** Plot of mean variance vs. neighborhood size to determine the fractal dimension of the shot-blasted surface (same image as **Figure 14.44**).*

An additional measure, which has units of length, is needed to characterize the magnitude. The intercept of the plot of the power spectrum has units of length and can be used for this purpose. So can the topothesy, defined as the horizontal distance over which the mean angular change in slope is 1 radian.

There are a variety of other measurement approaches that can be properly used with self-affine fractal surfaces. Two widely used techniques that deal with the range image of the surface directly are the covering blanket and the variogram. Both work correctly for isotropic surfaces, but they do not reveal anisotropy and can produce nonsense values in those cases rather than an average. The latter is simply a plot of the variance in elevation values as a function of the size of the measured region. Values from small areas placed systematically or randomly over the surface are averaged, and a single mean value obtained. This process is repeated at many different sizes, and a plot (**Figure 14.46**) is made that gives the dimension.

The covering-blanket or Minkowski method measures the difference (summed over the entire image) between an upper and lower envelope fitted to the surface as a function of the size of the neighborhood used. The minimum and maximum brightness rank operators discussed under image processing are applied with different-diameter neighborhoods, and the total difference between them is added up. This is analogous to the Minkowski dimension for a profile that was described in **Chapter 8**, obtained by using the Euclidean distance map to measure the area as a function of distance from the boundary line. The covering-blanket method produces a plot that gives a dimension, as shown in **Figure 14.47**. Notice that these three methods give only approximate agreement as to the numerical value of the dimension. Part of this is just the result of limited measurement precision, but part of the difference arises from the fact that all of these techniques measure something that is slightly different. These values are limits to the actual dimension and generally will not agree, so when comparisons are being made between

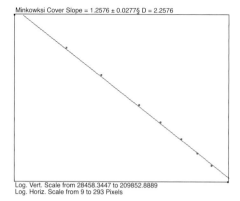

Minkowksi Cover Slope = 1.2576 ± 0.0277§ D = 2.2576

Log. Vert. Scale from 28458.3447 to 209852.8889
Log. Horiz. Scale from 9 to 293 Pixels

Figure 14.47 Plot of the Minkowski cover volume as a function of neighborhood size to determine the fractal dimension (same image as Figure 14.46).

surfaces, it is important to always use one technique for all of the measurements.

It is often attractive to perform measurements in a lower dimension, since a smaller number of data points are involved. Historically, much of the work with fractal measurement has been done with boundary lines, whose dimension lies between 1.0 (the Euclidean or topological dimension of a line) and 1.999... (a line whose irregularity is so great that it wanders across an entire plane). There is a way to do this with fractal surfaces, by intersecting the surface with a plane and then measuring the dimension of the line that is the intersection. It is vitally important, however, that this plane be parallel to the nominal surface orientation rather than a vertical cut. The vertical cut would produce the same profile as that obtained with a profilometer, but because the surface is self-affine and not self-similar, the proper measurement of this profile is complicated and the common techniques, such as the Richardson plot mentioned above, do not apply. Also, of course, the profile will be oriented in a particular direction and cannot be used with anisotropic surfaces.

The horizontal cut is called a slit-island method, and it corresponds exactly to the case Richardson was dealing with. The horizontal plane corresponds to sea level, and the outlines are the coastlines of the islands produced by the hills that rise above the sea. A plot of the length of these coastlines as a function of measurement scale produces a dimension that is exactly 1 less than the surface dimension (the difference between the topological dimensions of a surface and a line). Usually, it is not convenient to measure the length of a coastline on a digital image in a computer using the same procedure that Richardson did, by setting a pair of dividers to a particular scale length and "striding" around the coastline so that the boundary length was the divider setting times the number of strides. But there are a variety of other methods that are readily implemented in a computer.

The analog to the Minkowski blanket for the surface is a Minkowski sausage produced by thickening the boundary line by various amounts and plotting the area covered vs. the width of the stripe or sausage. The Euclidean distance map discussed in **Chapter 8** on binary image processing accomplishes this procedure very efficiently and without the directional variation that results from conventional pixel-based dilation. Another method is box-counting (**Figure 14.48**), in which a grid is placed on the image and the number of squares through which the boundary line passes is counted as a function of the size of the grids. While these methods are quite fast, they are only applicable to isotropic surfaces. Most real surfaces, and certainly the most interesting ones, are not isotropic.

It is beyond the scope of this text to discuss the relationships that have been found between fractal dimensions and various aspects of the history and properties of surfaces. In brief, most processes of surface formation that involve brittle fracture or deposit large amounts of energy in small regions tend to produce fractal surfaces, and the numerical value of the dimension is often a signature of the process that was involved (Russ 1997). Likewise, many surface-contact applications (electrical, thermal, etc.) depend upon the relationship between contact area and pressure, and fractal geometry is also pertinent to this case. Under some circumstances, friction and wear may also be related to the surface dimension. Fractal description of surfaces

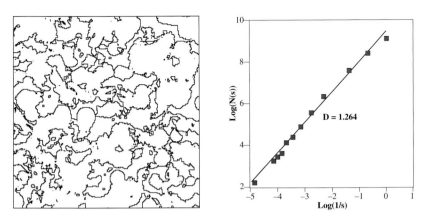

Figure 14.48 *Contour lines produced by thresholding the image from* **Figure 14.1d** *at 50% of its elevation range, and the plot from a box-counting measurement.*

is a new and somewhat "trendy" approach to surface characterization. While it clearly offers powerful methods that apply to some surfaces, it is inappropriate for other surfaces such as ductile deformation.

References

M. Abbasi-Dezfouli, T. G. Freeman (1994). Patch matching in stereo-images based on shape. *ISPRS Int. Arch. Photogrammetry Remote Sensing* 30: 1–8.

A. S. Abutaleb (1989). Automatic thresholding of gray level pictures using two-dimensional entropy. *Computer Vision Graphics Image Process.* 47: 22–32.

Agfa Compugraphic Division (1992). *Digital Color Prepress*, Vols. 1 and 2. Agfa Corp., Wilmington, MA.

M. Aguilar, E. Anguiano et al. (1992). Digital filters to restore information from fast scanning tunneling microscopy images. *J. Microscopy* 165(2): 311–324.

E. H. Aigeltinger, K. R. Craig, R. T. DeHoff (1972). Experimental determination of the topological properties of three-dimensional microstructures. *J. Microsc.* 95: 69–81.

H. Alto et al. (2005). Content-based retrieval and analysis of mammographic masses. *J. Electronic Imaging* 14: 023016.

M. R. Anderberg (1973). *Cluster Analysis for Applications*. Academic Press, New York.

Y. Anguy et al. (2005). Practical modelling of porous media from second-order statistics: the phase-retrieval problem and the interpretation of covariance. *J. Microscopy* 220(3): 140–149.

G. R. Arce, J. L. Paredes, J. Mullan (2000). Nonlinear filtering for image analysis and enhancement. In *Handbook of Image and Video Processing* (A. Bovic, Ed.). Academic Press, San Diego.

J. Arvo (Ed.) (1991). *Graphics Gems II*. Academic Press, San Diego, CA.

J. Astola, P. Haavisto, Y. Neuvo (1990). Vector median filters. *Proc. IEEE* 78: 678.

N. Baba, M. Naka, Y. Muranaka, S. Nakamura, I. Kino, K. Kanaya (1984). Computer-aided stereographic representation of an object constructed from micrographs of serial thin sections. *Micron Microscopica Acta* 15: 221–226.

N. Baba, M. Baba, M. Imamura, M. Koga, Y. Ohsumi, M. Osumi, K. Kanaya (1989). Serial section reconstruction using a computer graphics system: application to intracellular structures in yeast cells and to the periodontal structure of dogs' teeth. *J. Electron Microsc. Tech.* 11: 16–26.

J. V. Bacus, J. W. Bacus (2000). Method and Apparatus for Acquiring and Reconstructing Magnified Specimen Images from a Computer-Controlled Microscope. U.S. patents 6,101,265, 6,226,392, 6,272,235, 6,404,906, 6,522,774, 6,775,402.

J. W. Bacus, J. V. Bacus (2002). Method and apparatus for Internet, intranet and local viewing of virtual microscope slides. U.S. patents 6,396,941, 6,674,881.

A. J. Baddeley, H. J. G. Gundersen, L. M. Cruz-Orive (1986). Estimation of surface area from vertical sections. *J. Microsc.* 142: 259–276.

A. J. Baddeley, C. V. Howard, A. Boyde, S. Reid (1987). Three-dimensional analysis of the spatial distribution of particles using the tandem-scanning reflected light microscope. *Acta Stereol.* 6(Suppl. 2): 87–100.

Y. Balagurunathan, E. R. Dougherty (2003). Morphological quantification of surface roughness. *Optical Eng.* 42(6): 1795–1804.

R. Balasubramanian, C. A. Bouman, J. P. Allebach (1994). Sequential scalar quantization of color images. *J. Electronic Imaging* 3: 45–59.

D. Ballard (1981). Generalizing the Hough transform to detect arbitrary shapes. *Pattern Recognition* 13: 111–122.

D. H. Ballard, C. M. Brown (1982). *Computer Vision*. Prentice Hall, Englewood Cliffs, NJ.

D. H. Ballard, C. M. Brown, J. A. Feldman (1984). An approach to knowledge-directed image analysis. In *Computer Vision Systems* (A. R. Hanson and E. M. Riseman, Eds.). Academic Press, New York, pp. 271–282.

S. T. Barnard, W. B. Thompson (1980). Disparity analysis of images. *IEEE Trans. Pattern Anal. Machine Intelligence (PAMI)* 2: 333–340.

F. L. Barnes, S. G. Azavedo, H. E. Martz, G. P. Roberson, D. J. Schneberk, M. F. Skeate (1990). Geometric Effects in Tomographic Reconstruction. Rept. UCRL-ID-105130. Lawrence Livermore National Laboratory, Livermore, CA.

M. Barni (Ed.) (2006). *Document and Image Compression*. CRC Press, Boca Raton, FL.

M. F. Barnsley (1988). *Fractals Everywhere*. Academic Press, Boston.

M. F. Barnsley, et al. (1986). Solutions of an inverse problem for fractals and other sets. *Proc. Nat'l Acad. Sci.* 83: 1975–1977.

M. F. Barnsley, L. P. Hurd (1993). *Fractal Image Compression*, A. J. Peters, Wellesley, MA.

M. F. Barnsley, A. D. Sloan (1991). Method and Apparatus for Processing Digital Data. U.S. patent 5,065,447.

H. G. Barth, S.-T. Sun (1985). Particle size analysis. *Anal. Chem.* 57: 151.

A. Barty, K. A. Nugent, A. Roberts, D. Paganin (2000). Quantitative phase tomography. *Optics Communications* 175: 329–336.

S. Battiato et al. (2003). High dynamic range imaging for digital and still camera: an overview. *J. Electronic Imaging* 12: 459–469.

A. L. D. Beckers, A. W. M. Smeulders (1989). The probability of a random straight line in two and three dimensions. *Pattern Recognit. Let.* 11(4): 233–240.

J. K. Beddow, G. C. Philip, A. F. Vetter (1977). On relating some particle profiles characteristics to the profile Fourier coefficients. *Powder Technol.* 18: 15–19.

M. Beil et al. (2005). Quantitative analysis of keratin filament networks in scanning electron microscopy images of cancer cells. *J. Microsc.* 220: 84–95.

G. Bertrand, J.-C. Everat, M. Couprie (1997). Image segmentation through operators based on topology. *J. Electronic Imaging* 6: 395–405.

V. Berzins (1984). Accuracy of Laplacian edge detectors. *Computer Vision Graphics Image Process.* 27: 1955–2010.

P. J. Besl, N. D. McKay (1992). A method for registration of 3-D shapes. *IEEE Trans. Pattern Anal. Machine Intelligence (PAMI)* 14: 239–256.

S. Beucher, C. Lantejoul (1979). Use of watersheds in contour detection. In *Proc. Int. Workshop Image Process.* CCETT, Rennes, France.

G. B. Binnig, C. F. Quate, C. Gerber (1986). Atomic force microscope. *Phys. Rev. Lett.* 52: 930.

J. L. Bird, D. T. Eppler, D. M. Checkley, Jr. (1986). Comparisons of herring otoliths using Fourier series shape analysis. *Can. J. Fish. Aquat. Sci.* 43: 1228–1234.

W. J. Black (1986). *Intelligent Knowledge-Based Systems: An Introduction*. Van Nostrand Reinhold, London.

R. A. S. Blackie, R. Bagby, L. Wright, J. Drinkwater, S. Hart (1987). Reconstruction of three-dimensional images of microscopic objects using holography. *Proc. R. Microscopical Soc.* 22: 98.

F. Boddeke (1998). Quantitative Fluorescence Microscopy. ASCI Dissertation Series, Delft University Press, Delft, Netherlands.

F. R. Boddeke, L. J. van Vliet, H. Netten, I. T. Young (1994). Autofocusing in microscopy based on the OTF and sampling. *Bioimaging* 2: 193–203.

J. Bollmann et al. (2004). Automated particle analysis: calcareous microfossils. In *Image Analysis, Sediments and Paleoenvironments* (E. Francus, Ed.). Springer, Dordrecht, Netherlands, p. 229.

G. Borgefors (1996). On digital distance transforms in three dimensions. *Computer Vision Image Understanding* 64: 368–376.

G. Borgefors, I. Nystrom, G. Sanniti di Baja (1999). Computing skeletons in three dimensions. *Pattern Recognition* 32: 1225–1236.

S.-T. Bow (1992). *Pattern Recognition and Image Preprocessing*. Marcel Dekker, New York.

A. Boyde (1973). Quantitative photogrammetric analysis and quantitative stereoscopic analysis of SEM images. *J. Microsc.* 98: 452.

A. Boyde (2004). Improved depth of field in the scanning electron microscope derived from through-focus image stacks. *Scanning* 26: 265–269.

B. Bracegirdle, S. Bradbury (1995). *Modern Photomicrography*. Bios Scientific, Oxford, U.K.

R. N. Bracewell (1984). The fast Hartley transform. *Proc. IEEE* 72: 8.

R. N. Bracewell (1986). *The Hartley Transform*. Oxford University Press, Oxford, U.K.

R. N. Bracewell (1989). The Fourier transform. *Sci. Am.* June, 62–69.

S. Bradbury, B. Bracegirdle (1998). *Introduction to Light Microscopy*. Bios Scientific, Oxford, U.K.

M. von Bradke et al. (2004). Porosity determination of ceramic materials by digital image analysis — a critical examination. *Scanning* 27: 132–135.

G. Braudaway (1987). A procedure for optimum choice of a small number of colors from a large color palette for color imaging. In *Proc. Electronic Imaging '87*. San Francisco.

L. G. Briarty, P. H. Jenkins (1984). GRIDSS: an integrated suite of microcomputer programs for three-dimensional graphical reconstruction from serial sections. *J. Microsc.* 134: 121–124.

D. S. Bright, E. B. Steel (1986). Bright field image correction with various image processing tools. In *Microbeam Analysis* (A. D. Romig, Ed.). San Francisco Press, San Francisco, CA, pp. 517–520.

D. S. Bright, D. E. Newbury, R. B. Marinenko (1988). Concentration-concentration histograms: scatter diagrams applied to quantitative compositional maps. In *Microbeam Analysis* (D. E. Newbury, Ed.). San Francisco Press, San Francisco, pp. 18–24.

A. D. Brink, N. E. Pendcock (1989). Minimum cross-entropy threshold selection. *Pattern Recognition* 29: 179–188.

P. Brodatz (1966). *Textures: A Photographic Album for Artists and Designers.* Dover, New York.

L. G. Brown (1992). A survey of image registration techniques. *ACM Computing Surveys* 24: 325–376.

M. Brown, D. G. Lowe (2003). Recognizing panoramas. In *Proc. Int. Conf. Computer Vision*, Nice, France, pp. 1218–1225.

M. Brown et al. (2005). Multi-image matching using multi-scale oriented patches. In *Proc. Int. Conf. Computer Vision and Pattern Recognition*, San Diego, CA.

D. Bruton (2005). Available online at www.physics.sfasu.edu/astro/color.html.

R. K. Bryan, J. Skilling (1980). Deconvolution by maximum entropy, as illustrated by application to the jet of M87. *Mon. Notes R. Astron. Soc.* 191: 69–79.

M. A. Buena-Ibarra et al. (2005). Fast autofocus algorithm for automated microscopes. *Optical Eng.* 44: 3601.

M. Bueno et al. (2005). Polychromatic image fusion algorithm and fusion metric for automatized microscopes. *Optical Eng.* 44: 93201.

H-E. Bühler, H. P. Hougardy (1980). *Atlas of Interference Layer Metallography.* Deutsche Gesellschaft für Metallkunde, Oberursel, Germany.

V. Buzuloiu, M. Ciuc, R. M. Rangayyan, C. Vertan (2001). Adaptive-neighborhood histogram equalization of color images. *J. Electronic Imaging* 10: 445–459.

J. Canny (1986). A computational approach to edge detection. *IEEE Trans. Pattern Anal. Machine Intelligence (PAMI)* 8: 679–698.

A. S. Carasso (2001). Direct blind deconvolution. *SIAM J. Appl. Math.* 61: 1980–2007.

I. C. Carlsen (1985). Reconstruction of true surface topographies in scanning electron microscopes using backscattered electrons. *Scanning* 7: 169–177.

W. A. Carrington (1990). Image restoration in 3D microscopy with limited data. In *Bioimaging and Two Dimensional Spectroscopy*, Proc. SPIE (L. C. Smith, Ed.) 1205: 72–83.

J. E. Castle, P. A. Zhdan (1997). Characterization of surface topography by SEM and SFM: problems and solutions. *J. Phys. D: Appl. Phys.* 30: 722.

J. E. Castle et al. (1998). Enhanced morphological reconstruction of SPM images. *J. Phys. D: Appl. Phys.* 31: 3437–3445.

K. R. Castleman (1979). *Digital Image Processing.* Prentice Hall, Englewood Cliffs, NJ.

K. R. Castleman (1996). *Digital Image Processing.* Prentice Hall, Upper Saddle River, NJ.

R. L. T. Cederberg (1979). Chain-link coding and segmentation for raster scan devices. *Computer Graphics Image Process.* 10: 224–234.

Y. Censor (1983). Finite series expansion reconstruction methods *Proc. IEEE* 71:409–419.

Y. Censor (1984). Row-action methods for huge and sparse systems and their applications. *SIAM. Rev.* 23(4): 444–466.

D. Chappard et al. (2005). Microcomputed tomography for the study of hard tissues and bone biomaterials. *Microsc. Anal.* 5: 23–25.

Y-S Chen et al. (2005). Efficient fuzzy c-means clustering for image data. *J. Electronic Imaging* 14: 013017.

P. Chieco, A. Jonker, C. Melchiorri, G. Vanni, C. J. F. van Noorden (1994). A user's guide for avoiding errors in absorbance image cytometry. *Histochemical J.* 26: 1-19.

S. K. Chow et al. (2006). Automated microscopy system for mosaic acquisition and processing, *J. Microscopy* 22(2): 76–84.

C. K. Chui (1992). *An Introduction to Wavelets.* Academic Press, London.

F. Ciurea, B. Funt (2004). Tuning retinex parameters. *J. Electronic Imaging* 13: 58–64.

J. R. B. Cockett (1987). Decision expression optimization. *Fundamenta Informaticae* 10: 93–114.

L. Cohen (1991). On active contour models and balloons. *Computer Vision Graphics Image Process.* 53: 211–218.

M. L. Comer, E. J. Delp (1999). Morphological operations for color image processing. *J. Electronic Imaging* 8: 279–289.

J. Condeco, L. H. Christensen, S. F. Jorgensen, J. C. Russ, B.-G. Rosen (2000). A comparative study of image stitching algorithms for surface topography measurements. *Proc. X Int. Colloq. on Surfaces*, Chemnitz, Germany.

J. Cookson (1994). Three-dimensional reconstruction in microscopy. *Proc. R. Microscopical Soc.* 29: 3–10.

J. W. Cooley, J. W. Tukey (1965). An algorithm for the machine calculation of complex Fourier series. *Math. Comp.* 19: 279–301.

T. J. Cooper, F. A. Baqal (2004). Analysis and extensions of the Frankle-McCann retinex algorithm, *J. Electronic Imaging* 13: 85–92.

A. M. Cormack (1963). Representation of a function by its line integrals with some radiological applications. *J. Appl. Phys.* 34: 2722–2727.

A. M. Cormack (1964). Representation of a function by its line integrals with some radiological applications II. *J. Appl. Phys.* 35: 2908–2913.

T. N. Cornsweet (1970). *Visual Perception.* Academic Press, New York.

L. F. Costa, R. M. Cesar (2001). *Shape Analysis and Classification.* CRC Press, Boca Raton, FL.

L. Costaridou (Ed.) (2005). *Medical Image Analysis Methods.* CRC Press, Boca Raton, FL.

M. Coster, J.-L. Chermant (1985). *Précis D'Analse D'Images.* Éditions du Centre National de la Recherche Scientifique, Paris.

L.-M. Cruz-Orive (1976). Particle size-shape distributions: the general spheroid problem. *J. Microsc.* 107: 235; 112: 153.

L.-M. Cruz-Orive (1983). Distribution-free estimation of sphere size distributions from slabs showing over-projections and truncation, with a review of previous methods. *J. Microsc.* 131: 265.

L. M. Cruz-Orive (2005). A new stereological principle for test lines in three-dimensional space. *J. Microsc.* 219: 18–28.

P. E. Danielsson (1980). Euclidean distance mapping. *Computer Graphics Image Process.* 14: 227–248.

I. Daubechies (1992). Ten lectures on wavelets. In *CBMS-NSF Regional Conf. Series Appl. Math.* Philadelphia.

I. Daubechies (1996). Where do wavelets come from? A personal point of view. *Proc. IEEE* 84: 510–513.

D. G. Daut, D. Zhao, J. Wu (1993). Double predictor differential pulse coded modulation algorithm for image data compression. *Optical Eng.* 32: 1514–1523.

J. Davidson (1991). Thinning and skeletonization: a tutorial and overview. In *Digital Image Processing: Fundamentals and Applications* (E. Dougherty, Ed.). Marcel Dekker, New York.

E. R. Davies (1988). On the noise suppression and image enhancement characteristics of the median, truncated median and mode filters. *Pattern Recognition Lett.* 7: 87–97.

P. E. Debevec, J. Malik (1997). Recovering high dynamic range radiance maps from photographs. *Siggraph 1997,* Los Angeles.

H. W. Deckman, K. L. D'Amico, J. H. Dunsmuir, B. P. Flannery, S. M. Gruner (1989). Microtomography detector design. *Adv. X-Ray Anal.* 32: 641.

R. T. Dehoff, F. N. Rhines (1968). *Quantitative Microscopy.* McGraw Hill, New York.

D. DeMandolx, J. Davoust (1997). Multicolor analysis and local image correlation in confocal microscopy. *J. Microsc.* 185: 21–36.

D. R. Denley (1990a). Scanning tunneling microscopy of rough surfaces. *J. Vac. Sci. Technol.* A8(1): 603–607.

D. R. Denley (1990b). Practical application of scanning tunneling microscopy. *Ultramicroscopy* 33: 83–92.

P. A. Devijver, J. Kittler (1980). *Pattern Recognition: A Statistical Approach.* Prentice-Hall, Englewood Cliffs, NJ.

N. Dey et al. (2006). Richardson–Lucy algorithm with total variation regularization for 3D confocal microscope deconvolution. *Microsc. Res. Techn.* 69: 260–266.

G. Diaz, A. Zuccarelli, I. Pelligra, A. Griani (1989). Elliptic Fourier analysis of cell and nuclear shapes. *Comput. Biomed. Res.* 22: 405–414.

G. Diaz, D. Quacci, C. Dell'Orbo (1990). Recognition of cell surface modulation by elliptic Fourier analysis. *Computer Methods Programs Biomed.* 31: 57–62.

M. Dietzsch, K. Papenfuss, T. Hartmann (1997). The MOTIF method (ISO 12085): a suitable description for functional manufactural and metrological requirements. In *7th Int. Conf. Metrology and Properties of Engineering Surfaces* (B. G. Rosen, R. J. Crafoord, Eds.). Chalmers University, Göteborg, Sweden, pp. 231–238.

E. R. Dougherty, J. Astola (1994). *An Introduction to Nonlinear Image Processing.* SPIE, Bellingham, WA.

E. R. Dougherty, J. Astola (1999). *Nonlinear Filters for Image Processing.* SPIE, Bellingham, WA.

N. Draper, H. Smith (1981). *Applied Regression Analysis,* 2nd ed. Wiley, New York.

R. O. Duda, P. E. Hart (1972). Use of the Hough transform to detect lines and curves in pictures. *Commun. ACM* 15: 11–15.

R. O. Duda, P. E. Hart (1973). *Pattern Classification and Scene Analysis.* Wiley, New York.

F. Durand, J. Dorsey (2002). Fast bilateral filtering for the display of high dynamic range images. *ACM Trans. Graphics,* Proc. 2002 Siggraph Conf., San Antonio.

T. R. Edwards (1982). Two-dimensional convolute integers for analytical instrumentation. *Anal. Chem.* 54: 1519–1524.

M. Egmont-Petersen et al. (2002). Image processing with neural networks: a review. *Pattern Recognition* 35: 2279–2301.

R. Ehrlich, B. Weinberg (1970). An exact method for characterization of grain shape. *J. Sedimentation Petrol.* 40: 205–212.

R. Ehrlich, S. K. Kennedy, S. J. Crabtree, R. L. Cannon (1984). Petrographic image analysis: 1, analysis of reservoir pore complexes. *J. Sedimentation Petrol.* 54: 1365–1378.

P. A. van den Elsen, J. B. A. Maintz, E.-J. D. Pol, M. A. Viergever (1995). Automatic registration of CT and MR brain images using correlation of geometrical features. *IEEE Trans. Medical Imaging (MI)* 14: 384–396.

P. A. van den Elsen, E.-J. D. Pol, T. S. Sumanaweera, P. F. Hemler, S. Napel, J. R. Adler (1994). Grey value correlation techniques used for automatic matching of CT and MR brain and spine images. *SPIE Int. Conf. Visualization Biomedical Computing* 2359: 227–337.

P. A. van den Elsen, E.-J. D. Pol, M. A. Viergever (1993). Medical image matching: a review with classification. *IEEE Eng. Med. Biol.* 12: 26–39.

A. Engel, A. Massalski (1984). 3D reconstruction from electron micrographs: its potential and practical limitations. *Ultramicroscopy* 13: 71–84.

Y. Fahmy, J. C. Russ, C. Koch (1991). Application of fractal geometry measurements to the evaluation of fracture toughness of brittle intermetallics. *J. Mater. Res.* 6: 1856–1861.

C. Faloutsos, W. Equitz, M. Flickner, W. Niblack, D. Perkovic, R. Barber (1994). Efficient and effective querying by image content. *J. Intelligent Information Systems* 3: 231–262.

J. Feder (1988). *Fractals.* Plenum Press, New York.

L. A. Feldkamp, L. C. Davis, J. W. Kress (1984). Practical cone beam algorithm. *J. Opt. Soc. Am.* 1: 612.

S. F. Ferson, F. J. Rohlf, R. K. Koehn (1985). Measuring shape variation of two-dimensional outlines. *Systematic Zool.* 34: 59–68.

J. Fiala (2005). Reconstruct: a free editor for serial section microscopy. *J. Microsc.* 218: 52–61.

L. F. Firestone, K. Cook et al. (1991). Comparison of autofocus methods for automated microscopy. *Cytometry* 12: 195–206.

Y. Fisher, E. W. Jacobs, and R. D. Boss (1992). Fractal image compression using iterated transforms. In *Image and Text Compression* (J. A. Storer, Ed.). Kluwer Academic, Boston, pp. 35–61.

M. Flickner, H. Sawhney, W. Niblack, J. Ashley, Q. Huang (1995). Query by image and video content: the QBIC system. *IEEE Computer* 28: 23–32.

A. G. Flook (1978). Use of dilation logic on the Quantimet to achieve fractal dimension characterization of texture and structured profiles. *Powder Tech.* 21: 295–298.

A. G. Flook (1982). Fourier analysis of particle shape. In *Particle Size Analysis 1981–82* (N. G. Stanley-Wood, T. Allen, Eds.). Wiley Heyden, London.

J. D. Foley, A. Van Dam (1984). *Fundamentals of Interactive Computer Graphics.* Addison Wesley, Reading, MA.

J. D. Foley, A. Van Dam (1995). *Fundamentals of Interactive Computer Graphics*, 2nd ed. Addison Wesley, Reading, MA.

B. Forster et al. (2004). Complex wavelets for extended depth-of-field: a new method for the fusion of multichannel microscopy images. *Microsc. Res. Techn.* 65(1–2): 33–42.

I. France et al. (2004). Software aspects of automated recognition of particles: the example of pollen. In *Image Analysis, Sediments and Paleoenvironments* (E. Francus Ed.). Springer, Dordrecht, Netherlands, pp. 253–272.

E. Francus (Ed.) (2004). *Image Analysis, Sediments and Paleoenvironments*, Vol. 7. Springer, Dordrecht, Netherlands.

P. Francus, E. Pinard (2004). Testing for sources of errors in quantitative image analysis. In *Image Analysis, Sediments and Paleoenvironments*, Vol. 7 (E. Francus, Ed.). Springer, Dordrecht, Netherlands, p. 87.

J. Frank (Ed.) (1992). *Electronics Tomography.* Plenum Press, New York.

R. J. Frank, T. J. Grabowski, H. Damasio (1995). Voxelwise percentage tissue segmentation of human brain magnetic resonance images. In *Abstracts, 25th Annual Meeting, Soc. Neurosci.*, Washington, DC, p. 694; cited in M. Sonka, V. Hlavac, R. Boyle (1999). *Image Processing, Analysis and Machine Vision.* Brooks Cole, Pacific Grove, CA, p. 132.

M. Frederik, A. Collignon, D. Vandermeulen, P. Suetens, G. Marchal (1997). Multi-modality image registration by maximization of mutual information. *IEEE Trans. Medical Imaging (MI)* 16: 187–198.

H. Freeman (1961). On the encoding of arbitrary geometric configurations. *IEEE Trans. EC* 10: 260–268.

H. Freeman (1974). Computer processing of line-drawing images. *Computer Surveys* 6: 57–97.

H. Freeman, L. S. Davis (1977). A corner finding algorithm for chain-code curves. *IEEE Trans. Comput. (C)* 26: 297–303.

W. Frei (1977). Image enhancement by histogram hyperbolization. *Computer Graphics Image Process.* 6: 286–294.

W. Frei, C. C. Chen (1977). Fast boundary detection: a generalization and a new algorithm. *IEEE Trans. Comput. (C)* 26: 988–998.

B. R. Frieden (1988). A comparison of maximum entropy, maximum a posteriori and median window restoration algorithms. In *Scanning Microscopy*, Suppl. 2 (P. Hawkes et al., Eds.). Scanning Microscopy International, Chicago, pp. 107–111.

J. P. Frisby (1980). *Vision: Illusion, Brain and Mind*. Oxford University Press, Oxford, U.K.

K. S. Fu (1974). *Syntactic Methods in Pattern Recognition*. Academic Press, Boston.

K. S. Fu, J. K. Mui (1981). A survey on image segmentation. *Pattern Recognition* 13: 3–16.

K. S. Fu (1982). *Syntactic Pattern Recognition and Applications*. Prentice-Hall, Englewood Cliffs, NJ.

H. Fuchs, S. M. Pizer, L. C. Tsai, S. H. Bloomburg, E. R. Heinz (1982). Adding a true 3-D display to a raster graphics system. *IEEE Comput. Graphics Appl.* 2: 73–78.

K. Fukunaga (1990). *Statistical Pattern Recognition*, 2nd ed. Academic Press, Boston.

B. Funt et al. (2004). Retinex in MATLAB. *J. Electronic Imaging* 13: 48–57.

R. S. Gentile, J. P. Allebach, E. Walowit (1990). Quantization of color images based on uniform color spaces. *J. Imaging Technol.* 16: 12–21.

S. Geuna (2005). The revolution of counting "tops": two decades of the Disector principle in morphological research. *Microsc. Res. Tech.* 66: 270–274.

O. Ghita et al. (2005). Computational approach for depth from defocus. *J. Electronic Imaging* 14: 023021.

T. H. Goldsmith (2006). What birds see, *Scient. Amer.* 294(6): 68–75.

A. M. Gokhale et al. (2004). Design-based estimation of surface area in thick tissue sections of arbitrary orientation using virtual cycloids. *J. Microsc.* 216: 25–31.

O. Gomes, S. Paciornik (2005). Automatic classification of graphite in cast iron. *Microsc. Microanal.* 11: 363–371.

R. C. Gonzalez, P. Wintz (1987). *Digital Image Processing*, 2nd ed. Addison Wesley, Reading, MA.

R. C. Gonzalez, R. E. Woods (1993). *Digital Image Processing*. Addison Wesley, Reading, MA.

R. Gordon (1974). A tutorial on ART (algebraic reconstruction techniques). *IEEE Trans. NS* 21: 78–93.

A. Goshtasby (2005). *2-D and 3-D Image Registration for Medical, Remote Sensing and Industrial Applications*. Wiley, Hoboken, NJ.

Y. A. Gowayed, J. C. Russ (1991). Geometric characterization of textile composite preforms using image analysis techniques. *J. Computer Assisted Microsc.* 3: 189–200.

G. H. Granlund (1972). Fourier preprocessing for hand print character recognition. *IEEE Trans. Comput. (C)* 21: 195–201.

A. Grasselli (Ed.) (1969). *Automatic Interpretation and Classification of Images*. Academic Press, Boston.

C. Gratin, F. Meyer (1992). Morphological three-dimensional analysis. *Scanning Microsc.* Suppl. 6: 129–135.

F. C. A. Green, I. T. Young, G. A. Lighart (1985). A comparison of different focus functions for use in autofocus algorithms. *Cytometry* 6: 81–91.

S. Greenberg, D. Kogan (2005). Structure-adaptive anisotropic filter applied to fingerprints. *Optical Eng.* 44(12): 127004.

D. A. Grigg, P. E. Russell, et al. (1992). Probe characterization for scanning probe metrology. *Utramicroscopy* 42–44: 1616–1620.

W. Grimson (1981). *From Images to Surfaces*. MIT Press, Cambridge, MA.

S. Grossberg (Ed.) (1988). *Neural Computers and Natural Intelligence*. MIT Press, Cambridge, MA.

P. Gualtieri, P. Coltelli (1991). An automated system for the analysis of moving images. *J. Computer Assisted Microsc.* 3: 15–22.

H. J. G. Gundersen (1986). Stereology of arbitrary particles. *J. Microsc.* 143: 3–45.

H. J. G. Gundersen (2002). The smooth fractionator, *J. Microscopy* 207: 191–210.

H. J. G. Gundersen et al. (1988). Some new, simple and efficient stereological methods and their use in pathological research and diagnosis. *Acta Pathologica, Microbiologica Immunologica Scandinavica* 96: 857.

H. J. G. Gundersen, E. B. Jensen (1987). The efficiency of systematic sampling in stereology and its prediction. *J. Microsc.* 147: 229–263.

D.-P. Hader (Ed.) (1992). *Image Analysis in Biology*. CRC Press, Boca Raton, FL.

J. Hajnal et al. (2001). *Medical Image Registration*. CRC Press, Boca Raton, FL.

K. J. Halford, K. Preston (1984). 3-D skeletonization of elongated solids. *Computer Vision Graphics Image Process.* 27: 78–91.

Y. S. Ham (1993). Differential Absorption Cone-Beam Microtomography. Ph.D. thesis. North Carolina State University, Raleigh, NC.

D. J. Hand (1981). *Discrimination and Classification*. Wiley, New York.

R. Hanke (2003). Microanalysis by volume computed tomography. *GIT Imaging Microsc.* 4: 40–43.

R. M. Haralick (1978). Statistical and structural approaches to texture. In *Proc. 4th Int. Joint Conf. Pattern Recognition*, Kyoto, p. 45.

R. Haralick (1979). Statistical and textural approaches to textures. *Proc. IEEE* 67: 786–804.

R. M. Haralick, I. Dinstein (1975). A spatial clustering procedure for multi-image data. *Computer Graphics Image Process.* 12: 60–73.

R. M. Haralick, L. G. Shapiro (1988). Segmentation and its place in machine vision. *Scanning Microsc. Suppl.* 2: 39–54.

R. M. Haralick, L. G. Shapiro (1992). *Computer and Robot Vision*, Vol. I. Addison Wesley, Reading, MA.

R. M. Haralick, K. Shanmugam, I. Dinstein (1973). Textural features for image classification. *IEEE Trans. Syst. Manage. Cybern. (SMC)* 3: 610–621.

J. A. Hartigan (1975). *Clustering Algorithms.* John Wiley & Sons, New York.

R. V. L. Hartley (1942). A more symmetrical Fourier analysis applied to transmission problems. *Proc. IRE.* 30: 144–150.

S. Haykin (1993). *Neural Networks.* Macmillan, New York.

D. Hearn, M. P. Baker (1986). *Computer Graphics.* Prentice Hall, Englewood Cliffs, NJ.

J. Heath (2005). *Dictionary of Microscopy.* Wiley, New York.

M. Heath, S. Sarkar, T. Sanocki, and K. W. Bowyer (1997). A robust visual method for assessing the relative performance of edge-detection algorithms. *IEEE Trans. Pattern Anal. Machine Intelligence (PAMI)* 19: 1338–1359.

D. O. Hebb (1949). *The Organization of Behaviour.* John Wiley, New York.

P. Heckbert (1982). Color image quantization for frame buffer display. *Computer Graphics* 16: 297–307.

R. Hegerl (1989). Three-dimensional reconstruction from projections in electron microscopy. *European J. Cell Biol.* 48(Suppl. 25): 135–138.

H. Heijmans (1991). Theoretical aspects of grey-level morphology. *IEEE Trans. Pattern Anal. Machine Intelligence (PAMI)* 13: 568–582.

H. Heijmans (1994). *Morphological Image Operators.* Academic Press, New York.

C. Heipke (1992). A global approach for least-squares image matching and surface reconstruction in object space. *Photogrammetric Eng. Remote Sensing* 58: 317–323.

J. Van Helden (1994). CrestPathway algorithm. Personal communication.

L. Helfen et al. (2003). Determination of structural properties of light materials. *GIT Imaging Microsc.* 4: 55–57.

H. R. J. R. Van Helleputte, T. B. J. Haddeman, M. J. Verheijen, J.-J. Baalbergen (1995). Comparative study of 3D measurement techniques (SPM, SEM, TEM) for submicron structures. *Microelectronic Eng.* 27: 547.

G. T. Herman (1980). *Image Reconstruction from Projections: The Fundamentals of Computerized Tomography.* Academic Press, New York.

E. C. Hildreth (1983). The detection of intensity changes by computer and biological vision systems. *Computer Vision Graphics Image Process.* 22: 1–27.

K. Hoffmann et al. (2005). Simple tool for the standardisation of confocal spectral imaging systems. *GIT Imaging Microsc.* 3: 18–19.

H. Hogan (2005). Where's that picture? *Biophotonics Int.* July: 32–36.

T. J. Holmes, S. Bhattacharyya, J. A. Cooper, D. Hanzel, V. Krishnamurti (1995). Light microscopic images reconstructed by maximum likelihood deconvolution. In *Handbook of Biological Confocal Microscopy* (J. Pawley, Ed.). Plenum Press, New York, pp. 389–402.

T. J. Holmes, N. J. O'Connor (2000). Blind deconvolution of 3D transmitted light brightfield micrographs. *J. Microsc.* 200: 114–127.

B. J. Holt, L. Hartwick (1994). Visual image retrieval for applications in art and art history. In *Proc. Storage and Retrieval for Image and Video Databases II.* SPIE, San Jose, CA.

L. Holzer et al. (2004). Three-dimensional analysis of porous $BaTiO_3$ ceramics using FIB nanotomography. *J. Microsc.* 216: 84–95.

B. K. P. Horn (1970). Shape from Shading: A Method for Obtaining the Shape of a Smooth Opaque Object from One View. AI Tech Report 79, Project MAC. MIT, Cambridge, MA.

B. K. P. Horn (1975). Obtaining shape from shading information. In *Psychology of Computer Vision* (P. H. Winston, Ed.). McGraw Hill, New York, pp. 115–155.

P. Hough (1962). Method and Means for Recognizing Complex Patterns. U.S. patent 3,069,654.

C. V. Howard, M. G. Reed (1998). *Unbiased Stereology: Three Dimensional Measurements in Stereology.* BIOS Scientific, Oxford, U.K.

C. V. Howard, M. G. Reed (2005). *Unbiased Stereology: Advanced Methods.* BIOS Scientific Publ. Oxford, UK.

J. Hsieh (2003). *Computed Tomography.* SPIE Press, Bellingham, WA.

J. Huang, S. M. Dunn, S. M. Wiener, P. DeCosta (1994). A method for detecting correspondences in stereo pairs of electron micrographs of networks. *J. Computer Assisted Microsc.* 6: 85–102.

T. S. Huang (1979). A fast two dimensional median filtering algorithm. *IEEE Trans. ASSP* 27: 13–18.

D. H. Hubel (1988). *Eye, Brain, and Vision*. Scientific American Library, W. H. Freeman, New York.

H. E. Hurst, R. P. Black, Y. M. Simaika (1965). *Long Term Storage: An Experimental Study*. Constable, London.

C. Hwang, S. Venkatraman, K. R. Rao (1993). Human visual system weighted progressive image transmission using lapped orthogonal transform classified vector quantization. *Optical Eng.* 32: 1524–1530.

S. Inoué (1986). *Video Microscopy*. Plenum Press, New York.

S. Inoué, K. R. Spring (1997). *Video Microscopy — The Fundamentals*, 2nd ed. Plenum Press, New York.

B. Jahne (1997). *Practical Handbook on Image Processing for Scientific Applications*. CRC Press, Boca Raton, FL.

A. K. Jain (1989). *Fundamentals of Digital Image Processing*. Prentice Hall, London.

A. Jalba et al. (2004). Automatic segmentation of diatom images for classification. *Microsc. Res. Tech.* 65: 72–85.

M. James (1988). *Pattern Recognition*. Blackwell Scientific, London.

J. Jan (2005). *Medical Image Processing, Reconstruction and Restoration*. CRC Press, Boca Raton, FL.

J. R. Janesick (2001). *Scientific Charge-Coupled Devices*. SPIE Press, Bellingham, WA.

K. F. Jarausch, T. J. Stark, P. E. Russell (1996). Silicon structures for in-situ characterization of atomic force microscopy probe geometry. *J. Vac. Sci. Technol. B* 14: 3425.

E. T. Jaynes (1985). Where do we go from here? In *Maximum Entropy and Bayesian Methods in Inverse Problems* (C. R. Smith, W. T. Grandy, Eds.). D. Reidel Publishing, Dordrecht, Holland, pp. 21–58.

J. P. Jernot (1982). Thèse de Doctorat és Science, Université de Caen, France.

E. M. Johnson, J. J. Capowski (1985). Principles of reconstruction and three-dimensional display of serial sections using a computer. In *The Microcomputer in Cell and Neurobiology Research* (R. R. Mize, Ed.). Elsevier, New York, pp. 249–263.

L. R. Johnson, A. K. Jain (1981). An efficient two-dimensional FFT algorithm. *IEEE Trans. Pattern Anal. Machine Intelligence (PAMI)* 3: 698–701.

Q. C. Johnson, J. H. Kinney, U. Bonse, M. C. Nichols, R. Nusshardt, J. M. Brase (1986). *Micro-Tomography Using Synchrotron Radiation*. Preprint UCRL-93538A. Lawrence Livermore National Laboratory, Livermore, CA.

S. Joshi, M. I. Miller (1993). Maximum a posteriori estimation with good roughness for 3D optical sectioning microscopy. *J. Opt. Soc. Am. A* 10: 1078–1085.

M. Kaes, A. Witkin, D. Terzopoulos (1987). Snakes: active contour models. *J. Computer Vision* 1: 321–331.

A. C. Kak, M. Slaney (1987, 2001). *Principles of Computerized Tomographic Imaging*. SIAM, Philadelphia.

C. Kak, M. Slaney (1988). Principles of Computerized Tomographic Imaging. Pub. PC-02071. IEEE Computer Society Press, Washington, DC.

H. R. Kang (1997). *Color Technology for Electronic Imaging Devices*. SPIE Optical Engineering Press, Bellingham, WA.

H. R. Kang (1999). *Digital Color Halftoning*. SPIE Optical Engineering Press, Bellingham, WA.

L.-W. Kang, J.-J. Leon (2005). Fast indexing and searching strategies for feature-based image database systems. *J. Electronic Imaging* 14: 013019.

J. N. Kapur, P. K. Sahoo, A. K. C. Wong (1985). A new method for gray-level picture thresholding using the entropy of the histogram. *Computer Vision Graphics Image Process.* 29: 273–285.

N. Karssemeijer et al. (Eds.) (1998). *Digital Mammography*. Kluwer Academic, New York.

M. Kass, A. Witkin, D. Terzopoulos (1987). Snakes: active contour models. *Int. J. Computer Vision* 1: 321–331.

A. E. Kayaalp, R. C. Jain (1987). Using SEM stereo to extract semiconductor wafer pattern topography. *Proc. SPIE* 775: 18–26.

B. H. Kaye (1986). Image analysis procedures for characterizing the fractal dimension of fine particles. In *Proc. Particle Technol. Conf.*, Nuremberg, Germany.

B. H. Kaye (1989). *A Random Walk through Fractal Dimensions*. VCH Publishers, Weinheim, Germany.

B. H. Kaye, J. E. LeBlanc, G. Clark (1983). A study of physical significance of three-dimensional signature waveforms. In *Proc. Fine-Particle Characterization Conference*.

A. Keating (1993). Personal communication. Duke University, Durham, NC.

D. J. Keller (1991). Reconstruction of STM and AFM images distorted by finite-size tips. *Surf. Sci.* 253: 353–364.

D. J. Keller, F. S. Franke (1993). Envelope reconstruction of probe microscope images. *Surf. Sci.* 294: 409–419.

G. M. P. Van Kempen, L. J. Van Vliet, P. J. Verveer, H. T. M. Van der Voort (1997). A quantitative comparison of image restoration methods in confocal microscopy. *J. Microsc.* 185: 354–365.

M. R. Khadivi (1990). Iterated function system. In *Generating Fractal Fractures Models, Scaling in Disordered Materials: Fractal Structures and Dynamics*, Materials Research Society, Pittsburgh, PA, pp. 49–51.

D-W. Kim, K-S. Hong (2006). Real-time mosaic using sequential graph, *J. Electron. Imag.* 15(2): 023005.

S. Kim, J. Lee, J. Kim (1988). A new chain-coding algorithm for binary images using run-length codes. *Computer Vision Graphics Image Process.* 41: 114–128.

S. H. Kim, J. P. Allebach (2005). Optimal unsharp mask for image sharpening and noise removal. *J. Electronic Imaging* 14: 023005.

J. H. Kinney, Q. C. Johnson, M. C. Nichols, U. Bonse, R. A. Saroyan, R. Nusshardt, R. Pahl (1989). X-ray microtomography on beamline X at SSRL. *Rev. Sci. Instrum.* 60: 2471–2747.

J. H. Kinney, M. C. Nichols, U. Bonse, S. R. Stock, T. M. Breunig, A. Guvenilir, R. A. Saroyan (1990). Nondestructive imaging of materials microstructures using X-ray tomographic microscopy. *Proc. MRS Symposium on Tomographic Imaging*, Boston, p. 3.

R. Kirsch (1971). Computer determination of the constituent structure of biological images. *Comput. Biomed. Res.* 4: 315–328.

J. Kittler, J. Illingworth, J. Foglein (1985). Threshold selection based on a simple image statistic. *Computer Vision Graphics Image Process.* 30: 125–147.

V. Kober, M. Mozerov, J. Alvarez-Borrego (2001). Nonlinear filters with spatially connected neighborhood. *Optical Eng.* 40: 971–983.

L. P. Kok (1990). *100 Problems of My Wife, and Their Solution in Theoretical Stereology.* Coulomb Press, Leyden, Netherlands.

H. Kotera, H. Wang (2005). Multiscale image sharpening adaptive to edge profile. *J. Electronic Imaging* 14: 013002.

A. Kriete (Ed.) (1992). *Visualization in Biomedical Microscopies: 3-D Imaging and Computer Applications*, VCH, Weinheim, Germany.

C. Kubel et al. (2005). Recent advances in electron tomography: TEM and HAADF-STEM tomography for materials science and semiconductor applications. *Microsc. Microanal.* 11: 378–400.

L. Kubinova, J. Janacek (2001). Confocal microscope and stereology: estimating volume, number, surface area and length by virtual test probes applied to three-dimensional images. *Microsc. Res. Tech.* 53: 425–435.

F. P. Kuhl, C. R. Giardina (1982). Elliptic Fourier features of a closed contour. *Computer Graphics Image Process.* 18: 236–258.

K. J. Kurzydlowski, B. Ralph (1995). *The Quantitative Description of the Microstructure of Materials.* CRC Press, Boca Raton, FL.

M. Kuwahara, K. Hachimura, S. Eiho, and M. Kinoshita (1976). Processing of RI-angiocardiographic images. In *Digital Processing of Biomedical Images* (K. Preston and M. Onoe, Eds.). Plenum, New York, pp. 187–202.

R. L. Lagendijk, J. Biemond (1991). *Iterative Identification and Restoration of Images.* Kluwer Academic, Boston, MA.

L. Lam, S. Lee, C. Suen (1992). Thinning methodologies: a comprehensive survey. *IEEE Trans. Pattern Anal. Machine Intelligence (PAMI)* 14: 868–885.

C. Lantejoul, S. Beucher (1981). On the use of the geodesic metric in image analysis. *J. Microsc.* 121: 39.

R. S. Ledley, M. Buas, T. J. Golab (1990). Fundamentals of true-color image processing. *Proc. Int. Conf. Pattern Recognition* 1: 791–795.

D. L. Lee, A. T. Winslow (1993). Performance of three image-quality metrics in ink-jet printing of plain papers. *J. Electronic Imaging* 2: 174–184.

S. U. Lee, S. Y. Chung, R. H. Park (1990). A comparative performance study of several global thresholding techniques for segmentation. *Computer Vision Graphics Image Process.* 52: 171–190.

Z. Les, M. Les (2005). Shape understanding system: understanding of the complex object. *J. Electronic Imaging* 14: 023015.

P. E. Lestrel (Ed.) (1997). *Fourier Descriptors and Their Applications in Biology.* Cambridge University Press, Cambridge.

J. Y. Lettvin, R. R. Maturana, W. S. McCulloch, W. H. Pitts (1959). What the frog's eye tells the frog's brain. *Proc. Inst. Rad. Eng.* 47: 1940–1951.

S. Levialdi (1972). On shrinking binary picture patterns. *Commun. ACM* 15: 7–10.

H. Li, M. Novak, R. Forchheimer (1993). Fractal-based image sequence compression scheme. *Optical Eng.* 32: 1588–1595.

B. Lichtenbelt, R. Crane, S. Naqvi (1998). *Introduction to Volume Rendering.* Prentice Hall, Saddle River, NJ.

W. Lin, T. J. Holmes, D. H. Szarowski, J. N. Turner (1994). Data corrections for three-dimensional light microscopy stereo pair reconstruction. *I. Computer Assisted Microsc.* 6: 113–128.

M. Lineberry (1982). Image segmentation by edge tracing. *Appl. Digital Image Process,* IV, 359.

S. Lobregt, P. W. Verbeek, F. C. A. Groen (1980). Three-dimensional skeletonization: principle and algorithm. *IEEE Trans. Pattern Anal. Machine Intelligence (PAMI)* 2: 75–77.

R. L. Luck et al. (1993). Morphological Classification System and Method. U.S. patent 5,257,182.

E. Mach (1906). Über den Einfluss räumlich und zeitlich variierender Lichtreize auf die Gesichtswahrnehmung. *S.-B. Akad. Wiss. Wien, Math.-Nat. Kl.* 115: 633–648.

J. B. MacQueen (1967). Some methods for the classification and analysis of multivariate observations. *Proc. 5th Berkeley Symposium on Mathematical Statistics and Probability.* 1: 281–297.

E. Mainsah, K. J. Stout, T. R. Thomas (2001). Surface measurement and characterization. In *Metrology and Properties of Engineering Surfaces* (E. Mainsah, Ed.). Kluwer Academic, London, pp. 1–42.

S. G. Mallat (1989). A theory for multiresolution signal decomposition: the wavelet representation. *IEEE Trans. Pattern Anal. Machine Intelligence (PAMI)* 11: 674–693.

T. Malzbender, D. Gelb, D. Wolters (2001). Polynomial texture maps. In *Computer Graphics, Proc. Siggraph 2001,* Los Angeles, CA, pp. 519–528.

B. B. Mandelbrot (1967). How long is the coast of Britain? Statistical self-similarity and fractional dimension. *Science* 155: 636–638.

B. B. Mandelbrot (1982). *The Fractal Geometry of Nature.* W. H. Freeman, San Francisco.

B. B. Mandelbrot, D. E. Passoja, A. J. Paullay (1984). Fractal character of fracture surfaces of metals. *Nature* 308: 721.

R. Mann, S. Stanley, D. Vlaev, E. Wabo, K. Primrose (2001). Augmented reality visualization of fluid mixing in stirred chemical reactors using electrical resistance tomography. *J. Electronic Imaging* 10: 620–629.

P. Markiewicz, M. C. Goh (1994). Atomic force microscopy probe tip visualization and improvement of images using a simple deconvolution procedure. *Langmuir* 10: 5–7.

P. Markiewicz, M. C. Goh (1995). Atomic force microscope tip deconvolution using calibration arrays. *Rev. Sci. Instrum.* 66: 3186–3190.

D. Marr (1982). *Vision.* W. H. Freeman, San Francisco.

D. Marr, E. Hildreth (1980). Theory of edge detection. *Proc. R. Soc. Lond.* B207: 187–217.

D. Marr, T. Poggio (1976). Cooperative computation of stereo disparity. *Science* 194: 283–287.

M. De Marsicoi, L. Cinque, S. Levialdi (1997). Indexing pictorial documents by their content: a survey of current techniques. *Image Vision Computing* 15: 119–141.

C. G. Masi (2005). Dynamic structured light measures shapes. *Vision Systems Design* March 2005: 15–20.

G. A. Mastin (1985). Adaptive filters for digital image noise smoothing: an evaluation. *Computer Vision Graphics Image Process.* 31: 102–121.

Y. A. T. Mattfeldt (2005). Explorative statistical analysis of planar point processes in microscopy. *J. Microsc.* 220(3): 131–139.

A. D. McAulay, J. Wang, J. Li (1993). Optical wavelet transform classifier with positive real Fourier transform wavelets. *Optical Eng.* 32: 1333–1339.

J. J. McCann (2004). Capturing a black cat in shade: past and present of retinex color appearance models, *J. Electronic Imaging* 13: 36–47.

W. S. McCulloch, W. Pitts (1943). A logical calculus of the ideas immanent in nervous activity. *Bull. Math. Biophys.* 5: 115.

J. J. Mecholsky, D. E. Passoja (1985). Fractals and brittle fracture. In *Fractal Aspects of Materials.* Materials Research Society, Pittsburgh.

J. J. Mecholsky, T. J. Mackin, D. E. Passoja (1986). Crack propagation in brittle materials as a fractal process. In *Fractal Aspects of Materials II.* Materials Research Society, Pittsburgh.

J. J. Mecholsky, D. E. Passoja, K. S. Feinberg-Ringel (1989). Quantitative analysis of brittle fracture surfaces using fractal geometry. *J. Am. Ceram. Soc.* 72: 60.

G. Medioni, R. Nevatia (1985). Segment-based stereo matching. *Computer Vision Graphics Image Process.* 31: 2–18.

F. Melgani (2006). Robust image binarization with ensembles of thresholding algorithms, *J. Electron. Imag.* 15(2): 023010.

P. Miché et al. (2005). Passive 3-D shape recovery of unknown objects using cooperative polarimetric and radiometric stereo vision processes. *Optical Eng.* 44 (2): 027005.

D. L. Milgram (1975). Computer methods for creating photomosaics. *IEEE Trans. Comput. (C)* 24: 1113–1119.

D. L. Milgram, M. Herman (1979). Clustering edge values for threshold selection. *Computer Graphics Image Process.* 10: 272–280.

M. Minsky, S. Papert (1969). *Perceptrons: An Introduction to Computational Geometry.* MIT Press, Cambridge, MA.

M. W. Mitchell, D. A. Bonnell (1990). Quantitative topographic analysis of fractal surfaces by scanning tunneling microscopy. *J. Mater. Res.* 5: 2244–2254.

S. Mitra, T. Acharya (2003). *Data Mining. Multimedia, Soft Computing and Bioinformatics.* Wiley, Hoboken, NJ.

J. Modersitzki (2004). *Numerical Methods for Image Registration.* Oxford University Press, Oxford, U.K.

J. R. Monck, A. F. Oberhauser, T. J. Keating, J. M. Hernandez (1992). Thin-section ratiometric Ca^{2+} images obtained by optical sectioning of Fura-2 loaded mast cells. *J. Cell Biol.* 116: 745–759.

C. Montagne et al. (2006). Adaptive color quantization using the baker's transformation, *J. Electron. Imag.* 15(2): 023015

H. P. Moravec (1977). Towards automatic visual obstacle avoidance. *Proc. 5th IJCA* I: 584.

R. B. Mott (1995). Position-tagged spectrometry, a new approach for EDS spectrum imaging. In *Proc. Microscopy and Microanalysis.* Jones & Begall, New York, p. 595.

J. C. Mott-Smith (1970). Medial axis transformations. In *Picture Processing and Psychopictorics* (B. S. Lipkin and A. Rosenfeld, Eds.). Academic Press, New York.

P. Mouton (2002). *Principles and Practices of Unbiased Stereology: An Introduction for Bioscientists.* Johns Hopkins University Press, Baltimore.

H. R. Myler, A. R. Weeks (1993). *Pocket Handbook of Image Processing Algorithms in C.* Prentice Hall, Englewood Cliffs, NJ.

J. Nakamura (Ed.) (2006). *Image Sensors and Signal Processing for Digital Still Cameras.* CRC Press, Boca Raton, FL.

K. S. Nathan, J. C. Curlander (1990, February). Reducing speckle in one-look SAR images. *NASA Tech. Briefs,* 70.

F. Natterer (2001). *The Mathematics of Computerized Tomography.* SIAM, Philadelphia.

F. Natterer, F. Wubbeling (2001). *Mathematical Methods in Image Reconstruction.* SIAM, Philadelphia.

B. Neal, J. C. Russ, J. C. Russ (1998). A super-resolution approach to perimeter measurement. *J. Computer Assisted Microsc.* 10: 11–22.

B. Neal, J. C. Russ (2004). Principal components analysis of multispectral images. *Microsc. Today* 12(5): 36.

A. J. Nederbracht et al. (2004). Image calibration, filtering and processing. In *Image Analysis, Sediments and Paleoenvironments* (E. Francus, Ed.). Springer, Dordrecht, Netherlands, pp. 35–58.

C. V. Negoita, D. A. Ralescu (1975). *Applications of Fuzzy Sets to Systems Analysis.* Halsted Press, New York.

C. V. Negoita, D. A. Ralescu (1987). *Simulation, Knowledge-Based Computing, and Fuzzy Statistics.* Van Nostrand Reinhold, New York.

R. Nevatia, K. Babu (1980). Linear feature extraction and description. *Computer Graphics Image Process.* 13: 257–269.

W. Niblack (Ed.) (1993). Storage and retrieval for image and video databases. *SPIE Proc.* 1908.

A. Nicoulin, M. Mattavelli, W. Li, M. Kunt (1993). Subband image coding using jointly localized filter banks and entropy coding based on vector quantization. *Optical Eng.* 32: 1430–1450.

A. Nieminen, P. Heinonen, Y. Nuevo (1987). A new class of detail-preserving filters for image processing. *IEEE Trans. Pattern Anal. Machine Intelligence (PAMI)* 9: 74–90.

N. Nikolaidis, I. Pitas (2001). *3-D Image Processing Algorithms.* Wiley, New York.

J. F. O'Callaghan (1974). Computing the perceptual boundaries of dot patterns. *Computer Graphics Image Process.* 3: 141–162.

K. Oistämö, Y. Neuvo (1990). Vector median operations for color image processing. In *Nonlinear Image Processing* (E. J. Delp, Ed.). *SPIE Proc.* 1247: 2–12.

C. K. Olsson (1993). Image Processing Methods in Materials Science. Ph.D. thesis. Technical University of Denmark, Lyngby.

J. D. Ortiz, S. O'Connell (2004). Toward a non-linear grayscale calibration method for legacy photographic collections. In *Image Analysis, Sediments and Paleoenvironments* (E. Francus, Ed.). Springer, Dordrecht, Netherlands, pp. 125–141.

N. Otsu (1979). A threshold selection method from gray-level histograms. *IEEE Trans. Syst. Manage. Cybern. (SMC)* 9: 62; 377–393.

D. R. Overby, M. Johnson (2005). Studies on depth-of-field effects in microscopy supported by numerical simulations. *J. Microsc.* 220(3): 176–189.

I. Overington (1976). *Vision and Acquisition.* Pentech Press, London.

I. Overington (1992). *Computer Vision: A Unified Biologically Inspired Approach.* Elsevier, Amsterdam.\

Y. A. Ozkaya et al. (2005). Digital image processing and illumination techniques for yarn characterization. *J. Electr. Imaging* 14(2): 023001.

M. Pancorbo, E. Anguiano et al. (1991). New filtering techniques to restore scanning tunneling microscopy images. *Surface Sci.* 251/252: 418–423.

D. P. Panda, A. Rosenfeld (1978). Image segmentation by pixel classification in (gray level, edge value) space. *IEEE Trans. Comput. (C)* 27: 875–879.

Y.-H. Pao (1989). *Adaptive Pattern Recognition and Neural Networks.* Addison Wesley, Reading, MA.

J. Park et al. (2005). Fast disparity estimation algorithm using the property of stereo matching. *Optical Eng.* 44(6): 060501.

K. Parker et al. (2005). Color in medical imaging. *Biophotonics Int.* 1: 44–48.

J. R. Parker (1997). *Algorithms for Image Processing and Computer Vision.* John Wiley & Sons, New York.

T. Pavlidis (1977). *Structural Pattern Recognition.* Springer Verlag, New York.

T. Pavlidis (1980). A thinning algorithm for discrete binary images. *Computer Graphics Image Process.* 13: 142–157.

T. Pavlidis (1982). *Algorithms for Graphics and Image Processing.* Computer Science Press, Rockville, MD.

L. D. Peachey, J. P. Heath (1989). Reconstruction from stereo and multiple electron microscope images of thick sections of embedded biological specimens using computer graphics methods. *J. Microsc.* 153: 193–204.

D. M. Pearsall (1978). Phytolith analysis of archaeological soils: evidence for maize cultivation in formative Ecuador. *Science* 199: 177–178.

S. Peleg, J. Naor, R. Hartley, D. Avnir (1984). Multiple resolution texture analysis and classification. *IEEE Trans. Pattern Anal. Machine Intelligence (PAMI)* 6: 518.

A. P. Pentland (1983). Fractal-based description of natural scenes. *IEEE Trans. Pattern Anal. Machine Intelligence (PAMI)* 6: 661.

A. P. Pentland (Ed.) (1986). *From Pixels to Predicates.* Ablex, Norwood, NJ.

A. P. Pentland, R. W. Picard, S. Sclaroff (1994). Photobook: content-based manipulation of image databases. In *Proc. Storage and Retrieval Image and Video Databases II*, SPIE, San Jose, CA; *Int. J. Computer Vision* 18: 233–254.

E. Persoon, K.-S. Fu (1977). Shape discrimination using Fourier descriptors. *IEEE Trans. Syst. Manage. Cybern. (SMC)* 7: 170–179.

J. L. Pfalz (1976). Surface networks. *Geographical Analysis* 8: 77–93.

G. Piazzesi (1973). Photogrammetry with the scanning electron microscope, *J. Phys. E: Sci. Instrum.* 6: 392–396.

D. R. Piperno (1984). A comparison and differentiation of phytoliths from maize (*Zea mays* L.) and wild grasses: use of morphological criteria. *Am. Antiquity* 49: 361–383.

I. Pitas (2000). *Digital Image Processing Algorithms and Applications.* Wiley, New York.

E. Ponz et al. (2006). Measuring surface topography with scanning electron microscopy, *Microsc. Microanal.* 12: 170–177.

W. K. Pratt (1991). *Digital Image Processing*, 2nd ed. Wiley, New York.

T. Prettyman, R. Gardner, J. Russ, K. Verghese (1991). On the performance of a combined transmission and scattering approach to industrial computed tomography. *Appl. Radiat. Isot.* 44(10/11): 1327–1341.

J. M. S. Prewitt, M. L. Mendelsohn (1966). The analysis of cell images. *Annu. N.Y. Acad. Sci.* 128: 1035–1053.

L. Quam, M. J. Hannah (1974). Stanford Automated Photogrammetry Research. AIM-254. Stanford Artificial Intelligence Lab, Palo Alto, CA.

C. F. Quate (1994). The AFM as a tool for surface imaging. *Surf. Sci. (Netherlands)* 299–300: 980–995.

J. Radon (1917). Über die Bestimmung von Funktionen durch ihre Integralwerte längs gewisser Mannigfaltigkeiten. *Berlin Sächsische Akad. Wissen.* 29: 262–279.

Z. Rahman et al. (2004). Retinex processing for automatic image enhancement. *J. Electronic Imaging* 13: 100–110.

R. Ramanath (2000). Interpolation Methods for the Bayer Color Array. M.S. thesis. North Carolina State University, Raleigh, NC, Dept. of Electrical Eng.; available on-line at www4.ncsu.edu/~rramana/Research/Masters Thesis.pdf.

R. Rangayyan (2005). *Biomedical Image Analysis.* CRC Press, Boca Raton, FL.

M. Raspanti et al. (2005). A vision-based 3D reconstruction technique for scanning electron microscopy: direct comparison with atomic force microscopy. *Microsc. Res. Tech.* 67: 1–7.

B. S. Reddy, B. N. Chatterji (1996). An FFT-based technique for translation, rotation, and scale-invariant image registration. *IEEE Trans. Image Process.* 5: 1266–1271.

M. G. Reed, C. V. Howard, C. G. Shelton (1997). Confocal imaging and second-order stereological analysis of a liquid foam. *J. Microsc.* 185: 313–320.

M. G. Reed, C. V. Howard (1997). Edge corrected estimates of the nearest neighbor function for three-dimensional point patterns. *J. Microsc.* 186(2): 177–184.

A. A. Reeves (1990). Optimized Fast Hartley Transform with Applications in Image Processing. Masters thesis. Dartmouth College. Hanover. NH.

R. G. Reeves (Ed.) (1975). *Manual of Remote Sensing*. American Society of Photogrammetry, Falls Church, VA.

K. Rehm, S. C. Strother, J. R. Anderson, K. A. Schaper, D. A. Rottenberg (1994). Display of merged multimodality brain images using interleaved pixels with independent color scales. *J. Nucl. Med.* 35: 1815–1821.

E. Reinhard et al. (2002). Photographic tone reproduction for digital images. *ACM Trans. Graphics* 21(3): 267–276.

G. Reiss, J. Vancea et al. (1990). Scanning tunneling microscopy on rough surfaces: Tip-shape-limited resolution. *J. Appl. Phys.* 67(3): 1156–1159.

I. Rezanaka, R. Eschbach (Eds.) (1996). *Recent Progress in Ink Jet Technologies*, Society of Imaging Science and Technology, Springfield, VA.

H. Rheingold (1991). *Virtual Reality*. Touchtone Press, New York.

W. H. Richardson (1972). Bayesian-based iterative method of image restoration. *J. Opt. Soc. Am.* 62: 55–59.

J. P. Rigaut (1988). Automated image segmentation by mathematical morphology and fractal geometry. *J. Microsc.* 150: 21–30.

G. X. Ritter, J. N. Wilson (2001). *Handbook of Computer Vision Algorithms in Image Algebra*, 2nd ed. CRC Press, Boca Raton, FL.

L. Roberts (1982). Recognition of three-dimensional objects. In *The Handbook of Artificial Intelligence*, Vol. III (P. Cohen and E. Figenbaum, Eds.). Kaufmann, Los Gatos, CA.

L. G. Roberts (1965). Machine perception of three-dimensional solids. In *Optical and Electro-Optical Information Processing* (J. T. Tippett, Ed.). MIT Press, Cambridge, MA.

G. M. Robinson et al. (1991). Optical interferometry of surfaces. *Scientif. Amer.* 265(1): 66–71.

I. Rock (1984). *Perception*. W. H. Freeman, New York.

F. J. Rohlf, J. W. Archie (1984). A comparison of Fourier methods for the description of wing shape in mosquitoes (*Diptera: culicidae*). *Syst. Zool.* 33: 302–317.

F. J. Rohlf (1990). Morphometrics. *Annu. Rev. Ecol. Syst.* 21: 299–317.

D. W. Rolston (1988). *Principles of Artificial Intelligence and Expert System Development*. McGraw Hill, New York.

B. G. Rosen, R. J. Crafoord (Eds.) (1997). *Metrology and Properties of Engineering Surfaces*. Chalmers University, Göteborg, Sweden.

F. Rosenblatt (1958). The perceptron: a probabilistic model for information organization and storage in the brain. *Psych. Rev.* 65: 358–408.

A. Rosenfeld, A. C. Kak (1982). *Digital Picture Processing*, Vols. 1 and 2. Academic Press, New York.

F. S. Rosenthal, Z. A. Begum (2005). Image-based determination of chord lengths in air-dried lungs. *J. Microsc.* 219: 160–166.

I. Rovner (1971). Potential of opal phytoliths for use in paleoecological reconstruction. *Quaternary Res.* 1: 345–359.

Y. Rui, T. S. Huang, S.-F. Chang (1999). Image retrieval: current techniques, promising directions and open issues, *J. Visual Communication Image Representation* 10: 39–62.

J. Ruiz-Alzola et al. (2005). Landmark-based registration of medical image data. In *Medical Image Analysis Methods* (L. Costaridou, Ed.). CRC Press, Boca Raton, FL.

D. E. Rumelhart, G. E. Hinton, R. J. Williams (1986). Learning representations by back-propagating errors. *Nature* 323: 533–536.

J. C. Russ (1984). Implementing a new skeletonizing method. *J. Microsc.* 136: RP7.

J. C. Russ (1986). *Practical Stereology*. Plenum Press, New York.

J. C. Russ (1988). Differential absorption three-dimensional microtomography. *Trans. Am. Nucl. Soc.* 56: 14.

J. C. Russ (1990a). *Computer Assisted Microscopy*. Plenum Press, New York.

J. C. Russ (1990b). Surface characterization: fractal dimensions, Hurst coefficients and frequency transforms. *J. Computer Assisted Microsc.* 2: 161–184.

J. C. Russ (1990c). Processing images with a local Hurst operator to reveal textural differences. *J. Computer Assisted Microsc.* 2: 249–257.

J. C. Russ (1991). Multiband thresholding of images. *J. Computer Assisted Microsc.* 3: 77–96.

J. C. Russ (1993a). JPEG Image Compression and Image Analysis. *J. Computer Assisted Microsc.* 5: 237–244.

J. C. Russ (1993b). Method and application for ANDing features in binary images. *J. Computer Assisted Microsc.* 5: 265–272.

J. C. Russ (1994). *Fractal Surfaces*. Plenum Press, New York.

J. C. Russ (1995a). Computer-assisted manual stereology. *J. Computer Assisted Microsc.* 7: 35–46.

J. C. Russ (1995b). Median filtering in color space. *J. Computer Assisted Microsc.* 7: 83–90.

J. C. Russ (1995c). Thresholding images. *J. Computer Assisted Microsc.* 7: 41–164.

J. C. Russ (1995d). Designing kernels for image filtering. *J. Computer Assisted Microsc.* 7: 179–190.

J. C. Russ (1995e). Optimal greyscale images. *J. Computer Assisted Microsc.* 7: 221–234.

J. C. Russ (1995f). Segmenting touching hollow features. *J. Computer Assisted Microsc.* 7: 253–261.

J. C. Russ (1997). Fractal dimension measurement of engineering surfaces. In *7th Int. Conf. Metrology and Properties of Engineering Surfaces* (B. G. Rosen, R. J. Crafoord, Eds.). Chalmers University, Göteborg, Sweden, p. 170–174.

J. C. Russ (2001). Fractal geometry in engineering metrology. In *Metrology and Properties of Engineering Surfaces* (E. Mainsah et al., Eds.). Kluwer Academic, London, pp. 43–82.

J. C. Russ (2002). *Forensic Uses of Digital Imaging.* CRC Press, Boca Raton, FL.

J. C. Russ (2004). *Image Analysis of Food Microstructure.* CRC Press, Boca Raton, FL.

J. C. Russ, D. S. Bright, J. C. Russ, T. M. Hare (1989). Application of the Hough transform to electron diffraction patterns. *J. Computer Assisted Microsc.* 1: 3–77.

J. C. Russ, R. T. Dehoff (2001). *Practical Stereology,* 2nd ed. Plenum Press, New York.

J. C. Russ, I. Rovner (1987). Stereological verification of *Zea* phytolith taxonomy. *Phytolitharien Newsl.* 4(3): 10.

J. C. Russ, J. C. Russ (1988a). Automatic discrimination of features in grey scale images. *J. Microsc.* 148: 263–277.

J. C. Russ, J. C. Russ (1988b). Improved implementation of a convex segmentation algorithm. *Acta Stereologica* 7: 33–40.

J. C. Russ, J. C. Russ (1989a). Uses of the Euclidean distance map for the measurement of features in images. *J. Computer Assisted Microsc.* 1: 343.

J. C. Russ, J. C. Russ (1989b). Topological measurements on skeletonized three-dimensional networks. *J. Computer Assisted Microsc.* 1: 131–150.

J. C. Russ, H. Palmour III, T. M. Hare (1989). Direct 3-D pore location measurement in alumina. *J. Microsc.* 155(2): RP1.

P. Russell, D. Batchelor (2001 July). SEM and AFM: complementary techniques for surface investigations. *Microsc. Anal.,* 5–8.

M. R. Rutenberg et al. (2001). Automated Cytological Specimen Classification System and Method. U.S. patent 6,327,377.

F. F. Sabins, Jr. (1987). *Remote Sensing: Principles and Interpretation,* 2nd ed. W. H. Freeman, New York.

F. Sacerdotti et al. (2002). Closed regions: a proposal for spacing parameters for areal surface measurements. *Meas. Sci. Technol.* 13: 556–564.

P. K. Sahoo, S. Soltani, A. C. Wong, Y. C. Chen (1988). A survey of thresholding techniques. *Computer Vision Graphics Image Process.* 41: 233–260.

E. Sanchez, L. A. Zadeh (Eds.) (1987). *Approximate Reasoning in Intelligent System Decision and Control.* Oxford Press, New York.

J. Sanchez, M. P. Canton (1999). *Space Image Processing.* CRC Press, Boca Raton, FL.

L. J. Sartor, A. R. Weeks (2001). Morphological operations on color images. *J. Electronic Imaging* 10: 548–549.

S. Saunders (1991, Spring). Magellan: the geologic exploration of Venus. *Eng. Sci.* 15–27.

A. Savitsky, M. J. E. Golay (1964). Smoothing and differentiation of data by simplified least squares procedures. *Anal. Chem.* 36: 1627–1639.

R. J. Schalkoff (1991). *Pattern Recognition: Statistical, Syntactical and Neural Approaches.* Wiley, New York.

D. J. Schneberk, H. E. Martz, S. G. Azavedo (1991). Multiple energy techniques in industrial computerized tomography. In *Review of Progress in Quantitative Nondestructive Evaluation* (D. O. Thompson, D. E. Chimenti, Eds.). Plenum Press, New York.

H. P. Schwartz, K. C. Shane (1969). Measurement of particle shape by Fourier analysis. *Sedimentology* 13: 213–231.

H. Schwarz, H. E. Exner (1980). Implementation of the concept of fractal dimensions on a semi-automatic image analyzer. *Powder Technol.* 27: 107.

H. Schwarz, H. E. Exner (1983). The characterization of the arrangement of feature centroids in planes and volumes. *J. Microsc.* 129: 155.

C. Sciammarella et al. (2005). High accuracy contouring using projection moiré. *Optical Eng.* 44(9): 093605.

P. J. Scott (1995). Recent advances in areal characterization. In *IX Int. Oberflächenkolloq.* Technical University, Chemnitz-Zwickau, Germany, pp. 151–158.

P. J. Scott (1997). Foundations of topological characterization of surface texture. In *7th Int. Conf. Metrology and Properties of Engineering Surfaces* (B. G. Rosen, R. J. Crafoord, Eds.). Chalmers University, Göteborg, Sweden, pp. 162–169.

J. Serra (1982). *Image Analysis and Mathematical Morphology.* Academic Press, London.

M. Seul, L. O'Gorman, M. J. Sammon (2000). *Practical Algorithms for Image Analysis.* Cambridge University Press, Cambridge.

M. Sezgin, B. Sankur (2004). Survey over image thresholding techniques and quantitative performance evaluation. *J. Electronic Imaging* 13: 146–165.

M. Shao et al. (2005). Partition-based interpolation for color filter array demosaicking and super-resolution reconstruction. *Optical Eng.* 44(10): 107003.

L. G. Shapiro, R. M. Haralick (1985). A metric for comparing relational descriptions. *IEEE Trans. Pattern Anal. Mach. Intell.* PAI-7(1): 90–94.

G. Sharma (Ed.) (2003). *Digital Color Imaging Handbook.* CRC Press, Boca Raton, FL.

G. Sharma (2005). Imaging arithmetic: physics U math > physics + math. *SPIE Electronic Imaging Tech. Group Newsl.* 15(2): 1–10.

L. A. Shepp, B. F. Logan (1974). The Fourier reconstruction of a head section. *IEEE Trans. NS* 21: 21–43.

A. Shih, G. Wang, P. C. Cheng (2001). Fast algorithm for X-ray cone-beam microtomography. *Microsc. Microanal.* 7: 13–23.

D. Shuman (2005, May). Computerized image analysis software for measuring indents by AFM. *Microsc. Anal.* 15–17.

S. A. Sirr, J. R. Waddle (1999, May). The utility of computed tomography in the detection of internal damage and repair and the determination of authenticity of high quality bowed stringed instruments. *RadioGraphics* 203(801–805).

J. Skilling (1986). Theory of maximum entropy image reconstruction. In *Maximum Entropy and Bayesian Methods in Applied Statistics*, Proc. 4th Max. Entropy Workshop, University of Calgary, 1984 (J. H. Justice, Ed.). Cambridge University Press, Cambridge, pp. 156–178.

P. E. Slatter (1987). *Building Expert Systems: Cognitive Emulation.* Halsted Press, New York.

B. D. Smith (1990). Cone-beam tomography: recent advances and a tutorial review. *Optical Eng.* 29: 5.

P. W. Smith, M. D. Elstrom (2001). Stereo-based registration of range and projective imagery for data fusion and visualization. *Optical Eng.* 40(3): 352–361.

R. F. Smith (1990). *Microscopy and Photomicrography.* CRC Press, Boca Raton, FL.

B. Smolka, A. Chydzinski, K. W. Wojciechowski, K. N. Plataniotis, A. N. Venetsanopoulos (2001). On the reduction of impulse noise in multichannel image processing. *Optical Eng.* 40: 902–908.

D. L. Snyder, T. J. Schutz, J. A. O'Sullivan (1992). Deblurring subject to nonnegative constraints. *IEEE Trans. Signal Process. (SP)* 40: 1143–1150.

I. Sobel (1970). Camera Models and Machine Perception. AIM-21. Stanford Artificial Intelligence Lab, Palo Alto, CA.

R. Sobol (2004). Improving the retinex algorithm for rendering wide dynamic range photographs. *J. Electronic Imaging* 13: 65–74.

P. Soille (1999). *Morphological Image Analysis.* Springer Verlag, Berlin.

M. Sonka, V. Hlavac, R. Boyle (1999). *Image Processing, Analysis and Machine Vision*, 2nd ed. Brooks Cole, Pacific Grove, CA.

P. G. Spetsieris et al. (1995). Interactive visualization of coregistered tomographic images. In *Proc. Biomedical Visualization*, IEEE, Washington, D.C., p. 58.

S. Srinivasan, J. C. Russ, R. O. Scattergood (1990). Fractal analysis of erosion surfaces. *J. Mater. Res.* 5: 2616–2619.

J. A. Stark, W. J. Fitzgerald (1996). An alternative algorithm for adaptive histogram equalization. *Computer Vision Graphics Image Process.* 56: 180–185.

M. Stefik (1995). *Introduction to Knowledge Systems.* Morgan Kaufmann, San Francisco.

D. C. Sterio (1984). The unbiased estimation of number and sizes of arbitrary particles using the Disector. *J. Microsc.* 134: 127–136.

P. L. Stewart, R. M. Burnett (1991). Image reconstruction reveals the complex molecular organization of adenovirus, *Cell* 67: 145–154.

M. C. Stone, W. B. Cowan, J. C. Beatty (1988). Color gamut mapping and the printing of digital color images. *ACM Trans. Graphics* 7: 249–292.

J. A. Storer (1992). *Image and Text Compression.* Kluwer Academic, New York.

K. J. Stout, P. J. Sullivan, W. P. Dong, E. Mainsah, N. Luo, T. Mathia, H. Zahouani (1993). The Development of Methods for the Characterization of Roughness in Three Dimensions. Publication EUR 15178 EN of the Commission of the European Communities. University of Birmingham, Edgbaston, England.

R. G. Summers, C. E. Musial, P.-C. Cheng, A. Leith, M. Marko (1991). The use of confocal microscopy and stereocon reconstructions in the analysis of sea urchin embryonic cell division. *J. Electron Microscope Tech.* 18: 24–30.

Y. Sun et al. (2004). Autofocusing in computer microscope: selecting the optimal focus algorithm. *Microsc. Res. Tech.* 65: 139–149.

I. Sutherland (1965). The ultimate display. *Proc. IFIP 65* 2: 506–508, 582–583.

R. E. Swing (1997). *An Introduction to Microdensitometry.* SPIE Press, Bellingham, WA.

H. Talbot, T. Lee, D. Jeulin, D. Hanton, L. W. Hobbs (2000). Image analysis of insulation mineral fibers. *J. Microsc.* 200: 251–258.

L. Tang et al. (2005). Novel dense matching algorithm with Voronoi decomposition of images. *Optical Eng.* 44(10): 107201.

L. Tao, V. K. Asari, (2005). Adaptive and integrated neighborhood-dependent approach for nonlinear enhancement of color images. *J. Electron. Imag.* 14(4): 043006.

T. R. Thomas (1999). *Rough Surfaces*, 2nd ed. Imperial College Press, London.

M. M. Thompson (Ed.) (1966). *Manual of Photogrammetry*. American Society of Photogrammetry, Falls Church, VA.

M. von Tiedemann et al. (2006). Image adaptive point spread function estimation and deconvolution for *in vivo* confocal microscopy. *Microsc. Res. Techn.* 69: 10–20.

J. T. Tou, R. C. Gonzalez (1981). *Pattern Recognition Principles*. Addison Wesley, Reading, MA.

J. Trussell (1979). Comments on "Picture thresholding using an iterative selection method." *IEEE Trans. Syst. Manage. Cybern. (SMC)* 9: 311.

T.-M. Tu, S.-C. Su, H.-C. Shyu, P. S. Huang (2001). Efficient intensity-hue-saturation-based image fusion with saturation compensation. *Optical Eng.* 40: 720–728.

E. R. Tufte (1990). *Envisioning Information*. Graphics Press, Cheshire, CT.

E. R. Tufte (1997). *Visual Explanations: Images and Quantities, Evidence and Narrative*. Graphics Press, Cheshire, CT.

E. R. Tufte (2001). *The Visual Display of Quantitative Information*, 2nd ed. Graphics Press, Cheshire, CT.

J. N. Turner, D. H. Szaeowski, K. L. Smith, M. Marko, A. Leith, J. W. Swann (1991). Confocal microscopy and three-dimensional reconstruction of electrophysiologically identified neurons in thick brain slices. *J. Electron Microscope Tech.* 8: 11–23.

P. C. Twiss, P. C. E. Suess, R. M. Smith (1969). Morphological classification of grass phytoliths. *Soil Sci. Soc. Am. Proc.* 33: 109–115.

S. E. Umbaugh (1998). *Computer Vision and Image Processing*. Prentice Hall, Saddle River, NJ.

E. E. Underwood (1970). *Quantitative Stereology*. Addison Wesley, Reading, MA.

E. E. Underwood, K. Banerji (1986). Fractals in fractography. *Mater. Sci. Eng.* 80: 1.

J. G. Verly, R. L. Delanoy (1993). Some principles and applications of adaptive mathematical morphology for range imagery. *Optical Eng.* 32: 3295–3306.

H. Verschueren, B. Houben, J. De Braekeleer, J. De Wit, D. Roggen, P. De Baetselier (1993). Methods for computer assisted analysis of lymphoid cell shape and motility, including Fourier analysis of cell outlines. *J. Immunol. Meth.* 163: 99–113.

J. S. Villarrubia (1994). Morphological estimation of tip geometry for scanned probe microscopy. *Surf. Sci.* 321: 287–300.

J. S. Villarrubia (1996). Scanned probe microscope tip characterization without calibrated tip characterizers. *J. Vac. Sci. Technol.* B14: 1518–1521.

J. S. Villarrubia (1997). Algorithms for scanned probe microscopy image simulation, surface reconstruction and tip estimation. *J. Res. Natl. Inst. Stand. Tech.* 102: 425.

R. J. Wall, A. Klinger, K. R. Castleman (1974). Analysis of image histograms. In *Proc. 2nd Joint Int. Conf. Pattern Recognition*. IEEE 74CH-0885-4C, IEEE, Washington, D.C., pp. 341–344.

J. R. Walters (1988). *Crafting Knowledge-Based Systems: Expert Systems Made Easy*. Wiley, New York.

G. Wang, T. H. Lin, P. C. Cheng, D. M. Shinozaki, H. Kim (1991). Scanning cone-beam reconstruction algorithms for X-ray microtomography. *SPIE Scanning Microscope Instrumentation* 1556: 99.

G. Wang, M. Vannier (2001, July). Micro-CT scanners for biomedical applications. *Advanced Imaging*: 18–27.

Z. Wang (1990). *Principles of Photogrammetry (with Remote Sensing)*. Press of Wuhan Technical University of Surveying and Mapping, Beijing.

J. Wasen, R. Warren (1990). *Catalogue of Stereological Characteristics of Selected Solid Bodies*. Chalmers University, Goteborg, Sweden.

A. R. Weeks (1996). *Fundamentals of Electronic Image Processing*. SPIE Press, Bellingham, WA.

E. R. Weibel (1979). *Stereological Methods*, Vols. I and II. Academic Press, London.

S. Welstead (1999). *Fractal and Wavelet Image Compression Techniques*. SPIE Press, Bellingham, WA.

A. Wen, C. Lu (1993). Hybrid vector quantization. *Optical Eng.* 32: 1496–1502.

J. West, J. M. Fitzpatrick, M. Y. Wang, B. M. Dawant, C. R. Maurer, R. M. Kesler, R. J. Maciunas, C. Barillot, D. Lemoine, A. M. F. Collignon, P. A. van den Elsen, S. Napel, T. S. Sumanaweera, B. A. Harkness, P. F. Hemler, D. L. Hill, C. Studholme, J. B. A. Maintz, M. Viergever, G. Malandain, X. Pennec, M. E. Noz, G. Q. Maguire, M. Pollack, C. A. Pelizzari, R. A. Robb, D. Hanson, and R. P. Woods (1997). Comparison and evaluation of retrospective intermodality registration techniques. *J. Computer Assisted Tomography* 21: 540–566.

J. S. Weszka (1978). A survey of threshold selection techniques. *Computer Graphics Image Process.* 7: 259–265.

J. Weszka, C. Dyer, A. Rosenfeld (1976). A comparative study of texture measures for terrain classification. *IEEE Trans. Syst. Manage. Cybern. (SMC)* 6: 269–285.

J. S. Weszka, A. Rosenfeld (1979). Histogram modification for threshold selection. *IEEE Trans. Syst. Manage. Cybern. (SMC)* 9: 38–52.

D. J. Whitehouse (1994). *Precision: The Handbook of Surface Metrology.* Institute of Physics Publishing, Bristol, U.K.

H. K. Wickramasinghe (1989). Scanned-probe microscopes, *Scientif. Amer.* 261(4): 98–105.

H. K. Wickramasinghe (1991). Scanned probes old and new. *AIP Conf. Proc. (USA)* 241: 9–22.

B. Willis, B. Roysam, J. N. Turner, T. J. Holmes (1993). Iterative, constrained 3D image reconstruction of transmitted light bright field micrographs based on maximum likelihood estimation. *J. Microsc.* 169: 347–361.

R. Wilson, M. Spann (1988). *Image Segmentation and Uncertainty.* Wiley, New York.

G. Winstanley (1987). *Program Design for Knowledge-Based Systems.* Halsted Press, New York.

G. Wolf (1991). Usage of global information and a priori knowledge for object isolation. In *Proc. 8th Int. Congr. Stereology,* Irvine, CA, p. 56.

K. W. Wong (1980). Basic mathematics of photogrammetry. In *Manual of Photogrammetry,* 4th ed. American Society of Photogrammetry, Falls Church, VA, pp. 57–58.

R. J. Woodham (1978). Photometric stereo: a reflectance map technique for determining surface orientation from image intensity. *Proc. SPIE* 155: 136–143.

B. P. Wrobel (1991). Least-squares methods for surface reconstruction from images. *ISPRS J. Photogrammetry Remote Sensing* 46: 67–84.

H-S. Wu et al. (2005). Segmentation of intestinal gland images with iterative region growing. *J. Microsc.* 220(3): 190–204.

S. Wu, A. Gersho (1993). Lapped vector quantization of images. *Optical Eng.* 32: 1489–1495.

X. Wu et al. (2005). Novel fractal image-encoding algorithm based on a full binary tree searchless iterated function system. *Optical Eng.* 44(10): 107002.

Z. Q. Wu et al. (2005). Adaptive contrast enhancement based on highly overlapped interpolation. *J. Electronic Imaging* 14(3): 033006.

R. R. Yager (1979). On the measures of fuzziness and negation, part 1: membership in the unit interval. *Int. J. Gen. Syst.* 5: 221–229.

Y. Yakimovsky (1976). Boundary and object detection in real world images. *J. Assoc. Comput. Mach.* 23: 599–618.

G. J. Yang, T. S. Huang (1981). The effect of median filtering on edge location estimation. *Computer Graphics Image Process.* 15: 224–245.

N. Yang, J. Boselli, I. Sinclair (2001). Simulation and quantitative assessment of homogeneous and inhomogeneous particle distributions in particulate metal matrix composites. *J. Microsc.* 201: 189–200.

T. York (2001). Status of electrical tomography in industrial applications. *J. Electronic Imaging* 10: 608–619.

A. Yoshitaka, T. Ichikawa (1999). A survey on content-based retrieval for multimedia databases. *IEEE Trans. Knowledge Data Eng.* 11: 81–93.

R. W. Young, N. G. Kingsbury (1993). Video compression using lapped transforms for motion estimation/compensation and coding. *Optical Eng.* 32: 1451–1463.

L. A. Zadeh (1965). Fuzzy sets. *Information Control* 8: 338–353.

C. T. Zahn, R.Z. Roskies (1972). Fourier descriptors for plane closed curves. *IEEE Trans. Comput. (C)* 21: 269–281.

X. Zhou, E. Dorrer (1994). An automatic image matching algorithm based on wavelet decomposition. *ISPRS Int. Arch. Photogrammetry Remote Sensing* 30: 951–960.

Q. Z. Zhu, Z. M. Zhang (2005). Correlation of angle-resolved light scattering with the microfacet orientation of rough silicon surfaces. *Optical Eng.* 44(7): 073601.

T. G. Zimmerman, J. A. Lanier (1987). Hand gesture interface device. *CHI '87, Conf. Proc.*, ACM Press, New York, pp. 235–240.

H.-J. Zimmermann (1987). *Fuzzy Sets, Decision Making and Expert Systems.* Kluwer Academic, Boston, MA.

A. Zizzari (2004). *Methods on Tumor Recognition and Planning Target Prediction for the Radiotherapy of Cancer.* Shaker-Verlag, Aachen, Germany.

S. Zucker (1976). Region growing: childhood and adolescence. *Computer Graphics Image Process.* 5: 382–399.

O. Zuniga, R. M. Haralick (1983). Corner detection using the facet model. *Proc. IEEE Conf. Computer Vision Pattern Recognition,* 7: 30–37.

J. M. Zwier et al. (2004). Image calibration in fluorescence microscopy. *J. Microsc.* 216: 15–24.

Index

B

Background function fitting,
238–244
Background skeleton ("skiz"),
503–504, 509, 558
Background subtraction, 245–
247, 318
color images and, 251
correcting nonuniform
illumination, 236–237
division and automatic
scaling, 322
Back-projection, 635–637, 640,
658–659
Backscattering, 738, 740, 741
Balloons, 429, 439
Banding, 141–143
Band-pass filter, 373
Bar codes, 170, 599
Bayer pattern, 14
Bayes classifier, 611
Bayes' theorem, 641
Beam hardening, 646, 648, 660
Bially method, 383
Bicubic fitting, 261–263
Bilinear interpolation, 261, 263
Binary image processing, 443
boundary segmentation, 422
Euclidean distance map, *See*
Euclidean distance map
feature-level Boolean logic,
458–461
filling holes in features,
453–455, 494–495
foreground/background pixel
conventions, 443–444
grouping pixels into features,
452–458
image combination using
Boolean operations, *See*
Boolean operations
layer thickness measurement,
455–458
marker-based feature
selection, 458–461
double thresholding,
466–467
selection by location,
462–466
masks, 450–452
morphological operations
(erosion and dilation),
See Morphological
operations; *specific
operations*
separating waviness from
roughness, 760–761
skeletons, *See* Skeletons

superimposing labels, 452
surface composition maps,
746
template matching and
correlation, 482
thresholding, *See*
Thresholding
typical applications, 484–489
unsharp masking, 28, 95–96
watershed segmentation, 472,
493–496, 569
Binary image representation,
432–436
run-length encoding, 432–435
Birmingham measurement suite,
763–769
Bit shifting, 205
Blue channel noise, 15, 225
Blurring, 232, 382, 673
deconvolution, 377–382,
673–674
motion blur and, 386–389
point-spread function,
377–382, 698–699
Wiener deconvolution,
382–385
Fourier transform, 382,
636–637, 699
frequency-domain model, 377,
698
Gaussian model, 378, 382
isolation from power
spectrum, 384
Laplacian enhancement, 285
optical sectioning images,
385–386
smoothing operations, 205,
214
Boolean operations, 443–447, *See
also specific operations*
colocalization plots, 443–444
combining multiband
parameters, 412
combining operations,
447–450
erosion/dilation procedures
and, 487–489
feature-level logic, 458–466
grid or measurement template
superimposition,
455–458, 514
marker-based feature
selection, 458–461, 534
pixel ON/OFF conventions,
445–446
thresholding approaches, 404
Boundaries, *See also* Edges
automatic ridge-following, 429

centroid determination,
550–553
double thresholding, 466–467
edge finding, *See* Edge finding
enhancing, *See* Edge
enhancement; Image
enhancement
entropy-based method, 423
fractal dimension
determination, 479, *See
also* Fractal dimension
histogram modification and,
278
human vision and, 98, 102,
123–124
line-thickening, 505
line-thinning using
skeletonization,
504–505
local contrast equalization
and, 281
local inhibition and, 285–286
outlining and edge following,
428–429, 439
perimeter estimation, 579–581
pixels straddling, 21
selective histograms (ignoring
boundary pixels),
425–427
shape reconstruction using
harmonic analysis,
589–592, 726
snakes and balloons, 429, 439
superresolution measurement
technique, 580, 587
taut-string or rubber-band,
573
three-dimensional
measurement issues,
595, 725–726, *See also*
Surface measurement
applications
thresholding and
segmentation, 420–425
Bounding box, 550, 576
Bounding polygon, 573, 576
Brightness histogram, *See* Image
histogram
Brightness measurements,
543–548
Brightness values, 23–24, 57, 100,
543
area fraction measurement
and, 513
calibration and correction,
544–547
colocalization plot, 443–444
color calibration, 544, 547–
548

color image digitization problems, 547–548
compression algorithm, 147
computer display technology, 24–25
entropy, 232, *See also* Entropy-based methods
false color substitution in monochrome images, 33–35, *See also* Pseudocolor
measuring, 543–548
optical density vs., 544–547
range enhancement, 331–333
rank leveling, 244–247, 250–251, *See also* Rank-order filtering
significance of, 548
16-bit digitization, 24, 397
real number representation, 398, 543
visual adaptation to changing levels, 93, 105
visual contrast resolution, 92–95, 146–147
Broadcast television interlaced display, 19, 29
Brodatz textures, 606, 607
Buckytubes, 733, 744
Butterfly, 339
Butterworth filter, 358–359, 365

C

Caliper dimension, 553, 575, 576–578
Cameras
automatic gain system, 19, 544
CCD, *See* Charge-coupled device (CCD) cameras
CMOS, 17–18, 214
color, 12–15, 30, 37–38, 544, *See also* Color images
digital, *See* Digital still cameras
electronics and bandwidth limitations, 19
focusing, 18–19
HDTV applications, 30
high-depth images, 27–28
human visual performance vs., 29
pixels, 21–22
real-time imaging, 27
resolution, 15–17, 195–196
video, *See* Video cameras
voltage digitization, 5, 19–21, 23–24
width-to-height ratio, 21
Camouflage, 105
Carbon nanotubes, 733, 744
Cathode-ray tube (CRT) display, 24, 136
color displays, 56, 146
phosphor aging and color, 53
Cave-based virtual reality systems, 702
CCD cameras, *See* Charge-coupled device (CCD) cameras
CD storage media, 162–165
CD-R, 163, 165
CD-RW, 163
Center of gravity (centroid), 550–553
Center-surround comparisons, 99–102
Centroid, 550–553, 557–558, 584
Chain code, 435, 591, 626
perimeter estimation, 579
Change tree, 770
Charge-coupled device (CCD) cameras, 6–10
artifacts and limitations, 11–12
color imaging, 12–13, 548
miniaturization and performance, 9–10
noise sources, 12, 202
single-line systems, 29
spectral response, 8
Chemical maps, 411
Chessboard models, 489
Chi-squared statistics, 233, 642
Chord encoding, 432, 452, *See also* Run-length encoding
Chromosome karyotyping, 626
CIE chromaticity diagram, 44–45, 146, 183
threshold setting, 407
CIELab color space, 46–48
Circle fitting, 563–565
Circular size measures, 574–575
Circumscribed circle, 574–575
City-block models, 489
Classical stereology, 540–542
Classification, *See* Feature classification
Closing (dilation and erosion), 422
Euclidean distance map and, 491

feature measurement applications, 485–486
gray-scale, 245–246, *See also* Gray-scale morphological operations
noise filtering applications, 472
rank-based background leveling, 245–246
Cluster analysis, 619–622, 747
dendogram, 621
spanning tree, 621
CMOS cameras, 17–18, 214
CMY (cyan, magenta, yellow) color space, 42, 147
conversion to CMYK, 149
CMYK (cyan-magenta-yellow-black) system, 147–150
CMY conversion, 159
inks, 156
Coatings, compositional mapping, 741, 742
Coatings, thickness measurement, 455–458, 547, 758
Codec, 120, 192
Collage theorem, 191
Colocalization plot, 443–444
Colony counting, 461–462, 534–535
Color, surface characteristics and, 121–122
Color blindness, 103, 105
Color calibration, 52–53, 149–150
Color cameras, 12–15, 37–38, 544
HDTV applications, 30
Color correction and calibration, 51–55, 544, 547–548
automatic gain effects, 544
color standards, 545
tristimulus, 53–55
Color displays, 55–57, 146
projection devices, 56
Color filtering, 49–50
Color gamut, 44, 93–94, 146–149, 150, 156–157, 271
Color images, 31–39
blue channel noise, 15, 225
brightness leveling, 247–251
camera systems, 12–15
CCD cameras and, 548
compression, 36–37, 120, 180–181
contrast expansion and, 198
converting gray-scale to pseudocolor, 28
deconvolution and optical defect correction, 380
digital camera limitations, 41
digital video recording, 39
digitizing, 48–49, 547–548

display capabilities, 271
electron microscopy, 32
emission-rule volumetric
    images, 705
false color substitution in
    monochrome images,
    33–35, *See also*
    Pseudocolor
gray-scale interconversion,
    49–50
histogram equalization, 276
HTML documents, 160
human vision, 37, 90–91,
    93–94, 100–102, 325
hybrid median, 220–223
image enhancement using
    principal components
    analysis, 326
lighting conditions and, 51,
    91, 101–102, 121, 149
local or adaptive equalization,
    281
lookup tables, 180–181
median filter, 218, 220-223
moiré patterns, 227
MPEG moving picture
    standard, 193
multiple-channel images,
    32–33, 65–66, 404–406,
    692–694
multiple criteria thresholding,
    415
NTSC encoding scheme, 37,
    38
periodic noise filtering,
    365–366
photographing computer
    screen, 159
printing, 53, 146–153
realistic surface rendering,
    757
serial-section visualization,
    719
shading correction problems,
    247
16-bit, 543
stereoscopic applications, 72,
    697
storage requirements, 173
three-dimensional image
    visualization, 691–694,
    704, 719
transistor approach, 14–15
true color correspondences,
    271
vector ranking, 219
video, 12–13, 19, 36, 37–38
Color laser printers, 152–153
Color matching, 91, 149–150

Color separations, 150
Color spaces, 42–50, 100, *See also*
    specific types
    CIE chromaticity diagram,
        44–45, 146, 183
    compression optimization,
        183
    digitization, 48–49
    image analysis applications,
        49
    L*a*b model, 46–48
    lookup tables, 49, 270
    median filter and, 218
    subsampling, 36–37
    thresholding and
        segmentation, 404–409
Color television, 36
Color temperature, 47, 79, 121,
    149, 544
Colorization (artistic), 35–36
Compact disk (CD) storage
    media, 162–164, 165
Compactness, 582
Component video, 37–38
Compression, 119–121, 174–180
    assessing image quality,
        184–185
    audio, 193
    brightness values, 147
    color images, 36–37, 120,
        180–181
    color palette, 180–181
    delta compression, 175
    dictionary-based (Lempel-Ziv)
        techniques, 178–179
    digital camera limitations,
        39–41
    digital movies, 192–194
    entropy value, 177–178
    fractal approach, 120, 181,
        182, 190–192, 194
    high-frequency information
        loss, 189–190
    Huffman coding, 176–178
    human vision and, 119–121
    image quality and, 335–336
    lossless methods, 175, 180
    lossy techniques, 39–41, 120,
        181, 190, *See also* JPEG
        compression
    lower limit, 177–178
    noise and, 179
    optimal color space selection,
        183
    periodic noise and, 361
    problems for image analysis,
        41
    run-length encoding, 173,
        179–180

text, 176–177
unsuitability for scientific
    analysis, 120–121
variable-length coding,
    176–178
wavelet transform, 181
Computed tomography (CT),
    66, 631–632, *See also*
    Tomographic imaging
    isotropic virtual probes, 520
Computer-aided drafting (CAD),
    683, 711
Computer display monitors,
    24–25
    color displays, 55–57, 146,
        271
    photographing screen images,
        157–160
    representing three-
        dimensional structure,
        252–254
Concave surface, 532–534
Cone-beam geometry, 657, 663,
    694
Cones, 89–90, 326
Confocal scanning light
    microscope (CSLM),
    30, 527
    deconvolution and deblurring,
        385–386
    deconvolution and improving
        resolution, 675
    depth of field, 328, 330
    isotropic virtual probes, 520
    optical sectioning, 67,
        673–675
    reflection, 706, 708
    surface measurement
        applications, 736, 738
    surface-range images, 59–60
"Connectedness" rules, 435, 452
    voxels and, 594, 724
Connectivity, 532–533, 727
Constellations, 129, 560
Contact profilometers, 30
Content-based image retrieval
    (CBIR), 167
Context line, 610, 616
Contour maps, 430–432, 739, 748
Contouring, 218
Contrast expansion, 195–
    199, 270, *See*
    also Illumination
    nonuniformity
    correction
    brightness histogram, 196–197
    color images and, 198
    lookup tables, 270, 271
    noise and, 197, 199

Depth perception, 70, *See also* Stereoscopy

Derivatives-based image enhancement, 291–292
edge finding, 292–294, 298

Desert sub-sand mapping, 75

Detrending data, 61

Deuteranopia, 105

Difference of Gaussian (DoG), 288, 637, *See also* Laplacian of a Gaussian

Diffraction patterns, 1
frequency-domain representation, 347–348, 369
surface measurement applications, 740

Digital movies, 192–194, *See also* MPEG compression

Digital still cameras
CMOS technology, 18
color images, 14–15, 41
cooled circuitry, 16, 27
deconvolution applications, 386
focusing, 41
image compression, *See* Compression; JPEG compression
image resolution, 15–17, 386
image resolution, human visual performance vs., 29, 85
microscopy applications, 41
problems and limitations, 39–42
technical applications, 16
voltage digitization, 21
width-to-height ratio, 21

Digital-to-analog converter, 24

Digital video (DV) recording, 38–39, *See also* Video cameras

Digitization, 12–13
camera dynamic range, 195–196
camera voltage signals, 5, 19–21, 23–24
color images, 48–49, 547–548
photographic negatives, 31

Dilation, 245–246, 422, 438, 462, 468, 470–472, *See also* Closing; Morphological operations; Opening
anisotropic effects, 486
Boolean combinations, 487–489
boundary line thickening, 505
fate tables, 482

gray-scale, 228–229, 244–247, 479–480, 769, *See also* Gray-scale morphological operations
measurements using, 478–479
neighborhood isotropy and, 476–478
neighborhood parameters, 481–482
profile analysis applications, 769
scratch removal, 483
typical applications, 484–489

Discrete cosine transform (DCT), 120, 182

Disector, 465, 522, 529, 533–535, 727

Distance fade, 705

Distance standardization, 613

Dithering, 143

Dividing frequency transforms, 379, 382

Dividing images, 322

Dot-matrix printers, 136

Dots per inch (dpi), 136

Double stars, 96

Double thresholding, 466–467

Dry-ink printers, 155

Dual-energy tomography, 704

DVD storage media, 162–164

Dyadic operations, 390, *See also* *specific types*

Dye-sublimation, 135, 153–155

Dynamic ranging, 318

E

Edge enhancement, 455
difference of Gaussians, 288
directional derivatives, 291–294, 298
kernel operations and, 281–282
Laplacian, 282, 284–287
noisy images and, 307
Sobel operator, 297–299, 303, 317, 417–419, 426, 722
sombrero filter, 290
unsharp masking, 287–288

Edge finding, 100, 292–307, 455
Canny filter, 305
grain boundary discrimination, 305–306
kernel operations, 296–297, 304–305
Kirsch operator, 298
Laplacian, 292–293
local inhibition, 285–286

neighborhood size and, 303
oriented features and, 299–300, 303
Roberts' Cross operator, 293–296
Sobel operator, 297–299, 426
three-dimensional image processing, 722–723
usefulness of, 307

Edge following, 428–429, 439

Edges, *See also* Boundaries
frequency transforms and, 417
kernel operations and, 205, 281–282
Laplacian enhancement, 282, 284–287
median filtering and, 218
neighborhood operations implementation and, 317
selective histograms (ignoring boundary pixels), 425–427
sharpening using mode filter, 219
visual perception, 98, 123–124, 285–286

Eight-connected rule, 435, 452

Electrolytic etching, 676

Electromagnetic spectrum, 1, 16

Electron backscattering, 738

Electron diffraction patterns, 1
frequency-domain representation, 347–348, 369
surface measurement applications, 740

Electronic shuttering, 11–12, 27

Electron microscopy, *See* Scanning electron microscope; Transmission electron microscope

Electroplating, 731

Ellipse-based feature size description, 575

Ellipsometry, 741–742

Elongation, 582

Embossing effect, 292

Emission tomography, 651, 721

Entropy-based methods
automated thresholding, 403
boundary segmentation, 423
cross entropy, 234
image compression and, 177–178
maximum-entropy approach for artifact removal, 232–234

magnification effects, 574, 580
mean diameter and density measurement, 531–532
minimum and maximum limits, 550
morphological operations (erosion and dilation), 478–479, 485–486
neighbor relationships, 554–559
orientation determination, 553–554
shape description, 581–585, *See also* Shape
size, 540–542, 572–578
  area, 572–574
  bounding polygon, 573, 576
  caliper dimension, 553, 575
  ellipse-based description, 575
  equivalent circular diameter, 574–575
  fiber length and width, 577–578
  fractal perimeters, 585–588
  holes and, 573
  perimeter, 578, 579–581, 585–586
  real-world size correspondence, 574
  three-dimensional problems, 725–726
  three-dimensional, *See* Three-dimensional measurement
touching features, 493, 569–570, *See also* Watershed segmentation
ultimate eroded points, 496, 498
Feature orientation, *See also* Alignment; Anisotropy characterization
autocorrelation, 396
directional derivatives, 291–294, 298
edge finding and, 299–300
frequency transforms and, 345–348, 360
Feature recognition, 82, 599, 601–606, *See also* Feature classification; Optical character recognition
context or prior knowledge, 127–129

eyewitness descriptions, 117–119
facial recognition, 117–119, 172, 602–604, 624
fingerprint identification, 172, 190, 603–604
general problem, 439–441
grandmother cell, 87–88, 624
human vision, 86–89
military targets, 174, 601
object grouping or ordering, 129–131
shape and, 126–127
size and, 123–125
skeleton and, 499
surveillance videotape and, 116
syntactical models, 626–627
template matching and correlation, 390, 600–601, *See also* Template matching
threshold logic unit, 87–88, 624
Feature segmentation, *See* Segmentation
Feature selection, thresholding, *See* Thresholding
Feature shape, *See* Shape
Feature size distributions, 478, 540–542, 572–578
Feature skeleton, *See* Skeletons
Feret's diameter, maximum, 553, 576
Fiber analysis
  counting procedures, 568–569
  length and width, 577–578
  skeletons, 502–503, 569, 578
Fiducial marks, 257, 534, 550, 670, 672, 676, 684
File storage, *See* Image storage and file management
Film, photographic, *See* Photographic film
Filtered back-projection, 635–637, 640, 658–659
Fingerprint identification, 172, 190, 603–604
Firewire, 39
First-down line graphic, 550
Fixed-pattern noise (FPN), 18
Flash ADC, 4, 23
Flash memory, 164
Flatbed scanners, 31
  color calibration, 547–548
Flat-panel displays, 56
Flicker fusion, 686, 701
Flood fill algorithm, 765
Floppy disks, 164

Fluorescence light microscopy
  noise reduction, 203
  noise sources, 201
  significance of brightness values, 548
  three-dimensional data sets, 705
  use of image ratios, 322
Fluorescent lighting, 79
  noise sources, 201
Focus detection, 736
Focused-ion beam (FIB) machining, 68, 534, 676
Focusing, 18, *See also* Blurring
  automatic focus system, 18, 330
  digital camera problems, 41
  extended-focus images, 330–331, 391–392
  frequency transforms and astigmatism, 350–352
  video camera, 5–6
Fog level, 9
Football first-down line graphic, 550
Forgery and falsifications, 131–133
Form removal, 61–62
Formfactor, 582, 583, 604, 606, 610
Four-connected rule, 435, 452
Fourier descriptors (harmonic analysis), 589, 726
Fourier transform infrared (FTIR) spectroscopy, 741
Fourier transforms, 187, 335, 336–344, 360, *See also* Frequency-space image processing
  analyzing image resolution, 352–353
  blur removal, 383, 636–637, 699
  compression effects, 361
  confocal light microscope resolution and, 675
  correcting illumination nonuniformities, 242–244
  deconvolution and optical defect correction, 377–382
    Wiener deconvolution, 382–385
  diffraction pattern, 347–348, 369
  discrete transform, 182, 337, 338
  dividing, 379, 382

Gaussian point-spread function model, 378, 382
Gaussian smoothing, 206–211, 374
　blurring and, 205, 214
　separating waviness from roughness, 760–761
Geographical information system (GIS), 161–162, 170–171, 412, 684, 687
Geometrical distortion, 255–256
Global image measurements, 511, *See also* Stereology
Global positioning system (GPS), 171, 550
Google, 161
Gourard shading, 714, 755
Gradient characterization, 536–537, 554, 562
Grain-boundary images, 305–306, 309, 466–467, 505, 506
　ASTM grain size measurement, 521–522, 525
　length measurement, 525–526
Grain size, 521–522, 525
Grandmother cell, 87–88, 624
Gray-component replacement (GCR), 149
Gray scale
　banding or posterization, 141–143
　calibration, 544–547
　converting color image to, 49–50
　halftoning, *See* Halftoning
　human vision, logarithmic response, 141
　pseudocolor substitution, *See* Pseudocolor
Gray-scale morphological operations, 479–480, *See also* Morphological operations
　feature measurements, 480
　noise filtering applications, 228–229
　rank-based background leveling, 244–247
　surface analysis applications, 769
Gray-scale resolution, 23–26
　dim illumination and, 26
　high-dynamic-range images, 25
　human vision, 92, 271
Gray-scale skeletonization, 308
Gray-scale thinning, 426
Gray wedge, 545

Grid superimposition, 455–458, 513–514, 517
　cycloids, 526
　systematic random sampling, 528
Grinding, 676, 729
Guthrie, Arlo, 85, 127

H

Haar wavelet functions, 187–188
Halftone screen, 137
Halftoning, 136–140, 271
　artifact filtering, 365
　color images, 146
Hanning window function, 357
Harmonic analysis, 589–592
HDTV, *See* High-definition television
Head-mounted display, 702
Head phantom, 651, 652
Heat scale, 35
Heckbert algorithm, 49
Helical scanning, 657
Hierarchical data format (HDF), 180
High-definition television (HDTV), 13, 29–30, 193
High-depth images, 27–28
　HDTV, 29–30
　scanning technology and, 31
High-frequency information loss, 189–190, 213
High-pass filter, 147
　automatic focus system, 18
　Butterworth filter, 359
　digital camera problems, 41
　Laplacian, 286
　periodic noise filtering, 356–357, 359
High-speed photography, 109–110
Hillerman, Tony, 106
Hills and dales, 770
Histogram, *See* Image histogram
Hit-or-miss operator, 482
HLS (hue, lightness, saturation) color system, 45
Holes in features
　feature size measurement and, 573
　filling, 453–455, 494–495, 573
Holography, 1, 347, 700–701
Homomorphic range compression, 147
Horizontal cells, 97
Hough transform, 560–565
HSI (hue, saturation, intensity) color system, 45, 548

contrast expansion and, 198
histogram equalization, 276
image analysis applications, 49
median filter, 218
practical applications, 46
RGB conversion, 45–48
thresholding and, 405–409
HSV (hue, saturation, value) color space, 45
HTML documents, 160
Hubble telescope, 9, 378
Hue, 45, 100, 548
　computing, 49
　wrap-around modulo 360°, 247–251
Huffman coding, 176–178, 182
Human vision, 2, 83–86, 130
　acuity (spatial resolution), 94–96
　blind spot, 90, 110
　camera performance vs., 29
　color blindness, 103, 105
　color perception, 37, 90–91, 93–94, 100–102, 325
　comparison-based, 86–87
　computer-based image processing vs., 82
　contrast resolution, 9, 92–93, 146–147, 185, 240, 271
　cultural differences in image interpretation, 85–86
　depth perception, 70
　directional bias, 130
　edge or boundary perception, 98, 102, 123–124, 285–286
　　difference of Gaussians, 288
　eye–hand coordination, 112
　facial recognition, 117–119, 624
　gray-scale discrimination, 92, 141, 271
　how vs. what, 115–117
　illusions and, *See* Illusions
　image compression and, 119–121
　image resolution, 85, 89
　local to global hierarchies, 102–107
　motion perception, 105, 108–112
　neurophysiology, 96–99
　object grouping or ordering, 102–107, 129–131
　object recognition, 86–89
　rods and cones, 89–90, 97, 326

ion beam erosion, 676
marker-based feature
    selection, 461
morphological operations
    (erosion and dilation),
    484–485
mosaics, 78–79
multiple-channel images, 64
noise sources, 201
PCA applications, 325–326
pseudotopographic display,
    713
quantitative surface
    metrology, 759–760
significance of brightness
    values, 548
stereoscopy, 71–72, 677
sub-pixel resolution, 21
surface composition imaging,
    741
surface measurement
    applications, 71,
    738–739
thresholding multiband
    images, 410–411
undercuts and bridges, 743
very flat surfaces, 59
Scanning tunneling microscope
    (STM), 58, 62, 732–734
Scratch removal, 229, 470, 483
Sea bottom mapping, 75
Search engines, 161
Secondary ion mass spectrometry
    (SIMS), 67–69, 656, 669,
    676–677
    internal surface definition,
        710
    surface composition imaging,
        741
    volumetric rendering, 705–706
Second-order stereology, 537,
    539
Seed-fill technique, 438, 452
Segmentation, 443, See also
    Thresholding
    biases in area selection,
        132–133
    boundaries, 420–432, See also
        Boundaries
    fractal applications, 316
    general classification problem,
        439–441
    grouping pixels into features,
        452–458
    multiband images, 404–406,
        408–412
    noisy images and, 422–423
    region growing, 438

separating touching features,
    493, 569–570, See
    also Watershed
    segmentation
split-and-merge, 436–438
watershed segmentation, 472,
    493–496, 505, 569, 724
Seismic imaging, 66
    tomography, 632, 661–662
Self-affine image generation,
    190–192, See also
    Fractal compression
Self-avoiding distributions,
    556–557
Sequential removal, 675–677
Serial sections, 66–67, 530–531,
    596, 668, 669–673
    alignment, 256–258, 391, 393,
        597, 669–670, 684
    animation, 684
    color coding, 719
    combining multiple views,
        686
    depth dimension calibration,
        671
    interpolation between planes,
        685
    interpreting voxel values, 673
    optical sectioning, 67, See also
        Confocal scanning light
        microscope
    planar resectioning, 684–685,
        688–691
    section thickness control, 671,
        673
    sequential removal, 675–677
    SIMS technology, See
        Secondary ion mass
        spectrometry
    specimen distortion, 671
    stereological measurements,
        See Stereology
    surface area measurement,
        596–597
    surface rendering, 718–720
    three-dimensional data sets,
        682–684
    three-dimensional
        visualization issues, 129
    volume measurement,
        514–515, 596
Seurat, Georges, 136
Shading, 122, 236, See
    also Illumination
    nonuniformity
    correction
    color image correction
        problems, 247
Gourard shading, 714, 755

histogram equalization and,
    275
human perception, 98
image subtraction, 318–319
Phong shading, 714, 750, 755
pseudocolor lookup tables,
    240
surface rendering and, 714,
    750–752, 755
three-dimensional image
    visualization, 691–692
Shadow mask, 56
Shadows, 77
Shape, 126–127, 581–585
    classical stereology
        assumptions, 540–541
    descriptors and numerical
        parameters, 581–585
    feature classification and,
        604–606
    inconsistencies, 583
    location measures, 584–
        585
    fractals, 585–589, See also
        Fractal dimension
    harmonic analysis, 589–592,
        726
    illusions, 126–127
    skeleton, 126
    surface profile analysis, 760
    three-dimensional
        measurement problems,
        726
    topological parameters, See
        Topology
    unrolling, 589–592
Shape from shading, 122, 236,
    738, 751
Shepp and Logan head phantom,
    651, 652
Shot noise filtering, 214, 224
Shutter speed, 27
Shuttering, 11–12, 16, 27
Side-scan sonar, 59, 75
Signal-to-noise ratio (SNR), 23,
    26
    deconvolution and, 380
    neighborhood averaging and,
        203–213
Silicates, 322
Silicon lattice structure, 345
SIMS, See Secondary ion mass
    spectrometry
Single-photon emission
    tomography (SPECT),
    654–655
Sinogram, 633
16-bit images, 24, 397–398, 543,
    743

Suppression operators, 308
Surface area measurement,
        516–520
    area per unit volume, 523,
        725
    fractal perimeter and, 586
    image magnification and, 517
    problems of three-
        dimensional space, 595
    serial sections, 596–597
    voxel resolution and, 595
Surface characteristics, color and,
        121–122
Surface curvature, 532–534
    connectivity, 532–533
    Euler characteristic, 533
Surface image processing, 236,
        743–750
    compositional maps, 746–747
    convolution, 749–750
    profile measurements,
        760–763
    range images, 743–746
Surface imaging, 712, 729, 737,
        See also Range images;
        Three-dimensional
        imaging; specific
        methods
    compositional mapping,
        741–742
        processing, 746–747
    contact instruments, 732–
        735, 744–746, See
        also Atomic force
        microscope; Scanning
        tunneling microscope
    data presentation and
        visualization, 747–752
    deconvolution, 63
    diffraction patterns, 740
    illumination effects, 77
    interferometry, 712
    light probes, 736–737
        confocal optics, 736
        interferometry, 736–737
    measurement applications, See
        Surface measurement
        applications
    microscopic measurement,
        738–740, See also
        specific technologies
    multidimensional display
        issues, 746–747
    multiple-illumination
        orientation system, 122
    range image processing,
        743–746
    range imaging, 59–64, See also
        Range images

range-to-resolution ratios, 747
SEM applications, 71
stereoscopy, 739–740
surface reflectivity and, 713
very flat surfaces, 59
Surface measurement
    applications,
        758–760, See also
        Surface imaging;
        Three-dimensional
        measurements;
        specific measurement
        applications, methods,
        technologies
    autocorrelation function, 762,
        767–768
    dimensional measurement,
        759
    fractal-dimension
        measurement, 738,
        771–775
    human visual examination,
        755, 758
    Motif analysis, 762
    "peaks and valleys" definition,
        763, 765
    profile measurements,
        760–763
    proposed standard
        (Birmingham
        measurement suite),
        763–769
        amplitude parameters, 763,
            764–767
        functional parameters, 763,
            768–769
        hybrid parameters, 763,
            767–768
        spatial parameters, 763
    thickness measurement, 758
    topographic analysis, 770–771
Surface rendering, 711–716, See
        also Three-dimensional
        image visualization
    atomic force microscope
        imaging, 123
    color and, 757
    internal surfaces, 716, 719
    multi-ply connected surfaces,
        716–720
    range images, 710
    reflectivity characteristics, 750
    serial sections, 718–720
    shading, 714, 750–752, 755
    smoothing operations, 714
    splits and merges, 718–719
    stereo views, 715, 757
    surface relief, 749–750
    triangular facets, 714, 716

use of color, 719
visualization and, 752–757
    isometric presentation,
        753–754
    oblique view, 753
    perspective, 754
    realism, 754–757
Surface roughness, See also
        Texture
    autocorrelation, 396
    fractal dimension and, 316,
        354–355, 772, See also
        Fractal dimension
    microscopic measurement,
        738
    surface profile analysis,
        760–762
    waviness filtering, 760–761
Surfaces, 516, 711, 729
    defects, 731
    fractal boundaries, 588–589
    human vision and images on,
        729, 755, 758, 770
    production and modification
        methods, 729–731
    types or phases, 523–524
Surface waves, 741
Surveillance videotape, 116
    facial recognition, 602–604
S-video, 37–38
Synchrotrons, 659–660
Synesthesia, 128
Syntactical models, 626–627
Synthetic aperture radar, 59, 75,
        227, 710
Systematic random and uniform
        sampling, 527–529

T

Tagged image file format (TIFF),
        173, 180
Tape drives, 165
Taut-string boundary, 573
Template matching, 389, 482,
        600–601, See also Cross-
        correlation
    edge finding applications, 304
    three-dimensional image
        processing, 723
Teosinte, 618–619
Terrain classification, 322
Tessellation, 267, 309–310, 680
Text compression, 176–177
Text search, 172
Texture, See also Surface
        roughness

double thresholding
and Feature-AND
operations, 466–467
Euclidean distance map, 491
location-based feature
selection, 464–465
machine-vision systems,
401–402
manual adjustment, 400, 424
minimum area sensitivity,
423–424
multiband images, 404–406,
408–412
multiple criteria, 414–416
principal components
analysis, 410
16-bit images, 397–398
skeleton, *See* Skeletons
sparse-dot map, 422
split-and-merge vs., 438
textural characterization,
412–419
three-dimensional color
space, 405
three-dimensional image
processing, 724
two-dimensional thresholds,
406–408
using histogram, 397–400
selective histograms
(ignoring boundary
pixels), 425–427
Threshold logic unit, 87–88, 624
Thumbnail images, 171–172
TIFF, 173, 180
Time-lapse photography, 27
Tinting, 35–36
Toggle filter, 223
Tomographic imaging, 66, 69,
631–632, 667–668
beam hardening, 646, 648,
660
biomedical applications, 631–
632, *See also* Computed
tomography
head phantom, 651
resolution requirements,
663
cupping (deviation from
uniform density), 650
defects in reconstructed
images, 642–646
density measurement, 650
dosage problems, 659
electron microscopy, 657–658,
660–661
emission modality, 651
imaging geometries, 652–657

internal surface rendering,
716
inverse filter and, 636–637
linear attenuation coefficient,
632, 639
multienergy, 704–705
noise amplification, 644
ray tracing, 694
reconstruction mathematics,
632–637
algebraic reconstruction
technique, 639–641, 659
filtered back-projection,
635–637, 640, 658–659
frequency-space
reconstruction, 634–
635, 658
maximum-entropy
approach, 641–642
Radon transform, 561,
633–634
ray-integral equations, 633,
639–640
seismography, 632, 661–662
three-dimensional imaging,
656–662
depth resolution, 656–657
helical scanning, 657,
663–666
high-resolution
tomography, 663–666
view angles and detector
positions, 643
X-ray scattering effects, 648
Toner, 140
Top-hat filters, 100, 347–348
cross-correlation application,
390–391
frequency transforms,
363–365, 369–371
noise filtering applications,
229–230, 308, 363–365,
369–371
range imaging, 310
separating touching features,
569–570
Topographic analysis, 770–771
Topographic maps, 71, 432,
708–710, 739, *See also*
Contour maps
Topology, 593–594, 629
skeleton and, 126, 499–500,
593
three-dimensional, 596, 727
Topothesy, 773
Transfer functions, 271
modifying for contrast
manipulation, 273–274
Translation, 253–254

Transmission electron
microscope (TEM), 1,
57–58
aligning serial-section images,
672
binary image processing, 485
color images, 32
combining images with
different orientations,
328
depth of field, 680
frequency-domain
representation, 345
illumination issues, 236, 237
matching stereo pairs, 681
shadow applications, 77
three-dimensional imaging
geometries, 657–658
Transmission images, 57 58,
See also Transmission
electron microscope
Trapezoidal distortion, 255–256
Tree counting, 570–571
Tristimulus correction, 53–55,
101
Truncated median filter, 219
Trussell algorithm, 401–402
Tube-type camera, 5–6
Tubular structure volume
measurement, 529–530
"Typical" type image, 89, 127

U

Ultimate eroded points (UEPs),
493, 494, 496, 498,
569–570, 725
Ultrasound imaging, 706, 716
geometries, 654
Undercolor removal, 149
Unfolding (classical stereology),
540–542
Universal Product Code (UPC),
599
Unsharp masking, 28, 95–96, 100,
318, 386
edge enhancement, 287–288
Unsupervised classification, 606,
620
UPC bar codes, 599

V

Van Cittert iterative technique,
383, 699
Variance-based texture
extraction, 313–314
Variance equalization, 281

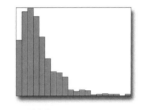

• *Fovea Pro*

Professional Image Analysis Tools

• I*mage* P*rocessing* T*ool* K*it*

Educational Image Processing Tools

• *Optipix*

Optimize your digital photos

Special 10% OFF!

When ordering use the coupon code "**IPH 5th Edition**" to receive a 10% discount on all Reindeer Graphics software.

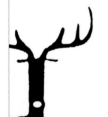

REINDEER
graphics

P O Box 2281
Asheville, NC 28802

http://www.reindeergraphics.com

Tel: 919 342 0209
Fax: 919 342 0210